ADVANCES IN THE PRECLINICAL STUDY OF ISCHEMIC STROKE

Edited by **Maurizio Balestrino**

Advances in the Preclinical Study of Ischemic Stroke
Edited by Maurizio Balestrino

Published by InTech

Janeza Trdine 9, 51000 Rijeka, Croatia

Publishing Process Manager Maja Bozicevic

Technical Editor Teodora Smiljanic

Cover Designer InTech Design Team

Additional hard copies can be obtained from orders@intechopen.com

Advances in the Preclinical Study of Ischemic Stroke, Edited by Maurizio Balestrino
p. cm.
ISBN 978-953-51-0290-8

For EU product safety concerns:
IN TECH d.o.o., Prolaz Marije Krucifikse Kozulić 3, 51000 Rijeka, Croatia,
info@intechopen.com or visit our website at intechopen.com.

Meet the editor

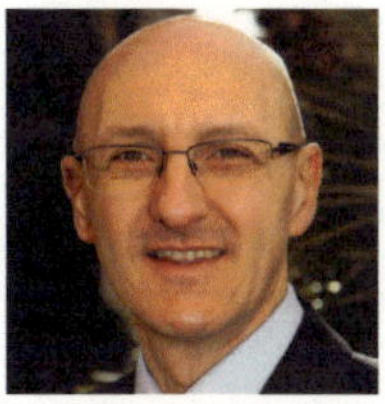

Maurizio Balestrino was born in Genoa, Italy, the birthplace of Christopher Columbus and of the blue jeans. He received there the Degree in Medicine and the Diploma of Specialist in Neurology. In 1983-1986 he was Research Associate in the Department of Physiology at Duke University, where he started an interest in ischemic brain damage. Back in Italy he has always combined clinical responsibilities as a neurologist and experimental research in brain anoxia or ischemia. He is currently Senior Researcher in the Stroke Unit of the University of Genoa, where he also directs the Laboratory of Experimental Neurophysiology. He has been partner or coordinator in national and international research projects aiming at bridging the gap between experimental research and clinical therapy.

Contents

Preface

In the last part of the 20th century scientists discovered drugs that made the brain more resistant to ischemia, to such an extent that cerebral tissue treated with them was only little damaged, or was not damaged at all, by an ischemic insult that badly damaged control, untreated tissue. It was the beginning of a very exciting era in neuroscience research, a period when academic and industrial scientists all pursued the research of a "neuroprotectant" that could defend the ischemic brain from irreversible damage. As most people know, the search turned out to be mostly unsuccessful because the drugs that in the animal models were effective were not so effective in the clinics. Frustratingly enough, one compound after another failed in clinical trials of stroke patients. The easiest and most common explanation given was that something was wrong with animal studies, and this is still the leading belief of mainstream neurologists. So, skepticism grew among clinicians, and nowadays it is very rare to find a clinician that gets excited by the idea of trying or studying a "neuroprotective" compound in stroke.

However, I think that such a dismissal is plain wrong. It is unconceivable that hundreds of scientists throughout the world have for 30 years all carried out flawed or even fraudulent research demonstrating that several compounds improve the resistance of the brain to ischemic damage. Granted, that may have happened sometimes, but hundreds of laboratories around the world cannot have been run during 30 years by incompetent or criminal scientists. At least, all successful animal research in neuroprotection must be seen as having provided a "proof-of-concept" demonstrating that it is possible to use drugs to protect the brain from ischemic damage. And in fact, that neuroprotection is indeed possible is demonstrated beyond doubt by the neglected survivor of that host of neuroprotectant agents: hypothermia. Hypothermia was demonstrated to be effective in a score of animal experiments, and it has now become recommended intervention in out-of-hospital cardiac arrest. Hypothermia is not a drug, but it demonstrates that neuroprotection is a reality, not a myth. Besides, it obviously shows that animal experiments were right, humans treated with hypothermia fare better than untreated ones, just like animal studies had predicted.

Thus, the fact that hypothermia is now successful in clinical practice, at least in out-of-hospital cardiac arrest, tells us one simple truth: neuroprotection is possible. Another demonstration that neuroprotection is possible may be edaravone, a neuroprotective compound that has been used for years in Japan and China, and that has been declared reasonably effective in ischemic stroke, at least pending larger trials, by a recent Cochrane Review (S. Feng, et al. Edaravone for acute ischaemic stroke. *Cochrane Database Syst. Rev.* 12:CD007230, 2011).

Why, then, have scores of drugs, previously found to be effective in animal models, failed clinical trials? The average clinician will answer this question by saying that animal experiments are useless, that they do not reflect the human situation, that they are badly designed and carried out, and so forth. Meetings and committees have even been celebrated to declare this truth, and to teach preclinical neuroscientists how to properly carry out their experiments, see for example the "STAIR" (Stroke Therapy Academic Industry Roundtable) meetings in the US.

Of course, there is some truth in this answer, and probably much more than "some". We are in the 21st century, and even animal experiments must be updated and modernized. I am perfectly convinced that preclinical scientists (among whom I proudly list myself) must learn, as they have done for a couple of centuries, new ways of designing and carrying out their experiments. "Blind" treatment and evaluation, use of older animals (more similar to stroke patients), reliance on permanent rather than on transient models of ischemia are just the simplest and most obvious improvements that should be implemented in the laboratory, at least for those experiments that are meant to build the foundation for a clinical translation of the treatment. All these modifications, and much more, will certainly improve the reliability and the usefulness of animal experiments, much in the same way as the use of statistics has greatly improved animal experimentation in the 20th century (remember those very old days when statistics were not required to publish an experiment?).

But I believe that other truths must be told, too.

First, clinicians have not been able to grasp the true conditions under which neuroprotection is possible. Clinicians (or maybe the drug industry?) have been blinded by the illusion that a simple cure to all ischemic strokes was at hand, and they simply treated all patients with stroke, irrespective, for example, of age, infarct size and comorbidity. Sometimes the neuroprotective treatment was administered one day after stroke onset, an obvious nonsense that was not justified by animal data. With these and other behaviors, clinicians lost the opportunity of neuroprotection by applying it to patients that were not apt to benefit from it. I was very happy in reading that this truth has finally been recognized even in published science: Reza et al. (Neuroprotection in acute ischemic stroke. *J Neurosurg Sci.* 55 (2):127-138, 2011) wrote that "Previous clinical studies have failed to show benefit [of neuroprotection] likely due to poor patient selection, altering time windows that had shown benefit in bench models and failure to link treatments with reperfusion". Alas, animal scientists must improve their work, but clinicians should finally understand how to properly exploit it.

Second, it should not be forgot that several neuroprotectant have failed not because they lacked efficacy, but because they revealed unexpected side effects. Many NMDA-receptor antagonists were discarded because in clinical trials they showed psychedelic unwanted effects. Tirilazad, an antioxidant belonging to the "lazaroid" class of antioxidants, unexpectedly worsened outcome of ischemic stroke, a fact very likely explained by some unexpected toxic action(s) that offset its neuroprotective ability.

So, the 21st century will hopefully favor the harmonization of basic research and of clinical neurology, two realities that were too distant from each other in the second half of the 20th century. Hopefully, preclinical scientists will learn how to carry out better experiments, **and** clinicians will learn how to best apply them to their patients. To do so, preclinical studies of stroke must be continued and improved. The Authors of this book have provided their expertise and experience in reporting ways how to do so.

The first section of this book collects studies of animal models of stroke. Advances in this area are needed because animal experiments, carried out with proper analgesia and respect for animal lives, will still be necessary for a long time. Although the 3 "R"s (reduction, refinement, replacement) have greatly decreased the need for in vivo animal experiments, the latter ones are still needed (cf. for example "Recommendations for Standards Regarding Preclinical Neuroprotective and Restorative Drug Development". *Stroke* 30 (12):2752-2758, 1999).

The second section of the book collects studies on pathophysiology of ischemic damage. This is an area where our knowledge has greatly advanced in the past decade, mainly due to the study of novel pathways of damage and of novel techniques to investigate them. Better knowledge of how brain tissue becomes damaged in stroke will hopefully lay the foundation for better therapies, be them recanalization (like thrombolysis) or neuroprotection (like hypothermia). Novel techniques like proteomics have greatly improved our capability to study and understand the pathological changes that are caused by ischemia.

The third section deals with neuroprotection. As we have discussed above, this has become a kind of Holy Grail for stroke scientists. Contributors to this section reviewed the state of the art in this quest or reported their experience in exploring novel ways of neuroprotection. Their work will be a useful addition to the store of knowledge that the modern Parsifal will exploit to finally find his Grail.

I am most grateful to the Authors of the various chapters, who have expertly written and patiently revised their very interesting work for this book. I also would like to thank the InTech publisher, who has invited me to edit this book and has provided me with the online tools and assistance that made the job possible. In particular I am most grateful to Ms. Ana Pantar, who was effective and determined in removing initial obstacles, thus making this project possible. And to Ms. Maja Bozicevic, without whose kind and efficient assistance this project could not have been successful. I hope readers will find our efforts useful.

Maurizio Balestrino, MD
Department of Neuroscience,
Ophthalmology and Genetics, University of Genova,
Italy

Part 1

Animal Models and Techniques

1

Ischemic Neurodegeneration in Stroke-Prone Spontaneously Hypertensive Rats and Its Prevention with Antioxidants Such as Polyphenols

Kazuo Yamagata
Laboratory of Molecular Health Science of Food,
Department of Food Bioscience and Biotechnology,
College of Bioresource Sciences, Nihon University (NUBS),
Japan

1. Introduction

Stroke involves cerebral infarction and hemorrhaging and is associated with very high mortality. Previous reports have indicated that ischemic stimulation such as the reoxygenation that occurs after hypoxia produces a large quantity of reactive oxygen species (ROS) that strongly induces neuronal death *in vivo* and *in vitro* (Negishi et al., 2001). Indeed, this is considered to be the factor that most strongly induces cell death in cerebral ischemia. In recent years, apoptosis has been suggested to be the mechanism responsible for ischemic neuronal death in animal stroke models (Tagami et al., 1998).

Stroke-prone spontaneously hypertensive rats (SHRSP) are widely used as a model of human stroke (Yamori et al., 1974). In this model, blood pressure is elevated as age increases, as is found in humans; and the rats eventually die of stroke. One feature of this model is that strokes develop spontaneously following severe hypertension (more than 150 mmHg). Therefore, in SHRSP, because strokes develop after the onset of elevated blood pressure, elevated blood pressure is considered to be the most critical factor for stroke induction. However, interestingly, the neuronal cells of this model exhibit a great vulnerability compared with normal control WKY/Izm rats during the reoxygenation conditions following hypoxia (Tagami et al., 1998; Yamagata et al., 2010c). In addition to the influence of blood pressure in SHRSP/Izm rats, the neuronal vulnerability of this model strongly contributes to stroke development. SHRSP/Izm rats are susceptible to apoptosis under conditions of hypoxia and reoxygenation (H/R) (Tagami et al., 1998). The expression of antioxidant enzymes in SHRSP/Izm rats is attenuated in comparison with that in WKY/Izm rats. We highlight that this attenuation of antioxidant enzymes is related to the vulnerability of neuronal cells (Yamagata et al., 2000b). Furthermore, an altered susceptibility to apoptosis was detected in the astrocytes of SHRSP/Izm rats compared with those of WKY/Izm rats (Yamagata et al., 2010a).

Epidemiologic study indicated the possibility of preventing stroke using antioxidants such as dietary polyphenols (Vita, 2005). Polyphenols are substances produced by plants via photosynthesis, and their structures contain many hydroxyl groups (-OH). Polyphenols are found in vegetables, fruit, and processed products. They are also found abundantly in red wine, tea, soybeans, and coffee. The preventive effects of polyphenols include the inhibition of blood pressure elevation, cholesterol-lowering activity, hypoglycemic activity, antioxidant activity, and antimutagen activity (Sies et al., 2010). The effects of polyphenols differ between substances, but most are capable of "antioxidation". It is considered that the antioxidative effects of polyphenols are advantageous in their roles as defensive substances that protect plant components from oxidation. Polyphenols are found in trace amounts in our diet and have been demonstrated to prevent degenerative diseases such as cancer and cardiovascular disease (Manach et al., 2004). This review describes the vulnerability of neuronal cells and susceptibility of astrocytes in SHRSP in stroke conditions. Furthermore, we describe the prophylactic effects of apigenin, epigallocatechin-3-gallate (EGCG), and resveratrol on endothelial cells as well as their stroke preventive effects.

2. Susceptibility of neuronal cells and astrocytes of SHRSP/Izm rats during cerebral ischemia

The reoxygenation after cerebral ischemia rapidly generates a large quantity of ROS. The following chain of events leads to neuronal cell injury (Love, 1999). Free radicals are generated early in the period of the reperfusion and cause neuronal damage (Bolli, 1991). Cerebral ischemia-reperfusion induced neuronal cell death is usually apoptotic (Rothstein et al., 1994). Here, we describe alteration in neuronal cells and astrocytes related to apoptosis in SHRSP/Izm rats during H/R.

2.1 Neuronal vulnerability of SHRSP during stroke and oxidative stress

Neuronal death because of cerebral ischemic stress strongly induces apoptosis (Rothstein et al., 1994). Reports indicate that the production of hydroxyl radicals is strongly induced in SHRSP/Izm rats during H/R (Negishi et al., 2001). SHRSP/Izm and WKY/Izm rats produce hydroxyl radicals in their hippocampi when subjected to reoxygenation after 20 minutes of hypoxia. However, SHRSP/Izm rats display significantly increased hydroxyl production when compared with normal WKY/Izm control rats (Tagami et al., 1998). In SHRSP/Izm rats the production of hydroxyl radicals is strongly induced during H/R (Negishi et al., 2001). The increased levels of hydroxyl radicals produced by SHRSP/Izm rats may induce neuronal injury. These findings suggest that capturing the hydroxyl radicals produced during H/R, in which the level of antioxidant substances is decreased, would be beneficial for preventing neuronal injury (Yamagata et al., 2010c).

2.2 The neuronal cells of SHRSP/Izm rats strongly induce apoptosis during H/R

Neuronal cells are easily damaged during H/R. We examined neuronal cells during hypoxia using SHRSP/Izm and WKY/Izm rats. After 24 hours of hypoxia, neuronal cell death was not observed in WKY/Izm or SHRSP/Izm rats. However, after 36 hours of hypoxia, neuronal cell death increased in SHRSP/Izm rats. This was not observed in WKY/Izm rats. The findings of a morphologic examination of SHRSP/Izm rats indicated that most neuronal cell death was apoptotic. About 41% of the WKY/Izm neurons died 1.5 hours after reoxygenation (necrosis = 12%, apoptosis = 29%). On the other hand, 78% of SHRSP/Izm neurons died (necrosis = 15%, apoptosis = 63%). Following three hours of reoxygenation, 99% of cells from both strains had died. In SHRSP/Izm rat neurons, fragmentation of DNA was strongly induced by 36 hours of hypoxia and reoxygenative stimulation for three hours (Tagami et al., 1998). The H/R induced apoptosis of neuronal cells in SHRSP/Izm rats (Yamagata et al., 2010c). The neuronal cells of SHRSP/Izm rats were strongly induced into apoptosis with 3 or 5 hours of reoxygenation following hypoxia. When DNA fragmentation was examined using a TUNEL method, few of the SHRSP/Izm rat neurons displayed DNA fragmentation when incubated under normal oxygen concentrations (data not shown). However, after 3 hours of reoxygenation following 36 hours of hypoxia, marked DNA fragmentation was seen. At the same time, many lipid droplets were detected in the cells (Tagami et al., 1998). We classified the apoptotic levels in H/R conditions via a morphologic analysis of neuronal death (Tagami et al., 1998, 1999). We demonstrated the criteria for neuronal apoptosis in the SHRSP/Izm rats in Table 1 and Figure 1. Neuronal axons and dendrites are lost in the early stages of apoptosis, and many lipid droplets are seen in the neuronal cell body (A, initial stage of apoptosis). Furthermore, cells shrink as apoptosis advances (B, second stage of apoptosis; C, third stage of apoptosis). The neuronal cell membrane is lost in the advanced stage of apoptosis, and the nucleus disappears (D). Figure 2 is considered to show the second stage of apoptosis (Tagami et al., 1998: Yamagata et al., 2010c). These processes eventually lead to cell death. From these results, it is suggested that the neuronal weakness of SHRSP/Izm rats is associated with stroke development (Fig. 4).

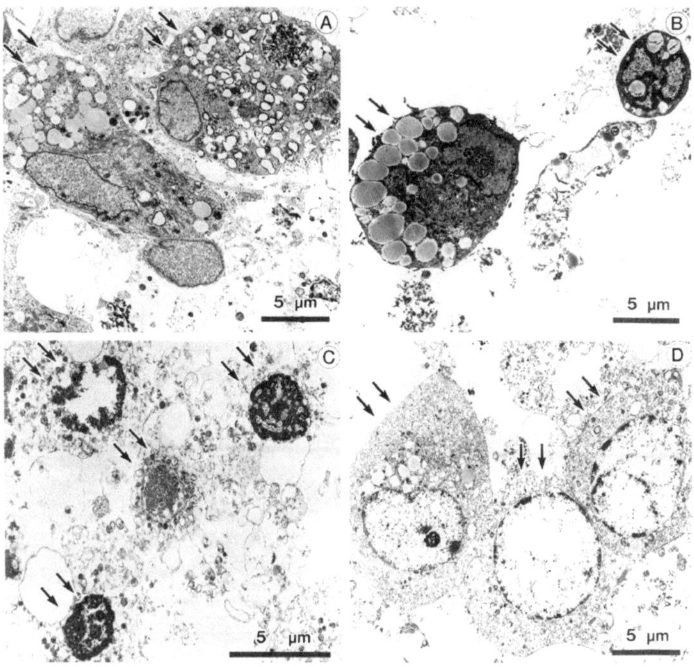

Fig. 1. Our criteria to determine apoptosis and necrosis in neurons during H/R in SHRSP/Izm rats.
A. initial stage, B, second stage, C. third stage and D necrosis (Tagami et al., 1998)

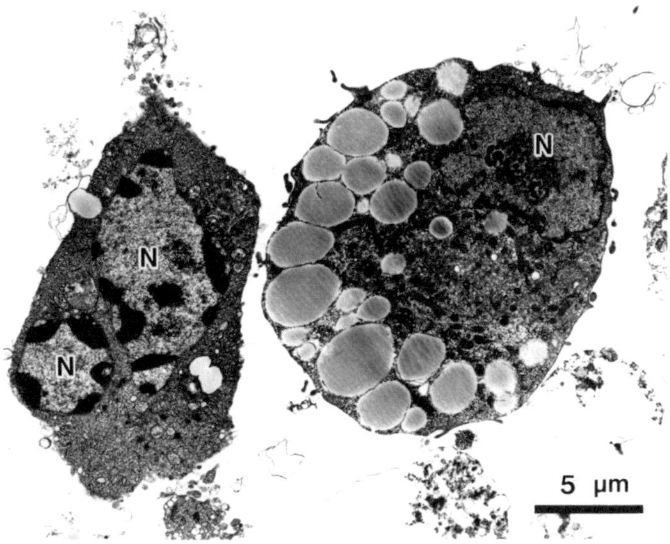

Fig. 2. Second stage of apoptosis in neurons during H/R in SHRSP/Izm rats. N: nucleus

Stage	Criteria of neuronal death	Features of morphological
1	Initial stage	The cells lose their axons and dendrites, and numerous lipid droplets appear in the cell bodies, although cell organelles remain intact
2	Second stage	The cells become round, small, and electron-dense, and their nuclei demonstrate prominent invagination
3	Advanced stage	The cells lose their cytoplasm and cell membrane, and their nuclei become small and dark before disappearing
4	Final stage	The cells become electron-lucent, organelles decrease in number, and nuclei contain abnormal clusters of chromatin (the cells lose their cytoplasm and cell membrane, and their nuclei become small and dark before disappearing)

Cited references (Tagami et al., 1998, 1999).

Table 1. The morphological criteria for neuronal apoptosis in the SHRSP/Izm rats.

2.3 Gene expression of Bcl_2 and thioredoxin II in neuronal cells of SHRSP/Izm rats during H/R

The apoptosis in neuronal cells of SHRSP/Izm is strongly induced by reperfusion after ischemia (Tagami et al., 1998). Simultaneously, oxidative stress can induce antioxidant enzymes in neuronal cells. Antioxidant enzymes can prevent the apoptosis caused by oxidation stress. Furthermore, the Bcl_2 gene is an oncogene related to human lymphoma and is able to inhibit the apoptosis induced by neurodegeneration stimuli (Akhtar et al, 2004). We highlight that the Bcl_2 gene expression in SHRSP/Izm rat neuronal cells is significantly attenuated after 30 minutes of reoxygenation following hypoxia in comparison with that in WKY/Izm rats (Yamagata et al., 2000b). The decrease in the expression of Bcl_2 leads to release of the cytochrome C from mitochondria. Thereafter, caspase activity increases and can strongly induce apoptosis. In SHRSP/Izm rat neurons, gene expression of thioredoxin II (Txn2) and mitochondrial cytochrome c oxidase III (CO III) decreased in a fashion similar to Bcl_2 30 minutes after reoxygenation following hypoxia (Yamagata et al., 2000b). Txn2 provides protection against ROS via its SH group. In addition, these proteins have many functions that contribute to intracellular signal transduction. Namely, CO III is associated with energy metabolism in mitochondria. It transfers electrons from the reduced form of cytochrome C to molecular oxygen. Vitamin E and CO III are present in mitochondria where they protect the cell from injury by free radicals (Yang & Korsmeyer, 1996). Attenuation of Bcl_2 and CO III gene expression in SHRSP/Izm rat neuronal cells may reduce energy metabolism and redox control during posthypoxic reoxygenation. The decrease of viability in SHRSP/Izm rat neurons, unlike that in WKY/Izm rat neurons, may be associated with their vulnerability.

2.4 Characteristics of SHRSP/Izm rat astrocytes during stroke

The functions of the astrocytes regulate outbreaks of cerebropathy (Chen & Swanson, 2003). In brain lesions, reactive astrocyte numbers increase and promote the development of stroke (Pekny & Nilsson, 2005). This characteristic of the astrocytes of SHRSP/Izm rats may be related to brain disease (Chen & Swanson, 2003). We separated astrocytes from the brain of fetal SHRSP/Izm rats and cultured them. We compared the proliferation of astrocytes from WKY/Izm with SHRSP/Izm rats under various culture conditions (Yamagata et al., 1995). The astrocytes isolated from fetuses are not influenced by blood pressure. We examined the characteristics of astrocytes from SHRSP/Izm rats in environments that were not influenced by blood pressure. We found that the growth of astrocytes from SHRSP/Izm rats was increased in comparison with those from WKY/Izm rats (Yamagata et al., 1995). We suggest that the numbers of astrocytes of the SHRSP/Izm rats are increased and that this strongly leads to the gliosis following damage. In the rat brain transient cerebral ischemia model, epidermal growth factor (EGF) receptor is related to mechanism of astrocyte reactivity. The details are not known, but astrocyte numbers of SHRSP/Izm rats may increase by cell division through EGF stimulation during the appearance of cerebral blood vessel pathogenesis. This proliferation of astrocytes is enhanced by vascular smooth muscle cells in SHRSP/Izm rats (Yamori et al., 1981). In fibrinoid necrosis degeneration by hypertension, the barrier function of endothelial cells diminishes and blood plasma components leak out of the circulation (Johansson, 1999). In SHRSP/Izm rats, there is denaturation of smooth muscle cells of the media, necrosis with a rise in blood pressure, and destruction of the blood–brain barrier (BBB) in perforating branch arteries (Tagami et al.,1987). We have indicated the possibility that attenuated endothelial barrier functions might be induced by comparing the astrocytic potency of SHRS/Izm rats (Yamagata et al., 1997b).

Glutamate is released as a neurotransmitter by nerve terminals and activates astrocytes. Furthermore, glutamate uptake via a glutamate transporter in the cell membrane is mediated by astrocytes. Glutamate produces lactate in astrocytes and the lactate produced by astrocytes is supplied as an energy source to neuronal cells (Pellerin & Magistretti 1994). Concurrently, the lactate supplied by astrocytes is important for the recovery of the neuronal cells after ischemia (Schurr et al., 1997; Dringen et al., 1995). We demonstrated that there is decreased lactate produced in cultured astrocytes from SHRSP/Izm rats when compared with that from WKY/Izm rat astrocytes during hypoxia (Yamagata et al., 2000a). The decreased lactate production by SHRSP/Izm rat astrocytes may cause neuronal cell death through reduced energy supply.

Furthermore, we examined characteristics of SHRSP/Izm rat astrocytes during stroke. In H/R, the expression levels of intercellular adhesion molecule-1 (ICAM1), monocyte chemotactic protein-1 (MCP1), and vascular cell adhesion molecule-1 (VCAM1) in astrocytes from SHRSP/Izm rats were increased in comparison with that in astrocytes from WKY/Izm rats (Yamagata et al., 2010a). In addition, production of glial cell line-derived neurotrophic factor (GDNF) by adenosine, H_2O_2, glutamate, sphingosine-1-phosphate (S1P) was decreased during H/R in astrocytes from SHRSP/Izm rats in comparison with that from astrocytes from WKY/Izm rats (Yamagata et al., 2002; 2003; 2007a) (Fig. 3). Moreover, production of l-serine by nitric oxide (NO) stimulation decreased in SHRSP/Izm rats in comparison with that in WKY/Izm rats (Yamagata et al., 2006). Not all of the differences seen in SHRSP/Izm rats compared with WKY/Izm rats may be related to the generation of neuronal dysfunction in SHRSP/Izm rats. However, decreased astrocytic lactate and GDNF production may worsen energy conditions and nutrition status of SHRSP/Izm rat neurons (Yamagata et al., 2008). We suggest that attenuation of astrocyte functions accelerates neuronal cell death during stroke and may participate in its appearance (Fig. 4).

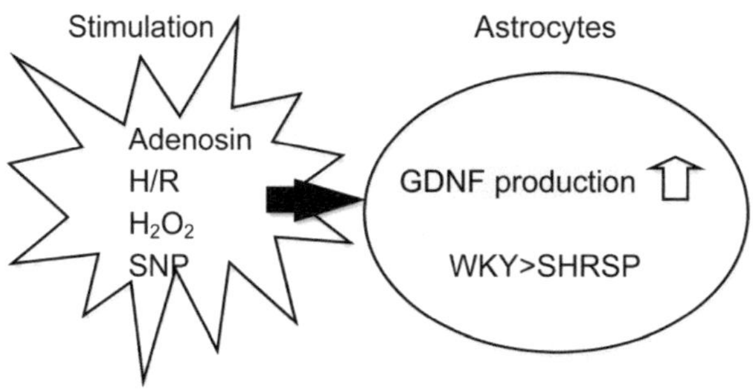

Fig. 3. Expression of GDNF in SHRSP/Izm rats by H/R stimulation.
H/R: hypoxia and reoxygenation: S1P: sphingosine-1-phosphate,
GDNF: glial cell line derived neurotrophic factor

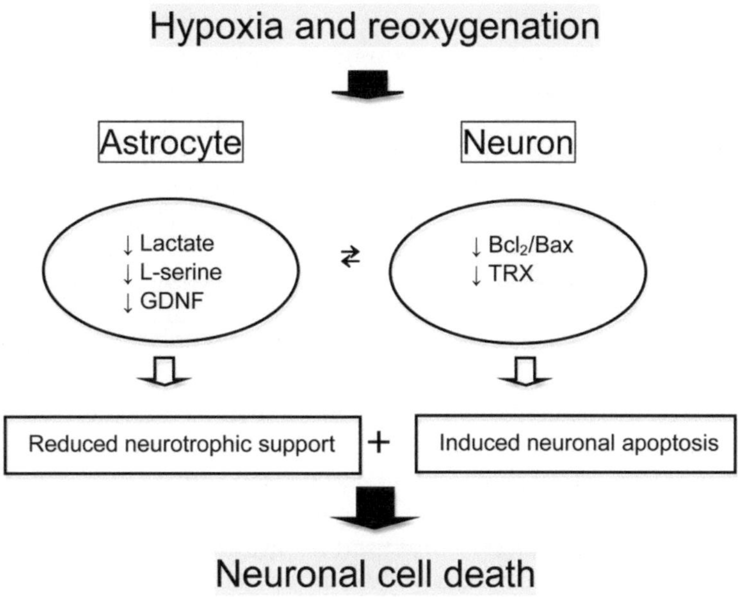

Fig. 4. Alteration of astrocytes and neuronal apoptosis by H/R stimulation.

3. Endothelial dysfunction and importance of stroke prevention through nutrition

The risk of stroke increases with the presence of arteriosclerosis in cerebral blood vessel endothelial cells. Here, we describe preventive action for endothelial cell disorders by food components. The secretion of cytokines by initial lesions strongly activates endothelial cells, vascular smooth muscle cells, and blood cells. For example, endothelial cells are strongly influenced by the effects of inflammatory cytokines such as tumor necrosis factor alpha (TNF-α) and interleukin beta (IL-1β) (Kofler et al., 2005). As a consequence, monocytic adhesion to endothelial cells is induced, which promotes various arteriosclerotic processes. Among these, the oxidative stress produced during the early period of the disorder triggers arteriosclerosis. When the various arteriosclerotic reactions begin simultaneously, they are very difficult to inhibit. Therefore, it is best to inhibit ROS production in the early stages of the disorder in order to avoid arteriosclerosis (Kondo et al., 2009). Indeed, the effects of nutritional components with antioxidant activity on the redox regulation of ROS in stroke conditions have been reported previously. It is considered to be possible to inhibit blood vessel disorders in the early stages and that the inhibition of ROS production using polyphenols prevents the development of arteriosclerosis (Manach et al., 2004). Therefore, it is very likely that arteriosclerosis prevention via the consumption of appropriate foods such as antioxidant nutrients can be used to reduce the risk of stroke.

3.1 Possible role of polyphenols against cerebral ischemia injury

Cerebral ischemia induces the rapid production of a large quantity of ROS and induces cell injury through self-perpetuating reactions. Free radicals are produced within several minutes of reoxygenation after cerebral ischemia and induce brain cell injury (Bolli, 1991). Cerebral ischemia elevates the intracellular level of calcium ions and activates calcium-dependent proteases. Moreover, these reactions activate xanthine dehydrogenase (XDH) and produce xanthine oxidase (XOD) (Thompson-Gorman & Zweier, 1990). It is considered that the superoxide anion radicals produced via this pathway cause neuronal death. However, the consumption of polyphenol-rich foods, such as fruits and vegetables, is beneficial for preventing vascular disorders (Manach et al., 2004). Epidemiological studies have indicated that an inverse correlation exists between polyphenolic consumption and the risk of having to undergo a cardiovascular procedure (Arts & Hollman, 2005). Polyphenols induce the production of vasodilatory factors such as NO (Auger et al., 2010) and prostacyclin (PGI_2) (Mizugaki et al., 2000) and inhibit the synthesis of endothelin-1, which induces vasoconstriction in endothelial cells (Reiter et al., 2010). On the other hand, the polyphenols present in the skin of grapes and in wine inhibit the proliferation and migration of smooth muscle cells (Lee et al., 2009). Polyphenols may eliminate the active oxygen produced by reoxygenation after cerebral ischemia via their antioxidative effects.

3.2 Vasorelaxant effects of polyphenols on endothelial cells

Epidemiological analysis has suggested that polyphenols have protective effects against heart disease. The polyphenols that protect against heart disease are found in foods including cocoa, wine, grape pips, berries, tea, tomatoes, soybeans, and pomegranates (Chong et al., 2010). The mechanisms by which polyphenols reduce the risk of heart disease are associated with the prevention of endothelial cell disorders. Endothelial cell disorders strongly induce arteriosclerosis, which subsequently progresses to heart disease and stroke. Therefore, the prevention of endothelial cell disorders by polyphenols is effective in preventing heart disease and stroke. Table 2 shows the effects of the typical polyphenols apigenin, EGCG, and resveratrol on endothelial cells. Jin et al. (2009) demonstrated that apigenin (0.5 – 72.0 μM) enhanced concentration-dependent relaxation in aortas. Apigenin action is mediated by weakening the oxidative stress and by NO reduction. On the other hand, it has been shown that stimulation of expression of endothelial NOS (eNOS) by apigenin occurs through phosphatidylinositol 3-kinase/Akt (PI3K/Akt) for Ca^{2+} dependence (Chen et al., 2010). Moreover, the blockade of adhesion of monocytes and cyclooxygenase (COX)-2 expression in endothelial cells by apigenin has been reported (Lee et al., 2007). We have shown that apigenin strongly inhibits high glucose- and TNF-α-induced VCAM1 expression and the adhesion of U937 in human endothelial cells (Yamagata et al., 2010b). These effects of apigenin are caused by the inhibition of Iionkinase (IKK) α and IKKε/IKKi. From these findings, we suggested that the mechanism by which apigenin inhibits the expression of adhesion molecules and the adhesion of monocytic U937 to endothelial cells involves nuclear factor kappa beta (NF-κβ). From the structure and inhibitory activity profiles of dietary flavonoids, it was recognized that the double bond found in the C-ring of flavonoids and the third hydroxyl group (A-ring) are required for the inhibition of VCAM1 gene expression (Yamagata et al., 2010b). Apigenin may inhibit monocytic adhesion caused by superoxide anions as well as block reductions in NO activity. From these reports, it is considered that apigenin reduces the levels of ROS, promotes NO activity, and inhibits cell adhesion. Moreover, apigenin strongly inhibited the TNF-α-stimulated expression of lectin-like oxidized low-density lipoprotein receptor-1 (LOX-1) (Yamagata et al., 2011) and the double bond of the C ring of apigenin is essential for this action (Fig. 5). As shown in Figure. 5, the inhibition of LOX-1 expression by apigenin requires a flavone frame, a double bond in the C-ring, and the absence of a third hydroxyl group in the B- and C-rings, which are not found in naringenin (not active) (Yamagata et al., 2011).

Polyphenol(s)	Effects on pathological condition(s)	Ref (authors and issue)
Apigenin	Endothelium-dependent vasorelaxant and antiproliferative effect	Zhang et al (2000)
	Inhibiton of VEGF	Osada et al., (2004)
	Inhibiton of laser-induced choroidal neovascularization	Zou and Chiou (2006)
	Inhibition of COX-2 expression and adhesion of monocytes	Lee et al., (2007)
	Inhibition of superoxide anion-mediated impairment	Ma et al., (2008)
	Inhibition of platelet adhesion and thrombus formation	Navarro-Nunez et al., (2008)
	Protection against the oxidative stress by the NO	Jin et al., (2009)
	Induction of calcium dependent activation of the NO	Chen et al., (2010)
	Inhibition of high glucose and TNFα-induced adhesion molecule expression	Yamagata et al., (2010b)
	Inhibition of TNFα-induced LOX-1 expression	Yamagata et al., (2011)
EGCG	Increase of the prostacyclin production	Mizugaki et al., (2000)
	Inhibition of the vascular-endothelial growth factor-induced intracellular signaling and mitogenesis	Neuhaus et al., (2004)
	Inhibits the angiotensin II-induced adhesion molecule expression	Chae et al., (2007)
	Inhibiton of MCP-1 expression	Hong et al., (2007)
	Improves endothelial function and insulin sensitivity, reduces blood pressure, and protects against myocardial I/R injury in SHR	Potenza et al., (2007)
	Inhibiton of TNFα-induced MCP-1 production	Ahn et al., (2008)
	Protection against linoleic-acid-induced endothelial cell activation	Zheng et al., (2009)
	Decrease of caveolin-1 expression	Li et al., (2009)
	Decrease of endothelin-1 expression and secretion	Reiter et al., (2010)
	Induction of the NO	Auger et al., (2010)
	Protection of against oxidized LDL-induced endothelial dysfunction	Lee et al., (2010)
	Protects against oxidized LDL-induced endothelial dysfunction by inhibiting LOX-1-mediated signaling	Ou et al., (2010)
	Decreases thrombin/ paclitaxel-induced endothelial tissue factor expression	Wang et al., (2010)
	inhibiton of angiotensin II-induced endothelial barrier dysfunction	Yang et al., (2010)

Resveratrol	Inhibition of angiogenesis, tumor growth, and wound healing	Brakenhielm et al., (2001)
	Prevention of superoxide-dependent inflammatory responses induced by I/R, PAF, or oxidants.	Shigematsu et al., (2003)
	Inhibition of VEGF-induced angiogenesis	Lin et al., (2003)
	Protection against peroxynitrite-mediated endothelial cell death	Brito et al., (2006)
	Attenuation of TNF alpha-induced activation; inhibition of NF-kappaB	Csiszar et al., (2006)
	Inhibition of MCP-1 synthesis and secretion	Cullen et al., (2007)
	Attenuates oxLDL-stimulated NADPH oxidase activity and protects endothelial cells from oxidative functional damages.	Chow et al (2007)
	Prevention of concentric hypertrophy and diastolic impairment	Juric et al., (2007)
	Induction of NO production by increasing estrogen receptor alpha	Klinge et al., (2008)
	Induction of NADPH oxidases 1 and 4 mediate cellular senescence	Schilder et al., (2009)
	Reduces oxidative stress by modulating the gene expression of SOD1, GPx1 and Nox4	Spanier et al (2009)
	Decrease of mitochondrial oxidative stress	Ungvari et al., (2009)
	Prevention of hyperglycemia-induced endothelial dysfunction	Xu et al., (2009)
	Decrease of oxidized LDL-evoked LOX-1 signaling	Chang et al., (2011)
	Protecton of H 2O2-induced oxidative stress	Kao et al., (2010)
	Protecton of oxidized LDL-induced breakage of the blood-brain barrier	Lin et al., (2010)

COX; cyclooxygenase, GPx1; glutathione peroxidase 1, I/R; ischemia/reperfusion, LDL; low density lipoprotein, LOX-1; lectin-like oxidized low-density lipoprotein receptor-1, MCP-1; monocyte chemotactic protein-1, NO; nitric oxide, Nox4; NADPH oxidase subunit, PAF; platelet-activating factor, SOD1; superoxide dismutase 1, SHR, spontaneously hypertensive rats, TNF; tumor necrosis factor, VEGF; vascular endothelial growth factor,

Table 2. Studies on the protective effects of apigenin, EGCG and resveratrol in endothelial cells

EGCG is a catechin that is found in green tea. The catechins found in tea include epicatechin (EC), epigallocatechin (EGC), epicatechin gallate (ECG), and epigallocatechin gallate

(EGCG), and the content order of these compounds is as follows: EGCG>EGC>ECG>EC. Catechins are also responsible for the bitter taste of green tea. Catechins account for around 13%–30% of the dry weight of tea leaves (Wolfram, 2007). EGCG suppresses the expression of adhesion molecules such as MCP1 (Ahn et al., 2008; Chae et al., 2007; Hong et al., 2007) and expression of endothelin-1 (Reiter et al., 2010). Like apigenin, EGCG inhibits the expression of monocyte adhesion molecules in endothelial cells stimulated with TNF-α (Ahn et al., 2008; Zheng et al., 2010) and it has been reported that EGCG inhibits the TNF-α-induced expression of activator protein-1 in endothelial cells and increased the expression of HO-1. These findings suggest that EGCG inhibits the expression of activator protein-1 and increases the expression of HO-1, both of which aid endothelial protection. Furthermore, a least one study demonstrated that EGCG downregulated the endothelial cell activation induced by linoleic acid via caveolin-1 (Zheng et al., 2009). Six hours of linoleate exposure induced the expression of caveolin-1 and COX-2 in caveolae. However, pretreatment with EGCG inhibited the expression of caveolin-1 and COX-2 induced by linoleic acid. Exposure to linoleic acid also increased the levels of several kinases (p38 MAPK, extracellular signal regulated kinase 1/2 8ERK1/2), and amino kinase terminal (Akt). According to these findings, EGCG activates several enzymes in endothelial cell caveolae and may have many preventive effects for vascular disorders.

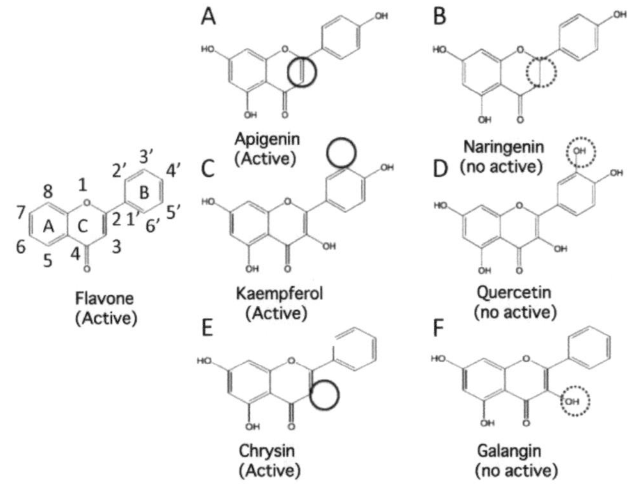

Fig. 5. Structures and LOX-1 inhibitory activities of apigenins.
○: active (indicates that the compound dose-dependently inhibited TNFα-induced LOX-1 gene expressions).

Many studies have demonstrated that ischemic heart disease is decreased by wine intake, and in particular, it has been shown that the antioxidative effects of the polyphenols found in red wine are important for cardioprotection. It was shown that this cardioprotective effect is caused by the actions of resveratrol. It has been confirmed that resveratrol displays various pharmacologic actions such as antioxidant activity in humans

(Brito et al., 2006; Chow et al., 2007; Spanier et al., 2009; Ungvari et al., 2009). Resveratrol is considered to decrease circulating low-density lipoprotein (LDL) cholesterol levels and thereby reduce the risk of cardiovascular disease (CVD) (Ramprasath & Jones, 2010). Resveratrol inhibits atherosclerosis and improves the function of endothelial cells in animal models. There have been many studies of resveratrol actions, which have shown that it has various effects on endothelial cells, as shown in Table 2. The effects of resveratrol and red wine on endothelial cells were investigated using experimental hypercholesterolemic rabbits (Zou et al., 2003). It was found that hypercholesterolemic rabbits displayed significant improvements in the functions of their endothelial cells after the administration of resveratrol (3 mg/kg/day), red wine (4 ml/kg/day), or nonalcoholic red wine (4 ml/kg/day) for 12 weeks. Moreover, they demonstrated decreased levels of plasma endothelin-1 and NO, which are increased by hypercholesterolemia. On the other hand, it was also shown that resveratrol protects against injury to the BBB caused by oxidized LDL (oxLDL) (Lin et al., 2010). It is considered that the mechanism behind these effects of resveratrol involves amelioration of the effects of oxLDL on the expression of occludin and ZO-1, which aids the stability of tight junctions. Resveratrol regulates the expression of tight junction proteins as a means of protecting against the disruption of the BBB induced by oxLDL. In a rat postischemic reoxygenation model, resveratrol decreased ROS generation (Shigematsu et al., 2003), and the effect of resveratrol on cerebral infarction was also examined in a rat middle cerebral artery occlusion (MCA) model (Sinha et al., 2002). In addition, after MCA and 2 hours of reperfusion, the rats were evaluated for motor disorders, malondialdehyde (MDA), reduced glutathione, and infarct volume. After MCA, increases in the frequency of functional motility disorders and the levels of MDA and reduced glutathione were observed. On the other hand, the administration of resveratrol prevented these increases and significantly decreased the infarct volume. These findings indicate that resveratrol inhibits the organ injuries produced by ischemia–reperfusion. The other polyphenols found in wine are not known to have this effect. Correspondingly, resveratrol prevents myocardial infarction by reducing peroxide levels. It is suggested that this effect can be attributed to the antioxidative effects of resveratrol (Dudley et al., 2008).

4. Preventive effects of antioxidant drugs and polyphenols for SHRSP rat neurons during stroke

We indicated that high dose vitamin E induced neutral gamma glutamylcystenyl synthase (γ-GCS), GSH levels, and strongly prevented neuronal death (Yamagata et al., 2009). Furthermore, we have shown that ebselen, a seleno–organic antioxidant (Yamagata et al., 2008), amlodipine, and carvedilol (Yamagata et al., 2004) prevented neuronal cell death in SHRSP/Izm rats. Another study demonstrated that the expression of VCAM1 by TNF-α in astrocytes isolated from SHRSP/Izm rats was increased compared with that in those from WKY/Izm rats. However, apigenin strongly attenuated TNF-α-induced VCAM1 mRNA and protein expression and suppressed the adhesion of U937 cells and SHRSP/Izm astrocytes (Yamagata et al., 2010a). It is suggested that apigenin regulates adhesion molecule expression in reactive astrocytes during ischemia and prevents neuronal death.

5. Conclusion

Endothelial cell dysfunction causes arteriosclerosis and promotes neuronal demise after stroke. Enhanced neuronal sensitivity to oxidative stress contributes to the neuronal death observed in SHRSP/Izm rats. Also, enhanced oxidative stress after hypoxia-reoxygenation is important in ischemic stroke. Polyphenols reduce oxidation stress and have a protective effect on endothelial and neuronal cells. Antioxidant nutrients such as polyphenols may prevent or reduce endothelial dysfunction and neuronal cell injury during cerebral ischemia.

6. Abbreviations

BBB; blood–brain barrier, CO III; cytochrome c oxidase III, COX; cyclooxygenase, CVD; cardiovascular disease, EC; epicatechin, ECG; epicatechin gallate, EGC; epigallocatechin, EGCG; epigallocatechin-3-gallate, EGF; epidermal growth factor, eNOS; endothelial NOS, γ-GCS; gamma glutamylcystenyl synthase, GDNF; glial cell line-derived neurotrophic factor, GSH: glutathione, HO-1; hemoxigenase-1, H/R; hypoxia and reoxygenation, ICAM1; intercellular adhesion molecule-1, IL-1β; interleukin beta, IKK; IIKKkinase, LDL; low-density lipoprotein, LOX-1; lectin-like oxidized low-density lipoprotein receptor-1, MCP1; monocyte chemotactic protein-1, NO; nitric oxide, NF-κβ; nuclear factor kappa beta, oxLDL; oxidized LDL, PGI_2; prostacyclin, PI3K/Akt; phosphatidylinositol 3-kinase/Akt, ROS; reactive oxygen species, SHRSP/Izm; spontaneously hypertensive rats/Izm, S1P; sphingosine-1-phosphate, TNF-α; tumor necrosis factor alpha, TRX; thioredoxin, VCAM1; vascular cell adhesion molecule-1, WKY/Izm; Wistar Kyoto rat/Izm, XDH; xanthine dehydrogenase, XOD; xanthine oxidase.
Keywords; Endothelial cells, Ischemic stroke, Polyphenol, SHRSP.

7. References

Ahn, H.Y., Xu, Y. & Davidge, S.T. (2008). Epigallocatechin-3-O-gallate inhibits TNFalpha-induced monocyte chemotactic protein-1 production from vascular endothelial cells. Life Sci 82 (17-18): 964-968.

Akhtar, R.S., Ness, J.M. & Roth, K.A. (2004). Bcl-2 family regulation of neuronal development and neurodegeneration. Biochim Biophys Acta 1644(2-3): 189-203.

Arts, I.C., & Hollman, P.C. (2005). Polyphenols and disease risk in epidemiologic studies. Am J Clin Nutr 81 (Suppl 1): 317S-325S.

Auger, C., Kim, J.H., Chabert, P., Chaabi, M., Anselm, E., Lanciaux, X., Lobstein, A. & Schini-Kerth, V.B. (2010). The EGCg-induced redox-sensitive activation of endothelial nitric oxide synthase and relaxation are critically dependent on hydroxyl moieties. Biochem Biophys Res Commun 393 (1): 162-167.

Bolli, R. (1991). Oxygen-derived free radicals and myocardial reperfusion injury: an overview. Cardiovasc Drugs Ther (Suppl 2): 249-268.

Bråkenhielm, E., Cao, R. & Cao, Y. (2001). Suppression of angiogenesis, tumor growth, and wound healing by resveratrol, a natural compound in red wine and grapes. FASEB J 15 (10): 1798-1800.

Brito, P.M., Mariano, A., Almeida, L.M. & Dinis, T.C. (2006). Resveratrol affords protection against peroxynitrite-mediated endothelial cell death: A role for intracellular glutathione. Chem Biol Interact 164 (3): 157-166.

Chae, Y.J., Kim, C.H., Ha, T.S., Hescheler, J. & Ahn, H.Y. & Sachinidis A. (2007). Epigallocatechin-3-O-gallate inhibits the angiotensin II-induced adhesion molecule expression in human umbilical vein endothelial cell via inhibition of MAPK pathways. Cell Physiol Biochem 20 (6); 859-866.

Chang, H.C., Chen, T.G., Tai, Y.T., Chen, T.L., Chiu, W.T. & Chen, R.M. (2011). Resveratrol attenuates oxidized LDL-evoked Lox-1 signaling and consequently protects against apoptotic insults to cerebrovascular endothelial cells. J Cereb Blood Flow Metab 31 (3): 842-854.

Chen, C.C., Ke, W.H., Ceng, L.H., Hsieh, C.W. & Wung, B.S. (2010). Calcium- and phosphatidylinositol 3-kinase/Akt-dependent activation of endothelial nitric oxide synthase by apigenin. Life Sci 87 (23-26); 743-739.

Chen, Y., & Swanson, R.A. (2003). Astrocytes and brain injury. J Cereb Blood Flow Metab 23 (2): 137-149.

Chong, M.F., Macdonald, R. & Lovegrove, J.A. (2010). Fruit polyphenols and CVD risk: a review of human intervention studies. Br J Nutr 104 (Suppl 3): S28-S39.

Chow, S.E., Hshu, Y.C., Wang, J.S. & Chen, J.K. (2007). Resveratrol attenuates oxLDL-stimulated NADPH oxidase activity and protects endothelial cells from oxidative functional damages. J Appl Physiol 102 (4): 1520-1527.

Csiszar, A., Smith, K., Labinskyy, N., Orosz, Z., Rivera, A. & Ungvari, Z. (2006). Resveratrol attenuates TNF-alpha-induced activation of coronary arterial endothelial cells: role of NF-kappaB inhibition. Am J Physiol Heart Circ Physiol 291 (4): H1694-H1699.

Cullen, J.P., Morrow, D., Jin, Y., Curley, B., Robinson, A., Sitzmann, J.V., Cahill, P.A. & Redmond, E.M. (2007). Resveratrol, a polyphenolic phytostilbene, inhibits endothelial monocyte chemotactic protein-1 synthesis and secretion. J Vasc Res 44 (1): 75-84.

Dringen R, Peters H, Wiesinger H, Hamprecht B. (1995). Lactate transport in cultured glial cells. Dev Neurosci 17 (2): 63-69.

Dudley, J.I., Lekli, I., Mukherjee, S., Das, M., Bertelli, A.A. & Das, D.K. (2008). Does white wine qualify for French paradox? Comparison of the cardioprotective effects of red and white wines and their constituents: resveratrol, tyrosol, and hydroxytyrosol. J Agric Food Chem 56 (20); 9362-9373.

Hong, M.H., Kim, M.H., Chang, H.J., Kim, N.H., Shin, B.A., Ahn, B.W. & Jung, Y.D. (2007). (-)-Epigallocatechin-3-gallate inhibits monocyte chemotactic protein-1 expression in endothelial cells via blocking NF-kappaB signaling. Life Sci 80 (21): 1957-1965.

Jin, B.H., Qian, L.B., Chen, S., Li, J., Wang, H.P., Bruce, I.C., Lin, J, & Xia, Q. (2009). Apigenin protects endothelium-dependent relaxation of rat aorta against oxidative stress. Eur J Pharmacol 616 (1-3): 200-205.

Johansson, B.B. (1999). Hypertension mechanisms causing stroke. Clin Exp Pharmacol Physiol 26 (7): 563-565.

Juric, D., Wojciechowski, P., Das, D.K. & Netticadan, T. (2007). Prevention of concentric hypertrophy and diastolic impairment in aortic-banded rats treated with resveratrol. Am J Physiol Heart Circ Physiol 292 (5): H2138-H2143.

Kao, C.L., Chen, L.K., Chang, Y.L., Yung, M.C., Hsu, C.C., Chen, Y.C., Lo, W.L., Chen, S.J., Ku, H.H. & Hwang, S.J. (2010). Resveratrol protects human endothelium from H(2)O(2)-induced oxidative stress and senescence via SirT1 activation. J Atheroscler Thromb 17 (9); 970-979.

Klinge, C.M., Wickramasinghe, N.S., Ivanova, M.M. & Dougherty, S.M. (2008). Resveratrol stimulates nitric oxide production by increasing estrogen receptor alpha-Src-caveolin-1 interaction and phosphorylation in human umbilical vein endothelial cells. FASEB J 22 (7): 2185-2197.

Kofler, S., Nickel, T. & Weis, M. (2005). Role of cytokines in cardiovascular diseases: a focus on endothelial responses to inflammation. Clin Sci (Lond) 108 (3): 205-513.

Kondo, T., Hirose, M. & Kageyama, K. (2009). Roles of oxidative stress and redox regulation in atherosclerosis. J Atheroscler Thromb 16 (5): 532-528.

Lee, B., Lee, E.J., Kim, D.I., Park, S.K., Kim, WJ. & Moon, S.K. (2009). Inhibition of proliferation and migration by piceatannol in vascular smooth muscle cells. Toxicol In Vitro 23 (7): 1284-1291.

Lee, J.H., Zhou, H.Y., Cho, S.Y., Kim, Y.S., Lee, Y.S. & Jeong, C.S. (2007). Anti-inflammatory mechanisms of apigenin: inhibition of cyclooxygenase-2 expression, adhesion of monocytes to human umbilical vein endothelial cells, and expression of cellular adhesion molecules. Arch Pharm Res 30 (10): 1318-1327.

Lee, Y.W., Lee, W.H. & Kim, P.H. (2010). Role of NADPH oxidase in interleukin-4-induced monocyte chemoattractant protein-1 expression in vascular endothelium. Inflamm Res 59 (9): 755-765.

Li, Y., Ying, C., Zuo, X., Yi, H., Yi, W., Meng, Y., Ikeda, K., Ye, X., Yamori, Y. & Sun, X. (2009). Green tea polyphenols down-regulate caveolin-1 expression via ERK1/2 and p38MAPK in endothelial cells. J Nutr Biochem 20 (12): 1021-1027.

Lin, M.T., Yen, M.L., Lin, C.Y. & Kuo, M.L. (2003). Inhibition of vascular endothelial growth factor-induced angiogenesis by resveratrol through interruption of Src-dependent vascular endothelial cadherin tyrosine phosphorylation. Mol Pharmacol 64 (5): 1029-1036.

Lin, Y.L., Chang, H.C., Chen, T.L., Chang, J.H., Chiu, W.T., Lin, J.W. & Chen. R.M. (2010). Resveratrol protects against oxidized LDL-induced breakage of the blood-brain barrier by lessening disruption of tight junctions and apoptotic insults to mouse cerebrovascular endothelial cells. J Nutr 140 (12): 2187-2192.

Love, S. (1999). Oxidative stress in brain ischemia. Brain Pathol 9 (1): 119-131.

Ma, X., Li, Y.F., Gao, Q., Ye, Z.G., Lu, X.J., Wang, H.P., Jiang, H.D., Bruce, I.C. & Xia, Q. (2008). Inhibition of superoxide anion-mediated impairment of endothelium by treatment with luteolin and apigenin in rat mesenteric artery. Life Sci 83 (3-4): 110-117.

Manach, C., Scalbert, A., Morand. C., Remesy, C. & Jimenez, L. (2004). Polyphenols: food sources and bioavailability. Am J Clin Nutr 79 (5): 727-747.

Mizugaki, M., Ishizawa, F., Yamazaki, T. & Hishinuma T. (2000). Epigallocatechin gallate increase the prostacyclin production of bovine aortic endothelial cells. Prostaglandins Other Lipid Mediat 62 (2): 157-164.

Navarro-Nunez, L., Lozano, M.L., Palomo, M., Martinez, C., Vicente, V., Castillo, J., Benavente-Garcia, O., Diaz-Ricart, M., Escolar, G. & Rivera, J. (2008). Apigenin inhibits platelet adhesion and thrombus formation and synergizes with aspirin in the suppression of the arachidonic acid pathway. J Agric Food Chem 56 (9): 2970-2096.

Negishi, H., Ikeda, K., Nara. Y. & Yamori, Y. (2001). Increased hydroxyl radicals in the hippocampus of stroke-prone spontaneously hypertensive rats during transient ischemia and recirculation. Neurosci Lett 306 (3): 206-208.

Neuhaus, T., Pabst, S., Stier, S., Weber, A.A., Schrör, K., Sachinidis, A., Vetter, H. & Ko, Y.D. (2004). Inhibition of the vascular-endothelial growth factor-induced intracellular signaling and mitogenesis of human endothelial cells by epigallocatechin-3 gallate. Eur J Pharmacol 483 (2-3): 223-227.

Osada, M., Imaoka, S. & Funae, Y. (2004). Apigenin suppresses the expression of VEGF, an important factor for angiogenesis, in endothelial cells via degradation of HIF-1alpha protein. FEBS Lett 575 (1-3): 59-63.

Ou, H.C., Song, T.Y., Yeh, Y.C., Huang, C.Y., Yang, S.F., Chiu, T.H., Tsai, K.L., Chen, K.L., Wu, Y.J., Tsai, C.S., Chang, L.Y., Kuo, W.W. & Lee, S.D. (2010). EGCG protects against oxidized LDL-induced endothelial dysfunction by inhibiting LOX-1-mediated signaling. J Appl Physiol 108 (6): 1745-1756.

Potenza, M.A., Marasciulo, F.L., Tarquinio, M., Tiravanti, E., Colantuono, G., Federici, A., Kim, J.A., Quon, M.J. & Montagnani, M. (2007). EGCG, a green tea polyphenol, improves endothelial function and insulin sensitivity, reduces blood pressure, and protects against myocardial I/R injury in SHR. Am J Physiol Endocrinol Metab 292 (5): E1378-E1387.

Pekny, M. & Nilsson, M. (2005). Astrocyte activation and reactive gliosis. Glia 50 (4): 427-434.

Pellerin, L. & Magistretti, J. (1994). Glutamate uptake into astrocytes stimulates aerobic glycolysis: a mechanism coupling neuronal activity to glucose utilization. Proc Natl Acad Sci USA 91 (22): 10625-10629.

Ramprasath, V.R. & Jones, P.J. (2010). Anti-atherogenic effects of resveratrol. Eur J Clin Nutr 64 (7): 660-668.

Reiter, C.E., Kim, J.A. & Quon, M.J. (2010). Green tea polyphenol epigallocatechin gallate reduces endothelin-1 expression and secretion in vascular endothelial cells: roles for AMP-activated protein kinase, Akt, and FOXO1. Endocrinology 151 (1): 103-114.

Rothstein, J.D., Bristol, L.A., Hosler, B., Brown, R.H. Jr. & Kuncl R.W. (1994). Chronic inhibition of superoxide dismutase produces apoptotic death of spinal neurons. Proc Natl Acad Sci USA 91 (10): 4155-4159.

Schurr, A., Payne, R.S., Miller, J.J. & Rigor, B.M. (1997). Glia are the main source of lactate utilized by neurons for recovery of function posthypoxia. Brain Res 774 (1-2): 221-224.

Schilder, Y.D., Heiss, E.H., Schachner, D., Ziegler, J., Reznicek, G., Sorescu, D. & Dirsch, V.M. (2009). NADPH oxidases 1 and 4 mediate cellular senescence induced by resveratrol in human endothelial cells. Free Radic Biol Med 46 (12): 1598-1606.

Shigematsu, S., Ishida, S., Hara, M., Takahashi, N., Yoshimatsu, H., Sakata, T. & Korthuis R.J. (2003) Resveratrol, a red wine constituent polyphenol, prevents superoxide-dependent inflammatory responses induced by ischemia/reperfusion, platelet-activating factor, or oxidants. Free Radic Biol Med 34 (7): 810-817.

Sies, H. Polyphenols and health: update and perspectives. (2010). Arch Biochem Biophys 501 (1): 2-5.

Sinha K, Chaudhary G, Gupta YK. (2002). Protective effect of resveratrol against oxidative stress in middle cerebral artery occlusion model of stroke in rats. Life Sci 71 (6): 655-665.

Spanier ,G., Xu, H., Xia, N., Tobias, S., Deng, S., Wojnowski, L., Forstermann, U. & Li, H. (2009). Resveratrol reduces endothelial oxidative stress by modulating the gene expression of superoxide dismutase 1 (SOD1), glutathione peroxidase 1 (GPx1) and NADPH oxidase subunit (Nox4). J Physiol Pharmacol 60 (Suppl 4): 111-116.

Tagami, M., Nara, Y., Kubota, A., Sunaga, T., Maezawa, H., Fujino, H. & Yamori, Y. (1987). Ultrastructural characteristics of occluded perforating arteries in stroke-prone spontaneously hypertensive rats. Stroke 18 (4): 733-740.

Tagami, M., Yamagata, K., Ikeda, K., Nara, Y., Fujino, H., Kubota, A., Numano, F, & Yamori, Y. (1998). Vitamin E prevents apoptosis in cortical neurons during hypoxia and oxygen reperfusion. Lab Invest 78 (11): 1415-1429.

Tagami, M., Yamagata, K., Ikeda, K., Fujino, H., Nara, Y., Nakagawa, K., Kubota, A., Numano, F. & Yamori, Y. (1999). Genetic vulnerability of cortical neurons isolated from stroke-prone spontaneously hypertensive rats in hypoxia and oxygen reperfusion. Hypertens Res 22 (1): 23-29.

Thompson-Gorman, S.L. & Zweier J.L. (1990). Evaluation of the role of xanthine oxidase in myocardial reperfusion injury. J Biol Chem 265 (12): 6656-6663.

Ungvari, Z., Labinskyy, N., Mukhopadhyay, P., Pinto, J.T., Bagi, Z., Ballabh, P., Zhang, C., Pacher, P. & Csiszar, A. (2009). Resveratrol attenuates mitochondrial oxidative stress in coronary arterial endothelial cells. Am J Physiol Heart Circ Physiol 297 (5): H1876-H1881.

Vita, J.A. (2005). Polyphenols and cardiovascular disease: effects on endothelial and platelet function. Am J Clin Nutr 81 (Suppl1): 292S-297S.

Wang, H.J., Lo, W.Y., Lu, T.L. & Huang, H. (2010). (-)-Epigallocatechin-3-gallate decreases thrombin/paclitaxel-induced endothelial tissue factor expression via the inhibition of c-Jun terminal NH2 kinase phosphorylation. Biochem Biophys Res Commun 391 (1): 716-721.

Wolfram, S. (2007). Effects of green tea and EGCG on cardiovascular and metabolic health. J Am Coll Nutr 26 (4): 373S-388S.

Xu, Q., Hao, X., Yang, Q. & Si, L. (2009). Resveratrol prevents hyperglycemia-induced endothelial dysfunction via activation of adenosine monophosphate-activated protein kinase. Biochem Biophys Res Commun 388 (2): 389-394.

Yang, D., Liu, J., Tian, C., Zeng, Y., Zheng, Y.H., Fang, Q. & Li, H.H. (2010). Epigallocatechin gallate inhibits angiotensin II-induced endothelial barrier dysfunction via inhibition of the p38 MAPK/HSP27 pathway. Acta Pharmacol Sin 31 (10): 1401-1406.

Yamagata, K., Nara, Y., Tagami, M. & Yamori, Y. (1995). Demonstration of hereditarily accelerated proliferation in astrocytes derived from spontaneously hypertensive rats. Clin Exp Pharmacol Physiol 22 (9): 605-609.

Yamagata, K., Tagami, M., Ikeda, K., Noguchi, T., Yamori, Y. & Nara, Y. (2000a). Reduced production of lactate during hypoxia and reoxygenation in astrocytes isolated from stroke-prone spontaneously hypertensive rats. Neurosci Lett 296 (2-3): 113-116.

Yamagata, K., Tagami, M., Ikeda, K., Yamori, Y. & Nara, Y. (2000b). Altered gene expressions during hypoxia and reoxygenation in cortical neurons isolated from stroke-prone spontaneously hypertensive rats. Neurosci Lett 284 (3): 131-134.

Yamagata, K., Tagami, M., Torii, Y., Takenaga, F., Tsumagari, S., Itoh, S., Yamori, Y. & Nara, Y. (2003). Sphingosine 1-phosphate induces the production of glial cell line-derived neurotrophic factor and cellular proliferation in astrocytes. Glia 41 (2): 199-206.

Yamagata, K., Tagami, M., Ikeda, K., Tsumagari, S., Yamori, Y. & Nara, Y. (2002). Differential regulation of glial cell line-derived neurotrophic factor (GDNF) mRNA expression during hypoxia and reoxygenation in astrocytes isolated from stroke-prone spontaneously hypertensive rats. Glia 37(1): 1-7.

Yamagata, K., Ichinose, S. & Tagami, M. (2004). Amlodipine and carvedilol prevent cytotoxicity in cortical neurons isolated from stroke-prone spontaneously hypertensive rats. Hypertens Res 27(4): 271-282.

Yamagata, K., Shoji, Y., Terashima, T. & Yokogoshi, H. (2006). Glutamate reduces secretion of l-serine in astrocytes isolated from stroke-prone spontaneously hypertensive rats. Neuroscience 143 (3): 729-737.

Yamagata, K., Hakata, K., Maeda, A., Mochizuki, C., Matsufuji, H., Chino, M. & Yamori Y. (2007a). Adenosine induces expression of glial cell line-derived neurotrophic factor (GDNF) in primary rat astrocytes. Neurosci Res 59 (4): 467-474.

Yamagata, K., Tagami, M., Nara, Y., Fujino, H., Kubota, A., Numano, F., Kato, T. & Yamori Y. (1997b). Faulty induction of blood-brain barrier functions by astrocytes isolated from stroke-prone spontaneously hypertensive rats. Clin Exp Pharmacol Physiol 24 (9-10): 686-691.

Yamagata, K., Tagami, M. & Yamori, Y. (2008). Nitric oxide reduces astrocytic lactate production and induces neuronal vulnerability in stroke-prone spontaneously hypertensive rats. Glia 56 (4): 387-393.

Yamagata, K. Ichinose, S., Tagawa, C. & Tagami, M. (2009). Vitamin E regulates SMase activity, GSH levels, and inhibits neuronal death in stroke-prone spontaneously hypertensive rats during hypoxia and reoxygenation. J Exp Stroke Transl Med 1 (2): 41-48.

Yamagata, K., Kitazawa, T., Shinoda, M., Tagawa, C., Chino, M. & Matsufuji. H. (2010a). Stroke status evoked adhesion molecule genetic alterations in astrocytes isolated from stroke-prone spontaneously hypertensive rats and the apigenin inhibition of their expression. Stroke Res Treat pii:386389. 1-11.

Yamagata, K., Miyashita, A., Matsufuji, H. & Chino, M. (2010b). Dietary flavonoid apigenin Inhibits high glucose and tumor necrosis factor alpha-induced adhesion molecule expression in human endothelial cells. J Nutr Biochem 21 (2): 116-124.

Yamagata, K., Tagami, M., & Yamori, Y. (2010c). Neuronal vulnerability of stroke-prone spontaneously hypertensive rats to ischemia and its prevention with antioxidants such as vitamin E. Neuroscience 170 (1): 1-7.

Yamagata, K., Miyashita, A., Chino, M. & Matsufuji, H. (2011). Apigenin inhibits tumor necrosis factor alpha plus high glucose-induced LOX-1 expression in human endothelial cells. Microvasc Res 81 (1): 60-67.

Yamori, Y. (1974). Importance of genetic factors in hypertensive cerebrovascular lesions: an evidence obtained by successive selective breeding of stroke-prone and-resistant SHR. Jpn Circ J 38 (12): 1095-1100.

Yamori, Y., Igawa, T., Kanbe, T., Kihara, M., Nara, Y. & Horie, R. Clin Sci (Lond) (1981). Mechanisms of structural vascular changes in genetic hypertension: analyses on cultured vascular smooth muscle cells from spontaneously hypertensive rats. 61 Suppl (7): 121s-123s.

Yang, E. & Korsmeyer, S.J. (1996). Molecular thanatopsis: a discourse on the BCL2 family and cell death. Blood 88 (2): 386-401.

Zhang, Y.H., Park, Y.S., Kim. T.J., Fang, L.H., Ahn, H.Y., Hong, J.T., Kim, Y., Lee, C.K. & Yun, Y.P. (2000). Endothelium-dependent vasorelaxant and antiproliferative effects of apigenin. Gen Pharmacol 35 (6): 341-347.

Zheng, Y., Lim, E.J., Wang, L., Smart, E.J., Toborek, M. & Hennig, B. (2009). Role of caveolin-1 in EGCG-mediated protection against linoleic-acid-induced endothelial cell activation. J Nutr Biochem 20 (3): 202-209.

Zheng, Y., Toborek, M. & Hennig, B. (2010). Epigallocatechin gallate-mediated protection against tumor necrosis factor-α-induced monocyte chemoattractant protein-1 expression is heme oxygenase-1 dependent. Metabolism 59 (10): 1528-1535.

Zou, Y., & Chiou, G.C. (2006). Apigenin inhibits laser-induced choroidal neovascularization and regulates endothelial cell function. J Ocul Pharmacol Ther 22 (6): 425-430.

Zou, J.G., Wang, Z.R., Huang, Y.Z., Cao, K.J. & Wu, J.M. (2003). Effect of red wine and wine polyphenol resveratrol on endothelial function in hypercholesterolemic rabbits. Int J Mol Med 11 (3): 317-320.

2

Frameless Stereotaxy in Sheep – Neurosurgical and Imaging Techniques for Translational Stroke Research

Antje Dreyer[1,2], Albrecht Stroh[3], Claudia Pösel[1], Matthias Findeisen[4], Teresa von Geymüller[1,2], Donald Lobsien[5], Björn Nitzsche[1] and Johannes Boltze[1,2]

[1]Fraunhofer Institute for Cell Therapy and Immunology, Department of Cell Therapy, Leipzig,
[2]Translational Centre for Regenerative Medicine, University of Leipzig, Leipzig,
[3]Institute of Neuroscience, Technical University Munich, Munich,
[4]Institute of Analytical Chemistry, University of Leipzig, Leipzig,
[5]Department of Neuroradiology, University of Leipzig, Leipzig, Germany

1. Introduction

The continuous pathologic reduction of cerebral blood flow is mainly caused by thromboembolic occlusion of a brain-supplying artery or cerebral blood vessel disruption. These events, representing the most important causes for ischemic or hemorrhagic strokes respectively, lead to an acute breakdown of neuronal function, secondary brain damage by numerous mechanisms and the loss of cerebral tissue. In industrialized nations, stroke accounts for every third case of death. Cerebral stroke furthermore represents the most frequent reason for permanent disability in adulthood (Kolominsky-Rabas et al., 2006) and is therefore considered to be one of the most dreaded diseases from a clinical, socio-economic and individual, patient-related perspective.

1.1 Current state of the art clinical stroke treatment and diagnosis

Intravenous thrombolysis by tissue plasminogen activator (tPA) is currently the only FDA-approved, effective and potentially curative treatment (Blinzler et al., 2011) for ischemic stroke. However, this approach is restricted to a narrow time window of 4.5 hours (Hacke et al., 2008). The approach is further limited by a sharply increasing number needed to treat (Hacke et al., 2008; Lansberg et al., 2009) and a significant risk for fatal adverse events (Shobha et al., 2011) at later stages of this time window. As a result, more than 95% of all stroke patients do not significantly benefit from systemic thrombolytic treatment (Barber et al., 2001). Alternatively, endovascular thrombolysis under thorough radiological surveillance can be applied in specialized centers, extending the therapeutic time window to up to 8.0 hours under optimal conditions (Natarajan et al., 2009).

Cerebral ischemia needs to be discriminated from hemorrhagic stroke by means of magnetic resonance imaging (MRI) or computer tomography (CT) prior to the start of therapy, as inducing thrombolysis after hemorrhagic strokes is fatal. The mentioned imaging modalities are also used to monitor disease progression and the beneficial, or eventually detrimental, impact of any therapeutic intervention.

Even though intracerebral hemorrhages are treated by multimodal strategies including neurosurgical interventions and diligent monitoring of blood pressure (Flower & Smith, 2011), the event is still associated with high morbidity and mortality rates (Rymer, 2011), leaving about 80% of patients dead or disabled. Repeated patient surveys by MRI or CT is therefore pivotal for early detection of complications after hemorrhagic stroke. In summary, imaging procedures are of utmost clinical importance for diagnosis, treatment and onward care after ischemic and hemorrhagic strokes.

1.2 Current recommendations for preclinical stroke research

Preclinical and translational stroke research aims to overcome the aforementioned therapeutic and prognostic limitations by the development of novel treatment strategies. The application of stem cell based therapies is currently among the most promising approaches in the field (Burns & Steinberg, 2011) and the first clinical trials have already been initiated (Sahota & Savitz, 2011). However, despite thorough research, the development of novel stroke therapies is so far characterized by continuous setbacks and the general failure to translate promising findings from animal models into effective clinical treatment paradigms (Del Zoppo, 1995). In particular this holds true for the development of neuroprotective therapies (O'Collins et al., 2006).

The inability to translate preclinical findings into clinical therapies has been a matter of debate for more than 15 years. International expert committees like the "Stroke Treatment Academic and Industry Roundtable" (STAIR) and "Stem Cell Therapies as an Emerging Paradigm in Stroke" (STEPS) consortia were formed to define, discuss and publish recommendations for adequate preclinical stroke research (The STAIR Participants, 1999; The STEPS Participants, 2009). Current guidelines for state of the art assessment of novel stroke treatment strategies comprise the design and application of relevant animal models (Fisher et al., 2009), the definition of the optimal route of administration for any therapeutic agent (Savitz et al., 2011; The STAIR Participants, 1999), as well as the choice of relevant imaging protocols to monitor therapeutic safety and efficacy (Savitz et al., 2011).

1.3 The role of large animal models in translational stroke research

Cerebral ischemia is mainly modeled by transient or permanent occlusion of the middle cerebral artery (MCA; Howells et al., 2010). Rodent models are widely available and represent experimental key systems for preclinical stroke research. These models offer many advantages such as well established methodology including surgical techniques, imaging procedures, histological techniques and protocols for molecular biology. Further, the availability of genetically modified strains and excellent tools to assess functional outcome favor the use of rodent stroke models.

However, the impact of a particular therapy in the gyrencephalic brain can only be assessed in large animals. Therefore, the use of a second, predominantly large animal species has been recommended by the STAIR and STEPS committees. Existing large animal models include rabbit (Amiridze et al., 2009), canine (Kang et al., 2007), feline (Garcia et al., 1977), and porcine (Imai et al., 2006) models for which middle cerebral artery occlusion (MCAO) techniques have been described. For anatomical reasons, most large animal models require enucleation and show high mortality rates (The STAIR Participants, 1999), rendering their applicability for long term safety and efficacy trials difficult.

Early models of cerebral hemorrhage were reported more than 45 years ago (Klintworth, 1965), using the application of mechanical force (e.g. balloon inflation) to induce cerebral hemorrhages. More contemporary models are often based on atlas-guided stereotaxic injections (Bullock et al., 1984) of autologous blood or bacterial collagenase into cerebral tissue, predominantly the rodent striatum (MacLellan et al., 2010). MR-guided application techniques have recently been reported in primates (Zhu et al., 2011) but are rarely used, presumable due to ethical and financial restrictions.

1.4 The ovine stroke model and its use for preclinical research

To compensate the above mentioned common limitations of large animal models an ovine model of ischemic stroke using permanent MCAO was developed by our group (Boltze et al. 2008). This model avoids enucleation and allows for long term observation of subjects due to minimal mortality rates.

Briefly, the method can be described as follows. A transcranial access is performed between the left eye and ear. Animals should be placed on the right side to avoid ventilation insufficiency due to a gaseous rumen edema during surgery. After superficial shaving and disinfection, the temporal muscle is incised at the Linea temporalis and temporally elevated from the parietal skull bone. Then, a trepanation of about 1 x 1 cm is performed right behind the orbital rim. After careful incision of the dura mater, the MCA is permanently electrocoagulated by a bipolar forceps. Occlusion of either one or two MCA branches or the entire cortical vessel allows a detailed control of lesion size and functional deficits (Boltze et al., 2008). The drill hole may be sealed by sterile bone cement after suturing of the dura. However, leaving the craniotomy open (only covered by the temporal muscle) avoids pathophysiological increase of intracerebral pressure in early post-stroke phases, significantly reducing post-stroke mortality. After refixation of the temporal muscle at the Linea temporalis and suturing the skin wound, the animals can be taken back to the stable and are allowed to recover. Adequate post stroke analgetic and antibiotic treatment has to be ensured. For any details regarding animal medication, behavioral phenotyping, advanced imaging and the surgical procedure itself, please refer to Boltze et al. (2008).

Species-appropriate housing can be realized with comparatively low efforts and over extended time periods. The price per sheep is relatively low and the species is broadly available. A special feature of the sheep stroke model is the control of lesion size and subsequent behavioral deficits by occlusion of the cortical MCA or a defined number of its branches. A protocol for testing and quantification of neurological functions is available to assess the impact of the MCAO modality and a potential therapeutic procedure. Moreover, the model is eligible for detailed MR, CT and positron emission tomography (PET) studies as well as the assessment of autologous cell therapies.

2. Stereotaxy and cell tracking for stroke-related applications

Stereotaxic concepts were developed as minimally invasive surgical approaches which use three-dimensional Cartesian or polar coordinate systems to localize small targets inside the body. The approach can be used for both diagnostic and therapeutic applications, as it allows the placement or the removal of a specimen from a certain location within the body with highest precision and minimal damage to the surrounding tissue. Stereotaxy is of particular importance in neurosurgery where the technique is routinely used for diagnosis and treatment of intracranial tumors (Willems et al., 2006), as well as for the application of deep brain stimulation electrodes in Parkinson's disease (Starr et al., 1998) and neuropathic pain (Stadler et al., 2011). The fibrinolytic evacuation of intracranial hemorrhages by a stereotaxic apporach has also been reported (Samadani & Rohde, 2009). Moreover, stereotaxic stem cell injections into the human brain are used in phase I and II clinical trials, as the local administration of therapeutic compounds close to the lesion is considered to be advantageous.

Albeit these concepts may have been strongly perpetuated towards clinical application clinical trials during the last years; the first reported results unfortunately resemble the translational failures that were known from past efforts. This holds true for experimental treatments in the field of stroke (Kondziolka et al., 2005) and Parkinson's disease (Gross et al., 2011) although these concepts were positively evaluated in preceding rodent studies. This emphasizes the relevance of large animal models as an important translational milestone. Whereas simplified stereotaxic devices based on brain atlases are widely available for rodents, the accuracy and complexity of human stereotaxic devices can currently only be modeled in primates. However, this complexity, including the individual, "lesion-specific" application of substances or the induction of phenotypically varying intacerebral hematomas may be critically needed in translational research to mimic the more heterogenic patient populations enrolled in clinical trials.

We expanded the sheep model to fill this methodological gap and to provide an additional large animal model for translational research in cell transplantation after ischemic stroke and intracerebral hemorrhages. Our model allows precise, MR-guided implantation of magnetically labeled, bone-marrow derived mesenchymal stem cells (stroke treatment) and autologous blood samples into the ovine brain (hemorrhage induction). The technique was developed using the Brainsight™ neuronavigation system (Rogue Research Inc., Quebec, Canada) and several modifications were applied to adapt the system to the ovine skull anatomy. Cell tracking can be performed reliably using clinical MR scanners with adequate resolution and sensitivity.

This chapter describes the methodology of image-guided frameless stereotaxic surgery in sheep with special emphasis on (i) the application of an autologous therapeutic cell population (e.g., the mesenchymal stem cells), (ii) the previous labeling and subsequent imaging protocols for MR-based cell tracking in sheep and (iii) the MR-guided induction of cerebral hemorrhage in the species.

3. Technical description of surgery

3.1 General information about the species and handling requirements

The neurosurgical approach for stereotaxy in sheep requires hornless subjects for easy accessibility of cranial structures. Merino sheep may be of advantage as many hornless strains can be found in this widely available race. Adult merino sheep weigh approximately 80 kilograms (ewe) to 130 kilograms (rams) and have a wither height of about 0.9 meter. This body size allows for relatively easy handling. Frequent and early contact to humans facilitates familiarization and improves the handling. Species appropriate housing, feeding as well as thorough medical inspections and blood screening, medication and vaccination ensure a significant reduction of postoperative complications and thereby enhance study quality (Boltze et al., 2008).

Anesthesia is performed as described elsewhere (Boltze et al., 2008). Animals should be intubated after induction of anesthesia and placed in a prone ("sphinx") position during surgery and imaging. Vital parameters (electrocardiogram, oxygen saturation, blood pressure, rectal body temperature) should be continuously monitored during any surgical intervention.

3.2 Frameless stereotaxy in sheep – preparation and data acquisition

The neuronavigation device, BrainSight™, is a frameless system that allows for MRI data set based planning of surgical approaches as well as for surveillance and precision control of the surgical intervention with an optical position sensor (Frey et al., 2004). An individual 3D-reconstruction of the head, especially the brain, is required for the precise planning and performance of the sterotaxic injections.

3.2.1 Fiducial marker positioning and imaging

The MR-compatible fiducial markers are attached to a maxillary splint (Fig. 1a). The use of the splint is different from neurosurgical approaches in human medicine, where fiducial markers can be fixed directly to cranial bones. This is not recommended in animals due to safety and welfare issues, especially when the animal is awake between MRI data set acquisition and surgery. The maxillary splint consists of a mouthpiece (Fig. 1a, 1) and two angled arms (Fig. 1a/b, 2) that hold the fiducial markers (Fig. 1a/b, 4). The mouthpiece is inserted carefully, avoiding damage to or constriction of the tracheal tube. It can be adapted to the individual shapes of the maxillary molars and the hard palate by using thermoplastic, which cures within a few minutes. The fiducial markers are usually placed in the area between the cheeks and the ears. The maxillary splint has to be adapted to each individual sheep to ensure maximum precision. The splint has to be inserted for imaging and surgery.

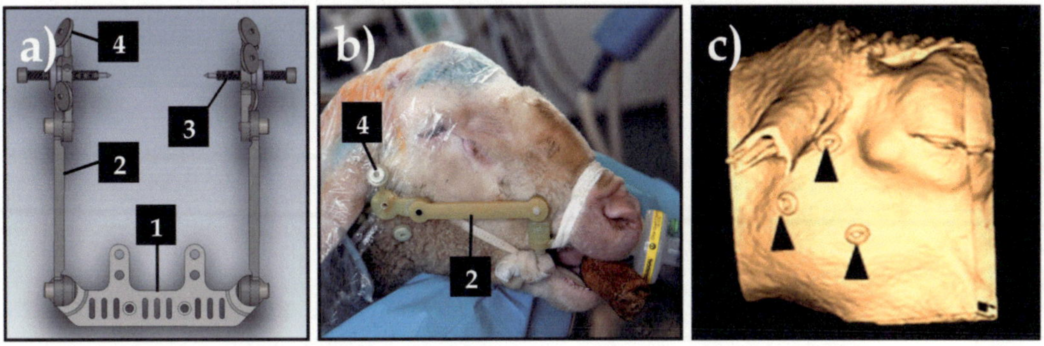

Fig. 1. Maxillary splint with fiducial marker
a) maxillary splint with mouthpiece (1), angeled arms (2), bar spacer to the skin (3) and fiducial marker (4); b) sheep before surgery, the maxillary splint is inserted and fixed with a bandage. The angeled arms (2) support the fiducial markers (4); c) 3D-MRI reconstruction of the skin illustrates the position of fiducial makers between cheek and ear (black arrow heads)

It should be fixed with bandages to ensure an accurate, stable and reproducible position. Otherwise, even minor displacements of the fiducial markers may lead to large divergences between planned and realized target.

A 1.5 T scanner is sufficient for MRI data set acquisition even though the use of a 3 T scanner is recommended. The optimal time span between data acquisition and surgery should be long enough for animal recovery from imaging anesthesia. However, for cell transplantation after MCAO, this time span must not be too long to stay within a potential therapeutic time window. Usually, a recovery phase of one day is sufficient, but longer recovery phases should be scheduled if permitted by the experimental design.

After initial anesthesia and transport, the sheep is placed on the scanner table and is fixed using adhesive tape (cloth tape tesa®, Tesa SE, Hamburg, Germany) on shoulder and hip, which can be easily removed from the wool. The sheep is covered by a drape which offers limited protection from cooling and prevents soiling of the scanner. For subsequent target planning, a high-resolution T1-weighted 3D sequence is acquired with a minimum resolution of 1 x 1 x 1 mm. Acquisition time depends on the number of averages, but usually does not exceed 30 minutes. Additionally, an acquisition of an angiographic sequence is recommended in order to avoid damaging major intracerebral vessels during surgery (see paragraph 3.2.2).

3.2.2 Planning of surgery

The BrainSight™ software (V2.1) consists of a graphical user interface with a tab based arrangement of modules (Fig. 2a, red rectangle). Pre-surgical image processing includes several steps that are explained in detail in the following paragraph.

After starting the software, the MRI data set has to be loaded. Therefore, click of the "Anatomical" tab (Fig. 2a, 1):

1. Select MRI 3D data set by pressing "Choose" and load the data.
2. Identify positioning of animal by clicking on "Show Image & Detail" (Fig. 2a, 2).
3. Choose the radio button which corresponds to the correct animal position (e.g. "actual" orientation → Sphinx Heads First; "scanner" orientation → supine head first)

To avoid accidental intrasurgical damage of major cerebral arteries, an overlay with an angiographic data set is recommended. Therefore, use the "Overlays" tab:

1. Implement the data set by clicking "Load Overlay".
2. Define the desired opacity by choosing the corresponding slider.

In the next step, anatomical structures can be defined by segmentation. While the skin reconstruction is performed automatically, other relevant anatomical structures like the brain and cranial bones have to be identified separately and on each slice. Select the "ROIs" (=region of interest) tab to perform this operation:

1. Press "New ROI from Region Paint".
2. Name the ROI (e.g. "brain").
3. Choose a threshold of grey value to localize the structure by moving the slider (Fig. 2b, 3).
4. The opacity of the selection can be changed by the corresponding slider (Fig. 2b, 4).
5. Start segmentation of the threshold areas in the middle of the brain by pressing on the "Seed Tool" icon (Fig. 2b, 5) and select the threshold area of the brain.
6. If necessary, correct the segmentation manually using the "Erase pencil". Cut the unwanted conjunction between target and non-target structures and clear all non-target structures using the "Erase Fill" tool (Fig. 2b, 5).

7. Choose the next slice.
8. Repeat points 5 to 7 for each MRI slice until all areas of the specific structure are completely selected.
9. Repeat steps 1 to 8 for any other target (e.g. bone, see below).

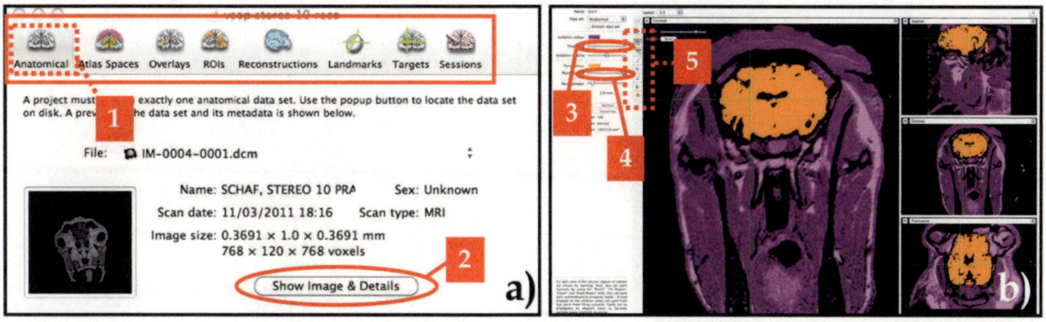

Fig. 2. BrainSight™ software applications I
a) Graphical user interface with tab based modules (red rectangle), "Anatomical" tab (1), "Show Image & Detail" button (2); b) "ROIs": reconstruction of the brain from MRI data set, slider of grey value threshold (3), slider of opacity (4), icon tools (5)

3D reconstructions are created after defining the ROIs. A skin reconstruction is necessary to register the fiducial markers. It is recommended to render 3D reconstructions from brain and bone. Use the "Reconstruction" tab as follows:

1. Skin reconstruction is performed automatically by choosing "Surface Skin". Use the threshold slider to suppress inclusion of air and/or wool in the skin rendering. Press "Compute skin" and subsequently name the reconstruction (e.g. "skin").
2. Bone and brain are calculated by selecting "Surface from ROIs". Label the generated surface as "bone" and "brain". Choose corresponding ROI from the "Select button" and press "Compute Surface".

The MRI-positive fiducial markers need to be relocalized manually in the MRI data set. The tagging of these pivotal landmarks requires maximum precision. Use the "Landmarks" tab:

1. Switch the layout to "1|3 windows".
2. Skin surface reconstruction should be opened in the large left window by choosing "Skin" of the select button (Fig. 3a, 1).
3. MRI data sets are now opened in three windows on the right side. Select "Inline & All Landmarks" in the upper, "Inline 90 & All Landmarks" in the middle and "Perpendicular & All landmarks" in the bottom window. You may wish to zoom out the fiducial marker for better view of their position.
4. Choose "sphere" from the select button (Fig. 3a, 2) as the shape of the fiducial markers. Coordinate system is "Brainsight" (preselected).
5. Press "New" (Fig. 3a, 3). The compiled landmarks will be named automatically.
6. Select a landmark position by choosing a fiducial marker in the skin reconstruction. It will be marked with a sphere. The crosshair in the MRI data now indicates the corresponding position in all views. Correct the relative position of the fiducial marker in each view using the sliders on the right hand side of the screen (Fig. 3a, 4). Position the cursor so that the crosshairs perfectly represents the middle of the fiducial marker in

the upper "Inline & All Landmark" frame and the "Inline 90 & All Landmarks" using the using the "AP" (anterior/posterior) and the "Lat" (medial/lateral) slider.

7. Press "New" for a new landmark and repeat step 6 until all fiducial markers are identified as landmarks by the software.

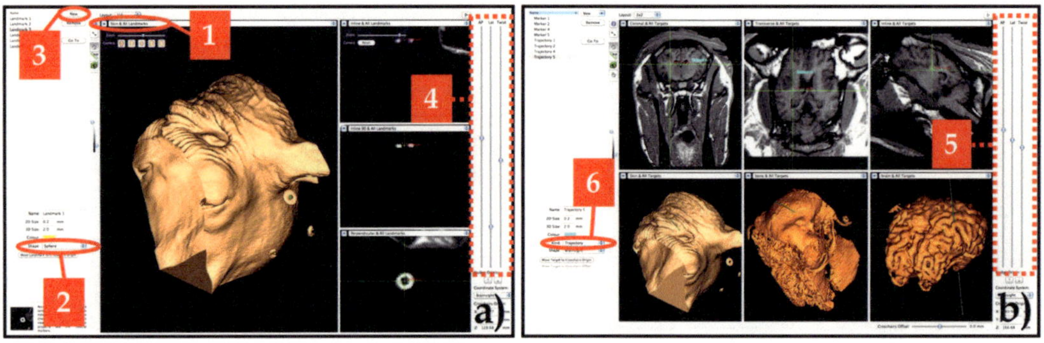

Fig. 3. BrainSight™ software applications II
a) identification of landmarks by MR images using the "landmarks" tab, select button of window view (1), select button of the shape of the fiducial marker (2), "New" button (3), sliders for positioning (4); b) definition of targets and trajectories in MRI and 3D reconstructions of skin, bone and brain, sliders for positioning (5), select button of marker or trajectory (6)

The last step of the planning procedure is the identification of the surgical targets according to the study design. In addition, optimal trajectories are planned during this step. The following recommendations for accessing the target should be considered to ensure a minimal invasive surgical procedure and to avoid surgical problems and complications:

i. Avoid the perforation of the horn plate, even hornless animals have one.
ii. Avoid the perforation of the frontal sinus.
iii. Avoid a trajectory that crosses major vessels (as identified by the angiographic overlay).
iv. Avoid cerebral sulci.

The route to the target (trajectory) and the target itself (marker) should be defined as follows using the "Targets" tab:

1. Switch to a 2 x 3 layout and arrange the frames as follows: MRI data are shown in the upper row and the reconstructed objects in the bottom row. Select "Coronal & All Targets" in the 1st, "Inline 90 & All Targets" in the 2nd and "Inline & All Targets" in the 3rd upper frame. Select "Skin & All Targets", "Bone & All Targets" and "Brain & All Targets" in the bottom row.
2. Coordinate system is "Brainsight" (preselected).
3. Place the crosshair at your target (since a homogeneous MRI signal from the target structure is preferred for the cell tracking experiments, the Corona radiata was used in this example).
4. Use the sliders (Fig. 3b, 5) to place the trajectory (arrow in the crosshair) and make sure it is chosen with respect to the aforementioned recommendations. Ascertain the position of the trajectory in each frame and correct the access using the "AP", "Lat" (lateral) and "Twist" sliders.
5. Choose "Trajectory" in the select button (Fig. 3b, 6) to confirm the planned trajectory. The trajectory is named automatically.

6. Choose "Marker" from the select button ("New" is preselect) to define the target point. The marker is named automatically.
7. Repeat steps 3 to 6 for more trajectories and markers.

Finally, the project should be saved to a specified folder (Menue → "File").

3.3 Frameless stereotaxy in sheep – surgical procedure

3.3.1 General surgery

The Brainsight™ hardware comprises an optical position sensor and a number of surgical devices (Fig. 4). During surgery the anesthetized sheep is placed in the prone position on the

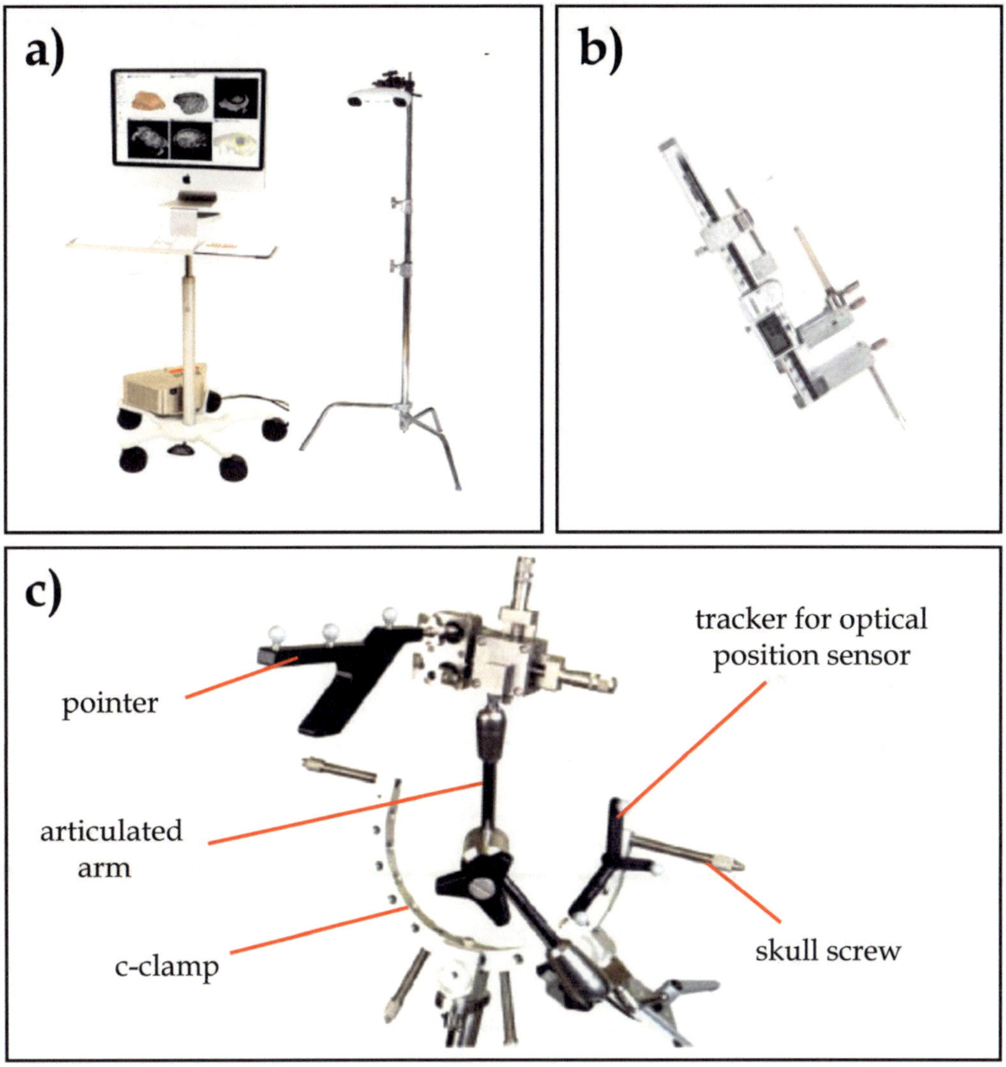

Fig. 4. Brainsight™ hardware
a) The peripheral hardware of Brainsight™ system comprises a computer and an optical position sensor (Polaris®); b) Additionally, a drill guide (not shown) and a ruler guide are available on request; c) The surgical instruments and hardware

operating table. On smaller tables, fix the animal with adhesive tape in the shoulder and hip region. The head rests on a foam rubber pad to ensure a stable and correct position. The upper head of the animal needs to be shaved and disinfected. Next, the maxillary splint has to be placed precisely in the mouth (ensure its correct position) and it should be fastened tightly with a bandage.

A rigid half-circular clamp (c-clamp) is used for fixation of the head and to provide support for the articulated arm. A similar holder system with skull pins is also used for neurosurgical procedures in humans (Olivier & Bertrand, 1983). The c-clamp is fixed to the skull bone by at least four adjustable skull screws. To avoid skull damage the screws are positioned at distinctive spots (e.g. beneath the Linea temporalis and ventral of the Protuberantia occipitalis externa, Fig. 6a). After fixing the c-clamp to the skull, the whole assembly is attached to the operating table using the adjustable mounting system. The system allows to lock the c-clamp, and thereby the skull in the appropriate position. Next the articulated arm is mounted at the c-clamp. Ensure that the entire field of surgery can be reached by the arm. Thereafter, the tracker (containing three track balls which can be recognized by the optical position sensor) is positioned at the c-clamp to act as a fixed optical reference for the coordination system. The system is now ready for merging the virtual MRI data with the spatial position of the sheep's head. The previously processed data sets (MR images, predefined landmarks and targets) have to be reopened by using the "File" option ("Open Project") in the menu. Choose the "Session" tab:

1. Choose "New Online Session" from the select button.
2. Select all "Targets in project" in the opened frame and move them to "Targets to sample in this session" via the drag and drop operations.
3. Press "Next Step" to enter the "Polaris" submodule in the "Session". A new frame will be opened automatically.

Next, the Polaris® optical position sensor has to be configured and adjusted:

1. Make sure the "Polaris status" is "ok" (Fig. 5a, 1) and that all tools (pointer, subject tracker) are located in the detection space (visible field). Otherwise press "Reset Polaris".
2. The tracker (fixed to the c-clamp) should be placed in the middle of the visible field by moving the Polaris camera. Ensure the correct position of the subject tracker in 3D, top, lateral and frontal view. Make sure that the visible field is wide enough to track the pointer when navigating in the periphery of the head. To check this move the Pointer in the 3D field of view).
3. Press "Next Step" (Fig. 5a, 2) to enter the "Registration" module.

Next steps require the spatial allocation of the surgical object (head) and MR images. Therefore, the registration of (physical) fiducial markers with the already defined virtual landmarks is performed as follows:

1. Switch the layout to 1|3 windows and use the same window allocation as during landmark tagging.
2. Perform manual registration update.
3. Select one landmark from the list. The correct selection will be confirmed acoustically. The specific landmark is now displayed and marked in each window.
4. Place the tip of the pointer in the divot of the corresponding fiducial marker. This is the most important step to ensure precision of the surgical approach. The pointer has to be placed orthogonally to the divot in each dimension. Avoid any pressure on the fiducial marker, which may alter its position. Make sure the pointer can be detected by the

optical position sensor. Make sure that the pointer does not move when recording the location of a fiducial markers.

5. Press "Sample & Go to next landmark".
6. Repeat Point 3 to 5 until all landmarks are co-registered with the fiducial markers.
7. Press "Next Step" to enter "Validation" procedure of the registration (see below).

The allocation of the landmarks and fiducial makers is validated as follows:

1. Arrange a 2 x 3 layout.
2. Place the pointer randomly in the divot of each fiducial marker. After ideal co-registration, the pointer tip should now precisely indicate the corresponding landmark. Check the distance of the pointer tip to the corresponding landmark. A vector drift of 1.6 mm can be tolerated, but a difference of <1.0 mm is strongly recommended while a deviation of <0.6 mm is optimal. Repeat the "Registration" in the case of >1.6 mm vector deviation or to ensure demanded precision.
3. To check for lateral deviation in registration of the subject's head, place the pointer on the skin surface at a virtual line between the eyes. Three points per side are recommended. Control the distance in the "Coronal" view, in the "Inline" view and in the "Skin" reconstruction. Repeat the registration in case a unilateral shift is noticed.
4. For longitudial deviation, place the pointer at several points on the skin (six are recommended) in the midline of the cranium. Control the distance in the "Sagital" view, in the "Inline" view and in the "Skin" reconstruction. Repeat the registration in case of a dorsoventral shift. NOTE: Skin thickness may be altered due to the animal being fixed in the c-clamp, causing the occipital skin to be pulled tautly or to bulge. This may alter the preceived skin thickness.
5. Press "Next Step" to continue with planning the surgery.

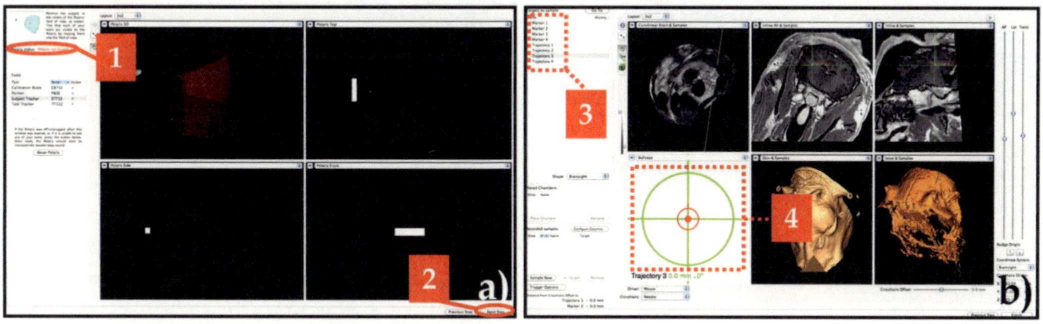

Fig. 5. BrainSight™ software applications III
a) Screenshots taken during the setting of the Polaris® optical position sensor. The tracker and the moveable pointer have to be located in the 3D field. Polaris status (1), "Next Step" button (2); b) For adjustment of trajectory and target (3) within the "Session" tab, the red "Bullseye" (4) has to overlap with the green crosshair as shown

Following this step, adjust the surgical access and the targets. Recall the planned targets in the software interface:

1. Arrange a 2 x 3 layout as follows: upper row comprises "Coronal & samples", "Inline 90 & samples" and "Inline & samples". Bottom row contains "Bullseye", "Skin & samples" and "Bone & samples".

2. Check that the coordinate system is "Brainsight", driver is "Pointer", and Crosshair is "Needle".
3. Select the first trajectory (Fig. 5b, 3).
4. Place the pointer in the articulated arm for adjustment of the trajectory (Fig. 6b). The pointer represents the needle to be inserted during surgery. Make sure the pointer is both locked in the chuck and located in the visible field.
5. Place the pointer tip next to the expected surgical access (drill hole) position by moving the articulated arm. After approximate adjustment, ascertain that the "Bullseye" (red circle) overlaps with the green crosshair.
6. Use the x-y stage to optimize the position. Make sure the red dot of the "Bullseye" aligns with the crosshair (Fig. 5b, 4).
7. Lock the articulated arm and place the stabilizing pin in the guide. Ensure that all hardware pieces are in the correct position and tightly locked now.
8. Measure the thickness of the cranial bone at the level of access in the "Inline 90 & samples" view on the computer. In order to avoid damage to the dura mater or the brain by drilling to deep you may wish to underestimate bone thickness by 0.5 mm.

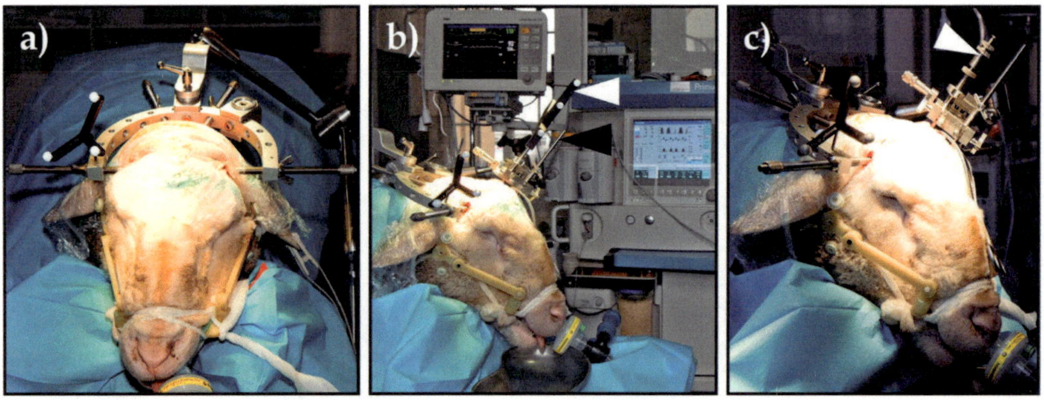

Fig. 6. Surgical set-up in sheep
a) Position of the c-clamp, fixed with 4 skull screws beneath the Linea temporalis and Protuberantia occipitalis externa, note the tracker on the right side of the c-clamp; b) The articulated arm is mounted on the c-clamp and additionally fixed by a sharp stabilizing pin (black arrow). The pointer (white arrow) is placed in the articulated arm at the desired trajectory. c) Drill guide (white arrow) for manual drilling is placed in the arm (Please note that the subject's head is not covered by surgical drape for better illustration)

The skin above the desired access is locally incised. The incision usually does not exceed one centimeter. The periosteum is removed using a Willigers raspartory. You may use small retractors for better accessibility. For skull trepanation, adjust the drill guide to the measured bone thickness, mount it at the end of the articulated arm and place it directly on the exposed skull surface. Drilling is performed at lower speed (10,000 rpm or less, for example using a Microspeed® uni, Aesculap AG, Tuttlingen, Germany). Since minor deviation between measured and real bone thickness can occur, the dura mater may not be reached after drilling. In that case, carefully continue with manual drilling (Fig. 6c). The correct position of the drill hole within the planned trajectory should be checked by placing the pointer tip in the drill hole. In case of minor deviation, the drill hole can be easily expanded during this step.

Next, the distance from the drill hole to the intracerebral target must be measured. Place the pointer tip in the drill hole at the level of the skull surface, not the level of the dura. The distance between the pointer tip and the target should now be displayed on the computer. Thereafter, a ruler guide with digital display is placed in the articulated arm. The instrument to be inserted into the brain, for example a filled Hamilton syringe (see 3.3.2), is mounted at the ruler guide. The tip of the instrument (e.g. a syringe cannula, Hamilton Company USA, Reno, USA) has to be positioned at the level of the skull surface, as done with the pointer tip for distance measuring. Now, set the digital display to zero for reference. The cannula can be inserted to the desired depth (Fig. 7).

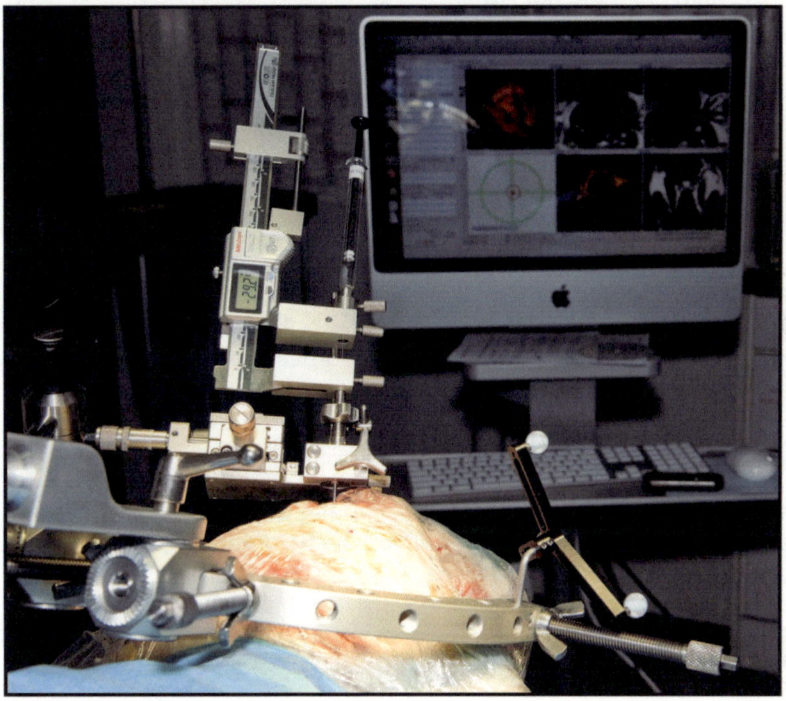

Fig. 7. Application equipment with ruler guide and Hamilton syringe. The syringe is inserted to a depth of 29.2 mm in the given example.

This should be done in a slow and steady manner to avoid microbleedings and injuries. Do not advance faster than 2 mm per minute. In case you want to inject any kind of substance or cell solution (as in the example given in 3.3.2) this should also be done slowly, ideally using a micropump at a maximum pump rate of 5 µl per minute. The cannula is left in position for another ten minutes to allow the injected substance to diffuse locally. The explantation of the cannula is done according to the implantation. Repeat all steps above for multiple insertions. Verify the trajectory for each individual injection. At the end of the surgery, the drill hole is plugged with sterile bone wax, the articulated arm and the c-clamp are removed carefully by detaching the screws, and the skin wounds are sutured. Before the animal awakes from the anesthesia, the maxillary splint is carefully removed and the sheep receives postoperative medication with antibiotics and analgesics for 5 days.

3.3.2 Exemplary applications

Exemplary application for stereotactically guided (cell or blood) depostions following stroke and other cerebral disorders are an emerging field of research in regenerative medicine. This route of administration is expected to be used in upcoming clinical trials. The sheep model allows the simulation of autologous cell therapies, in particular using intracerebral stereotactic cell delivery. This may be required for example when cell depots need to be placed next to a lesion site, which may vary between individual cases.

In the described stereotactic model, autologous bone marrow stromal cells (BMSC) were chosen as an example since these cells were reported to be benefical after stroke treatment and neurodegenerative diseases (Joyce et al., 2010). Also other cell types like neural or embryonic stem cells were used for local transplantation close to the infracted area border (Guzman et al., 2007) or into the contralateral hemisphere (Hoehn et al., 2002) in rodent models. After purification and cultivation (see 4.1.1), a defined cell number is suspended and stored in a Hamilton syringe with a 15.6 cm long cannula. The technique of stereotactic transplantation is described in 3.3.1. For post-translational tracking, the cells can be labeled with iron oxide nanoparticles such as VSOP (very small superparamagnetic ironoxide particles, Ferropharm, Germany) (see 4.1.1). The localization and migration of transplanted cells is monitored by MRI (see 4.1.2).

Alternatively, the stereotactic device can be used to model cerebral hemorrhage by application of blood into the sheep brain. For that purpose, autologous blood is collected from an arterial (preferred) or venous line in a heparinized syringe and is transferred to a Hamilton syringe before application. The steps are technically identical with the injection of cells (see 3.3.1). The injected blood volume depends on the planed region and the target dimensions, but should not exceed two milliliters in sheep (approx. weight of sheep brain: 120 g).

4. Application examples

4.1 Concept 1: Cell labeling for MRI-based tracking in vivo

4.1.1 Harvesting and processing of Bone Marrow Stromal Cells (BMSC)

Autologous cell harvest and cell processing

BMSC are commonly isolated from bone marrow aspirates. Bone marrow samples may be harvested from the iliac crest in humans and in sheep. Therefore, the puncture area on both iliac crests are shaved and disinfected while the anesthetized sheep is placed in a prone position. Samples of approximately 10 mL of bone marrow are taken from both sides by multiple punctures using a heparinized syringe. Higher aspiration volumes from single punctures may result in contamination with peripheral blood. In the next step, the mononuclear cells (MNC) are isolated by density gradient centrifugation, which should be done within one hour after bone marrow harvest. A protocol for the separation of ovine MNC is stated below.

1. Dilute bone marrow with phosphate buffer saline (PBS, Biochrom KG seromed®, Berlin, Germany) at a 1:1 (v/v) ratio.
2. Merge Biocoll (1.077 g/mL, Biochrom KG seromed®, Berlin, Germany) and Pancoll (1.091 g/mL, PAN-Biotech GmbH, Aidenbach, Germany) in a ratio of 1:1 (v/v) to obtain a density of 1.084 g/mL (separation medium). Add 7 mL of mixed separation medium into a 50 mL falcon tube.
3. Carefully place a layer of 10 mL of diluted bone marrow onto the gradient mixture. Avoid commixture between cell layer and the separation medium.

4. Centrifuge at 1,000 x g for 25 min.
5. Carefully transfer the interface layer of mononuclear cells to a sterile centrifuge tube by using a sterile pipette (Fig. 8a).
6. Wash cells twice in PBS.
7. Count MNC.

The BMSC population is isolated from MNC based on its ability to adhere to the cell culture flask. For that reason, MNC are seeded at a density of 5 x 10E4/cm^2 in a culture flask. Cells are cultivated with DMEM (high glucose, PAA Laboratories GmbH, Pasching, Austria), 10% FCS (Invitrogen GmbH, Darmstadt, Germany) and 1% penicillin/streptomycin (PAA Laboratories GmbH, Pasching, Austria) at 37°C and 5% CO_2 for 14 days. Two days after seeding, all non-adherent cells are removed by two washing steps with PBS.

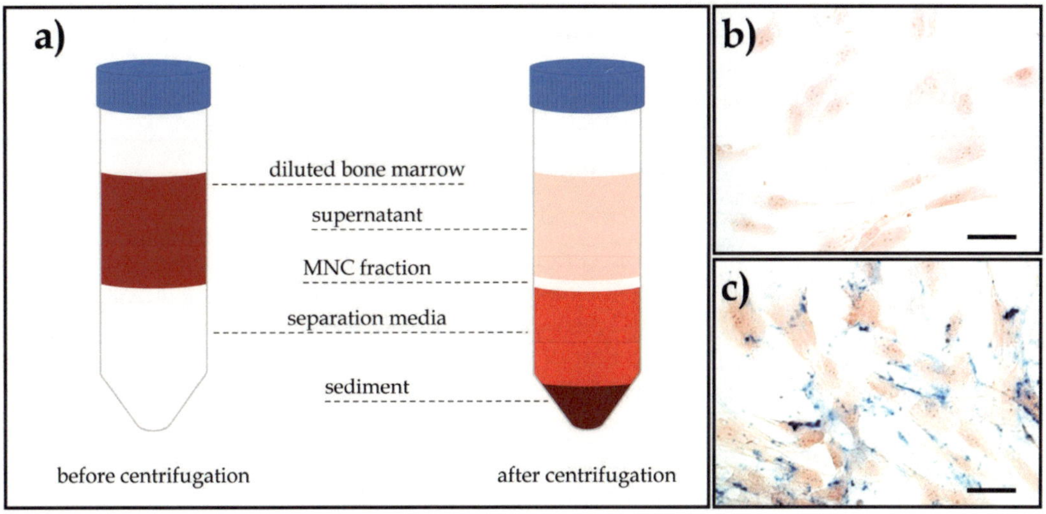

Fig. 8. Density gradient centrifugation of bone marrow and Prussian Blue staining of BMSC a) Density gradient centrifugation of diluted bone marrow: segmentation before and after centrifugation (supernatant: serum and platelets, sediment: erythrocytes and granulocytes) is displayed; b) cultivated, unlabeled, ovine BMSC stained with Prussian Blue (PB) and eosin; c) VSOP-labeled BMSC stained with PB and eosin; scale bar: 50 μm

Cell labeling

Very small superparamagnetic iron oxide particles (VSOP, Ferropharm, Teltow, Germany) are used for magnetic cell labeling. VSOP consist of a 5 nm iron oxide core coated by monomer citrate (total diameter of 9 nm) with a negative surface charge. Iron particle incorporation by the cells causes a strong decrease in the transverse relaxation time, which results in signal loss in T2*-weighted MR imaging (Arbab et al., 2003; Bowen et al., 2002; Renshaw et al., 1986). No apparent long-term cytotoxic effects were observed after using the particles both in vitro and in vivo (Fleige et al., 2002; Stroh et al., 2004 and 2009). For magnetic labeling sterile VSOP are added to the incubation medium. Addition of lipofection agents is not required for BMSC labeling. Cells are incubated with VSOP at 37°C and 5% CO_2 for 90 minutes. After incubation, the cells are washed three times with PBS to remove any remaining VSOP not endocytosed by cells. The cells are harvested by incubation with

trypsin (Invitrogen GmbH, Darmstadt, Germany) for 5 minutes and centrifugated at 350 x g. To visualize the incorporated iron oxide particles, Prussian Blue (PB) staining can be used (Fig. 8c). A protocol for PB staining is given in Table 1.
The cells can be labeled additionally using fluorescent dyes as GFP or PKH26, which may be helpful for histological examination after in vivo applications. This allows discrimination between initially labeled cells and cells that secondarily took up iron by endocytosis.

step	Prussian Blue staining	duration
1	Fixate in 4% paraformaldehyde	20 min
2	Stain with 2% potassium ferrocyanide, Trihydrate and 1% hydrochloride acid in a 1:1 ratio.	20 min
3	Wash in PBS	5 min
4	Stain in eosin	4 min
5	Wash in PBS	5 min
6	Conserve with glycerol (culture flasks) or mounting medium (slide)	

Table 1. Protocol for Prussian Blue staining of VSOP-labeled BMSC

Impact of VSOP labeling on cell viability and T2 relaxation time

The influence of 3.0 mM VSOP on cellular viability and magnetic labeling has been investigated for ovine BMSC in previous experiments. The viability was evaluated by the trypan blue dye exclusion test before labeling, immediately thereafter, as well as after 4 and 24 hours. Viability was compared to that of unlabeled cells. The transverse relaxation time (T2) was measured at 0.47 T/ 20 MHz (Minispec, Bruker, Ettlingen, Germany) immediately and 24 hours after VSOP-labeling to examine labeling efficacy.
Our own results show that cellular viability decreased to 86 ± 16 % immediately after labeling. At 4 hours after labeling, the cell viability rate remained unaltered (89 ± 14 %), but slightly declined to 75 ± 3 % after 24 hours (Fig. 9a). Relaxometry measurements resulted in T2 relaxation times of 1,888 ± 171 ms for unlabeled cells as compared to 434 ± 147 ms for VSOP-labeled cells ($p<0.01$), indicating a reduction of T2-time to 23 ± 8% after VSOP labeling (Fig. 9b, white). This result was reproduced 24 hours after labeling (Fig. 9b, black).

4.1.2 BMSC detection in vivo

Since VSOP shorten T2 relaxation time, the particles can be detected by MRI using gradient echo sequences, in particular T2* weighted imaging. Alternatively, susceptibility weighted imaging (SWI) can be used. The main difference to T2* is the inclusion of phase information into the image acquisition (Haacke et al., 2009). This is of particular advantage in case that dephasing particles such as iron-oxide particles are present in the respective voxel. The dephasing results in a hypointense signal at a given echo time. However, this signal loss is not specific, as there are a multitude of other sources of signal voids, such as blood and air.
The blooming effect is a well known phenomenon caused by iron oxide particles. Due to the augmented dephasing of proton spins, a major susceptibility artefact is depicted that exceeds the real dimension of the particle by a factor of up to 50. Hence, a small amount of

particles or labeled cells, or even single cells, can be detected by high field MRI (Dodd et al., 1999; Shapiro et al., 2005) taking advantage of the blooming effect.

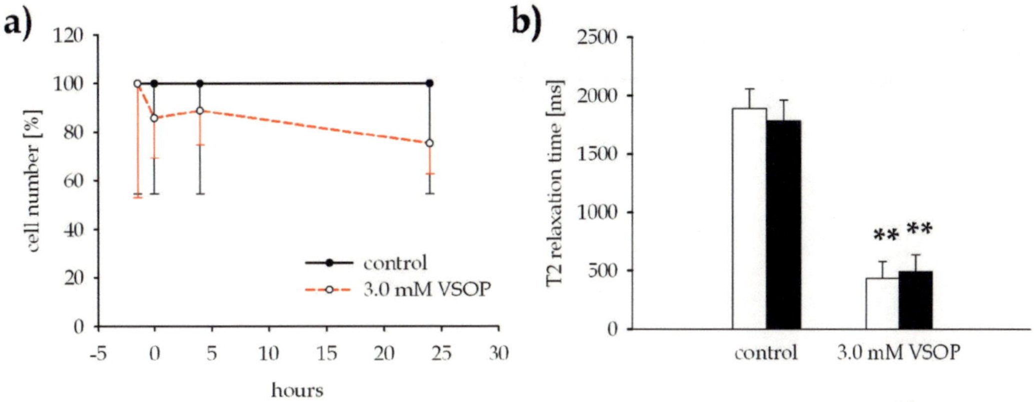

Fig. 9. Viability and relaxometry of VSOP-labeled BMSC
a) Viability during 24 hours after labeling, control treatment is set to 100%; b) Relaxometry of labeled and unlabeled BMSC. White bars: immediately; black bars: 24 hours after labeling (n=6 in each experiment)",**p<0.01.

sequence	resolution	TR	TE	duration
T2*	0.83 x 0.66 x 0.50 mm	620	20	2 h 07 min
SWI	0.56 x 0.39 x 0.25 mm	60	20	1h 29 min

Table 2. Parameters of MR imaging for detection of VSOP-labeled cells in ovine brain; TR – repetition time, TE – echo time

For in vivo detection of VSOP-labeled BMSC in the ovine brain a 3T MRI scanner (Magnetom Trio, Siemens AG, Munich, Germany) was used. After initial anesthesia the sheep was placed on the scanner table as described in 3.1.1 and shown in Fig. 10a. A flexible head coil (Siemens AG, Munich, Germany) was placed centrally above the brain (Fig. 10b). After a brief T2-weighted Turbo Spin Echo (TSE) sequence for anatomical orientation, SWI- and T2*-sequences were acquired with the field of view set to the region of transplantation. The sequence parameters are listed in Table 2. Two hours after transplantation, a distinct, ellipsoidal to circular hypointensity was detectable at all injection sites in T2* and SWI sequences (Fig. 11). This was not the case for control (saline) application without cells.

Histological examination allows discrimination of cellular signals to other sources of hypointense signal change (4.1.3).

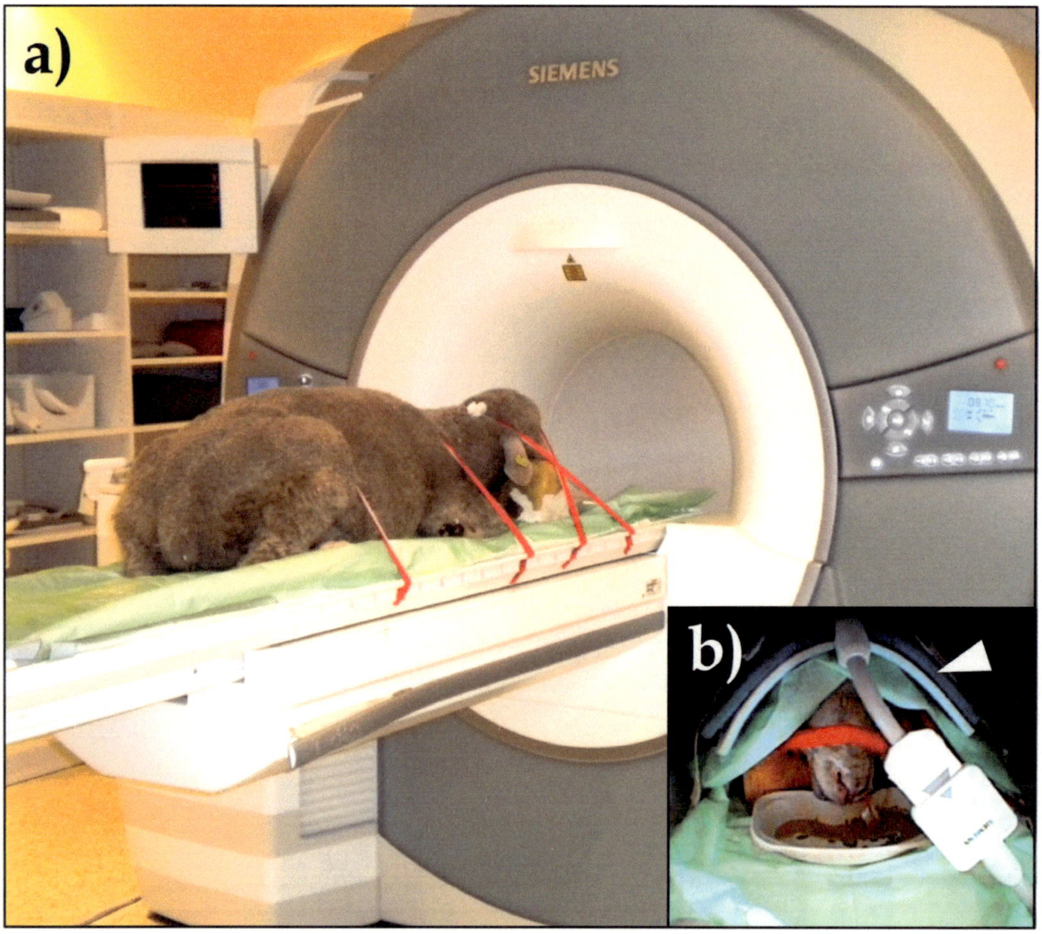

Fig. 10. MRI of sheep
a) Position of sheep in MR scanner. The animal is fixed with adhesive tap;
b) Image taken by the scanner's monitoring camera. The head is placed on a position pad and covered with folio drape and a flexible head coil is used (white arrow). Potentially excreted saliva and rumen fluid are collected by a plastic bowl placed directly below the animal's mouth

The non-invasive detection of the transplanted cells allows longitudinal studies for up to six months in the individual animal for precise detection of migration and localization of transplanted cells (Jendelova et al., 2004; Stroh et al., 2004 and 2005). It can also be combined with stroke related MR-examinations and allows tracing of migration processes towards the lesion.

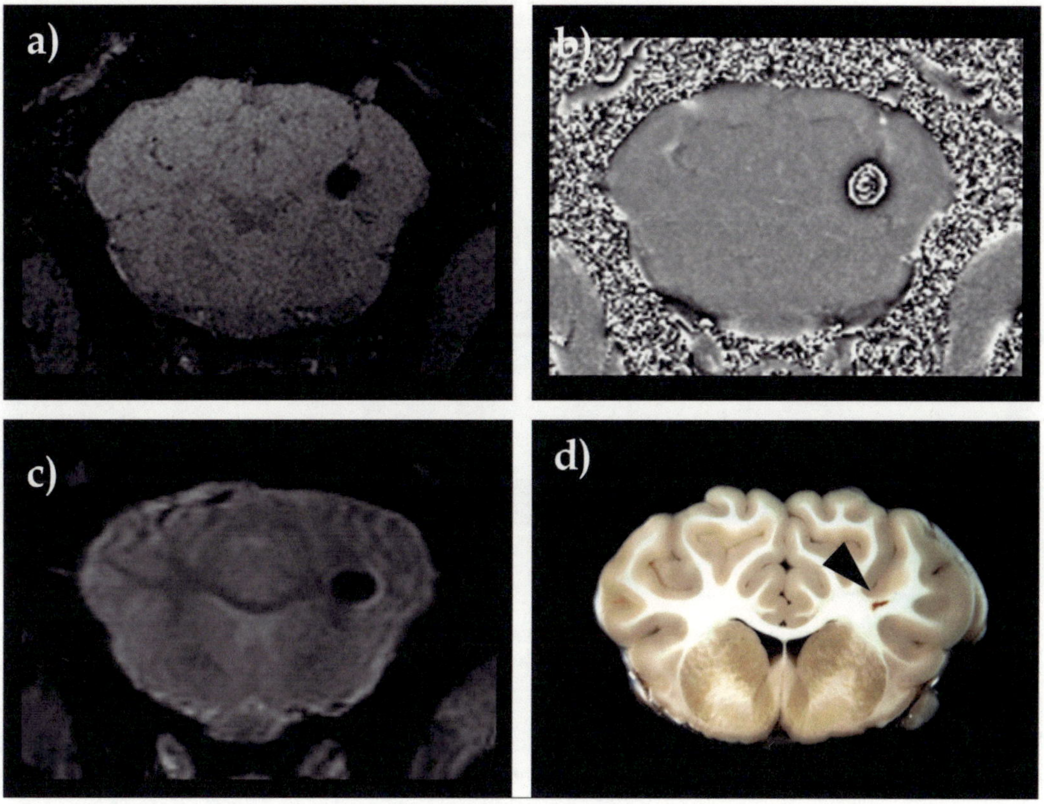

Fig. 11. MR and macroscopic view of 100,000 VSOP-labeled BMSC in the ovine brain
a) susceptibility weighted imaging (SWI), b) phase image of SWI, c) T2* image, d) macroscopic view on brain slice. Black arrow indicates the macroscopically visible BMSC graft

4.1.3 Neuropathology and ex vivo BMSC detection

Animals are sacrificed during deep anesthesia by a single, intravenously injection of 20 mL pentobarbital (Eutha 77, Essex Pharma LtD, Munich, Germany). After death is confirmed (abscence of cardiac, respiratory and reflexive activity over a period of at least two minutes) the sheep is rapidly decapitated at the atlanto-occipital junction. The carotid arteries are exposed for perfusion. Blunt perfusion cannulas are placed in each artery and are fixed with stout thread. Initially, the head is perfused with 3 L PBS followed by 20 L 4% paraformaldehyde (PFA, Carl Roth GmbH & Co. KG, Karlsruhe, Germany). A roller pump system (Roth Cyclo II, Carl Roth GmbH & Co. KG, Karlsruhe, Germany) can be used for that purpose. After removal of skin, muscles and adnexes by a sharp knife, the cranial cavity is opened using an oscillating saw (KM-40, Heraeus GmbH, Hanau, Germany). After careful removal of the dura, the open cranium is fixated in 4% PFA for at least 24 hours. Afterwards, the brain is removed for immersion fixation for another 48 hours in PFA.

Macroscopic examination of the brain comprises weighing, measuring of circumferences, and photographic documentation from all directions. Next, the brain is cut into 4 mm thick, coronal slices which are each photographed from rostral and occipital direction.

Usually, the transplantation procedure does not result in macroscopically visible brain tissue alterations. In a minor number of cases, a very small alteration is observable at the injection site (Fig. 12).

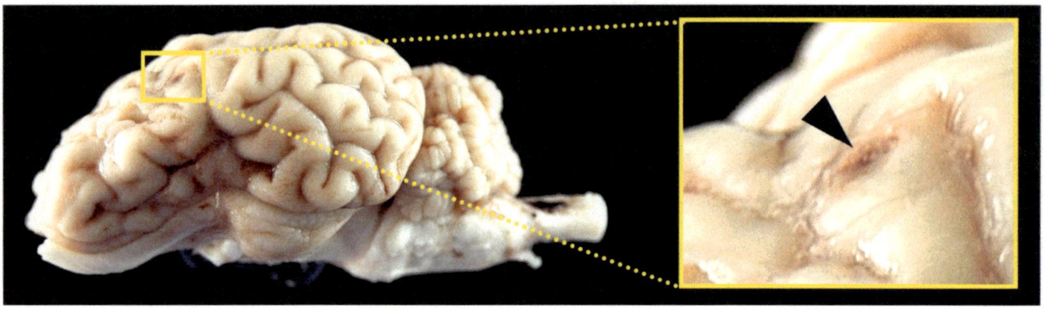

Fig. 12. Ovine brain after stereotatic transplantation
The insertion of the cannula may lead to a small alteration (black arrow) on the brain surface.

The transplantation area is cut out of the associated brain slice, embedded in paraffin and cut into 4 µm thick sections for histological analysis. Hematoxylin/eosin staining according to Table 3 is recommended for histological overview and exclusion of bleeding. Prussian Blue staining (according to Table 1, step 2 - 6) is used for detection of VSOP-labeled cells.

step	hematoxylin/eosin staining	duration
1	Stain in hematoxylin	2 min
2	Wash in piped water	2 min
3	Blue in warm piped water	10 min
4	Stain in eosin	4 min
5	Wash in pure water	5 min
6	Conservation (dehydrating, mounting)	

Table 3. Protocol for hematoxylin/eosin staining

Transplantation of 100,000 VSOP-labeled cells results in a brown spot at the transplantation site which was clearly visible in the coronal slice (Fig. 11d). Transplantation of PBS reveals no changes in the macroscopic view.
Histological investigation by hematoxylin/eosin staining usually reveals a small cavity containing the labeled cells with scattered mononuclear cells within the transplantation site 8 hours after transplantation. Occasionally, microbleedings may occur close to the injection site. In sheep transplanted with VSOP-labeled BMSC, PB-positive cells are clearly detected at the specified target region (Fig. 13). No migration of cells is observed 8 hours after transplantation.

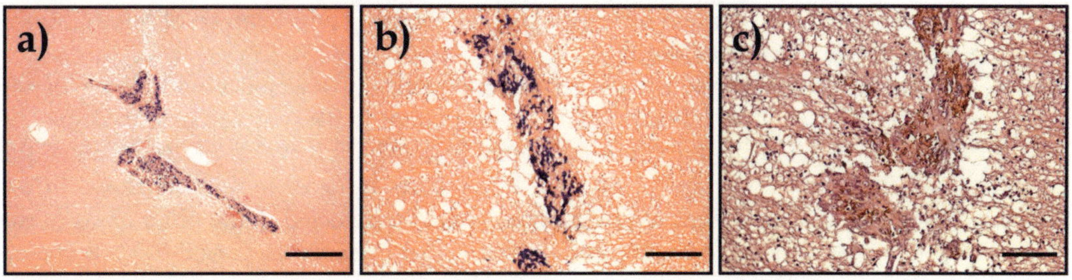

Fig. 13. Histological analysis of 100,000 transplanted, VSOP-labeled BMSC after striatal application
a) Overview of transplantation site stained with PB, scale bar: 500 µm; b) Magnification of PB staining, scale bar: 100 µm; c) hematoxylin/eosin staining of transplantation site, no microhemorrhages (e.g. due to cell injection) are detectable; bar: 100 µm

4.2 Concept 2: Hemorrhage model

4.2.1 Hemorrhage detection

T1-, T2- and T2*-weighted MR sequences can be used for hemorrhage detection. The injection of autologous blood into the sheep brain usually results in a spheric to ellipsoid-shaped blood clot, with the depot size depending on the injected blood volume. The MR signal characteristics of the hemorrhage differ depending on the temporal stage of the hemorrhage and the pulse sequence used (Kidwell & Wintermark, 2008). In the hyperacute stage, hemoglobin is still oxygenated and therefore diamagnetic, thus appearing iso- to hypointense in T1-weighted sequences (Fig. 14a) and hyperintense in T2-weighted MRI (Fig. 15a). A hypointense rim is observable in T2* sequence (Fig. 14b and c). In contrast, methemoglobin is present in the sub-acute stage. Methemoglobin is paramagnetic and generates a hyperintensive signal in T1-weighted and a hypointensive signal in T2-weighted MRI. Later, the signal changes become hypointensive in T1- and T2-weigthed MRI due to the progressive biodegradation of hemoglobin into superparamagnetic hemosiderin

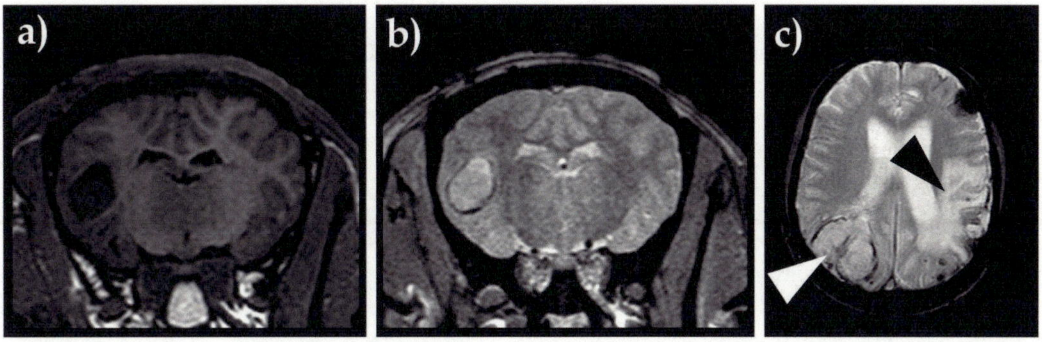

Fig. 14. Imaging of stereotactically placed blood clot (1.8 mL, 3 hours old) in ovine brain for simulation of intracerebral hemorrhage using T1 weighted (a) and T2* weighted sequences (b). An acute occipital intracerebral bleed in a human patient (T2*, 2 hours after onset of visual disturbances, white arrow) is shown in c) for direct comparison. For more details, please refer to main text. Note an old left temporal ischemia (secondary diagnosis) in this particular patient (black arrow)

towards the chronic phase of a hemorrhage. Also, a blooming effect can be observed by the high iron oxide content of hemosiderin (4.1.2).

Fig. 14 gives a direct comparison between a stereotactically injected blood depot in the sheep model and a hyperacute bleeding in a human patient (with symptom onset of approx. 2 h before MRI) in T2* MRI. A hyperintense signal is clearly observable in the center of the injected blood in the sheep brain (b) and the hyperacute intracerebral hemorrhage in the human patient (c), whereas a clear hypointense rim can be detected in the outer areas of the hemorrhage in both subjects. This difference in the signal intensity is caused by oxygenated hemoglobin in the central areas and deoxygenated hemoglobin in the peripheral areas of the hemorrhage. This signal behavior is typical for a hyperacute hemorrhage within a timeframe of approximately 3 to 9 h after symptom onset in human beings (Howells et al., 2010). In summary, the blood-induced MR signal 3 hours after autologous blood injection in the sheep model shows the same characteristics to the situation found in the human patient.

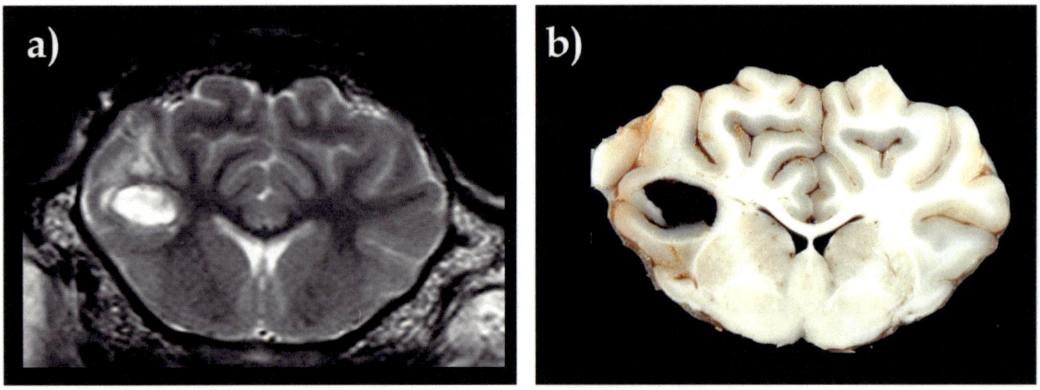

Fig. 15. MRI of induced, acute hemorrhage (1.5 mL) in the ovine brain
a) T2-weighted TSE sequence with a clearly observable, hyperintensive area (blood clot),
b) corresponding macroscopic view of brain slice

Tissue preparation for gross pathology after hemorrhage modeling can be performed according to 4.1.3. The clearly observable cavity in Fig. 15b indicates the injection site. The tissue around the injection site was compressed during blood injection. Similar findings are reported from autopsies of human patients who died from massive intracerebral hemorrhage in early stages.

5. Summary

Stereotactic neurosurgery is a routine technique in human medicine. Stereotaxy-based local treatments of stroke (and other diseases) were effectively tested in rodents using strain- and weight-adapted coordinates and approaches. Hence, it is expected that intracerebral administration paradigms will be evaluated in upcoming clinical trials. However, a proof of concept of such treatment paradigms may be demanded in translational research, preferentially using large animal models. However, similar techniques were so far only available for primate models which are restricted to highly specialized centers.

The described, frameless stereotaxy in sheep represents a novel and translational approach for neurosurgical applications in a widely available species. The used neuronavigation system BrainSight™ was successfully adapted to the ovine skull anatomy. It allows an individual and accurate planning as well as precise execution of stereotactic interventions. Next to a detailed description of the technique itself, two relevant applications of the experimental techniques are reported in this chapter. First, the magnetic labeling and stereotactic transplantation of a stem cell population into the ovine brain is described. The methodology allows for precise injection and tracking of autologous stem cell populations using a widely available 3T MRI scanner. Relatively simple but reliable pathohistological techniques for post-mortem brain assessment and detection of transplanted cells are also given. Thus, the reported methodology may be used for evaluation of cell-based treatment strategies of central nervous system disorders in the gyrencephalic brain. Second, the stereotactic technique can be used for precise modeling of intracerebral hemorrhages by autologous blood injection in sheep. The observed results are in good correlation to those seen in human patients, especially regarding relevant diagnostic findings in MRI. Summarizing, stereotactic interventions in sheep represent a well applicable and reliable approach for translational research with a wide spectrum of possible applications.

6. Acknowledgment

The authors thank Dr. Stephen Frey from Rogue Research Inc. for technical support and the staff of the Institute of Anatomy, Histology and Embrology, Faculty of Veterinary Medicine, University of Leipzig.

7. References

Amiridze, N., Gullapalli, R., Hoffman, G. & Darwish, R. (2009). Experimental model of brainstem stroke in rabbits via endovascular occlusion of the basilar artery. *J Stroke Cerebrovasc Dis.*, 18,4,281-287

Arbab, A.S., Bashaw, L.A., Miller, B.R., Jordan, E.K., Bulte, J.W. & Frank, J.A. (2003). Intracytoplasmic tagging of cells with ferumoxides and transfection agent for cellular magnetic resonance imaging after cell transplantation: methods and techniques. *Transplantation.*, 76, 7, 123-130

Barber, P.A., Zhang, J., Demchuk, A.M., Hill, M.D. & Buchan, A.M. (2001). Why are stroke patients excluded from TPA therapy? An analysis of patient eligibility. *Neurology*, 56, 8, 1015-1020

Blinzler, C., Breuer, L., Huttner, H.B., Schellinger, P.D., Schwab, S. & Köhrmann, M. (2011). Characteristics and outcome of patients with early complete neurological recovery after thrombolysis for acute ischemic stroke. *Cerebrovasc Dis.*, 31, 2, 185-190

Boltze, J., Förschler, A., Nitzsche, B., Waldmin, D., Hoffmann, A., Boltze, C.M., Dreyer, A.Y., Goldammer, A., Reischauer, A., Härtig, W., Geiger, K.D., Barthel, H., Emmrich, F. & Gille, U. (2008). Permanent middle cerebral artery occlusion in sheep: a novel large animal model of focal cerebral ischemia. *J Cereb Blood Flow Metab.*, 28, 12, 1951-1964

Bowen, C.V., Zhang, X., Saab, G., Gareau, P.J. & Rutt, B.K. (2002). Application of the static dephasing regime theory to superparamagnetic iron-oxide loaded cells. *Magn Reson Med.*, 48, 1, 52-61

Bullock, R., Mendelow, A.D., Teasdale, G.M. & Graham, D.I. (1984). Intracranial haemorrhage induced at arterial pressure in the rat. Part 1: Description of technique, ICP changes and neuropathological findings. *Neurol Res.*, 6, 4, 184-188

Burns, T.C. & Steinberg, G.K. (2011). Stem cells and stroke: opportunities, challenges and strategies. *Expert Opin Biol Ther.*, 11, 4, 447-461

Del Zoppo, G.J. (1995). Why do all drugs work in animals but none in stroke patients? 1. Drugs promoting cerebral blood flow. *J Intern Med.*, 237, 1, 79-88

Dodd, S.J., Williams, M., Suhan, J.P., Williams, D.S., Koretsky, A.P. & Ho, C. (1999). Detection of single mammalian cells by high-resolution magnetic resonance imaging. *Biophys J.*, 76, 1 Pt 1, 103-109

Fisher, M., Feuerstein, G., Howells, D.W., Hurn, P.D., Kent, T.A., Savitz, S.I., Lo, E.H. & STAIR Group. (2009). Update of the stroke therapy academic industry roundtable preclinical recommendations. *Stroke*, 40, 6, 2244-2250

Fleige, G., Seeberger, F., Laux, D., Kresse, M., Taupitz, M., Pilgrimm, H. & Zimmer, C. (2002). In vitro characterization of two different ultrasmall iron oxide particles for magnetic resonance cell tracking. *Invest Radio.l*, 37, 9, 482-488

Flower, O. & Smith, M. (2011). The acute management of intracerebral hemorrhage. *Curr Opin Crit Care.*, 17, 2, 106-114

Frey, S., Comeau, R., Hynes, B., Mackey, S. & Petrides, M. (2004). Frameless stereotaxy in the nonhuman primate. *Neuroimage*, 23, 3, 1226-1234

Garcia, J.H., Kalimo, H., Kamijyo, Y. & Trump, B.F. (1977). Cellular events during partial cerebral ischemia. I. Electron microscopy of feline cerebral cortex after middle-cerebral-artery occlusion. *Virchows Arch B Cell Pathol.*, 25, 3, 191-206

Gross, R.E., Watts, R.L., Hauser, R.A., Bakay, R.A., Reichmann, H., von Kummer, R., Ondo, W.G., Reissig, E., Eisner, W., Steiner-Schulze, H., Siedentop, H., Fichte, K., Hong, W., Cornfeldt, M., Beebe, K., Sandbrink, R. & Spheramine Investigational Group. (2011). Intrastriatal transplantation of microcarrier-bound human retinal pigment epithelial cells versus sham surgery in patients with advanced Parkinson's disease: a double-blind, randomised, controlled trial. *Lancet Neurol.*, 10, 6, 509-519

Guzman, R., Uchida, N., Bliss, T.M., He, D., Christopherson, K.K., Stellwagen, D., Capela, A., Greve, J., Malenko, R.C., Moslley, M.E., Palmer, T.D. & Steinerg, G.K. (2007). Long-term monitoring of transplanted human neural stem cells in developmental and pathological contexts with MRI. *Proc Natl Acad Sci U S A*, 104, 24, 10211-10216

Haacke, E.M., Mittal, S., Wu, Z., Neelavalli, J. & Cheng, Y.C. (2009). Susceptibility-weighted imaging: technical aspects and clinical applications, part 1. *AJNR Am J Neuroradiol.*, 30, 1, 19-30

Hacke, W., Kaste, M., Bluhmki, E., Brozman, M., Dávalos, A., Guidetti, D., Larrue, V., Lees, K.R., Medeghri, Z., Machnig, T., Schneider, D., von Kummer, R., Wahlgren, N., Toni, D. & ECASS Investigators (2008). Thrombolysis with alteplase 3 to 4.5 hours after acute ischemic stroke. *N Engl J Med.*, 359, 13, 1317-1329

Hoehn, M., Kustermann, E., Blunk, J., Wiedermann, D., Trapp, T., Wecker, S., S.,Föcking, M., Arnold, H., Heschler, J., Fleischmann, B.K., Schwind, W. & Bührle, C. (2002). Monitoring of implanted stem cell migration in vivo: a highly resolved in vivo magnetic resonance imaging investigation of experimental stroke in rat. *Proc Natl Acad Sci U S A*, 99, 25, 16267-16272

Howells, D.W., Porritt, M.J., Rewell, S.S., O'Collins, V., Sena, E.S., van der Worp, H.B., Traystman, R.J. & Macleod, M.R. (2010). Different strokes for different folks: the rich diversity of animal models of focal cerebral ischemia. *J Cereb Blood Flow Metab.*, 30, 8, 1412-1431

Imai, H., Konno, K., Nakamura, M., Shimizu, T., Kubota, C., Seki, K., Honda, F., Tomizawa, S., Tanaka, Y., Hata, H. & Saito, N. (2006). A new model of focal cerebral ischemia in the miniature pig. *J Neurosurg.*, 104, 2, 123-132

Jendelova, P., Herynek, V., Urdzikova, L., Glogarova, K., Kroupova, J., Andersson, B., Bryja, V., Burian, M., Hajek, M. & Sykova, E. (2004) Magnetic resonance tracking of transplanted bone marrow and embryonic stem cells labeled by iron oxide nanoparticles in rat brain and spinal cord. *J Neurosci Res.*, 76, 2, 232-243

Joyce, N., Annett, G., Wirthlin, L., Olson, S., Bauer, G. & Nolta, J.A. (2010) Mesenchymal stem cells for the treatment of neurodegenerative disease. *Regen Med.*, 5, 6, 933-946

Kang, B.T., Lee, J.H., Jung, D.I., Park, C., Gu, S.H., Jeon, H.W., Jang, D.P., Lim, C.Y., Quan, F.S., Kim, Y.B., Cho, Z.H., Woo, E.J. & Park, H.M. (2007). Canine model of ischemic stroke with permanent middle cerebral artery occlusion: clinical and histopathological findings. *J Vet Sci.*, 8. 4. 369-376

Kidwell, C.S. & Wintermark, M. (2008). Imaging of intracranial haemorrhage. *Lancet Neurol.*, 7, 3, 256-267

Klintworth, G.K. (1965). The pathogenesis of secondary brainstem hemorrhages as studied in an experimental model. *Am J Pathol.*, 47, 4, 525-536

Kolominsky-Rabas, P.L., Heuschmann, P.U., Marschall, D., Emmert, M., Baltzer, N., Neundörfer, B., Schöffski, O. & Krobot, K.J. (2006). Lifetime cost of ischemic stroke in Germany: results and national projections from a population-based stroke registry: the Erlangen Stroke Project. *Stroke*, 37, 5, 1179-1183

Kondziolka, D., Steinberg, G.K., Wechsler, L., Meltzer, C.C., Elder, E., Gebel, J., Decesare, S., Jovin, T., Zafonte, R., Lebowitz, J., Flickinger, J.C., Tong, D., Marks, M.P., Jamieson, C., Luu, D., Bell-Stephens, T. & Teraoka, J. (2005). Neurotransplantation for patients with subcortical motor stroke: a phase 2 randomized trial. *J Neurosurg.*, 103, 1, 38-45

Lansberg, M.G., Schrooten, M., Bluhmki, E., Thijs, V.N. & Saver, J.L. (2009). Treatment time-specific number needed to treat estimates for tissue plasminogen activator therapy in acute stroke based on shifts over the entire range of the modified Rankin Scale. *Stroke*, 40, 6, 2079-2084

MacLellan, C.L., Silasi, G., Auriat, A.M. & Colbourne, F. (2010). Rodent models of intracerebral hemorrhage. *Stroke*, 41, 10, 95-98

Natarajan, S.K., Snyder, K.V., Siddiqui, A.H., Ionita, C.C., Hopkins, L.N. & Levy, E.I. (2009). Safety and effectiveness of endovascular therapy after 8 hours of acute ischemic stroke onset and wake-up strokes. *Stroke*, 40, 10, 3269-3274

O'Collins, V.E., Macleod, M.R., Donnan, G.A., Horky, L.L., van der Worp, B.H. & Howells, D.W. (2006). 1,026 experimental treatments in acute stroke. *Ann Neurol.*, 59, 3, 467-477

Olivier, A., Bertrand, G. (1983). A new head clamp for stereotactic and intracranial procedures. Technical note. *Appl. Neuropyhsiol.*, 46, 5-6, 272-275

Renshaw, P.F., Owen, C.S., McLaughlin, A.C., Frey, T.G. & Leigh, J.S., Jr. (1986). Ferromagnetic contrast agents: a new approach. *Magn Reson Med.*, 3, 2, 217-225

Rymer, M.M. (2011). Hemorrhagic stroke: intracerebral hemorrhage. *Mo Med.*, 108, 1, 50-54

Sahota, P. & Savitz, S.I. (2011). Investigational therapies for ischemic stroke: neuroprotection and neurorecovery. *Neurotherapeutics*, 8, 3, 434-451

Samadani, U. & Rohde, V. (2009). A review of stereotaxy and lysis for intracranial hemorrhage. *Neurosurg Rev.*, 32, 1, 15-22

Savitz, S.I., Chopp, M., Deans, R., Carmichael, S.T., Phinney, D. & Wechsler, L. (2011). Stem Cell Therapy as an Emerging Paradigm for Stroke (STEPS) II. *Stroke*, 42, 3, 825-829

Shapiro, E.M., Skrtic, S. & Koretsky, A.P. (2005). Sizing it up: cellular MRI using micron-sized iron oxide particles. *Magn Reson Med.*, 53, 2, 329-338

Shobha, N., Buchan, A.M., Hill, M.D. & Canadian Alteplase for Stroke Effectiveness Study (CASES) (2011). Thrombolysis at 3-4.5 hours after acute ischemic stroke onset--evidence from the Canadian Alteplase for Stroke Effectiveness Study (CASES) registry. *Cerebrovasc Dis.*, 31, 3, 223-228

Stadler, J.A. 3rd, Ellens, D.J. & Rosenow, J.M. (2011). Deep brain stimulation and motor cortical stimulation for neuropathic pain. *Curr Pain Headache Rep.*, 15, 1, 8-13.

Starr, P.A., Vitek, J.L. & Bakay, R.A. (1998). Ablative surgery and deep brain stimulation for Parkinson's disease. *Neurosurgery*, 43, 5, 989-1013

Stroh, A., Zimmer, C., Gutzeit, C., Jakstadt, M., Marschinke, F., Jung, T., , Pilgrimm, H. & Grune, T. (2004). Iron oxide particles for molecular magnetic resonance imaging cause transient oxidative stress in rat macrophages. *Free Radic Biol Med.*, 36, 8, 976-984

Stroh, A., Faber, C., Neuberger, T., Lorenz, P., Sieland, K., Jakob, P.M., Webb, A., Pilgrimm, H., Schober, R., Pohl, E.E. & Zimmer, C. (2005). In vivo detection limits of magnetically labeled embryonic stem cells in the rat brain using high-field (17.6 T) magnetic resonance imaging. *Neuroimage*, 24, 3, 635-645

Stroh, A., Boltze, J., Sieland, K., Hild, K., Gutzeit, C., Jung, T., Kressel, J., Hau, S., Reich, D., Grune. T. & Zimmer, C. (2009). Impact of magnetic labeling on human and mouse stem cells and their long-term magnetic resonance tracking in a rat model of Parkinson disease. *Mol Imaging*, 8, 3, 166-178

The STAIR Participants. (1999). Recommendations for standards regarding preclinical neuroprotective and restorative drug development. *Stroke*, 30, 12, 2752-2758

The STEPS Participants. (2009) Stem Cell Therapies as an Emerging Paradigm in Stroke (STEPS): bridging basic and clinical science for cellular and neurogenic factor therapy in treating stroke. *Stroke*, 40, 2, 510-515

Willems, P.W., van der Sprenkel, J.W., Tulleken, C.A., Viergever, M.A. & Taphoorn, M.J. (2006). Neuronavigation and surgery of intracerebral tumours. J Neurol., 253, 9, 1123-1136

Zhu, H., Li, Q., Feng, M., Chen, Y.X., Li, H., Sun, J.J., Zhao, C.H., Wang, R.Z., Bezard, E. & Qin, C. (2011). A new cerebral hemorrhage model in cynomolgus macaques created by injection of autologous anticoagulated blood into the brain. *J Clin Neurosci.*, 18, 7, 955-960

3

A Master Key to Assess Stroke Consequences Across Species: The Adhesive Removal Test

Valentine Bouet and Thomas Freret
Université de Caen Basse-Normandie
France

1. Introduction

1.1 History of the adhesive removal test

Long-term consequences of stroke are often dramatically disabling for daily living but also costly for public health. Stroke research is therefore a priority for most industrialized countries. Therefore and paradoxically, the current situation is disappointing for the patients but stimulating for the researchers who have to figure out new therapies and assess their efficiency. The major initial problem to solve for clinicians when a stroke occurs is to rapidly distinguish between ischemia and hemorrhage to decide for the reperfusion of the brain or for the bleeding stop. Therefore, the first step of stroke treatment takes place within a very short-term and tiny time window (even if it was recently extended to 4 hours for thrombolysis). Next steps of the treatments are directed to avoid another stroke and to promote rehabilitation. For this latter, unfortunately, the treatments are scarce and although many different options have been tested (kinesiotherapy, speech therapy etc.), the situation is still unsatisfactory. News fields of research tried to find out new therapies aimed at improving neurogenesis, implanting stem cells or grafts, or stimulating trophic and growth factors, but in vain, transfer from animal to human is still disappointing. Another way to deal with treatment of stroke is to assess what happens in those patients who recover spontaneously. Indeed, around 33% of stroke patients spontaneously recover after stroke but the mechanisms involved in the recovery, not elucidated till now, could be interesting to promote. To assess these mechanisms, it is of a major importance to be able to measure long-term functional deficits in animal models of stroke, which is by the way a strong recommendation from the STAIR Roundtables (STAIR, 1999; STAIRIII, 2001).

According to the brain structures infracted, stroke induces many different symptoms affecting physiological, sensori-motor, and/or cognitive functions. In experimental studies, it is possible to induce different models of stroke and to assess with many different ways their consequences. However, given the extraordinary spontaneous recovery displayed by animals, especially rodents, it is not always possible to highlight long-term deficits. Indeed, small brain lesions induce deficits that either cannot be detected by global behavioral tests or only for a short term period after stroke (limb placing test, neurological score). That is the reason why news tests have been designed to assess functional recovery in animals. Among the various behavioral tests developed so far, the adhesive removal test and all its variations (sticky-tape test, bilateral asymmetry test) have been proved to be one of the most efficient to highlight tiny long term sensori-motor deficits. Originally brought back from bedside to

bench by Schallert *et al.* (Schallert et al., 1982), this test is derived from a neurologic exam routinely used by clinicians, namely the Double Simultaneous Stimulation (DSS). In fact, the DSS has been initially developed by clinicians to highlight the contralateral neglect syndrome which is observed in patients after damage to the parietal cortex (Heilman et al., 2000). During the DSS examination, the patient has to attend to and identify paired of sensory stimuli that are applied to both sides of the body at the same time. Stimuli can be visual, auditive or tactile. Extinction to double simultaneous tactile stimulation (tactile DSS) was first reported at the beginning of the 80's (Schallert et al., 1982). Tactile extinction is the failure to perceive and/or report tactile stimulation on the body side contralateral to a brain lesion when the homologous, ipsilesioned region is stimulated simultaneously; whereas no defect in tactile perception occurs with unilateral stimulation. Interestingly, tactile extinction showed to be promising as a predictor of post-stroke functional outcome (Rose et al., 1994).
In the way of improving the functional assessment in experimental stroke models, adhesive removal test has been first adapted to rats about a quarter of century ago (Schallert et al., 1982). The stimulus employed was then tactile, consisting of adhesive tapes applied to different parts of the animal body (forelimbs, hindlimbs and snout). It measures sensory functions, sensory neglect and motor functions independently for the left and the right side. Initially designed to highlight deficit induced by unilateral nigrostriatal damage, its range of application has been extended to several brain disorders (Parkinson disease, brain trauma, spinal cord lesion), including stroke. Giving advantage to assess sensory and motor deficits, free from postural bias and circling behaviors, the adhesive removal test has been highly used in rats to a large extent. Interestingly, long-term after stroke, while many tests are not sensitive enough to measure any deficit because of an apparent full recovery, the adhesive removal test is one of the rare tests powerful enough to give an objective score of the functional deficit. Besides, the deficits observed after stroke very well mimics the extinction to tactile double simultaneous stimuli reported in stroke patients (Schallert et al., 1982). Owing to its success in rats, the adhesive removal test has been afterward developed in other animal species. Thus, in the beginning of the 90's, the test was adapted to a nonhuman primate species, the marmoset (*Callithrix jacchus*) (Annett et al., 1992; Marshall &Ridley, 1996). Used then in gerbils (Ishibashi et al., 2003) and even dogs (Quaranta et al., 2004), it has been lastly developed in mice (Bouet et al., 2009; Bouet et al., 2007; Starkey et al., 2005). Thus, beyond its effectiveness to highlight long term, and consequently tiny, sensory and motor deficit, the adhesive removal test is adaptable to several animal models, which is a fundamental advantage to translate animal research to clinical application.
Convinced that this test could offer even more than it has already did, we will along this chapter give an overlook of the way it has to be performed and the results you may obtained in several animal models of stroke: mice, rats, and marmosets (Bouet et al., 2009; Bouet et al., 2010; Bouet et al., 2007; Freret et al., 2009; Freret et al., 2008; Freret et al., 2006; Freret et al., 2006), *i.e.* the most used species in neuroscience research.

2. Achievement of adhesive removal test across laboratory species

2.1 Species

As stated before, the adhesive removal test has been already developed in a wide range of animal species, from nonhuman primate to rodents (rats, mice, gerbils). This test can theoretically be performed in any species that is anatomically able to remove a piece of adhesive pasted on its body. However, according to the species concerned, technical details have to be adjusted, notably the size of adhesives tapes, but also the animal's body part that will be concerned by tactile stimulation depending on whether the species is purely a quadruped or not (see below).

2.2 Training and age

Although training sessions are not mandatory, they are highly recommended. Training decreases anxiety related to the test, and therefore decreases the probability that the animal will urinate and defecate during the subsequent test phase, allowing researchers to obtain an optimal level of performance. It is beside of prime importance to maintain consistency in the testing environment because small changes may impact on animals' emotional state and consequently on the functional outcome. Additionally, training allows indentifying any pre-operative asymmetries that would induce a bias in the interpretation of the data. Finally, training also decreases inter-individual variability, making performances homogenous. Once the animals display good performances, only deficits due to the insult are compared, without learning effect. Furthermore, it is important that sham-operated and experimental animals are trained to the task, because surgery itself could induce a slight change in performances. Besides, doing so allow to use each animal performance as its own control (training phase performances compared to those obtained after surgery).

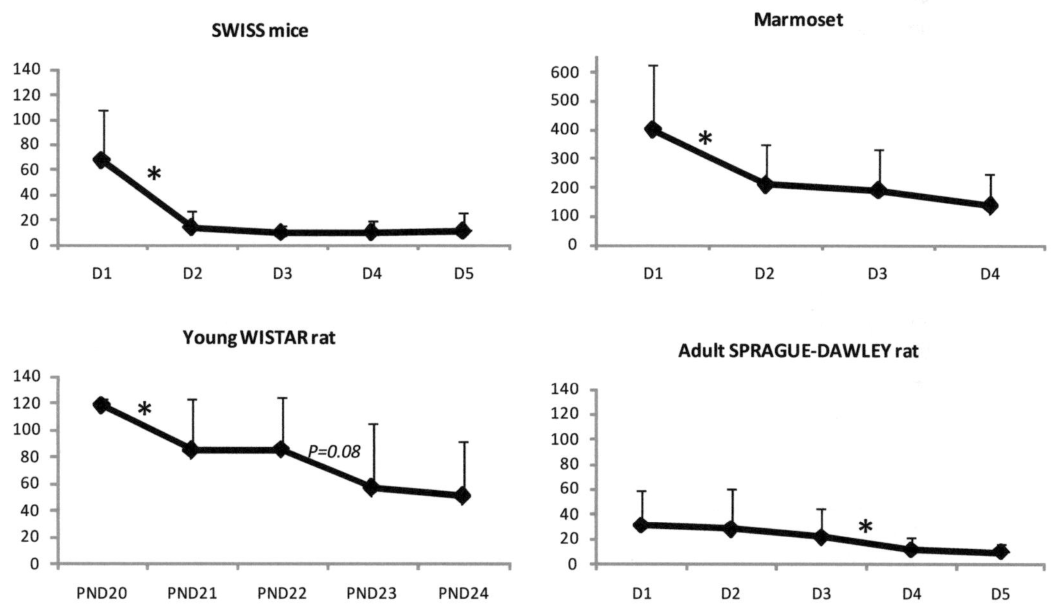

Fig. 1. Time to remove (s) an adhesive tape in four non-injured species during training. Data are expressed as mean (±SD). In all species, ANOVA indicates a significant decrease with time ($p<0.0001$ in NMRI mice, $p=0.0005$ in marmosets, $p=0.0015$ in young Wistar rats, $p<0.0001$ in adult Sprague Dawley rats). In most cases there is a decrease in performances between the first and the second day of training.

Even though adult animals are used in most studies, we recently showed that it is possible to perform the adhesive removal test in young rats (from post-natal day 20) (Bouet et al., 2010) - enlarging thus the range of application of the test to perinatal ischemic stroke. In this case, pups were submitted to a brain injury at the age of 7-days old. Thus, training to the task before injury was not feasible making confounding training and deficits related to the injury. We observed the first day that young rats (20 days old) were unable to perform the task within the given time. Afterwards, sham animals showed better and better performances with time while lesioned animals stayed on the plateau level. This indicates that in particular cases, it is possible to obtain satisfactory data even without training. Our data showed that one week of training (1 trial per day) is sufficient for adult rats, mice and marmosets to reach a plateau level (Figure 1), whereas it is not the case for rat pups (PND20). This increased duration of training with young animals is partly due to the fact that rearing is required to remove adhesive and at this age, hindlegs weight bearing is still unstable. Of note, in marmosets, the stress of the procedure induces high values in the time to remove the adhesive the first days that is the reason why the maximal time given to the animal to perform the task is of 10 min (2 min for rodents). However, the plateau is reached by the 3rd day of training.

2.3 Body parts

According to the species, adhesive removal is performed on different ways, related to the body parts on which adhesive tapes are placed, the parameters collected the place in which the test is performed… Concerning the body parts concerned, they often vary according to the location of the brain lesion and because of the differential sensitivity of different body parts of the species considered. For instance in rats, placing the adhesive on forepaws is the most efficient; indeed they do not really take care of adhesive placed on their back paws, probably because of weight support that induces a large stimulation of the plantar surface and strongly diminishes the discrimination. Additionally, sticking the adhesive tape on the forepaws of the animals will drive it to naturally remove the adhesive for its grooming. The same holds true for mice, in which adhesive test has been first described with positioning on the snout (Fleming et al., 2004), and then on forepaws (Bouet et al., 2009; Bouet et al., 2010; Bouet et al., 2007; Freret et al., 2009; Freret et al., 2006; Freret et al., 2006; Starkey et al., 2005), alike rats. In gerbils, and also in most of the studies performed in rats, the adhesive is placed on the wrist (Ishibashi et al., 2003). In primates, because of the role of hands in objects manipulation, adhesives are preferably placed around the feet (Annett et al., 1992; Freret et al., 2008; Marshall &Ridley, 1996).

Consequently, while removing an adhesive pasted on the forepaws seems quite easy to do for rodents after training, it seems to be more tricky for marmosets. Figure 2 shows that while rodent stand on their hindpaws to remove the adhesive with the mouth, the marmoset has to stand on his bottom and raise the leg to bring the foot to the mouth. Such postures are rather close to the grooming postures for rodents, but they are more scarse in marmosets. This is one of the reasons that explain the increase in time to remove the adhesive for marmosets compared to rodents. The other reason is due to the fact that for marmosets the adhesive tapes enroll all the foot, making hard, therefore time-consuming to unroll. Such a long adhesive tape unrolling the limb of the animal can also be done in rodents, making it even more difficult to remove (Komotar et al., 2007).

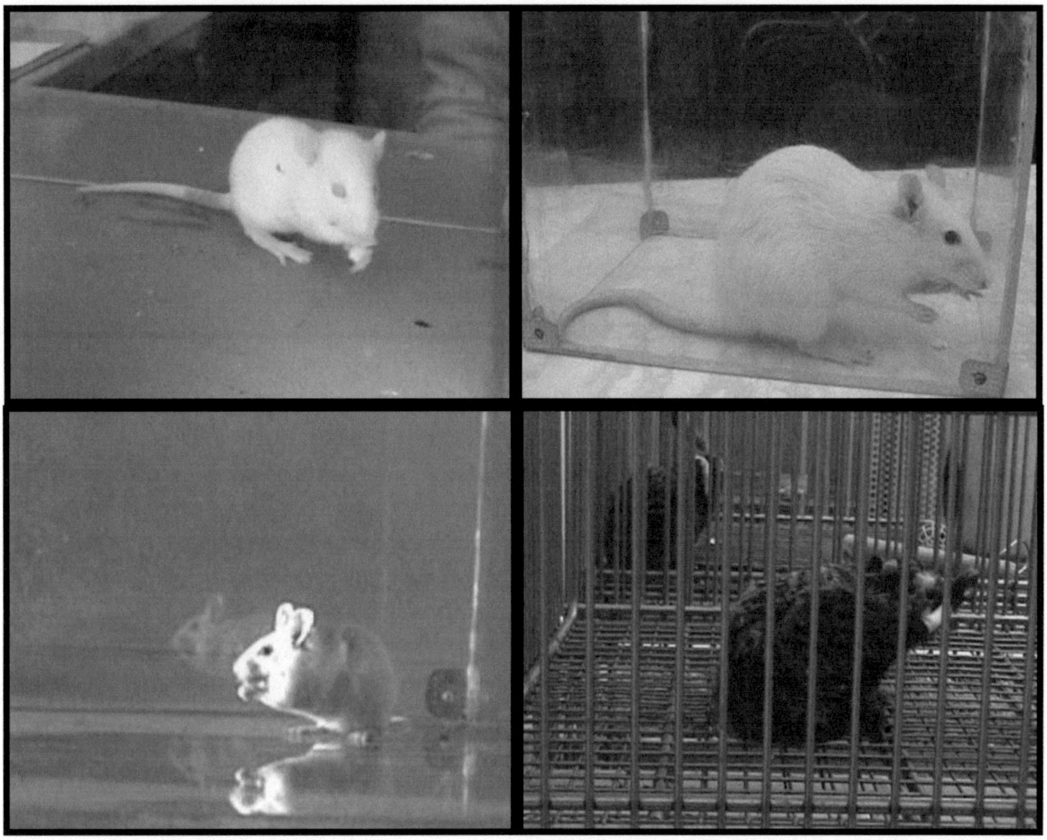

Fig. 2. Pictures depicting a young rat, an adult rat, a mouse and a marmoset being removing the adhesive tapes. All three species use the mouth to remove the adhesive. When very well trained, rats sometimes keep a three-feet posture to remove the tape. The training is very useful to render the animals accustomed to the procedure, and therefore to obtain homogenous data. When the training is not possible (for instance, if a brain injury is performed in young animals), the test is still possible, but the authors have to discuss the fact that the recovery and the learning of the task are mandatory overlapping.

2.4 Adhesive tape size

According to the species, the size of the tape has to be adapted and very tightly controlled. Indeed, Schallert and Whishaw (Schallert &Whishaw, 1984) showed that the size of the adhesive could strongly influence the performances. In rats, Komotar *et al.* (Komotar et al., 2007) advised to use very large adhesive tapes and pasted them around the wrist, in order to make a kind of sleeve that cannot be removed for the duration of 30 s (the main parameter is the time the animals attempts to remove the adhesive). Most of the times, in rats and mice adhesive tape is small and pasted on the paw with the aim to cover the three pads, thenar and hypothenar (size: 1x1cm in rats (Freret et al., 2006); 0.3x0.4cm in mice (Bouet et al., 2007)). In primates, the tape has to be rectangular and should roll up the foot (2x4.5 cm in marmosets, (Freret et al., 2008)). Unavoidably, there are many differences between labs in the achievement of this test, and therefore the most important things to keep in mind is to always have a control group, always apply the adhesive with the same pressure on the right and left hand (an experimenter blind to the treatment is an obvious necessity), and always buy the adhesive tape from the same supplier (same brand). Our experience is that the sewed-adhesives used for bandage are the best (from Sogiphar, Urgo or BSN Medicals in France for example).

2.5 Positioning of the adhesive

Adhesive positioning requires animal contention to ensure a very good precision (Figure 3). Contention has to be performed as gently as possible, because any increase in stress can totally biases the results by increasing the time to perform the task, and this is true whatever the species. For the rat and the marmoset, the animal can be held by the torso by an experimenter, while the other experimenter places the tapes (Bouet et al., 2010; Freret et al., 2008; Freret et al., 2006). For the mouse and the gerbil, the animal can be held by the back skin in order to let the forepaw free (about the same way used to make intraperitoneal injection) (Bouet et al., 2009; Ishibashi et al., 2003). The experimenters have to get used with the contention before starting the experiments, by a previous training if necessary. The contention has to be gentle but firm. Rodents have to be held by the back skin as close to the neck as possible to maintain the head and thus prevent any biting. Once the animal is quietly held, the experimenter has to place an adhesive on each paw (alternating right and left between days and between animals), in a way that the pressure is identical on both paws and that the same skin portion is covered on both paws. To avoid the experimenter who is in charge to place the adhesive to be bite, it is important to maintain the foreleg as extended as possible by pulling the fingers before placing the adhesive tape. For rodents, the adhesive is rectangular or squared, and for marmosets it is rectangular and has to be placed around the foot in order to make a small overlap of the tissue.

The animal is then placed back in his own cage (without congeners) or in an experimental box (if this last is used, a habituation period has to be performed before positioning the adhesive by giving to the animal 1 or 2 minute free exploration of the box). Indeed, the test can be either performed in the home cage or in a testing box, depending on the animals housing conditions. If animals are single-housed, the first solution should be preferred, since it avoids any supplementary stress for animal. As a contrary, carrying out the adhesive removal in a testing box rather than in the home cage, should be preferred when animal are group-housed to avoid interaction between individuals that can alter performances. Nevertheless, in the former case, a habituation period to the testing box should be respected.

2.6 Collecting the data

Once the animal is placed back in the cage with the two adhesive pasted on the paws, four different values have to be collected: time to contact and time to remove the adhesive for each paw.

- Tactile responses are measured by time to initial contact, which is related to the time taken by the animal to react to the presence of each adhesive. It is often considered as a sign of sensory system stimulation. The response of the animal to this stimulation is generally a shake of the paw of a touch with the mouth. For marmoset it can also be a scratching of the leg on the side of the adhesive.
- Time to remove is related to the time needed to completely take away each adhesive. Rodents as well as marmosets generally remove the adhesive with their mouth. Rodents

usually take a small piece between teeth and remove it in one movement (Figure 2), while marmosets often try several times to remove it by biting. The time to remove reflects as well as sensory and motor abilities, since it requires a correct dexterity.

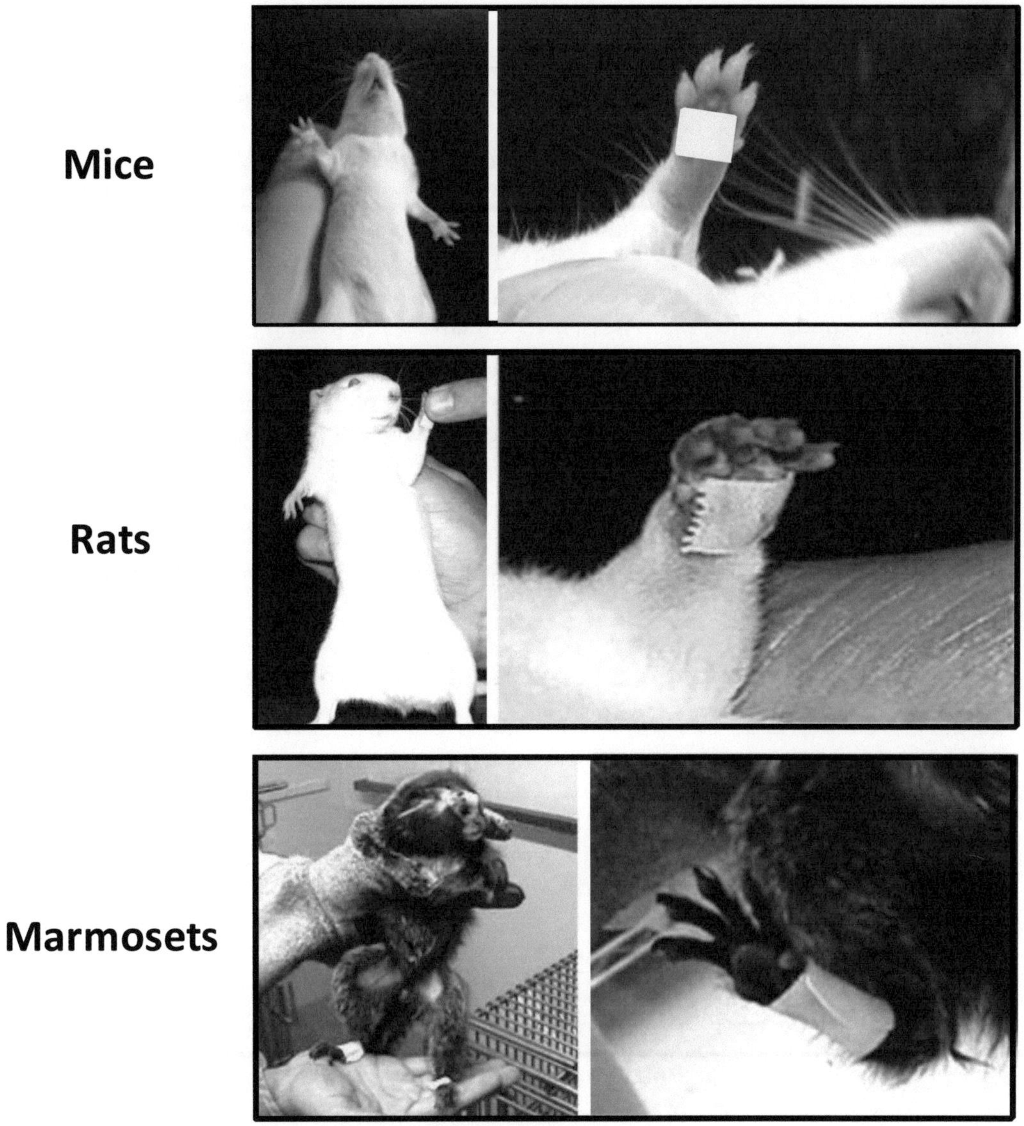

Fig. 3. Positioning of the adhesive tapes in mice, rats and marmosets. The piece of adhesive has to be positioned on fore paws for mice and rats, and on hind paws in marmosets (alternation between left and right for the first positioning and between trials should be achieved).

Overall, time to contact and time to remove crudely separate out sensory *versus* motor deficits (Schaar et al., 2010). On a side point, it should be noted that the adhesive removal test can also be used to measure animals sensory asymmetries. The magnitude of sensory asymmetry is measured by adjusting the ratio of the size of the adhesive tapes on each limb. This test can thus reveal asymmetrical biases in stimulus-directed activity after focal ischemia (Schallert et al., 2000).

2.7 Analyzing of the data collected

Statistical analyses have to be conducted on several parameters to check first some possible discrepancies but also to measure the intensity of the deficits and of the recovery. The first important point is to check, before any brain injury, if there is no initial asymmetry between left and right side. Indeed, it has been showed that for certain sensorimotor tasks, rodents could display an important asymmetry (Bulman-Fleming et al., 1997). The statistical analysis will therefore compare contralateral and ipsilateral removal and contact times. The second point concerns the appraisal of the deficit. To this, two different possibilities exist: data obtained after the injury could be compared to those obtained before the insult (this is also important in sham-operated animals to assess if surgery in itself induces or not any deficit). In this case, it is interesting to express data in percentages compared to pre-surgery. Otherwise, comparisons could also concern data obtained on the controlateral *versus* ipsilateral side. This allows comparing two measurements performed on the same animals within the same session. Moreover, this allows calculating an asymmetry index (contralateral - ipsilateral time).

As regards to number of animals per group, previous studies from the literature have proved that even a small number of animals per group allow to show statistical difference in the adhesive removal test (Freret et al., 2006; Zhang et al., 2011).

3. Deficits in adhesive removal test after stroke in rodents and marmosets

The adhesive-removal test is classically used to detect forepaw somatosensory - *time to contact* - and sensorimotor - *time to remove* - deficits that are not attributable to postural bias (Schallert et al., 1983). Its sensitivity to ischemia-induced deficits has already been reported in the literature (Modo et al., 2000) for every species in which it has been developed, and in most experimental models of cerebral ischemia. For best comparisons between species, most of the results presented here are related to the intra-luminal model of cerebral ischemia. This model has been chosen to illustrate our purpose, because it concerns the middle cerebral artery (MCA) - the most frequently affected artery in stroke patients, because duration of occlusion can be modified, but mostly because a reperfusion event is feasible and thus this closely mimics what happens in patients. In this model, the site of the occlusion of the MCA (MCAo) could either be proximal (close to the origin of the artery, p-MCAo) or distal (after the lenticulostriate branches, d-MCAo). In case of p-MCAo, behavioral deficits in the adhesive removal test are readily observable - even in mice, a species in which subtle behavioral changes are particularly difficult to detect. However, p-MCAo is not representative of all clinical situations because it leads to brain infarctions that are relatively larger than those observed in human stroke. As it induces smaller infarct, d-MCAo is more relevant to those clinical situations. Behavioral alterations after d-MCAo have been largely explored in rats or in marmosets, but, unfortunately, most of the studies using this model in mice considered time points early after surgery and mostly addressed lesion size. Only motor coordination difficulties, attentional deficits and a low increase in eye movement during the dark phase of sleep have been reported in mice (Baumann et al., 2006; Guegan et al., 2006; van Lookeren Campagne et al., 1999). The reason for this lack in literature is that long-term behavioral deficits (*i.e.*, several weeks after surgery) are difficult to detect in mice. Iadecola and colleagues even explained that they had to proximally occlude the artery "because dMCA occlusion produced no neurological deficits" in the mouse (Iadecola et al., 1997). This is presumably because of the low sensitivity of the behavioral testing available in the literature. Nevertheless, mice are of real interest in experimental studies because of their low cost and possible transgenic alterations. To further argue for the usefulness of the adhesive removal test, some data illustrating deficits observed in mice after d-MCAo are presented below (see figure 4). Surgical procedures used to induce stroke are described in Bouet et al., 2007, Bouet et al., 2010, Freret et al., 2008, Freret et al., 2009.

3.1 Expected results after cerebral ischemia across animals' species

As a rule, a highly significant impairment on the contralateral side is commonly observed, whereas the deficit is usually more or less important on the ipsilateral side. Besides, the contralateral deficit is often long-lasting with a delay that will vary according to the species considered and the duration of the occlusion of the middle cerebral artery, *i.e.* the severity of the injury (Figure 4). As regards to spontaneous recovery phenomenon, the ipsilateral deficit often disappears during the first stage after the insult. Quite a contrary, improvement of performances on the contralateral side is not always observed, once again according to the design of the study. This discrepancy of rate of recovery between ipsi- and controlateral side makes the adhesive removal test an efficient tool for assessing the kinetic of functional outcome after cerebral ischemia (acute and long-term phase). Thus, this task may be suitable for assessing both neuroprotective therapies which target early intervention as well as those aimed at the prevention of delayed damage and therapies which promote regeneration.

In rats, while no somatosensory impairment is observed after a 30-min duration of occlusion of the middle cerebral artery (MCAo), 60-min of occlusion induces a bilateral and long lasting deficit, as reflected by an increased time to contact (Figure 4; (Freret et al., 2006)). This deficit tends however to partially recover over time, as attested by the decreasing slope of the time to contact curves. To ensure any potent ischemia-induced somatosensory asymmetry, an index giving the difference between ipsi- and controlateral performances can be calculated (see Freret et al., 2006; Bouet et al., 2007). Thus, comparing contro- and ipsilateral side, it should be note that the rats display a preference towards the ipsilateral, thus non paretic side.

As regards to motor abilities estimated by the time to remove the adhesive, a unilateral and transient deficit can be observed after a 30-min MCAo (up to 1 week after surgery). By contrast, 60-min MCAo will drastically impact on motor functions; a bilateral motor coordination deficit - albeit only transient on the ipsilateral side - can be observed. This long-lasting deficit on the contralateral side reflects a failure to respond to a novel tactile stimulus.

In mice, considering a 60-min duration of occlusion of the MCA (p-MCAo), a bilateral somatensory deficit can be highlighted – as attested by the increased time to contact the adhesives (Bouet et al., 2009; Bouet et al., 2007). Besides, as regards to the time to remove the adhesives, a bilateral impairment can be observed after ischemia. Our group has observed that this deficit in motor coordination appears to be long lasting, longer time to remove the adhesive on the contralateral side of the lesion, since it is still observable up to 6 weeks after surgery (unpublished data).

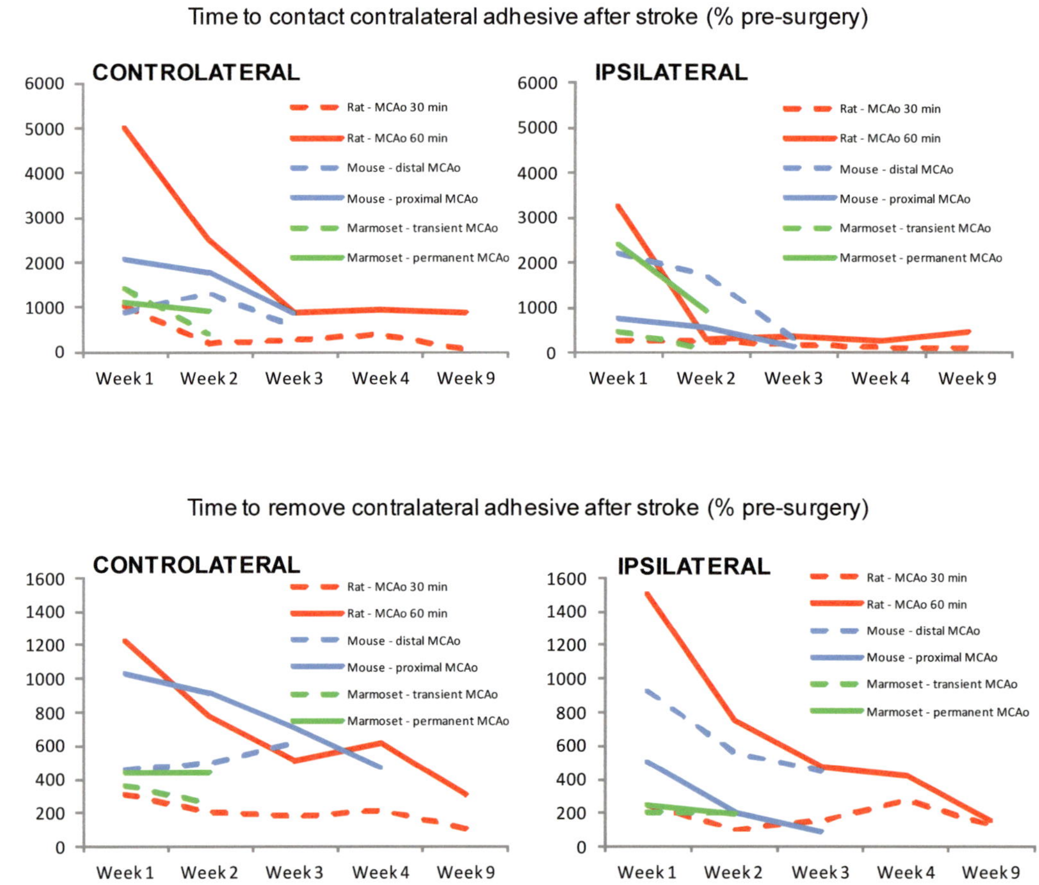

Fig. 4. Adhesive removal performances in rat, mouse and marmoset after stroke (% pre-surgical values). Mean percentage of time to contact the adhesive tapes (upper graphs), positioned on the controlateral side (left) and on the ipsilateral side (right). Time to remove the adhesive tapes (lower graphs), positioned on the controlateral side (left) and on the ipsilateral side (right). All stroke models presented concern the occlusion the middle cerebral artery (MCAo). For rats, stroke was induced by the intraluminal occlusion of the MCA (30 or 60 min). For mice, MCAo was occluded either by distal permanent electrocoagulation or by intraluminal occlusion (60 min - proximal). In marmosets, MCA was occluded by intraluminal approach either permanently of transiently (3 h).
Each point represents the mean of three trials performed on three consecutive days.

Take a look now at the impairments associated to relatively small brain lesion (d-MCAo), adhesive removal test is very useful to detect functional contralateral deficits, even 3 weeks after surgery (Freret et al., 2009). Whereas alteration in the somatosensory perception of the contralateral adhesive (time to contact) partially recovers within 3 weeks after ischemia, the sensorimotor contralateral impairment (time to remove) is still strongly present on the 3rd week after surgery.

In marmoset, an early bilateral somatosensory deficit (time to contact) (Freret et al., 2009) is induced by either transient (3h) or permanent proximal MCAo. This deficit is often transient on the ipsilateral side of the lesion and might be due, at least partly, to dizziness of the animal due to surgery and/or the anesthesia. With respect to the time to remove the adhesive, a bilateral motor coordination deficit is observed whatever the duration of the occlusion. Of note, it has been demonstrated in this same model of cerebral ischemia a spontaneous functional recovery on the ipsilateral side, while controlateral time to remove the adhesive remains hardly affected up to 4 weeks after surgery (Bihel et al.).

3.2 Correlations between brain histological damage and deficit in the adhesive removal test

Correlations between the cortical and striatal histological lesions and the ischemia-induced behavioral impairments in the adhesive removal test have been well investigated in the literature, mostly in rodents (Grabowski et al., 1991; Hudzik et al., 2000; Hunter et al., 1998; Rogers et al., 1997; Virley et al., 2000). We and other authors have demonstrated a close correlation between contralateral contact and removal latencies on this task and abnormal changes in the ipsilateral caudate putamen, lower parietal cortex and forelimb cortex following transient MCAo (30; 60 or 90 min; see Figure 5). Each of these regions of interest contributed to functional impairments on this task across an extended time course (up to several months post-ischemia) (Virley et al., 2000). As regards to the final cortical damage, it seems particularly correlated to both transient and long-lasting sensorimotor deficits measured by adhesive removal test. Conversely, the final striatal lesion appears to be consistently related to the adhesive removal motor deficits (time to remove) (Freret et al., 2006).

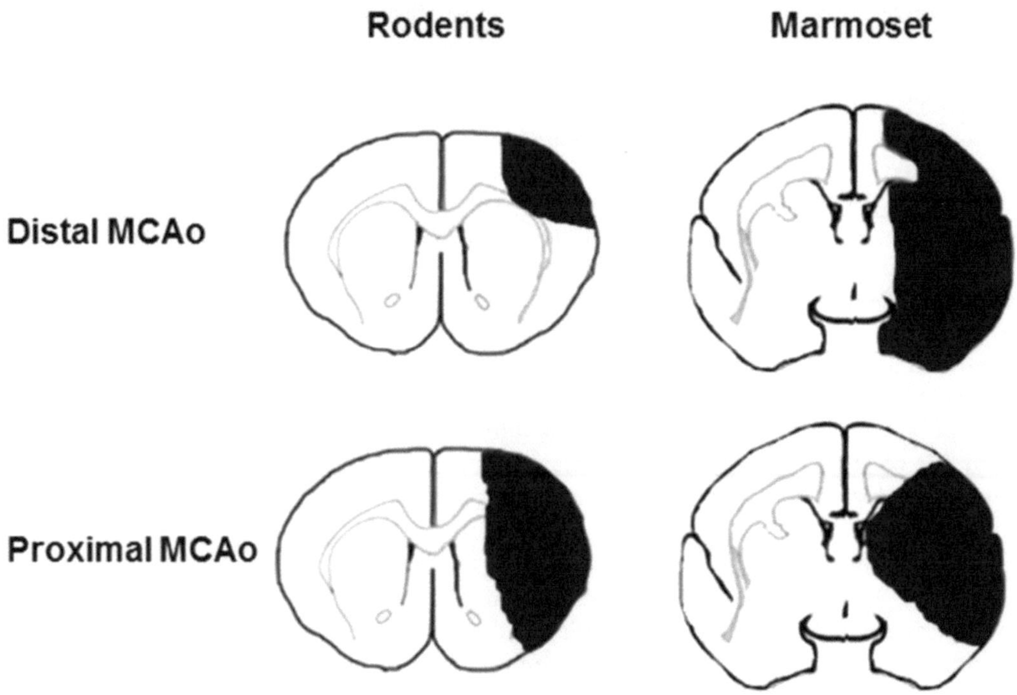

Fig. 5. Schemes showing extent of the lesion after distal and proximal models of Middle Cerebral Artery occlusion (MCAo) in rodents and marmoset. Distal MCAo refers to the occlusion of the artery in its distal portion, *i.e.* after lenticulostriate branches (usually

obtained by electrocoagulation or administration of pharmacological agent, *e.g.* endothelin-1 (Virley et al., 2004)), while proximal MCAo refers to an occlusion at the origin of the artery (intraluminal approach). Extent of the lesion has been drawn from our data and literature. Of note, these schemes are not fully representative of all experimental models of middle cerebral artery ischemia, but give an overview of most frequently obtained brain lesion.

On a side point, the potential relationship between impairments in the adhesive removal test and brain regions that undergo secondary degeneration has been less investigated so far. Indeed, ischemia is known to cause secondary degeneration in non-ischemic remote brain areas such as the ipsilateral thalamus (mostly the ventroposteromedial and ventroposterolateral nuclei (Iizuka et al., 1990)) as well as in the substantia nigra (Tamura et al., 1990). These regions that do not belong to the territory of the MCA, are connected to the primary lesion site. As regards to secondary thalamus shrinkage, retrograde as well as anterograde degeneration due, respectively, to cortical lesion (Iizuka et al., 1990) (Wallerian) and to basal ganglia lesion and/or extensive vasogenic edema (Dihne et al., 2002) are thought to be responsible. Whether the extent of these degenerative changes is or not directly correlated to the size of primary lesion is still under controversy (Freret et al., 2006; Iizuka et al., 1990). No matter how, in a rat stroke model, the final thalamic atrophy appears to be correlated with ischemia-induced deficits observed in the adhesive-removal test (especially its sensory component) (Freret et al., 2006). This correlation suggests that the thalamus makes, albeit moderately, a significant contribution to the ischemia-induced long-lasting somatosensory (ipsilateral bias) and sensorimotor deficits (dexterity alteration). These findings are in agreement with the known involvement of thalamic ventroposterior nuclei in the somatosensory pathways and sensory processing (Tracey &Waite, 1995). In addition, correlations appeared at the late chronic stage (*i.e.*, several weeks after ischemic insult, which is consistent with the delay of thalamic shrinkage development; (Fujie et al., 1990; Jones &Schallert, 1992). Regarding substantia nigra, damage to this brain structure is also correlated with contralateral deficits in the adhesive removal test (Virley et al., 2000).
Finally, talking about correlations between impairments in the adhesive removal test and brain damages in experimental models of focal ischemia, one must keep in mind that although the presence of such a correlation would make the interpretation of performances in this behavioral test easier, the absence of a linear relationship between both parameters does not mean the absence of involvement of the structure in the behavioral task. Indeed, one can imagine that beyond a single and direct relationship between one or several brain structures and the behavioral performances, those latter might depend upon the integrity of a cerebral network that can be influenced by others brain structures. If so, a lesion limited only to this cerebral network or to the related brain structures will have consequences on behavioral performances; even though the one or the other remains unaffected.

3.3 Sensitivity of the adhesive removal test to pharmacological treatment

In line with this consideration of a relationship between impairments in the adhesive removal test and brain damages in experimental models of focal ischemia, our group have demonstrated that a delayed and chronic administration of deferoxamine (an iron chelator) reduces the secondary thalamic atrophy and improves functional recovery in the adhesive removal test after focal ischemia in the rat (Freret et al., 2006). Similarly, a neuroprotective effect of D-JNKi (a peptide inhibitor of JNK (c-Jun-N-terminal kinase)) have been highlighted and corroborated with adhesive removal improvement in the rat (Esneault et al., 2008). This test has also proven to be useful for cellular therapies (Minnerup et al., 2011; Shen et al., 2007), or other pharmacological approaches (testosterone injection - (Morris et al., 2010)), Thymosin beta4 I - (Pan et al., 2005)). In mice, Rehni et al., 2007 (Rehni et al., 2007) showed that intracerebroventricular administration of stem cells derived from amniotic fluid is beneficial for adhesive removal after 60-min MCAo in mice. In marmosets, till now only few studies have assessed the effects of pharmacological agents on adhesive removal test after stroke, but much on Parkinson's disease (Annett et al., 1994).

Overall, those results argue in favor of the use of the adhesive removal test to accurately assess the effects of pharmacological agents on functional outcome. Indeed, this task is suitable for assessing both neuroprotective therapies which target early intervention as well as those aimed at the prevention of delayed damage and therapies which promote regeneration.

4. General overview and limitations of the adhesive removal test

Data reported here show that adhesive removal test *i.* can be easily performed in most species used in experimental research *ii.* is powerful to point out functional deficits on a long-term duration after brain injury. This is a particularly interesting point because it allows assessing efficiency of new therapeutic strategies. Those deficits are in human patients those for which no real efficient therapy exists, excepted rehabilitative strategies like kinesiotherapy. Measuring their importance in animals give models to go further in researches on brain injury recovery.

Contact and removal times give complementary information about the nervous system deficiency. Although the measurement of contact time is not a perfect reflect of sensory system functioning, because for obvious reasons it is related to a motor action (shaking paw, bringing paw to the mouth), it reflects nevertheless a sensory system stimulation. The animal feels or not that something is stuck on its paw and reacts by a movement. From experimental data obtained with adhesive removal, it is not possible to distinguish if the deficit in contact time is related to a primary somatosensory dysfunction (Ward et al., 1997), a sensory hemi-neglect (related to attentional deficit of a body part and involving striatum (Heilman et al., 2000; Reep et al., 2004)), or a tactile extinction phenomenon (related to bilateral stimulation (Schallert &Whishaw, 1984)).

Removal of the tape is a rather tricky task for all the animals presented here because it is not *per se* a natural situation. Rodents and marmosets use their mouth to do it, and amazingly after stroke rats often hold their deficient paw with the intact one to bring it to the mouth as if they were not able to maintain at the right position the deficient/controlateral hand.

The data presented here show that for equivalent brain lesions (parietal cortex and striatum affected by intraluminal model of stroke) all species tested display long-lasting deficits in removal time, at least at the dates tested, which is however rather long compared to delays usually assessed in stroke investigations. Time to contact the contralateral adhesive is also increased for few weeks after stroke, and comes back to normal levels for the less severe brain injury, while it stays abnormal for more severe injuries. It is important to note that the severity of the deficit is quite well related with the extent of the lesion, but also to the structures affected. When the parietal cortex alone is affected (30-min MCAo in rat, distal model in mouse), the deficit is less severe than when other structures are also involved in the lesioned area. Indeed, when the striatum is also affected (60-min MCAo in rat, proximal

model in mouse, both models in marmoset), the recovery is even longer and most of the time not complete within the delays tested.
Mechanisms implied in the recovery of the ability to remove the adhesive tape are not well determined but some of them have to be considered: structural modifications are undoubted (sprouting, synaptogenesis,..), functional modifications (synaptic plasticity, use of brain areas close to the lesion site to fulfill the roles of destroyed tissue…), sensory substitution (increasing role of deep cutaneous modality to replace for the superficial one…), or even behavioral strategies (as for instance, the rat holding the deficient paw with the intact paw to bring it to its mouth).

4.1 Sensory hemi-neglect or tactile extinction syndrome

In rats, a 60-min MCAo induces a long-lasting motor coordination deficit on the contralateral side, reflecting a failure to respond to a novel tactile stimulus. Whether this phenomenon reflects either a primary somatosensory dysfunction (Ward et al., 1997), a truly sensory hemi-neglect (*i.e.*, an attention deficit, as it is classically invoked in the clinic; (Heilman et al., 2000)), or a tactile extinction syndrome (*i.e.*, an interhemispheric perceptual interaction between both stimuli; (Schallert &Whishaw, 1984) is hard to say. Indeed, such duration of occlusion induces a lesion that includes the primary sensory cortical area (S1FL) and, in a secondary degenerative manner, part of the thalamus. These two regions are involved in the somatosensory information processing. On the other hand, it has been shown that unilateral lesions of the posterior parietal cortex and of the dorsocentral striatum (i.e., two structures that are at least partly affected by ischemia) result in multimodal neglect in the rat (Reep et al., 2004). Clinical studies on healthy subjects have reported that the vigilance component of attention to sensory stimuli involves, at least in part, the parietal cortex (Pardo et al., 1991). Thus, a lesion of the parietal cortex could also contribute to a sensory neglect syndrome in the rat after ischemia. An alteration of the cortical- basal-ganglia-thalamic network could lead to a sensory neglect syndrome in the rat. Nevertheless, a tactile extinction syndrome occurs frequently in stroke patients with right cerebral hemisphere damage (Rose et al., 1994), and the presence of neglect is not only debilitating for patient's ability for independent daily life but is also a significant predictor of poor outcome for recovery from hemiplegia in stroke patients (Denes et al., 1982). The long-lasting correlation described between the contralateral time to contact and the final cortical damage (Freret et al., 2006) reinforces the idea that this structure makes significant contribution to the sensory impairment observed after ischemia (Virley et al., 2000).

4.2 Facial and/or limb impairments

After d-MCAo in mice, even though the extension of the lesion is relatively limited, the adhesive removal test is efficient to highlight sensorimotor contralateral impairment (time to removal) 3 weeks after the surgery. This deficit may combine both sensory feedback alterations and motor coordination that are not attributable to postural bias (Schallert et al., 1983). Given the spatial distribution of the cerebral lesion (Figure 5), this impairment might also reflect in this case a face-related somatososensory perception alteration (*i.e.*, a difficulty for the animal to sense the adhesive with its ipsilateral whiskers when it approaches the tape to his face and/or with its tongue when he licks the adhesive in order to facilitate the removal) rather than a forelimb motor or sensory alteration (because the related brain region, *i.e.*, S1 FL, is mainly spared by ischemia). This hypothesis is in accordance with a study reporting the usefulness of the tongue protrusion test in a rat model of proximal cerebral ischemia (Gulyaeva et al., 2003). Furthermore, it suggests that permanent distal stroke could be a relevant model of oral and facial impairments, which are also tremendous problems in human stroke.

5. Conclusion

To conclude on the usefulness of the adhesive removal test, one must admit that this test:

1. is relevant because it was developed in relation to clinical evaluations,
2. is an accurate test to assess somatosensory and motor dysfunctions, even if they are very tiny,
3. is useful to assess recovery, since it is capable of measuring long-lasting deficits,
4. allows for longitudinal studies through adaptation of the size of the adhesive tape according to the age of the individual tested. Indeed, as previously described, we adapted the adhesive removal test to in 20 days old rat pups by reducing the size of the adhesive tape.
5. Finally, the adhesive removal test allows for interspecies comparison (marmosets, rats, dogs and mice), as strongly advised by the expert committees for preclinical studies.

6. References

Annett LE, Martel FL, Rogers DC, Ridley RM, Baker HF, Dunnett SB. Behavioral assessment of the effects of embryonic nigral grafts in marmosets with unilateral 6-OHDA lesions of the nigrostriatal pathway. Exp Neurol 1994;125(2):228-46.

Annett LE, Rogers DC, Hernandez TD, Dunnett SB. Behavioural analysis of unilateral monoamine depletion in the marmoset. Brain 1992;115 (Pt 3):825-56.

Baumann CR, Kilic E, Petit B, Werth E, Hermann DM, Tafti M, Bassetti CL. Sleep EEG changes after middle cerebral artery infarcts in mice: different effects of striatal and cortical lesions. Sleep 2006;29(10):1339-44.

Bihel E, Pro-Sistiaga P, Letourneur A, Toutain J, Saulnier R, Insausti R, Bernaudin M, Roussel S, Touzani O. Permanent or transient chronic ischemic stroke in the non-human primate: behavioral, neuroimaging, histological, and immunohistochemical investigations. J Cereb Blood Flow Metab;30(2):273-85.

Bouet V, Boulouard M, Toutain J, Divoux D, Bernaudin M, Schumann-Bard P, Freret T. The adhesive removal test: a sensitive method to assess sensorimotor deficits in mice. Nat Protoc 2009;4(10):1560-4.

Bouet V, Freret T, Ankri S, Bezault M, Renolleau S, Boulouard M, Jacotot E, Chauvier D, Schumann-Bard P. Predicting sensorimotor and memory deficits after neonatal ischemic stroke with reperfusion in the rat. Behav Brain Res 2010.

Bouet V, Freret T, Toutain J, Divoux D, Boulouard M, Schumann-Bard P. Sensorimotor and cognitive deficits after transient middle cerebral artery occlusion in the mouse. Exp Neurol 2007;203(2):555-67.

Bulman-Fleming MB, Bryden MP, Rogers TT. Mouse paw preference: effects of variations in testing protocol. Behav Brain Res 1997;86(1):79-87.

Denes G, Semenza C, Stoppa E, Lis A. Unilateral spatial neglect and recovery from hemiplegia: a follow-up study. Brain 1982;105 (Pt 3):543-52.

Dihne M, Grommes C, Lutzenburg M, Witte OW, Block F. Different mechanisms of secondary neuronal damage in thalamic nuclei after focal cerebral ischemia in rats. Stroke 2002;33(12):3006-11.

Esneault E, Castagne V, Moser P, Bonny C, Bernaudin M. D-JNKi, a peptide inhibitor of c-Jun N-terminal kinase, promotes functional recovery after transient focal cerebral ischemia in rats. Neuroscience 2008;152(2):308-20.

Fleming SM, Salcedo J, Fernagut PO, Rockenstein E, Masliah E, Levine MS, Chesselet MF. Early and progressive sensorimotor anomalies in mice overexpressing wild-type human alpha-synuclein. J Neurosci 2004;24(42):9434-40.

Freret T, Bouet V, Leconte C, Roussel S, Chazalviel L, Divoux D, Schumann-Bard P, Boulouard M. Behavioral deficits after distal focal cerebral ischemia in mice: Usefulness of adhesive removal test. Behav Neurosci 2009;123(1):224-30.

Freret T, Bouet V, Toutain J, Saulnier R, Pro-Sistiaga P, Bihel E, Mackenzie ET, Roussel S, Schumann-Bard P, Touzani O. Intraluminal thread model of focal stroke in the non-human primate. J Cereb Blood Flow Metab 2008;28(4):786-96.

Freret T, Chazalviel L, Roussel S, Bernaudin M, Schumann-Bard P, Boulouard M. Long-term functional outcome following transient middle cerebral artery occlusion in the rat - Correlation between brain damage and behavioral impairment. Behav Neurosci 2006:in press.

Freret T, Valable S, Chazalviel L, Saulnier R, Mackenzie ET, Petit E, Bernaudin M, Boulouard M, Schumann-Bard P. Delayed administration of deferoxamine reduces brain damage and promotes functional recovery after transient focal cerebral ischemia in the rat. Eur J Neurosci 2006;23(7):1757-65.

Fujie W, Kirino T, Tomukai N, Iwasawa T, Tamura A. Progressive shrinkage of the thalamus following middle cerebral artery occlusion in rats. Stroke 1990;21(10):1485-8.

Grabowski M, Nordborg C, Johansson BB. Sensorimotor performance and rotation correlate to lesion size in right but not left hemisphere brain infarcts in the spontaneously hypertensive rat. Brain Res 1991;547(2):249-57.

Guegan C, Braudeau J, Couriaud C, Dietz GP, Lacombe P, Bahr M, Nosten-Bertrand M, Onteniente B. PTD-XIAP protects against cerebral ischemia by anti-apoptotic and transcriptional regulatory mechanisms. Neurobiol Dis 2006;22(1):177-86.

Gulyaeva N, Thompson C, Shinohara N, Lazareva N, Onufriev M, Stepanichev M, Moiseeva Y, Fliss H, Hakim AM. Tongue protrusion: a simple test for neurological recovery in rats following focal cerebral ischemia. J Neurosci Methods 2003;125(1-2):183-93.

Heilman KM, Valenstein E, Watson RT. Neglect and related disorders. Semin Neurol 2000;20(4):463-70.

Hudzik TJ, Borrelli A, Bialobok P, Widzowski D, Sydserff S, Howell A, Gendron P, Corbett D, Miller J, Palmer GC. Long-term functional end points following middle cerebral artery occlusion in the rat. Pharmacol Biochem Behav 2000;65(3):553-62.

Hunter AJ, Mackay KB, Rogers DC. To what extent have functional studies of ischaemia in animals been useful in the assessment of potential neuroprotective agents? Trends Pharmacol Sci 1998;19(2):59-66.

Iadecola C, Zhang F, Casey R, Nagayama M, Ross ME. Delayed reduction of ischemic brain injury and neurological deficits in mice lacking the inducible nitric oxide synthase gene. J Neurosci 1997;17(23):9157-64.

Iizuka H, Sakatani K, Young W. Neural damage in the rat thalamus after cortical infarcts. Stroke 1990;21(5):790-4.

Ishibashi S, Kuroiwa T, Endo S, Okeda R, Mizusawa H. Neurological dysfunctions versus regional infarction volume after focal ischemia in Mongolian gerbils. Stroke 2003;34(6):1501-6.

Jones TA, Schallert T. Subcortical deterioration after cortical damage: effects of diazepam and relation to recovery of function. Behav Brain Res 1992;51(1):1-13.

Komotar RJ, Kim GH, Sughrue ME, Otten ML, Rynkowski MA, Kellner CP, Hahn DK, Merkow MB, Garrett MC, Starke RM, Connolly ES. Neurologic assessment of somatosensory dysfunction following an experimental rodent model of cerebral ischemia. Nat Protoc 2007;2(10):2345-7.

Marshall JW, Ridley RM. Assessment of functional impairment following permanent middle cerebral artery occlusion in a non-human primate species. Neurodegeneration 1996;5(3):275-86.

Minnerup J, Kim JB, Schmidt A, Diederich K, Bauer H, Schilling M, Strecker JK, Ringelstein EB, Sommer C, Scholer HR, Schabitz WR. Effects of neural progenitor cells on sensorimotor recovery and endogenous repair mechanisms after photothrombotic stroke. Stroke 2011;42(6):1757-63.

Modo M, Stroemer RP, Tang E, Veizovic T, Sowniski P, Hodges H. Neurological sequelae and long-term behavioural assessment of rats with transient middle cerebral artery occlusion. J Neurosci Methods 2000;104(1):99-109.

Morris DC, Chopp M, Zhang L, Lu M, Zhang ZG. Thymosin beta4 improves functional neurological outcome in a rat model of embolic stroke. Neuroscience 2010;169(2):674-82.

Pan Y, Zhang H, Acharya AB, Patrick PH, Oliver D, Morley JE. Effect of testosterone on functional recovery in a castrate male rat stroke model. Brain Res 2005;1043(1-2):195-204.

Pardo JV, Fox PT, Raichle ME. Localization of a human system for sustained attention by positron emission tomography. Nature 1991;349(6304):61-4.

Quaranta A, Siniscalchi M, Frate A, Vallortigara G. Paw preference in dogs: relations between lateralised behaviour and immunity. Behav Brain Res 2004;153(2):521-5.

Reep RL, Corwin JV, Cheatwood JL, Van Vleet TM, Heilman KM, Watson RT. A rodent model for investigating the neurobiology of contralateral neglect. Cogn Behav Neurol 2004;17(4):191-4.

Rehni AK, Singh N, Jaggi AS, Singh M. Amniotic fluid derived stem cells ameliorate focal cerebral ischaemia-reperfusion injury induced behavioural deficits in mice. Behav Brain Res 2007;183(1):95-100.

Rogers DC, Campbell CA, Stretton JL, Mackay KB. Correlation between motor impairment and infarct volume after permanent and transient middle cerebral artery occlusion in the rat. Stroke 1997;28(10):2060-5; discussion 6.

Rose L, Bakal DA, Fung TS, Farn P, Weaver LE. Tactile extinction and functional status after stroke. A preliminary investigation. Stroke 1994;25(10):1973-6.

Schaar KL, Brenneman MM, Savitz SI. Functional assessments in the rodent stroke model. Exp Transl Stroke Med 2010;2(1):13.

Schallert T, Fleming SM, Leasure JL, Tillerson JL, Bland ST. CNS plasticity and assessment of forelimb sensorimotor outcome in unilateral rat models of stroke, cortical ablation, parkinsonism and spinal cord injury. Neuropharmacology 2000;39(5):777-87.

Schallert T, Upchurch M, Lobaugh N, Farrar SB, Spirduso WW, Gilliam P, Vaughn D, Wilcox RE. Tactile extinction: distinguishing between sensorimotor and motor asymmetries in rats with unilateral nigrostriatal damage. Pharmacol Biochem Behav 1982;16(3):455-62.

Schallert T, Upchurch M, Wilcox RE, Vaughn DM. Posture-independent sensorimotor analysis of inter-hemispheric receptor asymmetries in neostriatum. Pharmacol Biochem Behav 1983;18(5):753-9.

Schallert T, Whishaw IQ. Bilateral cutaneous stimulation of the somatosensory system in hemidecorticate rats. Behav Neurosci 1984;98(3):518-40.

Shen LH, Li Y, Chen J, Cui Y, Zhang C, Kapke A, Lu M, Savant-Bhonsale S, Chopp M. One-year follow-up after bone marrow stromal cell treatment in middle-aged female rats with stroke. Stroke 2007;38(7):2150-6.

STAIR. Recommendations for standards regarding preclinical neuroprotective and restorative drug development. Stroke 1999;30(12):2752-8.

STAIRIII. Recommendations for clinical trial evaluation of acute stroke therapies. Stroke 2001;32(7):1598-606.

Starkey ML, Barritt AW, Yip PK, Davies M, Hamers FP, McMahon SB, Bradbury EJ. Assessing behavioural function following a pyramidotomy lesion of the corticospinal tract in adult mice. Exp Neurol 2005;195(2):524-39.

Tamura A, Kirino T, Sano K, Takagi K, Oka H. Atrophy of the ipsilateral substantia nigra following middle cerebral artery occlusion in the rat. Brain Res 1990;510(1):154-7.

Tracey DJ, Waite ME. Somatosensory System. In: Press A, editor. The rat nervous system 2nd Edition. Sydney: Academic Press; 1995. p 689-700.

van Lookeren Campagne M, Thibodeaux H, van Bruggen N, Cairns B, Gerlai R, Palmer JT, Williams SP, Lowe DG. Evidence for a protective role of metallothionein-1 in focal cerebral ischemia. Proc Natl Acad Sci U S A 1999;96(22):12870-5.

Virley D, Beech JS, Smart SC, Williams SC, Hodges H, Hunter AJ. A temporal MRI assessment of neuropathology after transient middle cerebral artery occlusion in the rat: correlations with behavior. J Cereb Blood Flow Metab 2000;20(3):563-82.

Ward NM, Sharkey J, Brown VJ. Assessment of sensorimotor neglect after occlusion of the middle cerebral artery in the rat. Behav Neurosci 1997;111(5):1133-45.

Zhang L, Li Y, Zhang C, Chopp M, Gosiewska A, Hong KW. Delayed administration of human umbilical tissue-derived cells improved neurological functional recovery in a rodent model of focal ischemia. Stroke 2011;42(5):1437-44.

4

Variations in Origin of Arteries Supplying the Brain in Rabbit and Their Impact on Total Cerebral Ischemia

David Mazensky, Jan Danko, Emil Pilipcinec,
Eva Petrovova and Lenka Luptakova
University of Veterinary Medicine and Pharmacy, Kosice
The Slovak Republic

1. Introduction

1.1 Laboratory animals

Animal testing, also known as animal experimentation, is the use of non-human animals in experiments. Worldwide it is estimated that the number of vertebrate animals—from zebrafish to non-human primates—ranges from the tens of millions to more than 100 million used annually (Cohn, 2010). The number of mice and rats used in the United States alone in 2001 was 80 million. Most animals are euthanized after being used in an experiment (Carbone, 2004).

It includes pure research such as genetics, developmental biology, behavioral studies, as well as applied research such as biomedical research, xenotransplantation, drug testing and toxicology tests, including cosmetics testing. Animals are also used for education, breeding and defense research. The practice is regulated to various degrees in different countries.

The earliest references to animal testing are found in the writings of the Greeks in the 2nd and 4th centuries BCE. Aristotle (384–322 BCE) and Erasistratus (304–258 BCE) were among the first to perform experiments on living animals (Cohen & Loew, 1984).

The ability of humans to change the genetics of animals took a large step forwards in 1974 when Rudolf Jaenisch was able to produce the first transgenic mammal, by integrating DNA from the SV40 virus into the genome of mice (Jaenisch & Mintz, 1974). This genetic research progressed rapidly and in 1996 Dolly the sheep was born, the first mammal to be cloned from an adult cell (Wilmut et al., 1997).

Toxicology testing became important in the 20th century. In the 19th century laws regulating drugs were more relaxed. For example, in the U.S. the government could only ban a drug after a company had been prosecuted for selling products that harmed customers. In the 1960s, in reaction to the Thalidomide tragedy, further laws were passed requiring safety testing on pregnant animals before a drug can be sold (Burkholz, 1997).

Albino rabbits are used in eye irritancy tests because rabbits have less tear flow than other animals and the lack of eye pigment in albinos make the effects easier to visualize. Rabbits are also frequently used for the production of polyclonal antibodies.

1.2 Cerebral ischemia

It is the deficiency of blood and metabolic substrates in the brain due to insufficient arterial supply or venous drainage, causing disruption of cerebral functions and partially reversible or irreversible damage to neurons.

Ischemia leads to alterations in brain metabolism, reduction in metabolic rates and energy crisis (Vespa et al., 2005).

There are two types of ischemia: focal ischemia, which is confined to a specific region of the brain; and global ischemia, which encompasses wide areas of brain tissue.

The main symptoms involve impairments in vision, body movement, and speaking. The causes of brain ischemia vary from sickle cell anemia to congenital heart defects. Symptoms of brain ischemia can include unconsciousness, blindness, problems with coordination, and weakness in the body. Other effects that may result from brain ischemia are stroke, cardiorespiratory arrest and irreversible brain damage.

An interruption of blood flow to the brain for more 10 seconds causes unconsciousness and an interruption in flow for more than a few minutes generally results in irreversible brain damage. In 1974, Hossmann and Zimmerman demonstrated that ischemia induced in mammalian brains for up to an hour can be at least partially recovered. Accordingly, this discovery raised the possibility of intervening after brain ischemia before the damage becomes irreversible.

Global brain ischemia occurs when blood flow to the brain is halted or drastically reduced. This is commonly caused by cardiac arrest. If sufficient circulation is restored within a short period of time, symptoms may be transient. However, if a significant amount of time passes before restoration, brain damage may be permanent. While reperfusion may be essential to protecting as much brain tissue as possible, it may also lead to reperfusion injury. Reperfusion injury is classified as the damage that ensues after restoration of blood supply to ischemic tissue.

1.3 Anatomy of the arteries supplying the brain in the rabbit

1.3.1 Aorta ascendens

The aorta ascendens arises almost linearly and dorsally in the midline. It extends from the cranial margin of the second rib cartilage to the cranial margin of the first rib cartilage. At first runs inside the pericard, left to beginning of the pulmonary trunk, to the left and cranially to the dorsal part of the right auricle and to the left and cranially to the right ventricle. Then it runs inside the thymus dorsally to the left side of the v. cava cranialis dextra (vena) and continues to the arcus aortae (Nejedlý, 1965).

1.3.2 Arcus aortae

The arcus aortae is running from the right to the left transversally and also a little caudally from the point of the second thoracic vertebra. Its dorsal wall is convex, the ventral wall is concave. It lies to the left from the v. cava cranialis dextra. The left part turns around the bronchus principalis sinister and ends on the left side of the third thoracic vertebra behind the v. cava cranialis sinistra. Very close to the midline of the body from its arise to the right the truncus brachiocephalicus and to the left the a. subclavia sinistra (arteria) (Popesko et al., 1990; Fig. 1). The truncus brachiocephalicus, the a. carotis communis sinistra and the a. subclavia dextra as branches of the arcus aortae were described by Nejedlý (1965). Nellie (1930) described the a. subclavia dextra and the a. subclavia sinistra as branches of the arcus aortae. Ding (2006) found the origin of the a. subclavia dextra in 1.5% of cases and the origin of the a. carotis communis sinistra in 4% of cases from the arcus aortae. White (1893) by studying 700 rabbits found in one case the a. carotis communis dextra et sinistra and the a. subclavia dextra et sinistra as independent branches of the arcus aortae.

1.3.3 Truncus brachiocephalicus

The truncus brachiocephalicus runs behind the cartilage of the first rib and the v. cava cranialis dextra on the left side of the trachea. Near the midline it courses to the right and then partly dorsally. Immediatelly after its origin gives off the a. carotis communis sinistra. The truncus brachiocephalicus is very short and divides into the a. carotis communis dextra and the a. subclavia dextra (Nejedlý, 1965). By other author the a. subclavia dextra was described as the first branch of the truncus brachiocephalicus (Popesko et al., 1990).

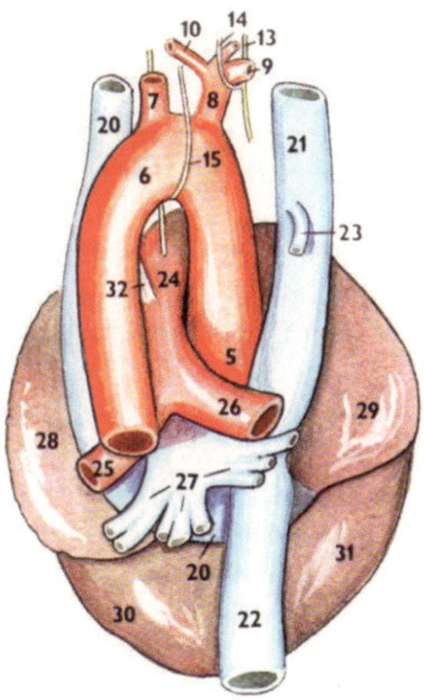

Fig. 1. Basis cordis
7. a. subclavia sinistra; 8. truncus brachiocephalicus; 9. a. subclavia dextra; 10. truncus bicaroticus; 13. n. vagus dexter; 14. n. recurrens dexter; 15. n. recurrens sinister; 20. v. cava cranialis sinistra; 21. v. cava cranialis dextra; 22. v. cava caudalis; 23. v. azygos dextra; 24. truncus pulmonalis; 25. a. pulmonalis sinistra; 26. a. pulmonalis dextra; 27. vv. pulmonales; 28. atrium sinistrum; 29. atrium dextrum; 30. ventriculus sinister; 31. ventriculus dexter; 32. ligamentum arteriosum; 33. lymphonodi thoracici aortici; 34. a. bronchalis. v. Vena. Vv. Venae. n. Nervus. a. Arteria. Dorsal view (Popesko et al., 1990)

1.3.4 Arteria carotis communis

In the neck region the a. carotis communis is covered by m. sternohyoideus (musculus), more cranially also by the m. sternothyroideus. It lies on the lateral surface of the trachea. The a. carotis communis lies dorsally to the esophagus, then laterally to the larynx. It reaches the maxillar angle laterally from the cranial end of the m. sternohyoideus and under the parotid gland. In this area it divides into the a. carotis interna and a. carotis externa (Nejedlý, 1965).

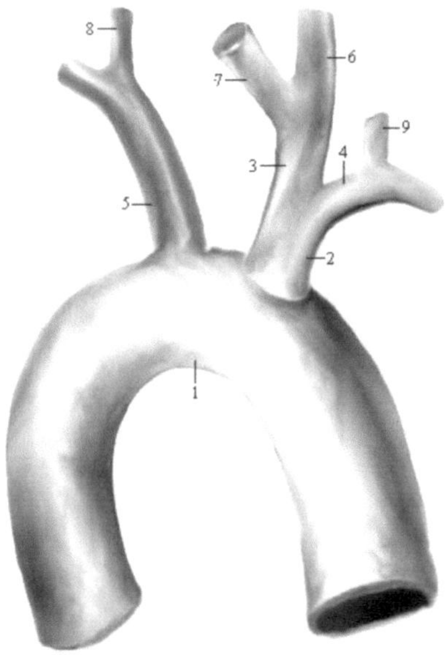

Fig. 2. Scheme of the origin of the large arteries supplying the brain in the rabbit
1. arcus aortae; 2. truncus brachiocephalicus; 3. truncus bicaroticus; 4. a. subclavia dextra; 5. a. subclavia sinistra; 6. a. carotis communis dextra; 7. a. carotis communis sinistra; 8. a. vertebralis sinistra; 9. a. vertebralis dextra. a. Arteria. Lateral view

1.3.5 Arteria carotis interna

The a. carotis interna as poorly developed artery it arises by the division of the a. carotis communis into the a. carotis externa and the a. carotis interna. From the a. carotis externa it is divided by m. styloglossus and m. stylopharyngeus. It is running dorsally on the medial side of the bulla tympanica ossis temporalis. It enters the canalis caroticus ossis temporalis and inside this canal continues into the skull cavity. It is running rostrally on the medial surface of the n. trigeminus (nervus) and on the lateral surface of the corpus ossis basisphenoidalis is directed into the sulcus caroticus. It turns dorsally on the medial surface on the place of the entrance of the n. oculomotorius into the fissura orbitalis. It crosses the n. oculomotorius to the right. In this way it makes three bends. After this it enters the ventral end of the canalis caroticus. Here it gives off the a. communicans caudalis and a. ophtalmica dorsalis and subsequently is divided into the a. carebri rostralis and a. cerebri media (Nejedlý, 1965).

1.3.6 Arteria subclavia

The a. subclavia runs caudally and dorsally to the v. subclavia, above the n. cervicalis VIII., behind the origin of the m. sternomastoideus and m. pectoralis superficialis. The branches of a. subclavia are: truncus costocervicalis, a. vertebralis, a. cervicalis superficialis, a. mammaria interna, a. intercostalis suprema, a. cervicalis profunda and a. transversa colli. The direct continuation is a. axillaris (Nejedlý, 1965).

1.3.7 Arteria vertebralis

The a. vertebralis enters the foramen transversarium of the sixth cervical vertebra. It gives off rr. musculares (rami) and rr. spinales. It continues inside the canalis transversarius of the cervical vertebrae cranially. It passes through the foramen tranversarium of the atlas, courses medially, then cranially and a little dorsally. It runs through the foramen vertebrale laterale of the atlas and gives off the a. spinalis dorsalis and ventralis. After this it penetrates the dura mater and continues to the cranial part of the medulla oblongata. On the caudal margin of the dorsal surface of the pars basilaris ossis occipitalis it is fused together with the contralateral a. vertebralis. This fusion forms the a. basilaris (Fig. 3). A. basilaris continues rostrally on the ventral surface of the medulla oblongata and pons. This artery gives off some branches which praticipate on the formation of the circle of Willis and by this way it participates on the arterial supplying of the brain (Nejedlý, 1965).

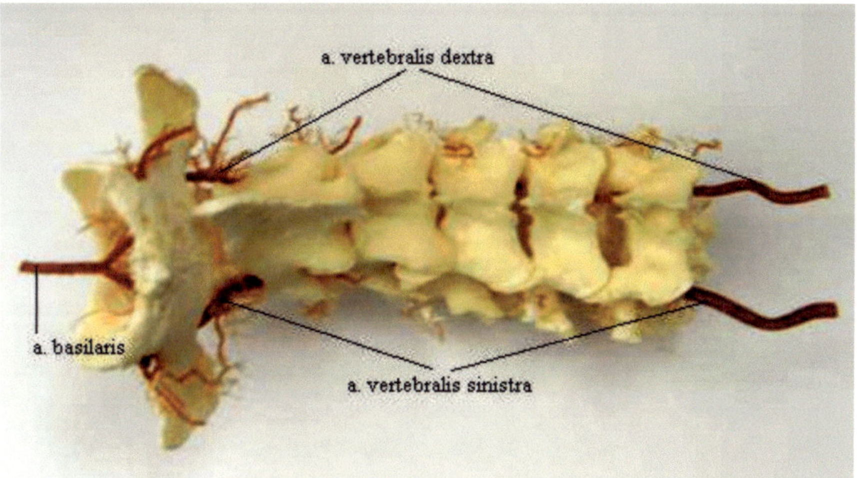

Fig. 3. Corrosion cast of the vertebral arteries

A. vertebralis dextra et sinistra located inside canalis transversarius of the cervical vertebrae. The fusion of the bilateral aa. vertebrales to the a. basilaris. a. Arteria. Dorsal view

1.3.8 The arteries of the brain

The arteries of the brain may be described on its ventral surface as follows:

a. A. cerebelli caudalis is the largest of the transverse branches arising from the a. basilaris on the ventral surface of the hindbrain. It originates about half way along the a. basilaris and passes laterally and up the side of the caudal part of the cerebellum
b. A. cerebri caudalis is a paired vessel formed at the level of the rostral margin of the pons by the bifurcation of the a. basilaris. It passes at each side laterally and dorsally to the caudal portion of the cerebral hemisphere, giving secondary branches to the diencephalon
c. A. cerebelli rostralis is a relatively large branch of the a. cerebri caudalis, arising near the origin of the latter and passing to the rostral portion of the cerebellum after giving branches to the midbrain
d. The end of the a. carotis interna lies on either side of the tuber cinereum. It turns forward, but is connected backwards with the a. cerebri caudalis by an a. communicans caudalis
e. A. cerebri media is given off from the a. carotis interna, branching over the middle portion of the hemispere to supply most of its lateral and dorsal surfaces

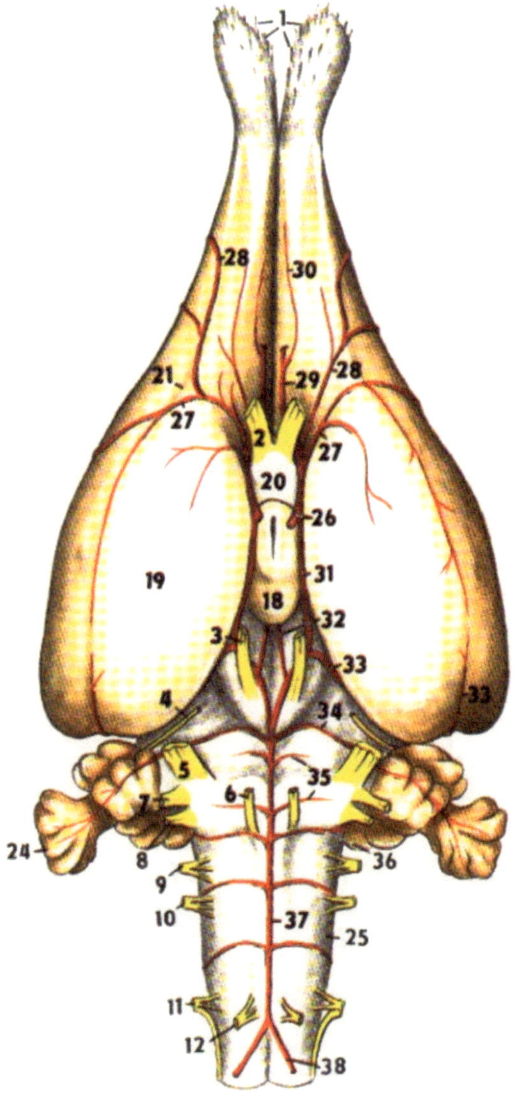

Fig. 4. The arteries of the brain
1. bulbus olfactorius; 2 n. opticus; 3. n. oculomotorius; 4. n. trochlearis; 5. n. trigeminus; 6. n. abducens; 7. n. facialis; 8. n. vestibulocochlearis; 9. n. glossopharyngeus; 10. n. vagus; 11. n. accessorius; 12. n. hypoglossus; 18. corpus mamillare; 19. lobus piriformis; 20. chiasma opticum; 21. sulcus rhinalis lateralis; 24. paraflocculus; 26. a. carotis interna; 27., 28. a. cerebri media; 27. r. caudalis; 28. r. rostralis; 29. a. cerebri rostralis; 30. a. ethmoidalis interna; 31. a. communicans caudalis; 32. r. corporis mamillaris; 33. a. cerebri caudalis; 34. a. cerebelli rostralis; 35. rami ad pontem; 36. a. cerebelli caudalis; 37. a. basilaris; 38. a. vertebralis. a. Arteria. r. Ramus. Ventral View (Popesko et al., 1990)

f. A. cerebri rostralis is the continuation of the a. carotis interna after the origin of the a. cerebri media. It passes to the rostral portion of the ventral surface of the cerebral hemisphere and to the olfactory bulb.

The a. cerebri rostralis unites with that of the other side to form a short common trunk between the hemispheres, which redivides into the paired vessels supplying the medial surfaces. A complete anastomic loop is thus formed round the hypothalamus by the a. carotis interna, a. cerebri rostralis, a. communicans caudalis and a. cerebri caudalis. This is the circle of Willis or the circulus arteriosus cerebri (Popesko et al., 1990). Nejedlý (1965) described the a. communicans rostralis as a connection between the bilateral aa. cerebri rostrales.

1.4 Rabbit as experimental animal of the brain ischemia

Over 20,000 rabbits were used for animal testing only in the UK in 2004. Examples include restricting blood flow to the brain to induce cerebral ischemia (Tolwani et al., 1999). This is most often carried out by ligation of major vessels, e.g. the truncus brachiocephalicus and the a. subclavia sinistra, in their place of origin (Hossmann 1998; Iwama et al., 2000; Pluta 1987). Harukuni and Bhardwaj (2006) reported ligation of the truncus brachiocephalicus and the a. subclavia sinistra as one way to induce total cerebral ischemia. Ischemia within the arteries branching from the vertebral arteries in the back of the brain may result in symptoms such as dizziness, vertigo, double vision, or weakness on both sides of the body. Other symptoms include, difficulty speaking, slurred speech and the loss of coordination (Beers et al., 2003). The aim of this study was to verify whether experimentally induced total cerebral ischemia in rabbits actually corresponds to total ischemia on the basis of the origin of certain vessels. We observed morphological variations in the origin and course of the arteries supplying the brain with blood in the rabbit.

2. Material and methods

2.1 Experimental animals

The study was carried out on 50 adult (age=140 days) New Zealand white rabbits (breed HY+), females (n=25) and males (n=25) of weight range 2.5-3 kg in an accredited experimental laboratory at the University of Veterinary Medicine in Kosice, Slovak Republic. The animals were kept in cages under standard conditions (temperature 15-20 °C, relative humidity 45 %, 12 hours light period) and fed granular mixed feed (O-10 NORM TYP, Spišské krmné zmesi, Spišské Vlachy, Slovak Republic). Drinking water was provided ad libitum.

2.2 Material

The Batson's No. 17 Plastic Replica and Corrosion Kit (Polysciences Europe GmbH, Germany) was used as a casting medium. This consist of Base Solution A (2-Propenoic acid, 2-methyl-, 1,2-ethanediyl 1 ester, Dibutyl phthalate, Methyl methacrylate, Polymethyl methacrylate), Catalyst (Acetone, Benzoyl peroxide, Dibutyl phthalate), Promoter C (Dibutyl 1 phthalate, N,N-Dimethyl-4-toluidine) and red pigment (1,2-Benzenedicarboxylic acid, bis[2-ethylhexyl ester], epoxidized soybean oil and 2-Naphthenecarboxylic acid).

2.3 Methods

2.3.1 Surgical preparation of the rabbit

The animals were injected intravenously with heparine (50, 000 UI/kg) 30 minutes before they were sacrified with intravenous injection of Embutramide (T-61, 0.3 mL/kg). The skin was subsequently removed as far as possible to prevent it from sticking to the corrosive cast in the maceration process. The thoracic cavity was opened from the left side by removing of the ribs. After the opening of the pericardial cavity a ligature was introduced to the ascending aorta. The aorta was cannulated through the left ventricle. The perfusion started after the fixation of the cannula in the ascending aorta with the ligature. The right vestibule was opened to lower the pressure in the vessels to ensure good injection. The vascular network was manually perfused through the fixed cannula in the ascending aorta for approximately 15-20 minutes with 2.5-3 l of warm (37 °C), 0.9 % NaOH in 0.01 M phosphate, pH 7.3 (Hossler & Monson, 1995).

2.3.2 Preparation of the casting medium

The red pigment was added to the Base solution A prior to mixing the catalyst and promoter. The pigment was added in the amount of 5 %. It was mixed and divided into two equal parts (each part=25 mL). To the first half Catalyst in amount of 12 mL was added and mixed. To the second half Promoter C in amount of 12 drops was added and mixed. Then these two parts were mixed together.

2.3.3 Application of the casting medium

The arterial network was filled with the casting medium manually through the same cannula inserted in the ascending aorta. Adequate filling was determined by the visualization of an even distribution of the casting medium (red) throughout the superficial vessels of the body. After the vascular casting is complete, the animals must not be manipulated for at least 30 minutes and then must be submersed in water at a temperature ranging from 40 °C to 60 °C for a period of 24 hours for full polymerization of the casting medium (Lametschwandtner et al., 1990).

2.3.4 Corrosion

The corrosion as the dissolution of tissues surrounding the cast was performed by potassium hydroxide (KOH) at the concentration of solution 2–4 % for a period of 2 days. For the corrosion to be faster, the solution must remain at a constant temperature of 40 °C (Lametschwandtner et al., 1990). The solution for the corrosion was changed every 12 hours. After the surrounding tissue was dissolved vascular castings were rinsed in running water for removing the rests of the soft tissues. Specimens were dried at the room temperature by air exposure (Flešárová et al., 2003).

3. Results and discussion

3.1 Variations in origin

3.1.1 A. carotis communis

Vascular corrosion cast of the rabbit aortic arch displaying the origin of the truncus brachiocephalicus and the a. subclavia sinistra from the arcus aortae in 92 % of cases (46 animals). a. Arteria. Ventral view. Macroscopic image

Vascular corrosion cast of the rabbit aortic arch displaying the origin of the truncus brachiocephalicus, the a. subclavia sinistra and the a. carotis communis sinistra from the arcus aortae in 6 % (3 animals). a. Arteria. Ventral view. Macroscopic image

In 92 % of cases (46 animals) the a. carotis communis sinistra originated as the first branch from the truncus brachiocephalicus. The a. carotis communis dextra arise together with the

a. subclavia dextra by terminal division of truncus brachiocephalicus (Fig. 5). The a. carotis communis sinistra originated from arcus aortae in 6 % (3 animals; Fig. 6).

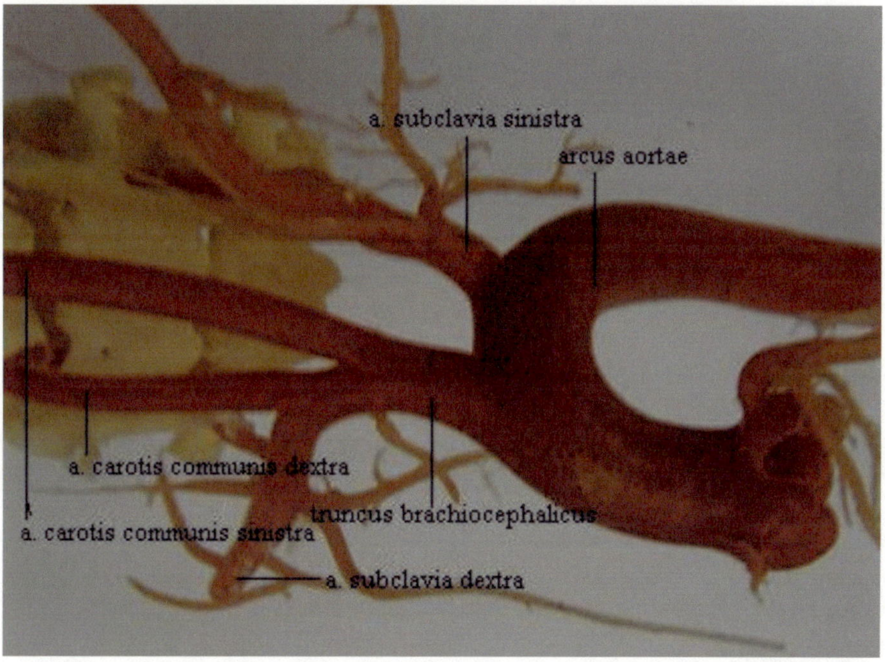

Fig. 5. Aortic arch of the rabbit without variations

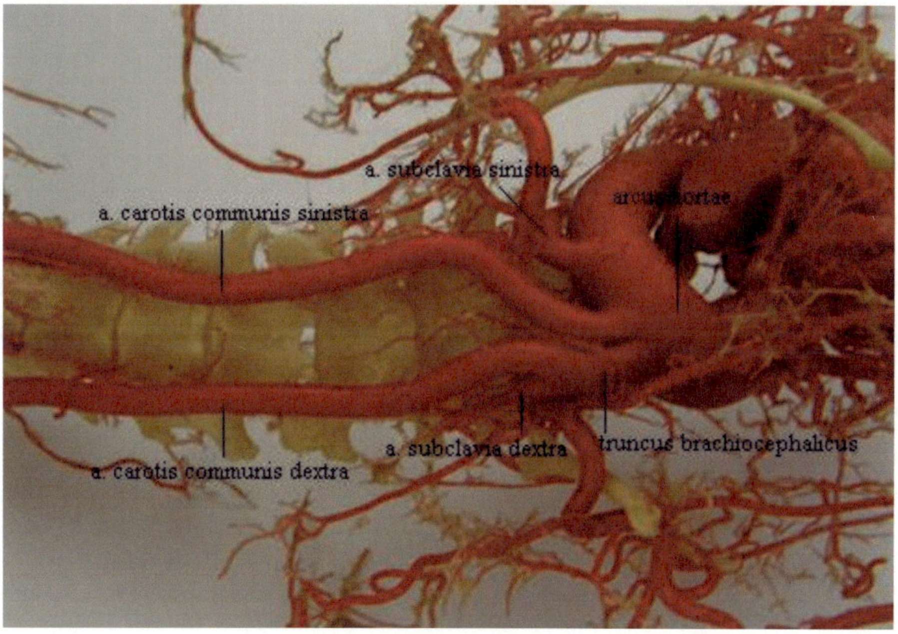

Fig. 6. Aortic arch of the rabbit with variation in origin of a. carotis communis sinistra

3.1.2 A. subclavia

In 98 % of cases (49 animals) the a. subclavia sinistra originated from the arcus aortae (Fig. 5). In 2 % (1 animal) originated from the arcus aortae the truncus bicaroticus, the a. subclavia dextra and the a. subclavia sinistra (Fig. 6).

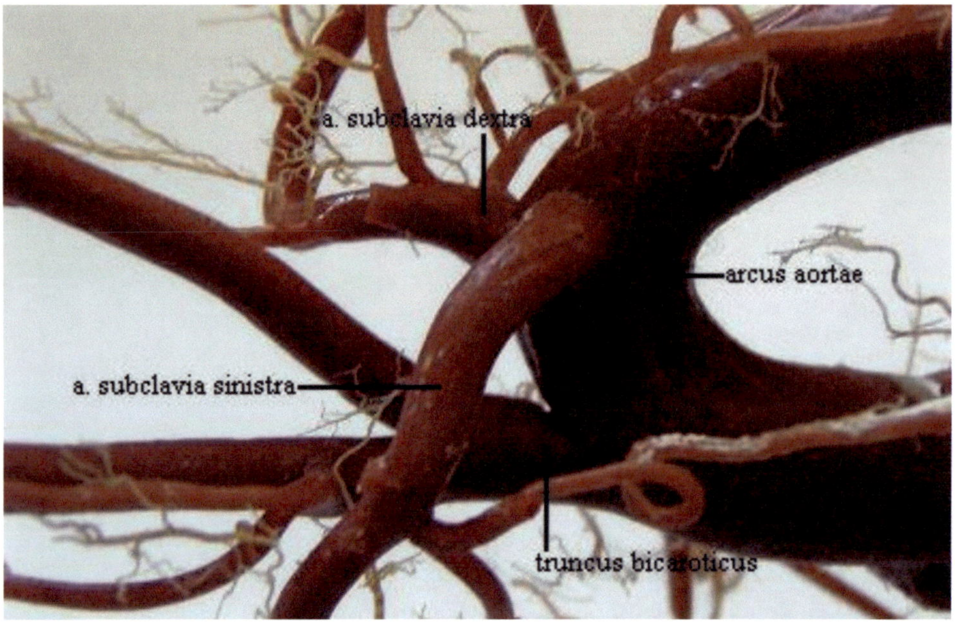

Fig. 7. Aortic arch of the rabbit with variation in origin of a. subclavia dextra

Vascular corrosion cast of the rabbit aortic arch displaying the origin of the truncus bicaroticus, the a. subclavia dextra and the a. subclavia sinistra from the arcus aortae in 2 % (1 animal). a. Arteria. Dorsolateral view. Macroscopic image

3.1.3 A. vertebralis

In 86 % of cases (43 animals) the a. vertebralis sinistra originated directly from the a. subclavia sinistra (Fig. 8) in 10 % of cases (5 animals) it originated from the arcus aortae as an independent branch (Fig. 9) and in 4 % of cases (2 animals) it arose from the arcus aortae as a common trunk with the a. scapularis descendens. The a. vertebralis dextra originated from the a. subclavia dextra in 98 % (49 animals) of cases. In that case we observed two aa. vertebralis dextrae (arteriae) with two different origins.
The a. vertebralis dextra I originated from the a. subclavia dextra and the a. vertebralis dextra II arose from the common trunk with the a. cervicalis superficialis dextra that originated from the a. carotis communis dextra.
After a short distance, they merged between the fifth and sixth cervical vertebrae into a single a. vertebralis dextra, which then entered the canalis transversarius at the level of the fifth cervical vertebra (Fig. 10). In summary, the origin of both aa. vertebrales varied in 16 % of cases (8 animals). In 8 % (4 animals) we found a bypass between the a. vertebralis sinistra and the a. basilaris (Fig. 11). This a. basilaris was also formed by the fusion of the a. vertebralis dextra et sinistra.

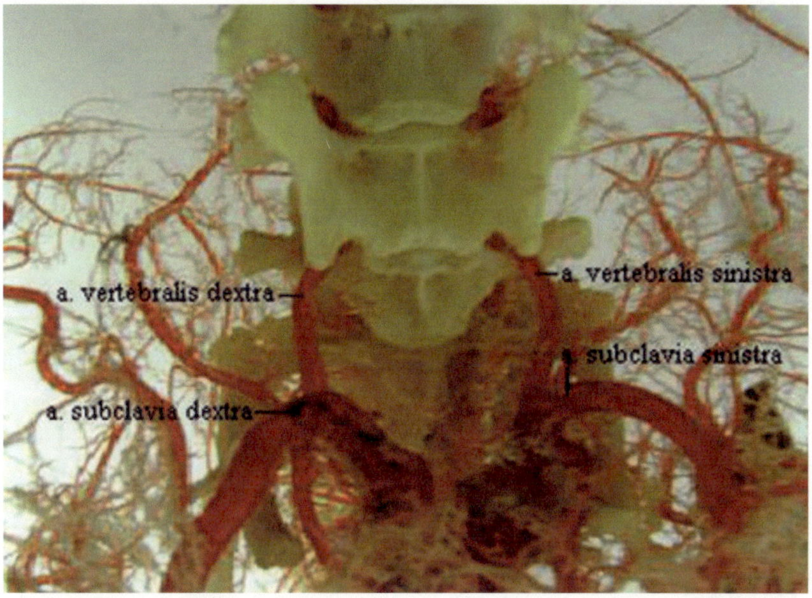

Fig. 8. A. vertebralis with its typical origin

Vascular corrosion cast displaying the origin of the a. vertebralis dextra et sinistra from the a. subclavia dextra et sinistra in 86 % of cases (43 animals). a. Arteria. Ventral view. Macroscopic image

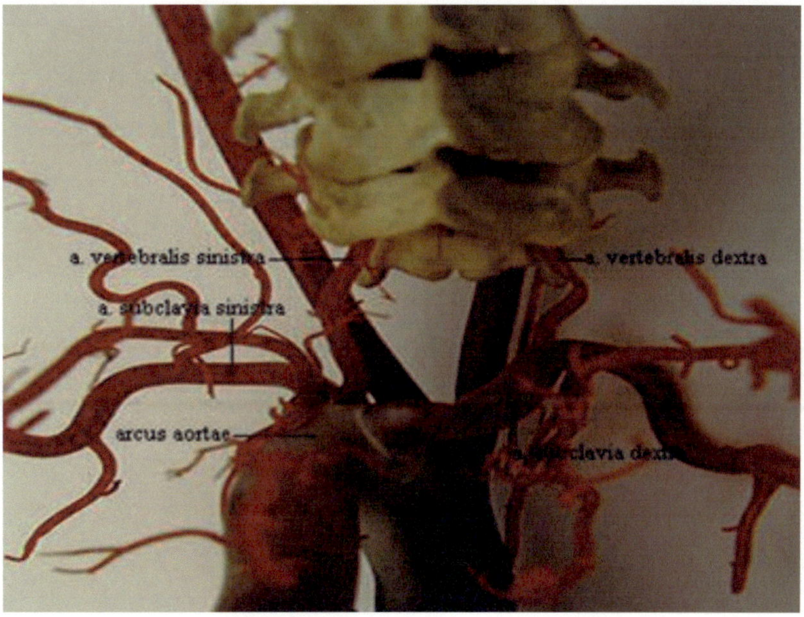

Fig. 9. Atypical origin of the a. vertebralis

Vascular corrosion cast displaying the origin of the a. vertebralis sinistra from the arcus aortae in 10 % of cases (5 animals). a. Arteria. Dorsal view. Macroscopic image

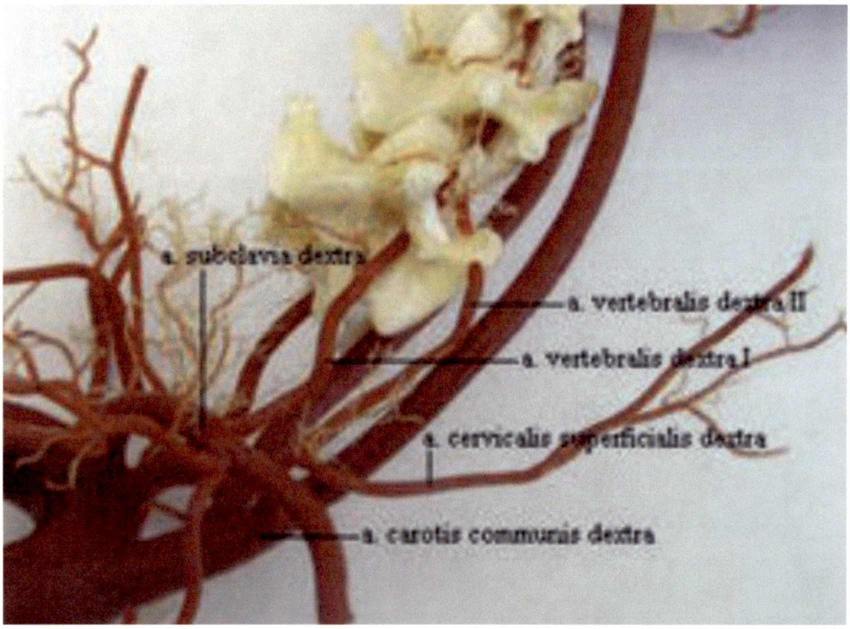

Fig. 10. Doubled a. vertebralis

Vascular corrosion cast displaying two aa. vertebrales dextrae. Note merging of the two arteriae into a single vessel. a. Arteria. aa. Arteriae. Lateral view. Macroscopic image

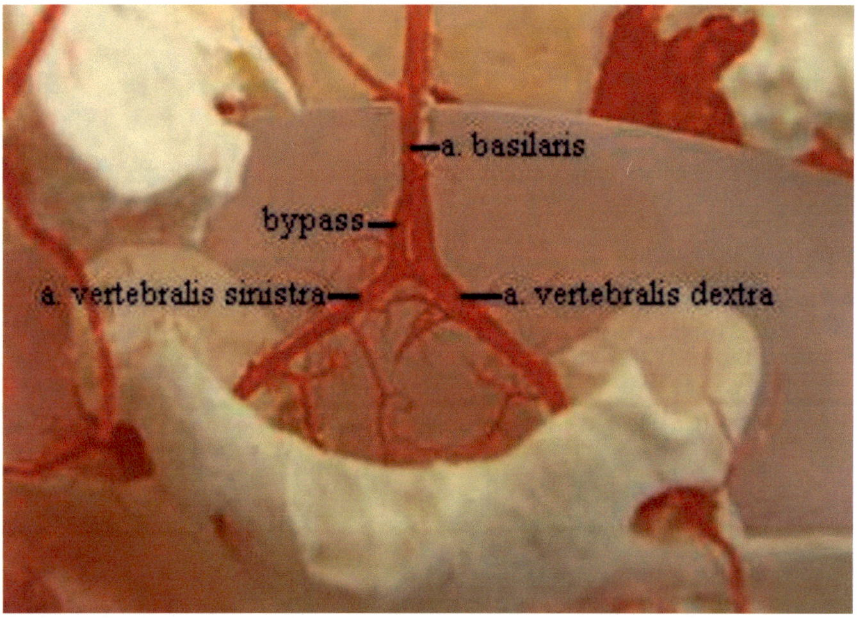

Fig. 11. Variation in formation of a. basilaris

Vascular corrosion cast displaying the bypass between the a. vertebralis sinistra and a. basilaris in 8 % (4 animals). a. Arteria. Dorsal view. Macroscopic image

3.1.4 A. carotis interna

Vascular corrosion cast of the cephalic and neck region displaying the origin of the a. carotis interna by the terminal division of the a. carotis communis together with the a. carotis externa in 94 % (47 animals). Note the entrance of the a. carotis interna to the canalis caroticus. a. Arteria. Ventrolateral view. Macroscopic image

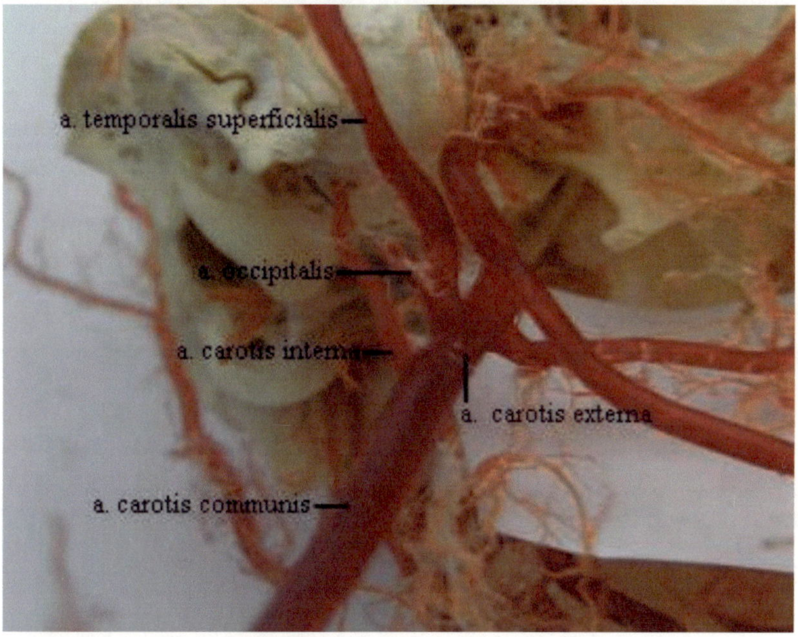

Fig. 12. Typical origin of a. carotis interna

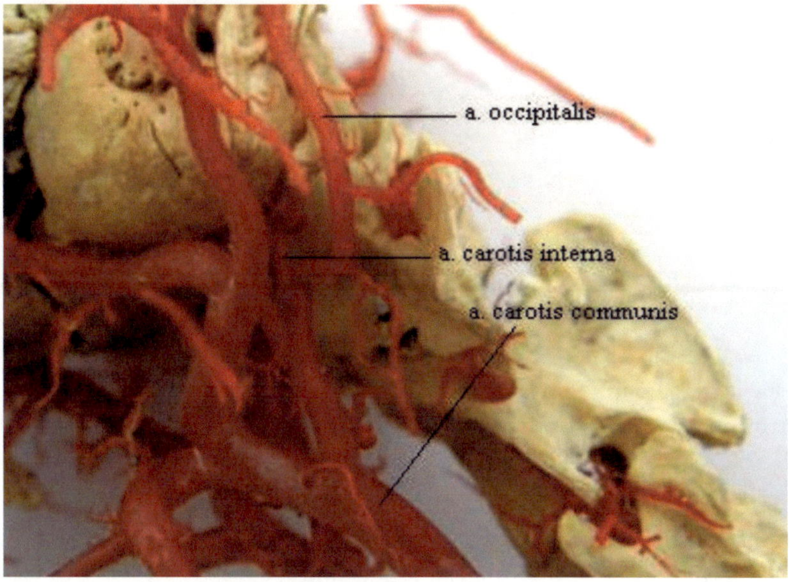

Fig. 13. Atypical origin of a. carotis interna

Vascular corrosion cast of the cephalic and neck region displaying the origin of the a. carotis interna from the common trunk with the a. occipitalis in 6 % (3 animals). a. Arteria. Caudoventral view. Macroscopic image

In 94 % (47 animals) the a. carotis interna arised by terminal division of the a. carotis communis together with the a. carotis externa (Fig. 12). In 6 % (3 animals) the a. carotis interna originated from a common trunk with the a. occipitalis (Fig. 13). The trunk is a branch of the a. carotis communis.

3.1.5 The arteries of the brain

In 40 % (20 animals) the a. cerebelli caudalis dextra et sinistra originated at the same level (Fig. 14). In 40 % (20 animals) the a. cerebelli caudalis dextra originated from the a. basilaris more rostrally than the a. cerebelli caudalis sinistra (Fig. 15). In 20 % (10 animals) the a. cerebelli caudalis sinistra originated more rostrally than the a. cerebelli caudalis dextra.

The a. cerebri caudalis dextra et sinistra originated from the a. basilaris at the same level in all studied animals (100 %).

The a. cerebri media dextra et sinistra originated from the a. carotis interna at the same level in all studied animals (100 %).

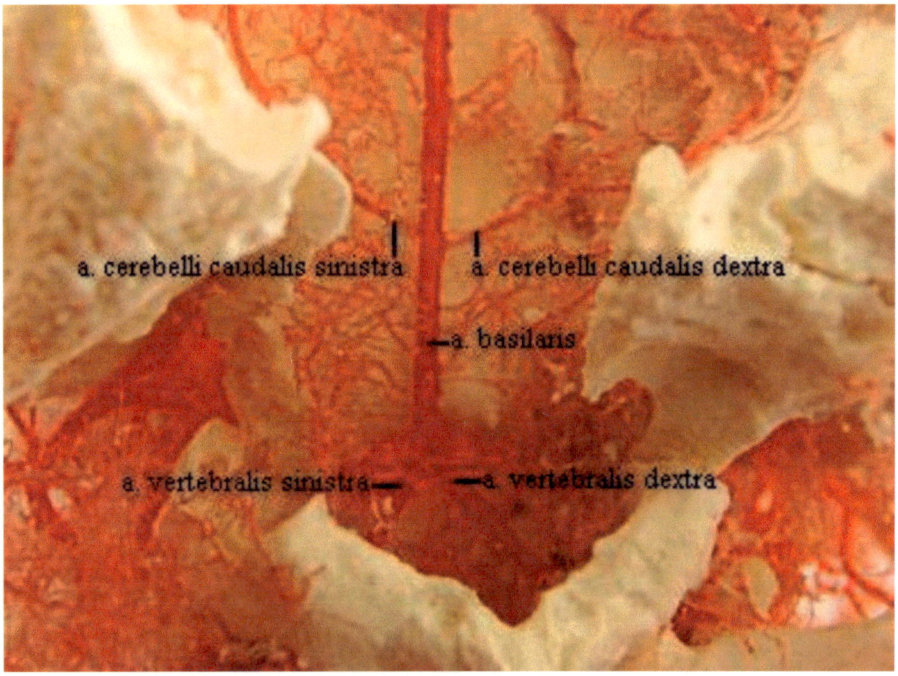

Fig. 14. Typical arrangement of a. cerebelli caudalis
Vascular corrosion cast. In 40 % (20 animals) the a. cerebelli caudalis dextra et sinistra originated at the same level from the a. basilaris. Dorsal view. Macroscopic image

The a. cerebri rostralis dextra et sinistra as the direct continuation from the a. carotis interna originated at the same level in all studied animals (100 %).

These all arteries were divided into the r. rostralis and r. caudalis. In 10 % (5 animals) the a. cerebri caudalis sinistra was divided into the r. rostralis, r. medius and r. caudalis.

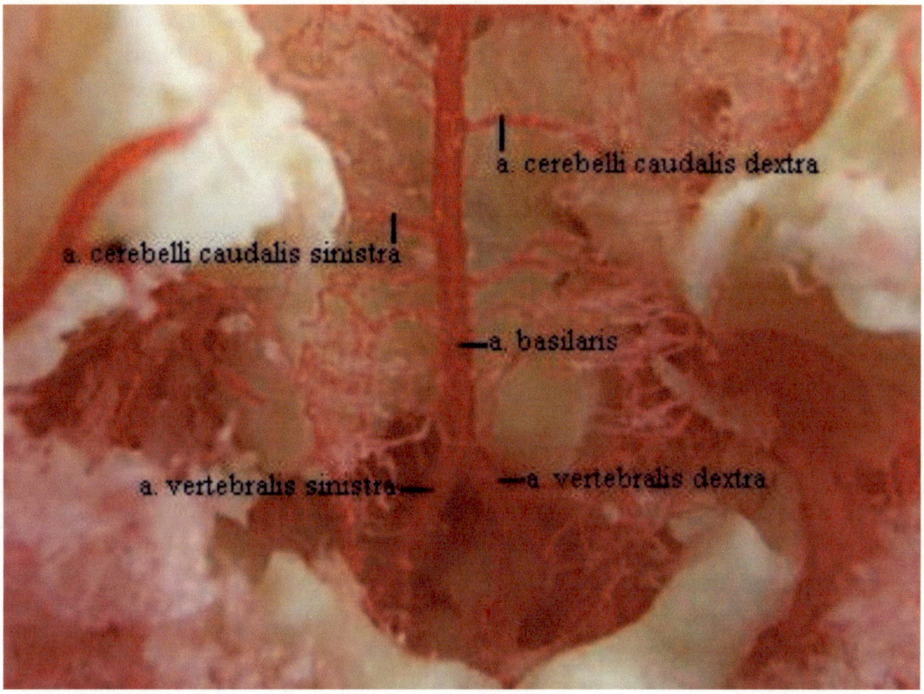

Fig. 15. Variation in arrangement of a. cerebelli caudalis
Vascular corrosion cast. The a. cerebelli rostralis dextra et sinistra originated from the a. basilaris at the same level in all studied animals (100 %). Dorsal view. Macroscopic image

3.2 Discussion

3.2.1 A. carotis communis

In 92 % of cases (46 animals) the a. carotis communis sinistra originated as first branch from the truncus brachiocephalicus. The a. carotis communis dextra arise together with the a. subclavia dextra by the terminal division of the truncus brachiocephalicus. Popesko et al. (1990) described a. carotis communis dextra et sinistra as branches arising from truncus bicaroticus by its terminal division. Truncus bicaroticus was described as the direct continuation of the truncus brachiocephalicus. The a. carotis communis sinistra as branch of the arcus aortae in 4 % (2 animals) was also described by Ding (2006). By Nejedlý (1965) the origin of the a. carotis communis sinistra from the arcus aortae was described as a typical arrangement of branches of the arcus aortae. In 2 % (1 animal) originated from the arcus aortae the truncus bicaroticus. Nellie (1930) described this arrangement in all studied animals. White (1893) by studying 700 rabbits found in one case the a. carotis communis dextra et sinistra as independent branches of the arcus aortae.

3.2.2 A. subclavia

In 98 % (49 animals) the a. subclavia dextra arise together with the a. carotis communis dextra by the terminal division of the truncus brachiocephalicus. By some authors the a.

subclavia dextra was described as the first branch arising from the truncus brachiocephalicus (Popesko et al., 1990). Nellie (1930) described the a. subclavia dextra and the a. subclavia sinistra as branches of the arcus aortae. Ding (2006) found the origin of the a. subclavia dextra in 1.5% of cases from the arcus aortae and Nejedlý (1965) described it as typical arrangement of the branches of the arcus aortae. White (1893) by studying 700 pieces rabbits found in one case a. subclavia dextra et sinistra as independent branches of the arcus aortae.

3.2.3 A. vertebralis

Until now the scientific literature has cited almost exclusively the uniform origin of the a. vertebralis from the a. subclavia (Nejedlý, 1965; Popesko et al., 1990). It was not described independent origin from the arcus aortae or the doubled a. vertebralis like in our cases. In 8 % (4 animals) we found the bypass between the a. vertebralis sinistra and the a. basilaris at the place of fusion of the a. vertebralis dextra et sinistra to the a. basilaris.

3.2.4 A. carotis interna

We found the origin of the a. carotis interna and the a. carotis externa by the terminal division of the a. carotis communis in 92 % (46 animals). The same origin was described by Nejedlý (1965) and Popesko et al. (1990). But we found except this typical arrangement the origin of the a. carotis interna from the a. occipitalis in 8 % (4 animals).

3.2.5 The arteries of the brain

Until now the origin of the bilateral a. cerebri rostralis et caudalis and a. cerebelli rostralis et caudalis was described at the same level from the a. basilaris and the a. carotis interna (Nejedlý, 1965; Popesko et al., 1990). We found that in 40 % (20 animals) the a. cerebelli caudalis dextra originated from the a. basilaris more rostrally than the a. cerebelli caudalis sinistra. In 20 % (10 animals) the a. cerebelli caudalis sinistra originated more rostrally than the a. cerebelli caudalis dextra.

These all arteries were divided into the r. rostralis and r. caudalis (Nejedlý, 1965; Popesko et al., 1990). In 10 % (5 animals) the a. cerebri caudalis sinistra was divided into the r. rostralis, r. medius and r. caudalis.

The bilateral aa. cerebri rostrales are fused together. The same arrangement was described by Popesko et al. (1990). The a. communicans rostralis as a connection between bilateral aa. cerebri rostrales was described by Nejedlý (1965).

4. Conclusion

The effect of various chemical substances (Cantu & Hegsted, **1970**) on the brain nerve tissue damaged by ischemia as well as various pathological and pathophysiological changes induced by the total cerebral ischemia in rabbits and other laboratory animals are the subject of many studies (Ishiyama et al., 2010).

The place of origin of the truncus brachiocephalicus and the a. subclavia sinistra are most commonly used to induce the total cerebral ischemia by ligation (Hossmann 1998; Iwama et al., 2000; Pluta, 1987). Harukuni and Bhardwaj (2006) present also the ligation of the truncus brachiocephalicus and the a. subclavia sinistra as a possible way to induce the total cerebral ischemia. The question is, whether this method of induction of the total cerebral ischemia is correct.

The variations in the origin of arteries supplying the brain which we found point to the possibility of induction only a partial brain ischemia in a given set of animals. The probability of causing the partial brain ischemia may be the same as the percentage of the occurrence of found variations.

One way to avoid obtaining of distorted results is the ligation of the arteries before their entering to the target organ, in this case to the brain. These arteries can be the a. basilaris or the a. carotis interna. The best results probably would have been achieved by ligation of the arteries on the ventral surface of the brain that are directly involved in the blood supply of the nerve tissue. However, this method is time consuming and surgically very difficult in. Another possibility is the detailed preparation of arteries in the place of their origin to avoid possible variations.

With this work we tried to emphasize the need for more detailed knowledge of the circulatory system of the rabbit, which is one of the ways to achieve more objective results also in a smaller number of animals used in experiments.

5. References

Beers, M.; Fletcher, A.; Jones, T. & Porter, R. (2003). *The Merck Manual of Medical Information.* New York: Merck & Co. Inc., ISBN 0743477340, New York, USA

Burkholz, H. (1997). Giving Thalidomide a Second Chance. In: *FDA Consumer* (US Food and Drug Administration). 06 Jun 2011. Available from: http://findarticles.com/p/articles/mi_m1370/is_n6_v31/ai_19903511/

Cantu, R.C. & Hegsted, D.M. (1970). Comparison of cerebrovascular perfusion after ischemia in normal and atherosclerotic rabbits. *Journal of Surgical Research,* Vol. 10, No. 3, pp. 129-131, ISSN 0022-4804

Carbone, L. (2004). *What Animals Want.* Oxford University Press. ISBN 9780195161960, Oxford, USA

Cohen, B.J. & Loew F.M. (1984). *Laboratory Animal Medicine: Historical Perspectives in Laboratory Animal Medicine.* (eds J.G. Fox, B.J. Cohen and F.M. Loew) Academic Press, Inc., ISBN 0122639510, Orlando, Florida, USA

Cohn, M. (2010). *Alternatives to Animal Testing Gaining Ground.* The Baltimore Sun. ISBN 978-0-230-60014-0, Baltimore, USA

Ding, Y.H.; Dai, D.; Layton, K.F.; Lewis, D.A.; Danielson, M.A.; Kadirvel, R.; Cloft, H.J. & Kallmes, D.F. (2006). Vascular Anatomic Variation in Rabbits. *Journal of Vascular and Interventional Radiobiology,* Vol.17, No.6, pp. 1031-1035, ISSN 0345-8865

Flešárová, S.; Tesfaye, A.; Danko J, Bátor, R.; Dorko, F. & Barta, A. (2003). Morphological variations of arcus aortae in rabbits. *Acta Veterinaria Brno,* Vol. 72, No. 7, pp. 116, ISSN 0001-7213

Harukuni, I. & Bhardwaj, A. (2006). Mechanisms of Brain Injury after Global Cerebral Ischemia. *Neurological Clinic,* Vol.24, No.1, pp. 1-21, ISSN 0733-8619

Hossler, F.E. & Monson, F.C. (1995). Microvasculature of the rabbit urinary bladder. *The Anatomical Record,* Vol.243, No.4, pp. 438-448, ISSN 1932-8486

Hossmann, K-A. (1998). Experimental models for the investigation of brain ischemia. *Cardiovascular Research,* Vol.39, No.1, pp. 106-120, ISSN 0008-6363

Ishiyama, T.; Shibuya, K.; Ichikawa, M.; Masamune, T.; Kiuchi, R.; Sessler, D.I. & Matsukawa, T. (2010). Cerebral pial vascular changes under propofol or sevoflurane anesthesia during global cerebral ischemia and reperfusion in rabbits. *Journal of neurosurgical anesthesiology,* Vol. 22, No. 3, pp. 207-213, ISSN 0898-4921

Iwama, H.; Akama, Y. & Tase, C. (2000). Global brain ischemia produced by clamping left subclavian artery and bicarotid trunk in the rabbit. *American Journal of Emergency Medicine,* Vol.18, No.1, pp. 31-35, ISSN 0263-1933

Lametschwandtner, A.; Lametschwandtner, U. & Weiger, T. (1990). Scanning electron microscopy of vascular corrosion casts.technique and aplications: uptade review. *Scanning microscopy,* Vol.4, No.4, pp. 889-941, ISSN 0891-7035

Nejedlý, K. (1965). *Biology and systematic anatomy of laboratory animals,* SPN, ISBN 16-924- 65, Praha, Czech Republic

Nellie, B.E. (1930). Note on an abnormality in the blood vascular system of the rabbit. *Journal of Anatomy,* Vol.65, No.1, pp. 152-153, ISSN 0021-8782

Pluta, R. (1987). Resuscitation of the rabbit brain after acute complete ischemia lasting up to one hour: pathophysiological and pathomorphological observations. *Resuscitation,* Vol.15, No.4, pp. 267-287, ISSN 0300-95721987

Popesko, P.; Rajtová, V. & Horák, J. (1990). *Anatomic atlas of small laboratory animals.* Príroda, ISBN 80-07-00040-2, Bratislava, Slovak Republic

Tolwani, R.J.; Jakowec, M.W.; Petzinger, G.M.; Green, S. & Waggie, K. (1999). Experimental models of Parkinson's disease: insights from many models. *Laboratory animal science,* Vol.49, No.4, pp. 363–371, ISSN 0023-6772

Vespa, P.; Bergsneider, M.; Hattori, N.; Wu, H-M.; Huang, S-CH.; Martin, N.A.; Glenn, T.C.; McArthur, D.L. & Hovda, D.A. (2005). Metabolic crisis without brain ischemia is common after traumatic brain injury: a combined microdialysis and positron emission tomography study. *Journal of Cerebral Blood Flow & Metabolism,* Vol.25, No.6, pp. 763–774, ISSN 0271-678X

White, P.J. (1893). Unusual Origin of Arteries in the Rabbit. *Nature,* Vol.47, No.1216, pp. 365, ISSN 0028-0836

Wilmut, I.; Schnieke, A.E.; McWhir, J.; Kind, A.J. & Campbell, K.H. (1997). Viable offspring derived from fetal and adult mammalian cell. *Nature,* Vol.385, No.6619, pp. 810–813, ISSN 0028-0836

Part 2

Pathophysiology of Ischemic or Anoxic Damage

5

Cerebral Ischemia Induced Proteomic Alterations: Consequences for the Synapse and Organelles

Willard J. Costain[1], Arsalan S. Haqqani[2], Ingrid Rasquinha[1], Marie-Soleil Giguere[2] and Jacqueline Slinn[3]
[1]*Glycosyltransferases and Neuroglycomics, Institute for Biological Sciences, National Research Council, Ottawa, ON,*
[2]*Proteomics, Institute for Biological Sciences, National Research Council, Ottawa, ON,*
[3]*Cerebrovascular Research, Institute for Biological Sciences, National Research Council, Ottawa, ON,*
Canada

1. Introduction

The synapse is the focal point for neuronal communication and neuron-glia interactions. Synaptic structure and function are intimately related and many of the proteins that provide structure to the synapse also regulate synaptic function (Abe et al. 2004, Couchman 2003, Ehlers 2002, Passafaro et al. 2003). The synaptic structure - function relationship is highly apparent during pathological conditions. This is exemplified in neurodegenerative disorders, such as Alzheimer's disease, where synaptic function is positively correlated with neuronal function (Gasic & Nicotera 2003) and viability (Deisseroth et al. 2003), with synaptic pathology preceding cell death (Gasic & Nicotera 2003).

Maintenance of synaptic structure and functionality is a process that is highly energy dependent. Studies of synaptosomal morphology and metabolism have indicated that the synapse is highly susceptible to ischemic damage (Pastuszko et al. 1982, Rafalowska et al. 1980, Sulkowski et al. 2002, Enright et al. 2007, Zhang & Murphy 2007). This exceptional requirement for energy necessitates the localization of numerous mitochondria proximal to the synaptic bouton and mitochondria are a commonly observed feature in synaptosomal preparations (Costain et al. 2008). Synaptosomal metabolic activity (Rafalowska et al. 1980) and the rate of neurotransmitter re-uptake (Pastuszko et al. 1982) are decreased following acute hypoxia. Furthermore, Sulkowski *et al* (2002) observed that ischemia decreases synaptosomal oxygen consumption and metabolic capacity for a period of 24 hours.

Cerebral ischemia induces a marked depletion in synaptic vesicle content and increases the number of damaged mitochondria (Sulkowski et al. 2002, Costain et al. 2008). Importantly, ischemia-induced alterations in synaptosomal morphology are indistinguishable from that of brain slices (Sulkowski et al. 2002). Ischemia-like conditions (hypoxic stress or excitotoxicity) induce dramatic and rapidly reversible structural/morphological changes in dendritic spines (Hasbani et al. 2001, Mattson et al. 1998, Park et al. 1996, Enright et al. 2007,

Zhang & Murphy 2007). The structural (Park et al. 1996) and biochemical alterations (Martone et al. 1999) at the synapse rapidly return to normal following cessation of ischemic stressors. This initial period of apparent recovery is followed by a period of morphological and biochemical alterations that persist for upwards of 24 hours (Martone et al. 1999). Similarly, dysregulation of synaptic adhesion is observed prior to the onset of neuronal cell death and continues thereafter (Costain et al. 2008). These studies indicate that the synapse is highly responsive to ischemia and is an important modulator of post-ischemic neuronal fate. Signals triggered at the synapse propagate toward the cell body and instigate delayed post-ischemic neuronal death in a process termed as ***synaptic apoptosis*** (Mattson et al. 1998).

Synaptically localized signals, either anti- or pro-apoptotic, can be propagated to the cell body in both an anterograde and retrograde manner (Mattson & Duan 1999). Apoptotic stimuli have been shown to induce caspase-3 activation, mitochondrial membrane depolarization and phospholipid asymmetry in isolated synaptosomes (Mattson et al. 1998). Similarly, trophic factor withdrawal increases axonal caspase-3 activity, but not within the neuronal soma (Mattson & Duan 1999). In hippocampal neurons, apoptotic signals initiated at the dendrites have been shown to subsequently spread toward the cell body (Mattson & Duan 1999). Synaptic apoptosis may be a mechanism that is necessary for synaptic remodeling under non-pathological conditions as well as contributing to or initiating neuronal apoptosis during pathological conditions. Pro-apoptotic proteins have been found to play a role in non-pathological processes such as neurogenesis, neurite outgrowth and synaptic plasticity (Mattson & Gleichmann 2005). This suggests that signals triggered at the synapse may propagate toward the cell body and instigate post-ischemic neuronal death.

Cellular protein levels are determined by the balance between the rates of synthesis and degradation, and cerebral ischemia has a pronounced effect on these processes. The transcriptional response to cerebral ischemia has been studied using high throughput methods under a variety of experimental conditions (Gilbert et al. 2003, MacManus et al. 2004). Similarly, cerebral ischemia-induced protein degradation has been examined for a variety of individual proteins. Activation of a variety of proteases, such as members of the caspase, calpain and cathepsin families, is a well-described consequence of cerebral ischemia (Vanderklish & Bahr 2000, Kagedal et al. 2001). Complicating this is the observation that cerebral ischemia causes proteosomal (DeGracia et al. 2002), lysosomal (Costain et al. 2010), mitochondrial (Costain et al. 2010) and endoplasmic reticulum dysfunction (Ge et al. 2007). Thus, it is almost impossible to predict post-ischemic cellular protein levels from gene expression data alone. When focusing on a subcellular structure, such as the synapse, an additional mechanism will impact protein levels. Intracellular transport mechanisms can target a protein to a specific region or be involved in sequestering proteins away from their original location (Zhao et al. 2005, Vanderklish & Bahr 2000). As a result of these factors, the best approach for determining post-ischemic synaptic protein levels is to perform a direct assessment using proteomic methodologies.

An understanding of the cell death processes that are precipitated by exposure to cerebral ischemia is necessary for designing rational therapeutic intervention. Considering that cell death can be mediated by multiple inter-related mechanisms, it is perhaps unsurprising that the majority of single target small molecules have failed in clinical trials for stroke (Ginsberg 2008). The role of apoptotic cell death in cerebral ischemia has long been studied (Hou &

MacManus 2002), and more recently ischemia induced autophagy has become an active area of interest (Liu et al. 2010). While necrotic cell death is well known to occur in cerebral infarcts, the recent identification of programed necrosis, or 'necroptosis', has reinvigorated research in ischemia-induced necrotic cell death.

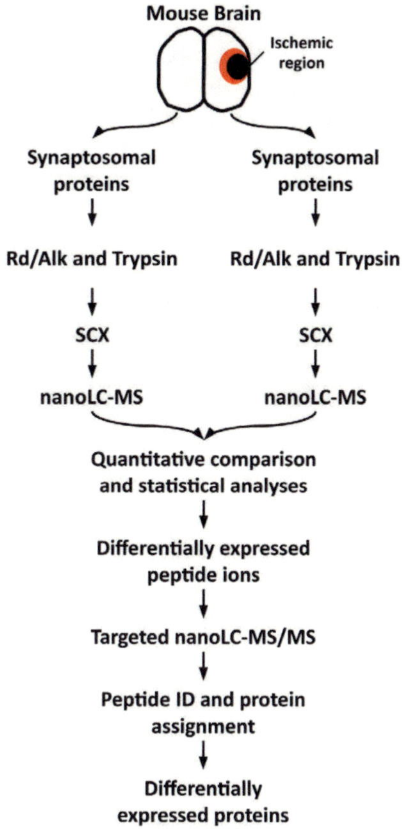

Fig. 1. Outline of the ischemic synaptosomal proteomic analysis procedure. Focal ischemia was performed 20 hours prior to the isolation of the ipsilateral (ischemic) and contralateral (non-ischemic) mouse brain hemispheres. Synaptosomes were isolated from the entire forebrain hemispheres and processed as described in the diagram.

While cell death mechanisms are typically viewed as pathways involving multiple proteins and organelles, neuronal pathology can also be examined from an organelle centric perspective. Organelle dysfunction can precipitate the initiation of cell death pathways, rather than simply being relay points for signaling events. The essence of this distinction is the difference between extrinsic activation of cell death and internal/intrinsic activation. The primary route of activation of cell death following cerebral ischemia is through intrinsic pathways involving the mitochondria, lysosomes endoplasmic reticulum, and nucleus (Yamashima & Oikawa 2009, Chen et al. 2010, Ankarcrona et al. 1995). Thus, a strategy that involves examining the interaction between organelles during pathological conditions may enable the identification of new targets that can be exploited as therapies for cerebral ischemia.

The effects of cerebral ischemia are often, by necessity, described from a highly reductionist point of view, with most studies focusing on specific signaling pathways or individual molecules. Conversely, genomic and proteomic datasets offer the opportunity to expand the scope of understanding and enable the interpretation of systematic responses. While there is a wealth of data available describing neuronal proteins localized in synaptosomes as well as pre-synaptic and post-synaptic preparations, to date studies on the effects of cerebral ischemia on the synaptic proteome are limited (Costain et al. 2008). The aim of this chapter is to integrate new and existing genomic and proteomic datasets to provide a comprehensive understanding of the effect of cerebral ischemia on the function of neuronal organelles, as well as their role in mediating cell death and / or neuroprotection.

2. Materials and methods

2.1 Animal care

A local committee for the Canadian Council on Animal Care approved all procedures using mice. The C57B mice were purchased from Charles River Canada (St-Constant, PQ). Under temporary isoflurane anesthesia, the mice (20-23 g) were subjected to occlusion of the left middle cerebral artery (MCAO) using an intraluminal filament as previously described (Costain et al. 2008). After 1 hr of ischemia, the animals were briefly reanesthetized, the filament withdrawn and wounds sutured. After 20 hrs of reperfusion, mice were briefly anesthetized with isoflurane and the brain rapidly excised and dissected on ice.

2.2 Synaptosome preparation

Contralateral (CT) and ischemic (IS) hemispheres from one mouse were manually homogenized in 2 ml of HM buffer (0.32 M sucrose, 1 mM EDTA, 0.25 mM DTT, 1 U/ml RNasin (Promega)) using a dounce homogenizer, 800 rpm 13 strokes at 4 °C. The homogenates were centrifuged (1000 g for 10 min at 4 °C) and the supernatant retained. The pellet was homogenized and centrifuged (as before) a second time. The first and second supernatants were transferred to 2 ml polycarbonate tubes and centrifuged at 20,000 g for 20 min at 4 °C. The resultant pellet was resuspended in 2 ml HM buffer using a dounce homogenizer. Discontinuous sucrose:percoll gradients were prepared by layering 2 ml each, in order, of 25% (percoll in HM buffer), 15%, 10% and 3% into 10 ml polycarbonate centrifuge tubes. One ml of the sample was then layered on top of a gradient and centrifuged at 32,000 g for 5 min at 4 °C. Five fractions were collected following centrifugation: F1 - 3% percoll (cytoplasm), F2 - interface between 3% and 10% percoll (myelin), F3 - interface between 10% and 15% percoll (small synaptosomes, myelin & mitochondria), F4 - interphase between 15% and 25% percoll (intact synaptosomes), and F5 - pellet (mitochondria). Fractions F1 - F4 were made up to 3 ml with HM buffer and centrifuged at 12,000 g for 20 min at 4 °C. The supernatant was removed and the pellet washed with 1 x PBS, twice (each time spinning at 12000 x g for 10min). The final pellet was resuspended in either HM buffer or 50 mM Tris pH 8.5, 0.1% SDS. The physical and biochemical characteristics of the synaptosome preparation used here are described in further detail in Costain *et al.* (2008).

2.3 Protein preparation, digestion and ion exchange chromatography

Proteins from each synaptosome sample were precipitated by adding 10 volumes of cold acetone and incubating at 1 h at -20 °C followed by centrifugation at 5000×g for 5 min. Pellets

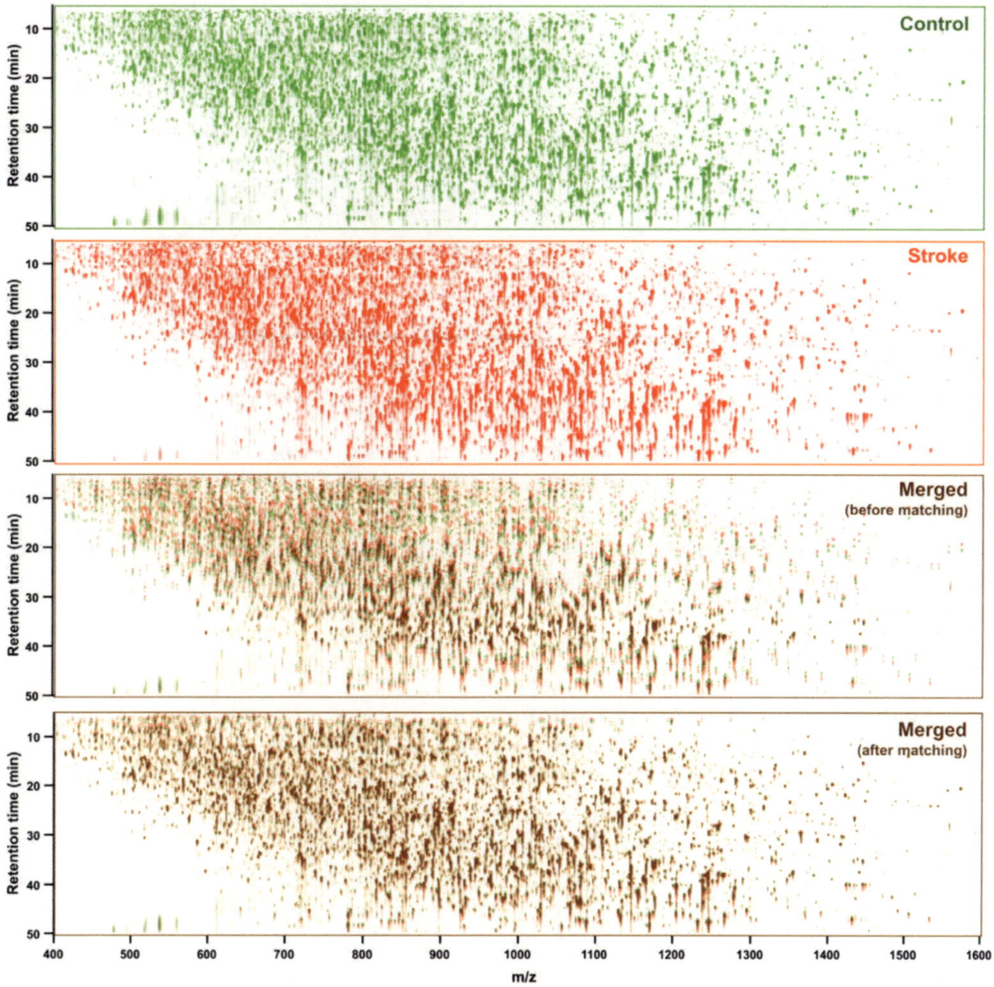

Fig. 2. NanoLC-MS analysis of contralateral (control) and ipsilateral (stroke) samples. Shown are images representing the nanoLC-MS data from each sample, where each spot represents a peptide ion. MatchRx software was used to extract peptide data, align the control and stroke datasets and correct retention time variations. Shown are the merged images before and after MatchRx-dependent correction. More than 5000 ions were detected per sample.

were dissolved in an appropriate volume of denaturing buffer (50 mM Tris-HCl, pH 8.5, 0.1% SDS) to a final protein concentration of 2 mg/mL. One hundred µg of each protein was transferred to a fresh tube. The proteins were reduced using dithiothrietol (4 mM, 10 min at 95 °C), alkylated using iodoacetamide (10 mM, 20 min at room temperature in dark), and digested using 5 µg of MS-grade trypsin gold (Promega, 12-18 h at 37 °C). The digested peptides were diluted 10-fold in 10 mM KH_2PO_4, pH 3.0, 25% acetonitrile and loaded onto a cation exchange column (POROS® 50 HS, 50-µm particle size, 4.0 mm x 15 mm, Applied Biosystems) for separation. Five fractions were eluted using step-gradient of 0-350 mM KCl. Each fraction was evaporated to dryness and dissolved in 5% acetronitrile, 1% acetic acid for analysis by mass spectrometry (MS).

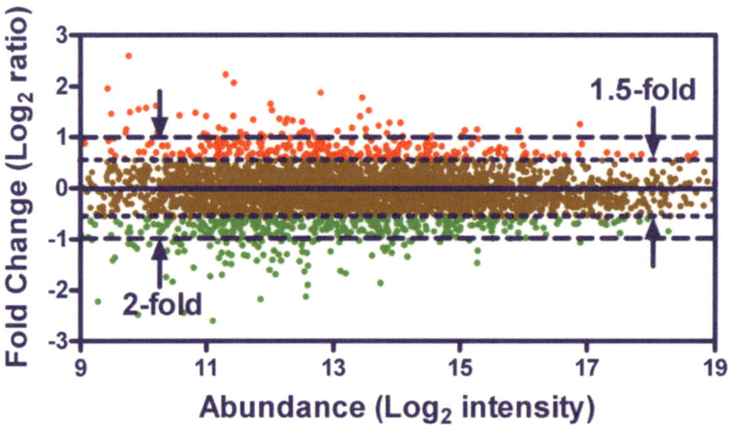

Fig. 3. Scatter plot showing relative expression of peptides in stroke and control synaptosomes. Peptide intensities were extracted from nanoLC-MS runs using MatchRx and ratio-intensity plots of stroke-vs-control samples after global median normalization were plotted. Peptides showing up (red) or down (green) regulation by 1.5-fold in stroke relative to control samples and showing a p <0.05 were considered differentially expressed. These corresponded to ~27% of the peptides and were used for targeted identification using nanoLC-MS/MS.

2.4 MS analysis and protein identification

A hybrid quadrupole time-of-flight MS (Q-TOF Ultima, Waters, Millford, MA) with an electrospray ionization source (ESI) and with an online reverse-phase nanoflow liquid chromatography column (nanoLC, 0.075 mm × 150 mm PepMap C18 capillary column, Dionex/LC-Packings, San Francisco, CA) was used for all analyses. Samples were separated on the nanoLC column using a gradient of 5-75% acetonitrile and 0.2% formic acid in 90 min, at 350 nL/min supplied by a CapLC HPLC pump (Waters). Five percent of each sample was first analyzed by nanoLC-MS in a survey (MS-only) mode for quantitation using MatchRx software as described recently (Haqqani et al. 2008). Briefly, each scan was background-subtracted, Savitzky-Golay-based smoothed, and centroided using Masslynx software v4.0 (Waters) and exported as an mzXML file (Pedrioli et al. 2004). Using MatchRx software, isotopic distribution pattern, charge state, and quantitative abundance of peptides in each nanoLC-MS run were determined. The peptides were then aligned across multiple nanoLC-MS runs through a neighboring-peak finding algorithm (Haqqani et al. 2008) followed by quantitatively comparing the levels of each peptide in the ipsilateral and contralateral fractions to identify differentially expressed peptides. Peptides showing consistent $\log_2$ fold-change of >1.5 or <-1.5 among biological replicates and showing significant difference from mean expression levels ($p < 0.05$, Wilcoxon matched pairs test) were considered differentially expressed. Images of each run were also generated to visually validate the differentially expressed peptides using MatchRx (**Fig. 4**). To sequence the differentially expressed peptides, they were included in a 'include list'. Another 5% of each sample was then re-injected into the mass spectrometer, and only the peptides included in the 'include list' were sequenced in MS/MS mode (targeted nanoLC-MS/MS). All MS/MS spectra were obtained on 2+, 3+, and 4+ ions. Peak lists were submitted to a probability-based search engine, Mascot version 2.2.0 (Matrix Science Ltd., London, U.K.) (Hirosawa et al. 1993). The initial database utilized was a composite of forward and reverse Uniprot-Swiss-Prot *Mus musculus* protein database (Aug 2011 containing 16,390 sequences). Unmatched peptides were subsequently searched against the remaining Uniprot-Swiss-Prot database (Aug 2011 containing 531,473 sequences). Searches were performed with a specified trypsin enzymatic cleavage with one possible missed cleavage. The false-positive rates (FPR) in database searching by Mascot were calculated as described earlier (Peng et al. 2003): FPR = (2 × Nrev)/(Nrev + Nfwd), where Nrev is the number of peptides identified (after filtering) from the reverse-database, and Nfwd is the number of peptides identified (after filtering) from the forward database. To maximize the number of peptides and keep the FPR < 0.5%, ion scores > 20, parent ion tolerance of < 0.1 Da, fragment ion tolerance of < 0.2 Da, and minimal number of missed cleavages were chosen. As an independent statistical measure of peptide identification, Peptide Prophet probabilities were also measured. All identified peptides had $p \geq 0.90$. The MS/MS spectrum of each differentially expressed peptide pair was manually examined and confirmed.

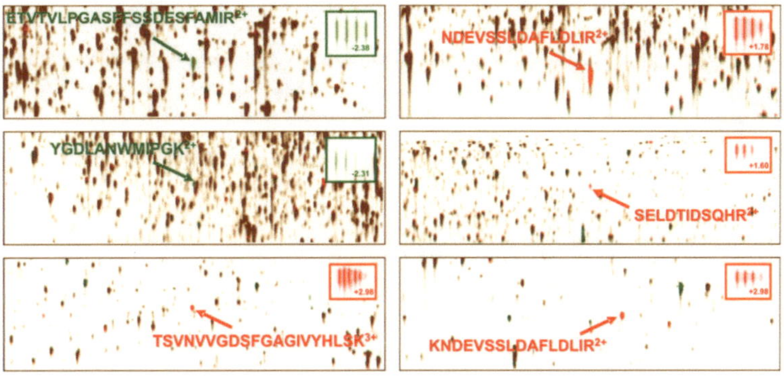

Fig. 4. Examples of differentially expressed proteins on nanoLC-MS images. Shown are merged images representing nanoLC-MS data of control (green image) and stroke (red image) samples. The two down-regulated peptides (green) are from 3-Oxoacid CoA Transferase 1 (Q9D0K2, Oxct1) and the four up-regulated peptides (red) are from glial high affinity glutamate transporter (P43006, Slc1a2). Peptides were identified by targeted nanoLC-MS/MS. In each image, *inset* shows a close-up image of the indicated peptide and the fold-change in stroke sample relative to control. For detailed list see **Tables 1** and **2**.

3. Results

3.1 Label-free proteomic analysis of ischemic synaptosomes

An outline of the experimental procedure is provided in **Fig. 1**. Following cerebral ischemia, the ipsilateral and contralateral hemispheres were separated and synaptosomal proteins isolated. The proteins from each sample were digested into sequenceable peptides, separated into 4 cation exchange chromatography fractions and analyzed by nanoLC-MS to quantify the level of each peptide. Each cation exchange fraction contained more than 12,000 peptide peaks as identified by nanoLC-MS analysis (**Fig. 2**). MatchRx software was thus used to identify quantitative differences in the nanoLC-MS runs between all the ipsilateral and contralateral fractions. The software extracts peptide-peak intensities and enables correction of retention time variations amongst multiple nanoLC-MS runs (**Fig. 2**), thus allowing accurate peptide alignment and quantitative comparison of the samples. Statistical analyses were carried out to identify differentially expressed peaks, resulting in the determination that 27% of the peaks showed differential expression (≥ 1.5 fold difference) between the two hemispheres (**Fig. 3**). As the variability between two biological synaptosomal preps was found to be about 10% (unpublished data), the observed differences were primarily attributable to the effects of cerebral ischemia and much less due to biological variability.

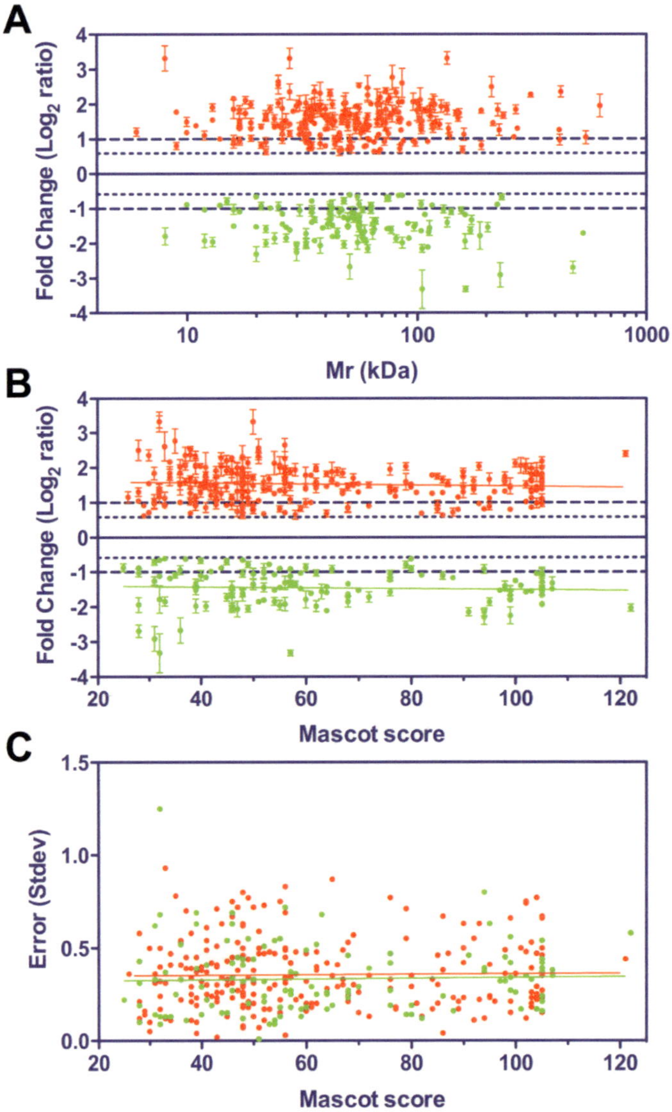

Fig. 5. Linear regression analysis of bias in label-free proteomics data. Expression data were plotted against protein mass and mascot score in panels A and B, respectively. Error values were plotted against mascot score in panel C. Linear regression analyses were performed on the up (red)- and down (green)-regulated proteins independently. Regression lines are plotted in panels B and C. Analyses of the regression slopes did not detect significant

departures from zero, indicating that there was no correlation between expression and protein size / mascot score or error and mascot score. A runs test indicated that there was no departure from linearity in the regression analysis of error versus mascot score. Furthermore, no significant differences were detected between the up and down regulated proteins in any of the analyses.

The differentially expressed peaks were then sequenced by re-injecting each fraction and analyzing with targeted nanoLC-MS/MS using an include list containing the masses and retention times of each targeted peak. The sequenced peptides were used to generate a list of ischemia-responsive proteins. A total of 371 proteins were identified as responsive to cerebral ischemia (hereafter referred to as either the IS dataset or IS proteins) (**Tables 1** and **2**). Two-thirds (68%) of these proteins were up-regulated and the remaining were down-regulated. Examples of up- and down-regulated proteins are shown in **Fig. 4**. A series of linear regression analyses were performed to ensure that the expression data was free of systematic bias. The results of the linear regression analyses indicate that the expression values were not correlated to protein mass (**Fig. 5A**) or Mascot score (**Fig. 5B**). Similarly, the measurement error was not correlated to Mascot score (**Fig. 5C**). These results indicate that the observed expression and error values are due to biological effects.

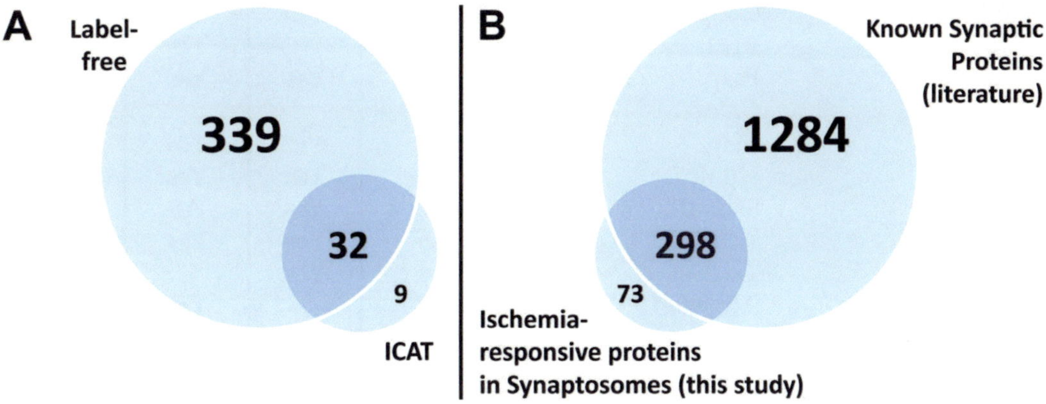

Fig. 6. (A) Venn diagram showing the number of differentially expressed proteins identified by label-free proteomics, ICAT proteomics (Costain et al. 2010) and both methods. (B) Venn diagram showing the overlap between the IS dataset using label-free proteomics (this study, 371 proteins) and the known synaptosomal proteins (1582 proteins) in the literature (Cheng et al. 2006, Morciano et al. 2005, Phillips et al. 2005, Schrimpf et al. 2005, Witzmann et al. 2005, Jordan et al. 2004, Peng et al. 2004, Stevens et al. 2003, Li et al. 2004).

To validate the purity of our synaptosomal preps, the IS proteins were searched against a known collection of synaptic protein datasets from recent literature that had been identified by proteomics. More than 80% of the IS proteins were found in these datasets (**Fig. 6B**), demonstrating that our preps are consistent with other synaptosomal datasets. However, the IS proteins corresponded to only about 23% of all the known synaptic proteins (**Fig. 6B**), which is also consistent with the fact that < 30% of the peaks were found as differentially expressed (**Fig. 3**). Literature mining through PubMed search identified that 56 proteins are known to be associated with middle cerebral artery occlusion model of ischemia (**Tables 1** and **2**).

Accession	Symbol	Exprs	Mito	synDB	MCAO
Q9CR67	Tmem33	3.3 ± 0.5		Yes	
Q06185	Atp5i	3.3 ± 0.7	Yes	Yes	
O54774	Ap3d1	3.3 ± 0.4		Yes	
P41216	Acsl1	2.8 ± 0.8	Yes	Yes	
XP_618960		2.7 ± 0.3	Yes	Yes	
Q5NCP0	Rnf43	2.6 ± 0.9	Yes	Yes	
O08709	Prdx6	2.6 ± 0.6	Yes	Yes	2
Q8BWF0	Aldh5a1	2.5 ± 0.2	Yes	Yes	
Q64487	Ptprd	2.5 ± 0.6		Yes	
Q68FF7	Slain1	2.5 ± 0.5		Yes	
Q8K2B3	Sdha	2.4 ± 0.4	Yes	Yes	
P16858	Gapdh	2.4 ± 0.6	Yes	Yes	5
P20108	Prdx3	2.4 ± 0.5	Yes	Yes	
P11531	Dmd	2.4 ± 0.5			
Q9QYB8	Add2	2.3 ± 0.4		Yes	
P15105	Glul	2.3 ± 0.5	Yes	Yes	8
Q9QYA2	Tomm40	2.3 ± 0.6	Yes	Yes	
Q8VE33	Gdap1l1	2.3 ± 0.3	Yes	Yes	
P11881	Itpr1	2.3 ± 0.4		Yes	
Q61207	Psap	2.3 ± 0.5	Yes	Yes	3
Q921L8	Galnt11	2.2 ± 0.4			
P10637	Mapt	2.2 ± 0.7		Yes	4
Q9CR61	Ndufb7	2.2 ± 0.1	Yes	Yes	
Q8BH59	Slc25a12	2.1 ± 0.8	Yes	Yes	
Q7TPR4	Actn1	2.1 ± 0.5	Yes	Yes	
P97493	Txn2	2.1 ± 0.4	Yes		9
Q9Z1G4	Atp6v0a1	2.1 ± 0.8		Yes	
P42228	Stat4	2.1 ± 0.1			
NP_001074599	Ogdhl	2.1 ± 0.5	Yes	Yes	
Q8BMS1	Hadha	2.1 ± 0.7	Yes	Yes	
Q9JLZ3	Auh	2 ± 0.4	Yes	Yes	
P81066	Irx2	2 ± 0.6			
Q3TRM8	Hk3	2 ± 0.4		Yes	
P09671	Sod2	2 ± 0.6	Yes	Yes	3
Q60931	Vdac3	2 ± 0.8	Yes	Yes	
Q8BMF4	Dlat	2 ± 0.6	Yes	Yes	
Q9Z2W1	Stk25	2 ± 0.5			1
P48318	Gad1	2 ± 0.6	Yes	Yes	5
P06745	Gpi	2 ± 0.2		Yes	1
O55143	Atp2a2	2 ± 0.7	Yes	Yes	
O08599	Stxbp1	2 ± 0.4	Yes	Yes	
Q9DCX2	Atp5h	2 ± 0.5	Yes	Yes	
P35486	Pdha1	2 ± 0.7	Yes	Yes	
P13595	Ncam1	2 ± 0.8		Yes	6
Q8R4N0	Clybl	2 ± 0.2	Yes		2

Accession	Symbol	Exprs	Mito	synDB	MCAO
P35803	Gpm6b	2 ± 0.8		Yes	
Q09666	Ahnak	2 ± 0.5			
Q61792	Lasp1	2 ± 0.8		Yes	
P20152	Vim	1.9 ± 0.4	Yes	Yes	9
Q99P72	Rtn4	1.9 ± 0.5		Yes	
P62874	Gnb1	1.9 ± 0.5	Yes	Yes	
Q08460	Kcnma1	1.9 ± 0.5		Yes	5
Q9CPP6	Ndufa5	1.9 ± 0.3	Yes	Yes	
Q8BIZ0	Pcdh20	1.9 ± 0.2			
Q9CR62	Slc25a11	1.9 ± 0.3	Yes	Yes	
Q8BVE3	Atp6v1h	1.9 ± 0.4	Yes	Yes	
P14094	Atp1b1	1.9 ± 0.9		Yes	
NP_444473	PRSS1	1.9 ± 0.7			
P18872	Gnao1	1.9 ± 0.8		Yes	
P60879	Snap25	1.9 ± 0.5		Yes	8
Q8VEA4	Chchd4	1.9 ± 0.5	Yes		
P57776-1	Eef1d	1.9 ± 0.4			
P14873	Map1b	1.8 ± 0.8		Yes	4
Q01279	Egfr	1.8 ± 0.6			5
Q9ERS2	Ndufa13	1.8 ± 0.5	Yes		
Q8VDD5	Myh9	1.8 ± 0.4		Yes	
Q80Z24	Negr1	1.8 ± 0.5		Yes	
Q925N0	Sfxn5	1.8 ± 0.3	Yes	Yes	
Q9UPR5	SLC8A2	1.8 ± 0.5	Yes	Yes	
Q8BFR5	Tufm	1.8 ± 0.4	Yes	Yes	
Q68FD5	Cltc	1.8 ± 0.7	Yes	Yes	
P17426	Ap2a1	1.8 ± 0.4		Yes	
P12960	Cntn1	1.8 ± 0.5		Yes	
Q9CR68	Uqcrfs1	1.8 ± 0.3	Yes	Yes	
Q91VD9	Ndufs1	1.8 ± 0.3	Yes	Yes	
Q62425	Ndufa4	1.8 ± 0.2	Yes	Yes	
Q8CAA7	Pgm2l1	1.8 ± 0.5		Yes	
P50516	Atp6v1a	1.8 ± 0.3	Yes	Yes	
Q9Z2I0	Letm1	1.8 ± 0.2	Yes	Yes	
Q96PV0	Syngap1	1.7 ± 0.5		Yes	
Q80TJ1	Cadps	1.7 ± 0.5		Yes	
P17742	Ppia	1.7 ± 0.3	Yes	Yes	1
P14231	Atp1b2	1.7 ± 0.6		Yes	
E9Q6J4	Ceacam3	1.7 ± 0.4			
Q9D6M3	Slc25a22	1.7 ± 0.4	Yes	Yes	
O55131	Sept7	1.7 ± 0.7		Yes	
P62761	Vsnl1	1.7 ± 0.6		Yes	
Q9D051	Pdhb	1.7 ± 0.3	Yes	Yes	
P14824	Anxa6	1.6 ± 0.3	Yes	Yes	
Q9QY06	Myo9b	1.7 ± 0.3			

Accession	Symbol	Exprs	Mito	synDB	MCAO
Q61644	Pacsin1	1.7 ± 0.3		Yes	
Q9D2G2	Dlst	1.7 ± 0.3	Yes	Yes	
Q9DBL1	Acadsb	1.7 ± 0.4	Yes	Yes	
P17182	Eno1	1.7 ± 0.5		Yes	
P63038	Hspd1	1.7 ± 0.7	Yes	Yes	10
Q9ULD0	OGDHL	1.7 ± 0.3	Yes	Yes	
Q8BKZ9	Pdhx	1.6 ± 0.3	Yes	Yes	
P62748	Hpcal1	1.6 ± 0.2		Yes	
P14211	Calr	1.6 ± 0.4		Yes	
P62482	Kcnab2	1.6 ± 0.5			
P40142	Tkt	1.6 ± 0.3		Yes	
P99029	Prdx5	1.6 ± 0.5	Yes	Yes	2
Q8VEM8	Slc25a3	1.6 ± 0.4	Yes	Yes	
P23818	Gria1	1.6 ± 0.4		Yes	5
O35526	Stx1a	1.6 ± 0.5		Yes	
P51830	Adcy9	1.6 ± 0.4		Yes	
XP_927453		1.6 ± 0.2			
P53994	Rab2a	1.6 ± 0.4	Yes	Yes	
P60710	Actb	1.6 ± 0.4	Yes	Yes	12
P31650	Slc6a11	1.6 ± 0.7		Yes	1
Q9Z2Q6	Sept5	1.6 ± 0.7	Yes	Yes	
Q99KI0	Aco2	1.6 ± 0.5	Yes	Yes	5
P46460	Nsf	1.6 ± 0.5		Yes	
Q6IFX4	Krt39	1.6 ± 0.5	Yes		
Q8R404	Qil1	1.6 ± 0.1	Yes	Yes	
O09111	Ndufb11	1.5 ± 0.7	Yes	Yes	
Q9DC69	Ndufa9	1.5 ± 0.3	Yes	Yes	
O88741	Gdap1	1.5 ± 0.5		Yes	
P07477	PRSS1	1.5 ± 0.4		Yes	
P17751	Tpi1	1.5 ± 0.3	Yes	Yes	
Q91V61	Sfxn3	1.5 ± 0.3	Yes	Yes	
P57780	Actn4	1.5 ± 0.5	Yes	Yes	
P97300	Nptn	1.5 ± 0.4		Yes	
Q99LC3	Ndufa10	1.5 ± 0.1	Yes	Yes	
P63017	Hspa8	1.5 ± 0.5	Yes	Yes	
Q99104	Myo5a	1.5 ± 0.5		Yes	1
Q9CQ69	Uqcrq	1.5 ± 0.4	Yes	Yes	
P46096	Syt1	1.5 ± 0.4		Yes	
Q8CAQ8	Immt	1.5 ± 0.3	Yes	Yes	
Q91WF3	Adcy4	1.5 ± 0.3			
Q64133	Maoa	1.5 ± 0.3	Yes	Yes	3
P97807	Fh	1.5 ± 0.2	Yes	Yes	1
Q9Z2I9	Sucla2	1.5 ± 0.2	Yes	Yes	
Q63810	Ppp3r1	1.5 ± 0.3			
O94925	GLS	1.5 ± 0.7	Yes	Yes	

Accession	Symbol	Exprs	Mito	synDB	MCAO
Q9R1T4	Sept6	1.5 ± 0.3		Yes	
P61922	Abat	1.5 ± 0.3	Yes	Yes	
Q61206	Pafah1b2	1.5 ± 0.4			
P06151	Ldha	1.5 ± 0.2	Yes	Yes	
P54227	Stmn1	1.5 ± 0.3		Yes	3
P31648	Slc6a1	1.4 ± 0.5		Yes	1
P28652	Camk2b	1.4 ± 0.3		Yes	
Q61548	Snap91	1.4 ± 0.2	Yes	Yes	
P48962	Slc25a4	1.4 ± 0.2	Yes	Yes	
P68254	Ywhaq	1.4 ± 0.2	Yes	Yes	
P50518	Atp6v1e1	1.4 ± 0.1	Yes	Yes	
Q8VHW2	Cacng8	1.4 ± 0.4		Yes	
O55125	Nipsnap1	1.4 ± 0.3	Yes	Yes	
O70566	Diaph2	1.4 ± 0.2	Yes	Yes	
P20936	RASA1	1.4 ± 0.2			
Q9ES97	Rtn3	1.4 ± 0.3		Yes	
P50114	S100b	1.4 ± 0.2		Yes	7
O08553	Dpysl2	1.4 ± 0.4	Yes	Yes	2
Q60930	Vdac2	1.4 ± 0.5	Yes	Yes	
Q02053	Uba1	1.4 ± 0.2		Yes	
Q9R0P9	Uchl1	1.4 ± 0.2		Yes	2
P10126	Eef1a1	1.4 ± 0.6	Yes	Yes	
Q60932	Vdac1	1.4 ± 0.3	Yes	Yes	
P06837	Gap43	1.4 ± 0.3		Yes	14
P62835	Rap1a	1.4 ± 0.2	Yes	Yes	
Q9D0F9	Pgm1	1.3 ± 0.2		Yes	
P62204	Calm1	1.3 ± 0.2		Yes	25
P47753	Capza1	1.3 ± 0.4		Yes	
P52480	Pkm2	1.3 ± 0.4	Yes	Yes	
Q9QZD8	Slc25a10	1.3 ± 0.4	Yes	Yes	
Q9EQF6	Dpysl5	1.3 ± 0.5	Yes		1
Q5SUA5	Myo1g	1.3 ± 0.2	Yes	Yes	
Q9D0S9	Hint2	1.3 ± 0.3	Yes	Yes	
Q62261	Sptbn1	1.3 ± 0.2		Yes	
Q8BVI4	Qdpr	1.3 ± 0.2	Yes	Yes	
O70443	Gnaz	1.3 ± 0.2	Yes	Yes	
P18760	Cfl1	1.3 ± 0.3	Yes	Yes	
Q62315	Jarid2	1.3 ± 0.2			
Q03963	Eif2ak2	1.3 ± 0.2			
P35802	Gpm6a	1.3 ± 0.4		Yes	
Q9D6R2	Idh3a	1.3 ± 0.2	Yes	Yes	1
O08749	Dld	1.3 ± 0.4	Yes	Yes	
P38647	Hspa9	1.3 ± 0.4	Yes	Yes	1
O88737	Bsn	1.3 ± 0.3		Yes	
P70268	Pkn1	1.3 ± 0.3			

Accession	Symbol	Exprs	Mito	synDB	MCAO
Q61879	Myh10	1.3 ± 0.3		Yes	
P62814	Atp6v1b2	1.3 ± 0.2		Yes	
P07901	Hsp90aa1	1.3 ± 0.3	Yes	Yes	
P63328	Ppp3ca	1.3 ± 0.3	Yes	Yes	
P56382	Atp5e	1.2 ± 0.2	Yes	Yes	
P99028	Uqcrh	1.2 ± 0	Yes	Yes	
P05201	Got1	1.2 ± 0.2	Yes	Yes	
P16277	Blk	1.2 ± 0.3		Yes	
Q9CQA3	Sdhb	1.2 ± 0.3	Yes	Yes	
P07146	Prss2	1.2 ± 0.2			
Q9WV55	Vapa	1.2 ± 0.3		Yes	
P28663	Napb	1.2 ± 0.2		Yes	
O35658	C1qbp	1.1 ± 0.2	Yes	Yes	
Q9CZW5	Tomm70a	1.1 ± 0.2	Yes	Yes	
Q9Z0J4	Nos1	1.1 ± 0.3	Yes	Yes	66
Q80XN0	Bdh1	1.1 ± 0.2	Yes	Yes	
P34884	Mif	1.1 ± 0.2		Yes	3
Q8K314	Atp2b1	1.1 ± 0.3		Yes	
Q640R3	Hepacam	1.1 ± 0.1		Yes	
Q5SWU9	Acaca	1.1 ± 0.1	Yes	Yes	
Q00690	Sele	1.1 ± 0			26
A2AJ76	Hmcn2	1 ± 0.3			
Q9JI46	Nudt3	1 ± 0.2		Yes	
Q6PCP5	Mff	1 ± 0.1	Yes	Yes	
O70283	Wnt2b	1 ± 0.2			
P70295	Aup1	1 ± 0.2			
Q80Y86	Mapk15	1 ± 0.2		Yes	
Q9CQ54	Ndufc2	1 ± 0.2	Yes	Yes	
P00405	Mtco2	1 ± 0.3	Yes	Yes	
P63082	Atp6v0c	1 ± 0.2			
Q9D8W7	Ociad2	1 ± 0.2	Yes		
XP_922613	Spnb5	1 ± 0.3			
P43006	Slc1a2	1 ± 0.2		Yes	10
Q9R111	Gda	1 ± 0.2		Yes	
Q9CQI3	Gmfb	0.9 ± 0.3		Yes	
XP_922643		0.9 ± 0.1			
O35857	Timm44	0.9 ± 0.2	Yes		
Q8BM92	Cdh7	0.9 ± 0.1		Yes	
P56564	Slc1a3	0.8 ± 0.2	Yes	Yes	
O54983	Crym	0.9 ± 0.1	Yes		
NP_082646	Pot1b	0.9 ± 0.2			
Q9JKR6	Hyou1	0.9 ± 0.2			
Q9CQH3	Ndufb5	0.9 ± 0.2	Yes		
P48320	Gad2	0.9 ± 0.1		Yes	1
Q61735	Cd47	0.9 ± 0.1			1

Accession	Symbol	Exprs	Mito	synDB	MCAO
Q9H4G0	EPB41L1	0.9 ± 0.2		Yes	
P08228	Sod1	0.9 ± 0.2	Yes	Yes	10
P62137	Ppp1ca	0.9 ± 0.3		Yes	
Q62277	Syp	0.9 ± 0.2		Yes	30
Q9QZ83	Actg1	0.9 ± 0.2	Yes	Yes	
A8E4K7	Pcdhb8	0.8 ± 0.1			
Q8K183	Pdxk	0.8 ± 0.2			2
P08556	Nras	0.8 ± 0.2	Yes	Yes	
Q61194	Pik3c2a	0.8 ± 0.3			
Q9DCS9	Ndufb10	0.8 ± 0.1	Yes	Yes	
Q62420	Sh3gl2	0.8 ± 0.2		Yes	
P48771	Cox7a2	0.8 ± 0.3	Yes		
O35728	Cyp4a14	0.8 ± 0.1			
Q6GQS1	Slc25a23	0.8 ± 0.3	Yes		
Q9CWZ7	Napg	0.7 ± 0.1	Yes	Yes	
Q99JY0	Hadhb	0.7 ± 0.1	Yes	Yes	
Q8K0T0	Rtn1	0.7 ± 0.2		Yes	
P0CG49	Ubb	0.7 ± 0	Yes	Yes	17
P84091	Ap2m1	0.7 ± 0.1	Yes	Yes	
P70335	Rock1	0.7 ± 0.2			
O09112	Dusp8	0.7 ± 0.1			
Q3UK37		0.7 ± 0.1			
Q8BLF1	Nceh1	0.7 ± 0.2			
Q76MZ3	Ppp2r1a	0.6 ± 0	Yes	Yes	
Q8BGZ1	Hpcal4	0.6 ± 0.2		Yes	
B9EJA4	Clasp2	0.6 ± 0.1			
P05202	Got2	0.3 ± 1.6	Yes	Yes	1

Table 1. List of up-regulated proteins in the IS dataset. The expression (Exprs) of each proteins is provided (mean ± SD, n = 3), as well as their presence in the mitochondria (Mito) or synapse (SynDB). The number of citations in PubMed that have associated each proteins with stoke (MCAO) are also provided.

To further characterize the IS dataset, the proteins were categorized into biological processes and subcellular localizations using a combination of Panther, Uniprot and other datasets (Taylor et al. 2003). Categorization by biological processes showed that the majority of the IS proteins are involved in transport, signal transduction, intracellular trafficking and carbohydrate metabolism (**Fig. 7A**). Additionally, up-regulated proteins were involved in the processes of immunity/defense, cell adhesion and neurogenesis. Subcellular classification mainly categorized the proteins into mitochondrial, cell membrane, cytoplasmic and membrane/cytoplasmic localizations (**Fig. 7B**). Consistent with our previous report (Costain et al. 2010), approximately half (51%) of the IS dataset were mitochondrial proteins (**Fig. 7B**), whereas < 25% of known synaptosomal proteins are mitochondrial. These changes were mainly due to mitochondrial oxidoreductases involved in electron transport and proteins involved in the TCA cycle, suggesting severe deficits in the capacity of the mitochondria to produce energy. About 20% of the identified ischemic

Accession	Symbol	Exprs	Mito	SynDB	MCAO
Q920I9	Wdr7	-3.3 ± 0.2		Yes	
Q8R1B4	Eif3c	-3.3 ± 1.3		Yes	
P42356	PI4KA	-2.9 ± 0.6		Yes	
Q8R071	Itpka	-2.7 ± 0.5		Yes	
P67778	Phb	-2.3 ± 0.4	Yes		
P19783	Cox4i1	-2.3 ± 0.8		Yes	
Q4U256	Ank3	-2.2 ± 0.6		Yes	
Q9DBG3	Ap2b1	-2.2 ± 0.5	Yes	Yes	
P51881	Slc25a5	-2.1 ± 0.5	Yes		
Q3V1U8	Elmod1	-2.1 ± 0.5	Yes	Yes	
P58281	Opa1	-2.1 ± 0.3		Yes	
Q64516	Gyk	-2.1 ± 0.4		Yes	
Q99LY9	Ndufs5	-2 ± 0.6			
P54285	Cacnb3	-2 ± 0.7	Yes	Yes	
Q8VD37	Sgip1	-2 ± 0.5		Yes	
P49615	Cdk5	-2 ± 0.4	Yes	Yes	
Q62159	Rhoc	-2 ± 0.6	Yes	Yes	2
Q9DB77	Uqcrc2	-2 ± 0.6		Yes	
Q9DCT2	Ndufs3	-2 ± 0.3	Yes	Yes	
P21803	Fgfr2	-1.9 ± 0		Yes	
Q7TQD2	Tppp	-1.9 ± 0.5	Yes	Yes	
Q64521	Gpd2	-1.9 ± 0.6	Yes	Yes	
P08249	Mdh2	-1.9 ± 0.2		Yes	
Q91WS0	Cisd1	-1.9 ± 0.7		Yes	
Q5DU25	Iqsec2	-1.9 ± 0.4			
Q03265	Atp5a1	-1.9 ± 0.2	Yes	Yes	
Q9CPQ1	Cox6c	-1.8 ± 0.5	Yes		
Q04447	Ckb	-1.8 ± 0.3	Yes	Yes	
P61161	Actr2	-1.8 ± 0.2	Yes	Yes	
Q9D6J6	Ndufv2	-1.8 ± 0.5	Yes		
Q5NVN0	PKM2	-1.8 ± 0.4			
Q6PIC6	Atp1a3	-1.7 ± 0.4			
Q8QZT1	Acat1	-1.7 ± 0.6			
O08539	Bin1	-1.7 ± 0.7			
Q9JHU4	Dync1h1	-1.7 ± 0.3	Yes	Yes	
Q91VR2	Atp5c1	-1.7 ± 0.4	Yes	Yes	
P14618	PKM2	-1.7 ± 0.5		Yes	
O88935	Syn1	-1.6 ± 0.4			
Q9D0K2	Oxct1	-1.6 ± 0.5	Yes	Yes	
Q61330	Cntn2	-1.6 ± 0.7	Yes	Yes	
Q91XV3	Basp1	-1.6 ± 0.5		Yes	
Q3V1L4	Nt5c2	-1.6 ± 0.3	Yes	Yes	
Q8BG39	Sv2b	-1.6 ± 0.4			
P61982	Ywhag	-1.6 ± 0.3	Yes	Yes	
Q80ZF8	Bai3	-1.6 ± 0.4		Yes	

Accession	Symbol	Exprs	Mito	SynDB	MCAO
P17427	Ap2a2	-1.6 ± 0.3	Yes	Yes	
Q9DBF1	Aldh7a1	-1.6 ± 0.4	Yes	Yes	8
P39053	Dnm1	-1.5 ± 0.2	Yes	Yes	
P70404	Idh3g	-1.5 ± 0.1	Yes	Yes	
P99024	Tubb5	-1.5 ± 0.3	Yes	Yes	
P12787	Cox5a	-1.5 ± 0.3	Yes	Yes	
Q8CI94	Pygb	-1.5 ± 0.6		Yes	
XP_001006010		-1.5 ± 0.1	Yes	Yes	
Q9QXV0	Pcsk1n	-1.5 ± 0.3		Yes	
P68368	Tuba4a	-1.5 ± 0.3		Yes	
Q2EMV9	Parp14	-1.5 ± 0.3	Yes	Yes	1
P05064	Aldoa	-1.5 ± 0.3		Yes	
NP_031573	Sirpa	-1.4 ± 0.4		Yes	
O88342	Wdr1	-1.4 ± 0.4	Yes	Yes	
Q9D0M3	Cyc1	-1.4 ± 0.2		Yes	
Q9QWI6	Srcin1	-1.4 ± 0.5			
Q69ZK9	Nlgn2	-1.4 ± 0.2		Yes	
P56480	Atp5b	-1.4 ± 0.2		Yes	
Q8CIV2	ORF61	-1.4 ± 0.3	Yes	Yes	
Q3UM45	Ppp1r7	-1.4 ± 0.5	Yes	Yes	
O55100	Syngr1	-1.4 ± 0.2	Yes	Yes	
P97797	Sirpa	-1.3 ± 0.3	Yes	Yes	
P51174	Acadl	-1.3 ± 0.3			
Q9CZ13	Uqcrc1	-1.3 ± 0.4			
BAE40217	Tubb5	-1.3 ± 0.3		Yes	5
AAA40509	Tubb4	-1.3 ± 0.4		Yes	
Q9WUM5	Suclg1	-1.3 ± 0.3			
Q8CHC4	Synj1	-1.3 ± 0.4	Yes	Yes	
P14152	Mdh1	-1.3 ± 0.2	Yes	Yes	
P17710	Hk1	-1.2 ± 0.2			
P23116	Eif3a	-1.2 ± 0.1		Yes	
O43837	IDH3B	-1.2 ± 0.4	Yes	Yes	
Q9CZU6	Cs	-1.2 ± 0.3		Yes	
XP_889898		-1.1 ± 0.3	Yes	Yes	
Q6NXI6	Rprd2	-1.1 ± 0.2	Yes	Yes	
NP_001013813	Gm5468	-1.1 ± 0.1	Yes	Yes	
P11627	L1cam	-1.1 ± 0.3	Yes	Yes	
O77784	IDH3B	-1.1 ± 0.4	Yes	Yes	
Q9CPU4	Mgst3	-1.1 ± 0.1	Yes	Yes	
Q8R570	Snap47	-1.1 ± 0.3		Yes	
Q8TCB6	OR51E1	-1.1 ± 0.2		Yes	
NP_082221	Csl	-1.1 ± 0.4	Yes	Yes	
Q9WUM4	Coro1c	-1.1 ± 0.1	Yes	Yes	
P10649	Gstm1	-1.1 ± 0.2		Yes	
Q9DB20	Atp5o	-1 ± 0.2	Yes		

Accession	Symbol	Exprs	Mito	SynDB	MCAO
Q9R0N5	Syt5	-1 ± 0.3	Yes	Yes	
Q9QXY2	Srcin1	-1 ± 0.2		Yes	
Q9CQY6	LOC675054	-1 ± 0.2	Yes	Yes	
Q3TC72	Fahd2	-1 ± 0.4	Yes	Yes	
Q8BK30	Ndufv3	-1 ± 0.2		Yes	1
Q9EQ20	Aldh6a1	-1 ± 0.3		Yes	
P30275	Ckmt1	-1 ± 0.2	Yes	Yes	1
Q8CHU3	Epn2	-1 ± 0.3	Yes	Yes	
O35643	Ap1b1	-0.9 ± 0.2	Yes	Yes	
O35874	Slc1a4	-0.9 ± 0.2		Yes	
P56391	Cox6b1	-0.9 ± 0.1	Yes	Yes	
A2AGT5	Ckap5	-0.9 ± 0.2	Yes	Yes	
P19536	Cox5b	-0.9 ± 0.1		Yes	
Q60597	Ogdh	-0.9 ± 0.3		Yes	
Q3TMW1	Ccdc102a	-0.9 ± 0.2		Yes	4
NP_570954	IDH3B	-0.9 ± 0.4		Yes	
P61205	Arf3	-0.9 ± 0.2	Yes	Yes	
Q9DC70	Ndufs7	-0.9 ± 0.3	Yes	Yes	
Q61124	Cln3	-0.8 ± 0.2	Yes	Yes	
Q99LC5	Etfa	-0.8 ± 0.1			
P63040	Cplx1	-0.8 ± 0.1	Yes	Yes	
Q8BH44	Coro2b	-0.7 ± 0.1	Yes	Yes	6
Q9CXZ1	Ndufs4	-0.7 ± 0.1		Yes	
P49025	Cit	-0.7 ± 0.1	Yes	Yes	
Q7TQF7	Amph	-0.7 ± 0.2	Yes	Yes	
P48678	Lmna	-0.7 ± 0.1	Yes	Yes	
O89053	Coro1a	-0.6 ± 0.1		Yes	
Q8BUV3	Gphn	-0.6 ± 0.1		Yes	
P35831	Ptpn12	-0.6 ± 0.1			

Table 2. List of down-regulated proteins in the IS dataset. The expression (Exprs) of each proteins is provided (mean ± SD, n = 3), as well as their presence in the mitochondria (Mito) or synapse (SynDB). The number of citations in PubMed that have associated each proteins with stoke (MCAO) are also provided.

proteins were classified as membrane/cytoplasmic, i.e., they exist in both cell membranes and cytoplasm. These 73 proteins consist of membrane trafficking proteins, transfer/carrier proteins, calcium-binding proteins, cytoskeletal proteins and transporters and are known to be involved in the processes of vesicle trafficking and synaptic transmission. Of the remaining identified ischemic proteins, 11% were classified as membrane-only and 9% as cytoplasm-only (**Fig. 7B**). The membrane-only proteins consist of transporters, adhesion molecules and cytokine receptors, which are known to be involved in the processes of cell adhesion, cell communication, signal transduction, neurogenesis and transport. The cytoplasm-only proteins consist of cytoskeletal proteins, enzymes (e.g., hydrolases, kinases, phosphatases) and G-proteins and are involved in the processes of signal transduction, cell structure maintenance and cell motility.

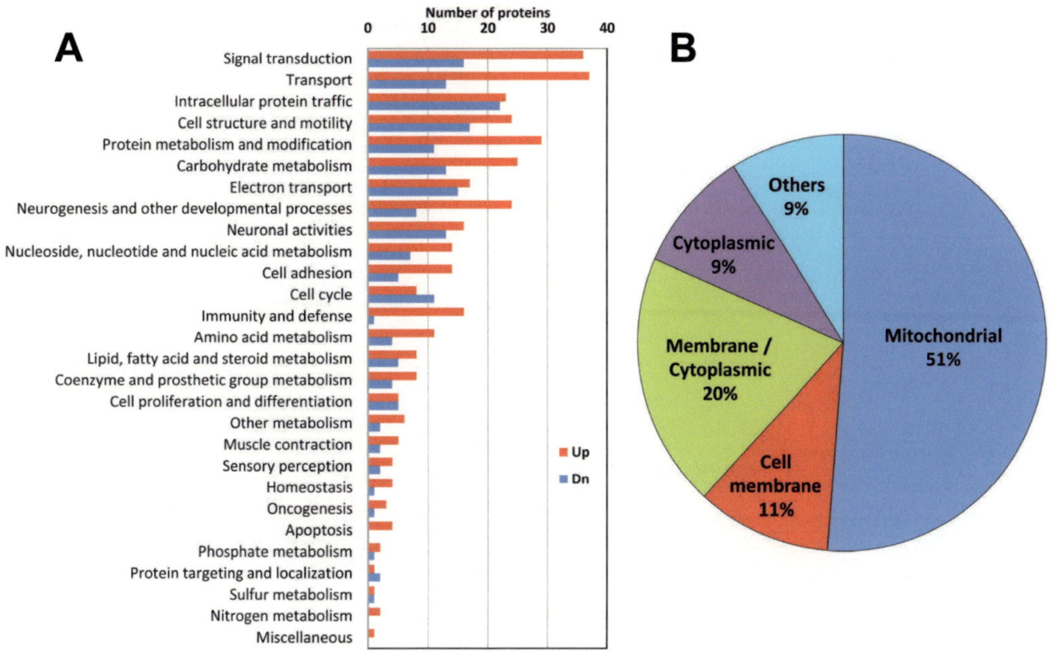

Fig. 7. Classification of differentially expressed proteins after targeted identification using nanoLC-MS/MS. (A) Protein classification by biological processes using the Panther classification system. (B) Protein classification by subcellular localizations using Panther, Uniprot and a dataset from Taylor et al. (2003).

3.2 Statistical analysis of Gene Ontology meta data

Graphical and statistical analyses of the Gene Ontology (GO) annotations were performed using the BiNGO 2.4.4 plugin for Cytoscape 2.8.2. This analysis involves gathering the GO meta data associated with the IS proteins, and determining if any annotations are statistically over-represented for each annotation category. BiNGO makes use of the hierarchical structure of the GO database to produce a graphical representation of the significantly over-represented ontologies, enabling the depiction of the parent-child relationships of the annotations. **Fig. 8** is the graphical representation of the relative positions of the terms in the GO hierarchy, with the degree of significance indicated according to color (white nodes are not significant). The size of each node (area) is proportional to the number of proteins annotated to each node. The major, significant *cellular component* ontologies (**Fig. 8A**) are cytoplasm, mitochondrion, cytoskeleton, plasma membrane, cytoplasmic membrane-bounded vesicle, Golgi apparatus, endoplasmic reticulum and vacuole. This list indicates that cerebral ischemia induces dramatic alterations in the proteomes of organelles that are involved in regulating cell death/survival processes. This is further supported by the *molecular function* ontologies (**Fig. 8C**) that are significantly enriched in terms such as kinase activity, transporter activity, antioxidant activity, electron carrier activity and nucleotide binding. Additionally, the enriched *biological process* ontologies (**Fig. 8B**) are dominated by a variety of metabolic processes, as well as transport, cellular component organization, cellular homeostasis, response to stress and response to external stimulus. Taken together, the gene ontology information paints a picture of a dynamic proteome that is responding to highly stressful injury.

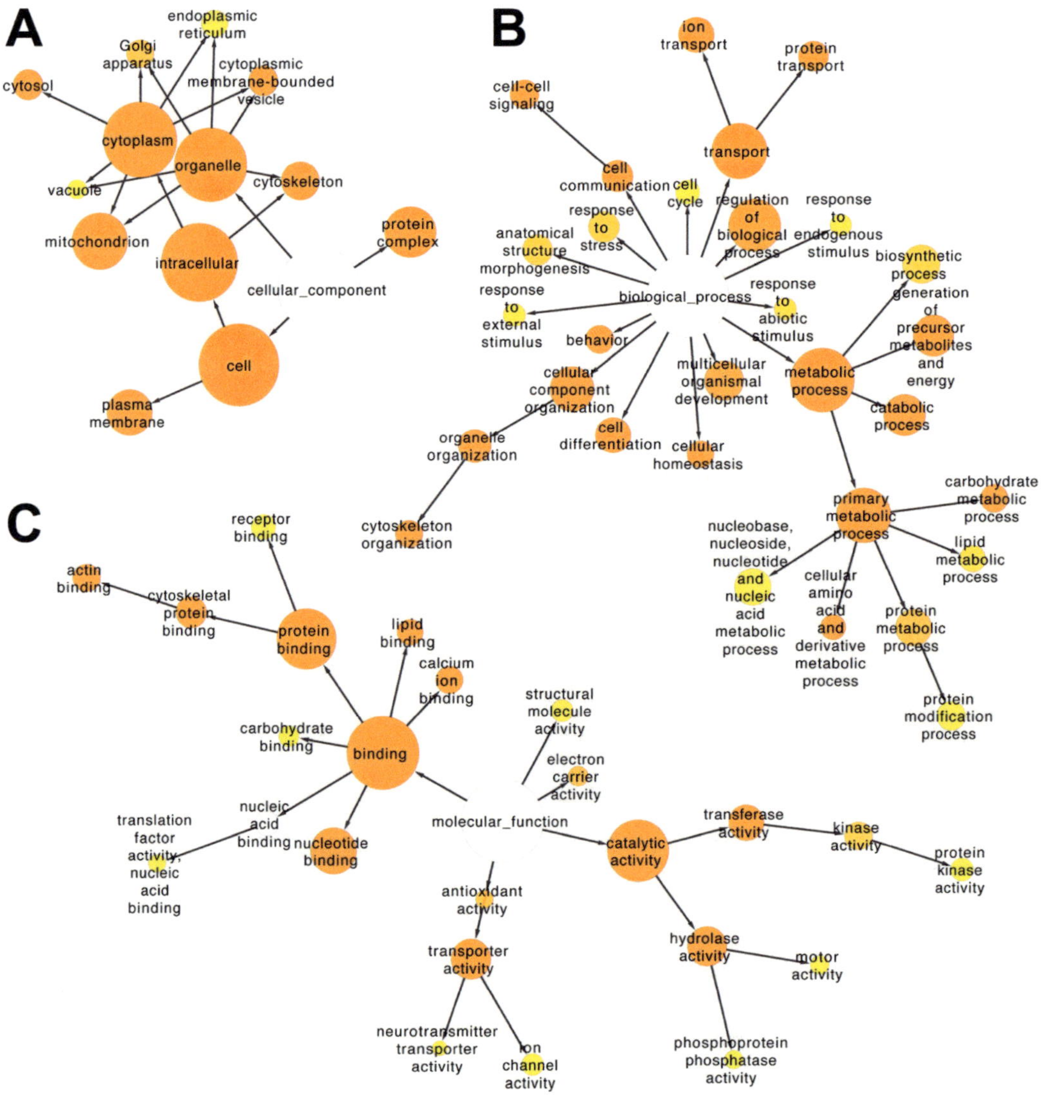

Fig. 8. Statistical analysis of Gene Ontology meta data. Statistical analysis of the Gene Ontology classification of the IS dataset was performed using the BiNGO plugin in Cytoscape. Graphical representations of significantly enriched ontologies are presented for cellular component (A), biological process (B) and molecular function (C).

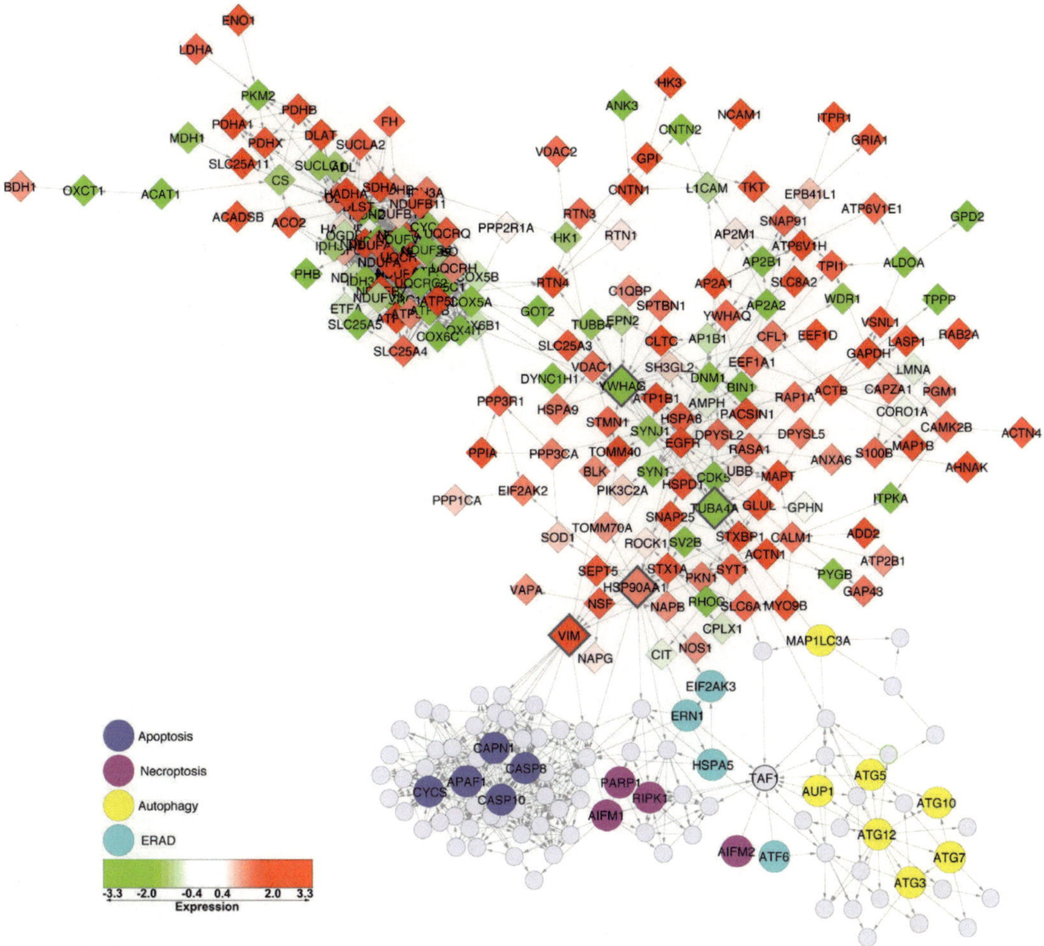

Fig. 9. Identification of therapeutic targets using a network of interactions between the IS dataset and key proteins involved in cell death mechanisms. Networks were constructed with MiMI from regulators of cell death pathways for apoptosis (Map3k14, Endog, Aifm1, Apaf1, Cycs, Capn1, Casp8, Casp10), autophagy (Aup1, Map1lc3a, Atg3, Atg5, Atg7, Atg10, Atg12), necroptosis (Aifm1, Aifm2, Parp1, Ripk1) and ER stress (ERAD; Ern1, Ern2, Hspa5, Atf6, Eif2ak3). These networks were joined with an ischemia network constructed of interacting proteins in the IS dataset (diamonds). The expression of the ischemic synaptic proteins is mapped onto the nodes according to the scale provided, with red and green representing up- and down-regulation, respectively. Key proteins (highlighted with bold node borders) for joining the cell death networks to the ischemia network (Hsp90aa1, Tuba4a, Vim) as well as highly integrated proteins (Ywhag and Taf1) were identified.

3.3 Comparison with ischemic-responsive proteins identified by ICAT

We recently identified 41 ischemia-responsive synaptosomal proteins at 20 h using ICAT-based nanoLC-MS/MS proteomics. While the ICAT-based method exhibited a high quantitative reproducibility, quantitative accuracy, and a wide dynamic range (Costain et al. 2010), it did not provide a very comprehensive analysis of the proteins. A comparison between the label-free and ICAT methods is shown in **Table 3**. While both methods have high quantitative reproducibility, the label-free method identified about 5-times more proteins and peptides in a synaptosome prep than the ICAT method. In addition, the number of peptides per protein and proteome coverage was significantly higher using the label-free method. The label-free method also showed higher peptide scores and identified several cysteine-free proteins. The label-free method identified 32 of the proteins that were also identified by ICAT (**Fig. 6A**) and the majority (80%) of their expressions values (i.e., fold change in response to MCAO) were in agreement between the two methods. Thus, while both methods are quantitatively comparable, the label-free approach provided a much more comprehensive coverage of the proteome and addressed some of the limitations of ICAT, including the detection of cysteine-free proteins.

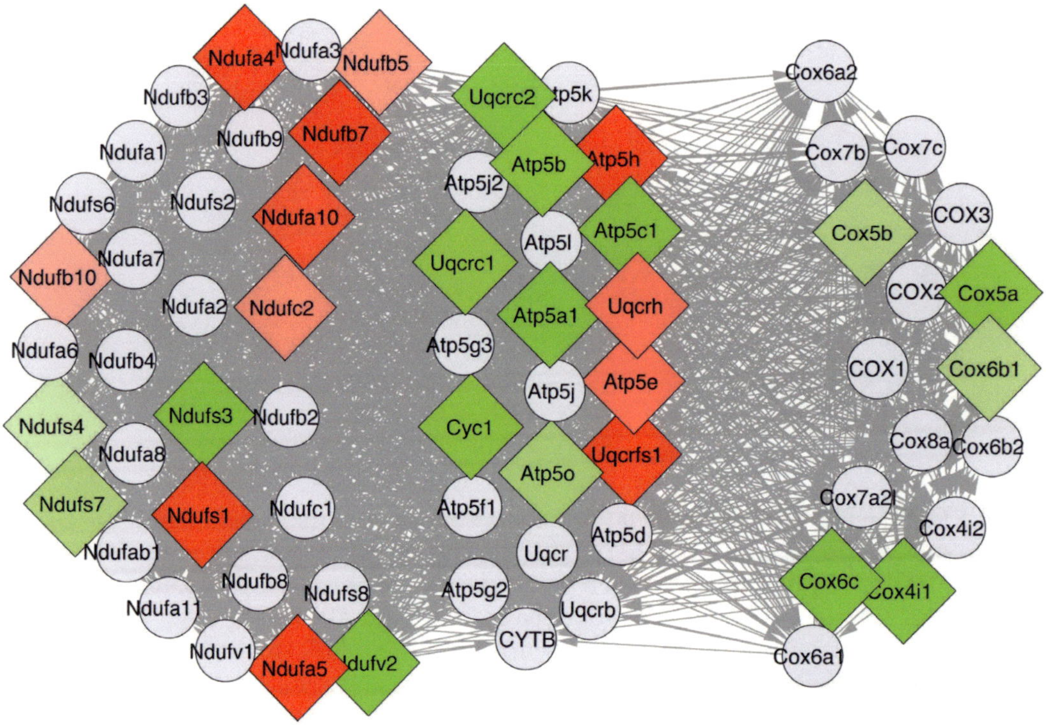

Fig. 10. Cerebral ischemia disrupts synaptosomal oxidative phosphorylation. An interaction network was constructed from proteins involved in oxidative phosphorylation using MiMI. The network segregated into proteins from 3 groups: complex I (NADH dehydrogenase (ubiquinone), complex IV (cytochrome-C oxidase) and complex V (ATP synthesis).

	Label-free	ICAT	*t-test*
Mean number of ions detected by nanoLC-MS per sample	>12,000	<4,000	$p<0.0001$
Quantitative reproducibility (mean coefficient of variance)	10%	9%	*ns*
Total unique proteins identified	371	41	
Peptides per protein	3.9	1.2	$p<0.0001$
Protein coverage (%)	15%	4.4%	$p<0.0001$
Peptide scores	71	32	$p<0.0001$
Number of cysteine-free proteins	13	N/A	

Table 3. Statistical comparison of label-free and ICAT based nanoLC-MS proteomics.

3.4 Protein interaction analysis

In an effort to identify proteins that are important in mediating ischemia-induced cell death, interaction networks were constructed using the MiMI plugin in Cytoscape. Key proteins involved in initiating the four major active cell death mechanisms were identified and stringent interaction networks were individually constructed. Additionally, a network of interactions among the proteins in the IS dataset was constructed, which resulted in the generation of a network consisting of 203 proteins (IS network). The cell death networks were merged with the IS network, resulting in the identification of a number of proteins that are likely to be important mediators of synaptic pathology and cell death (**Fig. 9**). This analysis revealed a strong degree of association between apoptosis and necroptosis, but little direct interaction with autophagy. In comparison, ER associated degradation (ERAD) was associated with both necroptosis and autophagy. **Fig. 9** indicates that the IS network is connected to apoptosis primarily through the vimentin (Vim) protein, whereas the necroptosis and ERAD networks are connected to the IS network in large part due to Hsp90aa1. In comparison, the autophagy network was connected to the IS network through Tuba4a. Additionally, the 14-3-3 protein Ywhag was revealed to be a highly connected protein within the IS network and the transcription factor Taf1 is a point of convergence for the ERAD, autophagy and necroptosis pathways.

As mentioned, many of the IS proteins are involved in a group of activities that are of obvious importance to cellular metabolism and signaling. These functionalities are highly important in maintaining cellular homeostasis as well as in deciding cellular fate during injurious conditions. **Fig. 10** is a graphical representation of the interactions among the proteins involved in the process of oxidative phosphorylation. The proteins segregated into three groups with related functions: cytochrome-C oxidase activity, NADH dehydrogenase (ubiquinone) activity and hydrogen ion transmembrane transporter activity. The expression of the proteins reveals that the Cox proteins were universally down-regulated, whereas proteins in the other groups exhibited more varied effects. **Fig. 11A** is a network of the proteins involved in glycolysis - gluconeogenesis. The figure demonstrates that there is widespread up-regulation of glycolytic proteins, with down-regulation of only two proteins. Similarly, **Fig. 11B** indicates that there is widespread up-regulation of proteins with anti-oxidant activity. Interestingly, two of the proteins identified in **Fig. 9**, Hsp90aa1 and Taf1, are also involved in the antioxidant response. The results depicted in **Fig. 11** clearly demonstrate that the ischemic synaptosomal proteome is actively engaged in an attempt to counteract the effects of cerebral ischemia, namely energy depletion and oxidative damage.

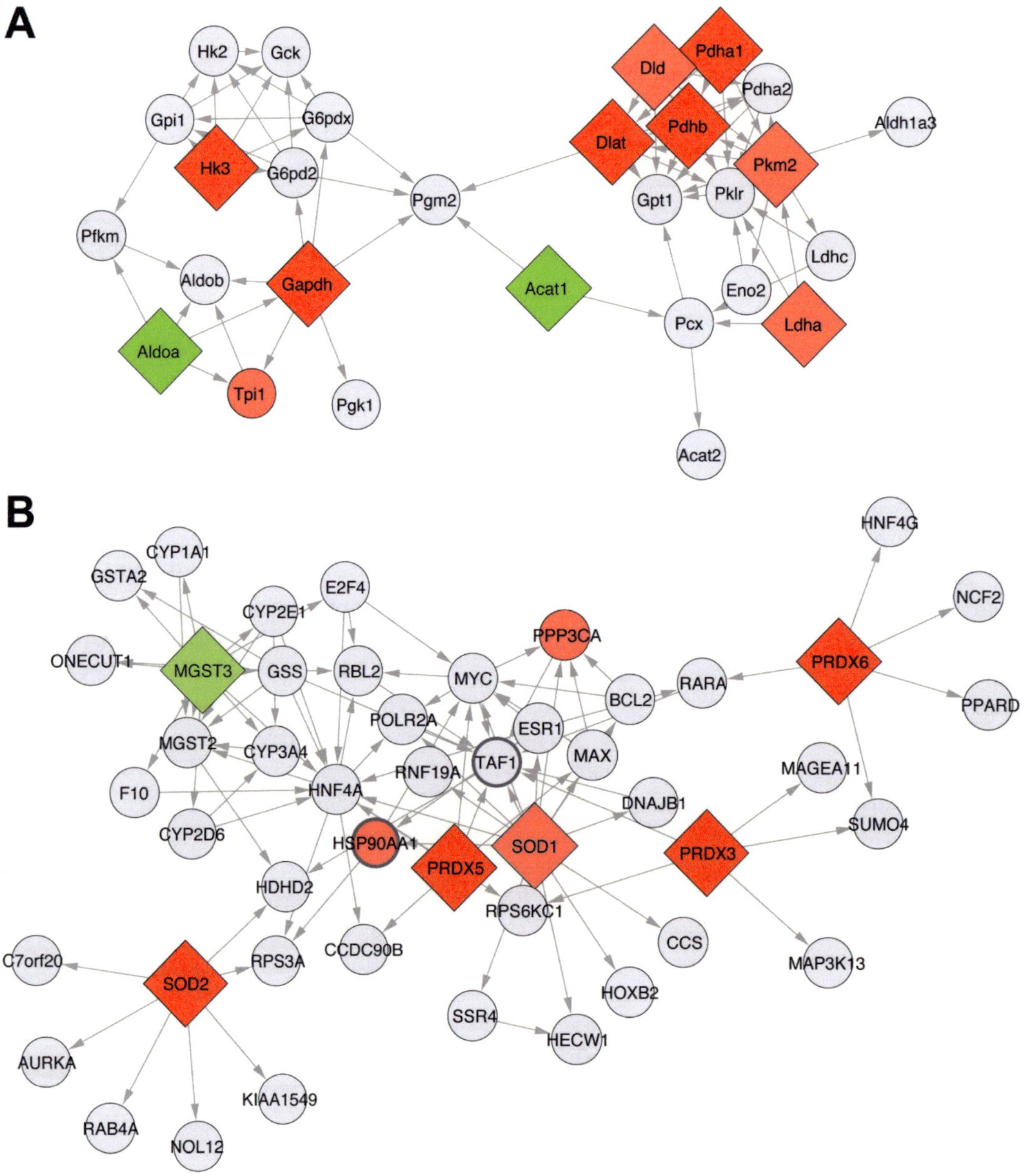

Fig. 11. Interaction network analysis demonstrates cellular responses to energy depletion and oxidative stress. Panel A is a network of proteins involved in glycolysis - gluconeogenesis, showing the up-regulation of proteins involved in this process. Panel B is a network showing the up-regulation of proteins with anti-oxidative properties.

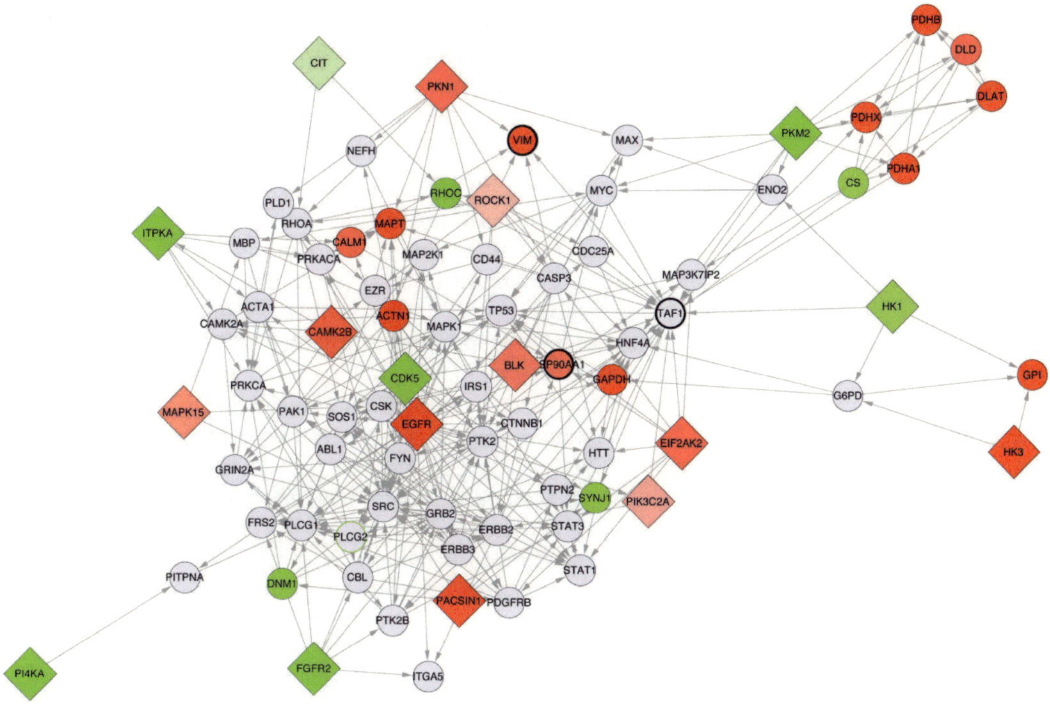

Fig. 12. Interaction network of ischemia regulated protein kinases. The network shows the regulated kinases (diamonds) interact with a subset of 16 other proteins in the IS dataset.

Actively regulated cell death processes rely on a variety of cellular signaling cascades, typically involving specific protein kinases. We found that the expression of 24 protein kinases were altered in post-ischemic synaptosomes and constructed an interaction network from this subset of proteins (**Fig. 12**). The resultant kinase network included 17 of the 24 kinases as well as 16 non-kinase synaptosomal proteins that were in the IS dataset. Interestingly, three of the key proteins identified in **Fig. 9** were present in the kinase network (Hsp90aa1, Vim and Taf1), supporting a broad role for these proteins in ischemic pathology. Interestingly, a group of proteins constituting the pyruvate dehydroxylase complex (Pdhb, Pdha1, Pdhx, Dld and Dlat), which links glycolysis and the tricarboxylic acid (TCA) cycle, were up-regulated, while citrate synthase (Cs) was down-regulated. The figure confirms that a wide variety of signaling pathways are affected by cerebral ischemia.

4. Discussion

The aim of this study is to characterize the effects of cerebral ischemia on the synaptic proteome and to examine the functional consequences of these alterations with particular emphasis on their relevance to neuronal cell death processes. As outlined, cellular protein levels are determined by the balance between synthesis and degradation, which is affected by a multitude of factors including: transcription, translation, proteases activity, and post-translational modifications. Ischemic conditions complicate the matter by causing dysfunction in the proteosome (DeGracia et al. 2002) and endoplasmic reticulum (Ge et al. 2007). Thus, gene expression data alone is a poor indicator of post-ischemic cellular protein levels. Furthermore focusing on the synapse adds the prospect of intracellular transport mechanisms and localized translation further blurring the association between transcription and synaptic protein levels (Zhao et al. 2005, Vanderklish & Bahr 2000, Havik et al. 2003). As a result of these factors, the best approach for determining post-ischemic synaptic protein levels is to perform a direct assessment using proteomic methodologies.

4.1 Cerebral ischemia-induced alterations in the synaptic proteome

Here, we determined the proteomic response of the mouse brain synapse to cerebral ischemia by performing an analysis of mouse brain synaptosomes. Using a label-free nanoLC-MS/MS method, we identified 371 synaptosomal proteins that were altered 20 hrs after cerebral ischemia (**Table 3**), representing ≈ 27% of the total peaks detected. Linear regression analysis was used to exclude the possible influence of systemic bias on expression due to protein size and MASCOT score (**Fig. 5**). The purity of the synaptosomal prep was validated by the determination that > 80% of the IS dataset were previously characterized as being localized in the synapse (**Fig. 6**). Consistent with our previous study, the majority of the IS proteins were localized in the mitochondria (Costain et al. 2010), and the localization of the remaining proteins was consistent with the synaptic compartment. Furthermore, literature mining of PubMed indicated that only ≈ 15% of the IS proteins were associated with the MCAO model of cerebral ischemia. A statistical analysis of the ontological classification of the IS dataset revealed a number of important details (**Fig. 8**). Firstly, the significant enrichment of proteins located in the mitochondria, endoplasmic reticulum and Golgi apparatus indicate the importance of these structures in mediating post-ischemic neuronal function. Secondly, significantly enriched molecular function ontologies include kinase, transport, antioxidant and electron carrier activity. These functions are related to metabolism, and are consistent with tissues responding to catastrophic energy depletion. Lastly, the significantly enriched biological process ontologies were also associated with metabolism and stress responses. The present results, obtained using label-free nanoLC-MS/MS, are largely in agreement with our previous ICAT-based proteomics study (**Table 3**). The consistency between these datasets reflects the reproducibility and purity of synaptosomal preparations, as well as the proteomic methodologies. Furthermore, the label-free method produced a more comprehensive dataset than the ICAT method, exhibiting greater protein coverage, peptide scores and the ability to identify cysteine-free proteins.

4.2 Interaction network analysis

In an effort to place the observed alterations in the IS dataset into biological context, a variety of protein interaction analyses were performed. Interaction networks can be constructed from a variety of data types, such as protein-protein, protein-DNA and genetic interactions. The value of examining such interactions is that the overall biochemical function of proteins or DNA is a product of the interactions in which they participate. Thus, analyzing functional interactions enables the construction of signaling pathways or interaction networks that are capable of modeling a system or interpreting systematic responses to a given perturbation. In the present study, we used our observed systematic alterations in synaptosomal protein expression, and protein-protein interaction analyses to aid in interpreting the net effect of ischemia on the biological system (synapses and neurons). Furthermore, we integrated our observations in IS synaptosomes with key proteins in cell death pathways that are highly predictive of cell fate. Lastly, we focused on certain subsets of proteins to produce interaction networks that provided insight into the key biological processes.

BiNGO and MiMI are valuable analysis tools that are integrated into the Cytoscape framework. The GO networks created by BiNGO identify the statistically overrepresented ontologies associated with a given gene or protein dataset. This enables rapid identification and characterization of ontologies (biological process, molecular function, cellular location) that are specific to a given dataset, as well as the hierarchical nature of the ontologies. MiMI, on the other hand, gathers interaction information from various public databases and constructs an interaction network based on a list of proteins of interest. In these interaction networks, lines drawn between entities (proteins) can represent a variety of interactions, such as binding, phosphorylation, or other biologically relevant modifications. Such analyses allow for the identification of intermediary proteins that are important to the network, but are not directly identified by either biochemical analysis or literature mining. Importantly, interaction networks can be used to identify highly integrated 'hubs', which are likely to represent key factors in a given biological process or pathology.

Cell death can occur either in an unregulated or a regulated manner. Apoptosis is a well-studied regulated cell death mechanism, and awareness of regulated necrosis (necroptosis) has been increasing (Ankarcrona et al. 1995, Baines 2010, Hitomi et al. 2008). Additionally, autophagy and ER associated degradation (ERAD) are regulated processes that are vital to cell fate decisions during injurious conditions (Liu et al. 2010, Petrovski et al. 2011). Importantly, Liu et al. (2010) recently reported that cerebral ischemia induces protein aggregation, leading to multiple organelle damage that is likely to be responsible for delayed neuronal death. We constructed an IS protein interaction network that enabled the identification of five proteins that appear to be critical in linking the consequences of synaptic ischemia to regulated cell death processes (**Fig. 9**). Of the proteins identified, Vim appeared to provide the strongest association with apoptosis, whereas Hsp90aa1 was the protein that provided a link to necroptosis and ERAD. Although Vim is an intermediate filament protein expressed in glia that may not be expected to be found in the synapse, it is common to find proteins such as Vim and Gfap in synaptosomal preparations (Costain et al. 2008) and is likely to be due to the intimate association between glia and synaptic structures. Nonetheless, up-regulation of Vim following cerebral ischemia has been frequently reported, and is thought to represent the activation of astrocytes and the reactive gliosis process. Furthermore, genetic ablation of Vim has been shown to counteract neuronal pathology, indicating that Vim is relevant to ischemic synaptosomal function (Pekny & Pekna 2004). Similarly, up-regulation of heat shock proteins, such as Hsp27 and Hsp70, in response to cerebral ischemia is a well-documented finding (Franklin et al. 2005, Currie & Plumier 1998). The Hsp90 family of molecular chaperones are involved in a variety of cellular processes, such as signal transduction, protein folding and protein degradation. Hsp90aa1 is the inducible cytoplasmic form of Hsp90 and aids in the folding of a wide variety of proteins. While other ischemia-responsive heat shock proteins that are associated with MCAO were identified in the present study (**Table 1** and **2**; Hspd1, Hspa9), Hsp90aa1 has not previously been associated with cerebral ischemia and is therefore a good candidate for further examination of its role in ischemia-induced necroptosis and ERAD.

The IS network analysis indicated that autophagy was associated with the IS dataset though the cytoskeletal protein Tuba4a (**Fig. 9**). Tuba4a has previously been identified as a synaptic protein, but has not been associated with MCAO. Alterations in cellular cytoskeletal proteins, such as Map2, are known to occur following exposure to ischemic injury (Kharlamov et al. 2009) and the observed reduction in Tuba4a expression is consistent with disruption of cytoskeletal structures. Reduced expression in other tubulin/tubulin related proteins (Tubb4, Tubb5, Tppp) was also observed, indicating an autophagy-mediated failure in the microtubule system and collapse of the synaptic structure function relationship.

Another interesting finding to arise from the IS network analysis is the prominence of the transcription factor Taf1 in connecting the autophagy, ERAD and necroptosis sub-networks. While Taf1 is involved in basal transcription, it has recently been found to be an important factor in certain neurodegenerative conditions (Davidson et al. 2009, Sako et al. 2011). Similarly, the down-regulated protein Ywhag was a highly integrated protein within the IS network, whereas the related protein Ywhaq was up-regulated with fewer interconnections (**Fig. 9**). There is growing interest in Ywhag as a mediator of neuroprotection in cerebral ischemia (Dong et al. 2010) and the observed decrease in its expression is consistent with the activation of cell death pathways. Additionally, up-regulation of Ywhaq has been observed in amyotrophic lateral sclerosis patients (Malaspina et al. 2000), and has been found to be necessary for autophagy (Wang et al. 2010). These findings suggest that the 14-3-3 proteins are likely to be playing an important role in mediating post-ischemic neuronal cell death and are good targets for therapeutic intervention in stroke.

The role of mitochondria in the pathology of ischemic neuronal death (apoptotic and necrotic) is well established (Iijima 2006, Tsujimoto & Shimizu 2007). Cerebral ischemia results in a sustained increase in intracellular Ca^{++} that is buffered by the mitochondria. The increased Ca^{++} levels disrupt the mitochondrial membrane potential and induce the formation of the permeability transition pore, thereby activating the intrinsic apoptosis pathway (Tsujimoto & Shimizu 2007). In the synaptosome, hypoxia induces mitochondrial membrane potential disruption (Aldinucci et al. 2007) and Brown *et al* (2006) have demonstrated that synaptic mitochondria are more sensitive to Ca^{++} overload than non-synaptic mitochondria. Our present findings confirm our previous observation that widespread alterations in protein expression occur in post-ischemic synaptic mitochondria (Costain et al. 2010). An interaction network was constructed from the large number of IS proteins that are involved in oxidative phosphorylation (**Fig. 10**). This interaction network clearly demonstrates that cerebral ischemia induces an imbalance in oxidative phosphorylation, with down-regulation of complex IV components and more variable effects on complex I and V. While oxidative phosphorylation is clearly disrupted, there is evidence that the cells are attempting to compensate by up-regulating glycolytic enzymes (**Fig. 11A**) as well as proteins with anti-oxidative activity (**Fig. 11B**). Unfortunately, glycolysis cannot produce the same amount of ATP that is derived from oxidative phosphorylation.

A wide variety of protein kinases are involved in mediating regulated cell death, and we identified a subset of 24 protein kinases within the IS dataset. An interaction network was constructed from the IS kinases subset (**Fig. 12**) and the kinase network independently identified three of the key proteins singled out in the IS network analysis (**Fig. 9**), supporting the contention that these proteins are involved in post-ischemic cell signaling pathways. Hsp90aa1, Taf1 and Vim were essential for connecting the four cell death mechanisms to the IS dataset, and their association with alterations in protein kinase levels further confirms their importance in mediating synaptic pathology.

5. Conclusion

In closing, this study has demonstrated that the synapse is highly responsive to cerebral ischemia and is highly informative about cerebral ischemia-induced cell death mechanisms at the organelle level. We have used interaction network analyses of the IS dataset to clarify the effects cerebral ischemia on metabolic function, as well as to identify five proteins that are integral to cell death pathways and are potential targets for therapeutic intervention. This report also confirms that cerebral ischemia induces marked aberrations in synaptic mitochondria, lysosomes, endoplasmic reticulum and golgi apparatus, thereby emphasizing the interplay between organelles during oxidative damage.

6. References

Abe, K., Chisaka, O., Van Roy, F. & Takeichi, M. (2004) Stability of dendritic spines and synaptic contacts is controlled by alpha N-catenin. *Nature Neuroscience,* 7, 357-363.

Aldinucci, C., Carretta, A., Ciccoli, L., Leoncini, S., Signorini, C., Buonocore, G. & Pessina, G. P. (2007) Hypoxia affects the physiological behavior of rat cortical synaptosomes. *Free Radical Biology and Medicine,* 42, 1749-1756.

Ankarcrona, M., Dypbukt, J. M., Bonfoco, E., Zhivotovsky, B., Orrenius, S., Lipton, S. A. & Nicotera, P. (1995) Glutamate-induced neuronal death: a succession of necrosis or apoptosis depending on mitochondrial function. *Neuron,* 15, 961-973.

Baines, C. P. (2010) Role of the mitochondrion in programmed necrosis. *Front Physiol,* 1, 156.

Brown, M. R., Sullivan, P. G. & Geddes, J. W. (2006) Synaptic mitochondria are more susceptible to Ca2+overload than nonsynaptic mitochondria. *Journal of Biological Chemistry,* 281, 11658-11668.

Chen, X., Karnovsky, A., Sans, M. D., Andrews, P. C. & Williams, J. A. (2010) Molecular characterization of the endoplasmic reticulum: insights from proteomic studies. *Proteomics,* 10, 4040-4052.

Cheng, D., Hoogenraad, C. C., Rush, J. et al. (2006) Relative and absolute quantification of postsynaptic density proteome isolated from rat forebrain and cerebellum. *Molecular and Cellular Proteomics,* 5, 1158-1170.

Costain, W. J., Haqqani, A. S., Rasquinha, I., Giguere, M. S., Slinn, J., Zurakowski, B. & Stanimirovic, D. B. (2010) Proteomic analysis of synaptosomal protein expression reveals that cerebral ischemia alters lysosomal Psap processing. *Proteomics,* 10, 3272-3291.

Costain, W. J., Rasquinha, I., Sandhu, J. K., Rippstein, P., Zurakowski, B., Slinn, J., Macmanus, J. P. & Stanimirovic, D. B. (2008) Cerebral ischemia causes dysregulation of synaptic adhesion in mouse synaptosomes. *Journal of Cerebral Blood Flow and Metabolism,* 28, 99-110.

Couchman, J. R. (2003) Syndecans: proteoglycan regulators of cell-surface microdomains? *Nature Reviews Molecular Cell Biology,* 4, 926-937.

Currie, R. W. & Plumier, J. C. (1998) The heat shock response and tissue protection. In: *Delayed preconditioning and adaptive cardioprotection,* (G. F. Baxter and D. M. Yellon eds.), Vol. 207, pp. 135-153. Kluwer Academic Publishers, Dordrecht ; Boston.

Davidson, M. E., Kerepesi, L. A., Soto, A. & Chan, V. T. (2009) D-Serine exposure resulted in gene expression changes implicated in neurodegenerative disorders and neuronal dysfunction in male Fischer 344 rats. *Archives of Toxicology,* 83, 747-762.

DeGracia, D. J., Kumar, R., Owen, C. R., Krause, G. S. & White, B. C. (2002) Molecular pathways of protein synthesis inhibition during brain reperfusion: implications for neuronal survival or death. *Journal of Cerebral Blood Flow and Metabolism,* 22, 127-141.

Deisseroth, K., Mermelstein, P. G., Xia, H. & Tsien, R. W. (2003) Signaling from synapse to nucleus: the logic behind the mechanisms. *Current Opinion in Neurobiology,* 13, 354-365.

Dong, Y., Zhao, R., Chen, X. Q. & Yu, A. C. (2010) 14-3-3gamma and neuroglobin are new intrinsic protective factors for cerebral ischemia. *Molecular Neurobiology,* 41, 218-231.

Ehlers, M. D. (2002) Molecular morphogens for dendritic spines. *Trends in Neurosciences,* 25, 64-67.

Enright, L. E., Zhang, S. & Murphy, T. H. (2007) Fine mapping of the spatial relationship between acute ischemia and dendritic structure indicates selective vulnerability of layer V neuron dendritic tufts within single neurons in vivo. *Journal of Cerebral Blood Flow and Metabolism,* 27, 1185-1200.

Franklin, T. B., Krueger-Naug, A. M., Clarke, D. B., Arrigo, A. P. & Currie, R. W. (2005) The role of heat shock proteins Hsp70 and Hsp27 in cellular protection of the central nervous system. *International Journal of Hyperthermia,* 21, 379-392.

Gasic, G. P. & Nicotera, P. (2003) To die or to sleep, perhaps to dream. *Toxicology Letters,* 139, 221-227.

Ge, P., Luo, Y., Liu, C. L. & Hu, B. (2007) Protein aggregation and proteasome dysfunction after brain ischemia. *Stroke,* 38, 3230-3236.

Gilbert, R. W., Costain, W. J., Blanchard, M. E., Mullen, K. L., Currie, R. W. & Robertson, H. A. (2003) DNA microarray analysis of hippocampal gene expression measured twelve hours after hypoxia-ischemia in the mouse. *Journal of Cerebral Blood Flow and Metabolism,* 23, 1195-1211.

Ginsberg, M. D. (2008) Neuroprotection for ischemic stroke: past, present and future. *Neuropharmacology,* 55, 363-389.

Haqqani, A. S., Kelly, J. F. & Stanimirovic, D. B. (2008) Quantitative protein profiling by mass spectrometry using label-free proteomics. *Methods in Molecular Biology,* 439, 241-256.

Hasbani, M. J., Schlief, M. L., Fisher, D. A. & Goldberg, M. P. (2001) Dendritic spines lost during glutamate receptor activation reemerge at original sites of synaptic contact. *Journal of Neuroscience,* 21, 2393-2403.

Havik, B., Rokke, H., Bardsen, K., Davanger, S. & Bramham, C. R. (2003) Bursts of high-frequency stimulation trigger rapid delivery of pre-existing alpha-CaMKII mRNA to synapses: a mechanism in dendritic protein synthesis during long-term potentiation in adult awake rats. *European Journal of Neuroscience,* 17, 2679-2689.

Hirosawa, M., Hoshida, M., Ishikawa, M. & Toya, T. (1993) MASCOT: multiple alignment system for protein sequences based on three-way dynamic programming. *Computer Applications in the Biosciences,* 9, 161-167.

Hitomi, J., Christofferson, D. E., Ng, A., Yao, J., Degterev, A., Xavier, R. J. & Yuan, J. (2008) Identification of a molecular signaling network that regulates a cellular necrotic cell death pathway. *Cell,* 135, 1311-1323.

Hou, S. T. & MacManus, J. P. (2002) Molecular mechanisms of cerebral ischemia-induced neuronal death. *International Review of Cytology,* 221, 93-148.

Iijima, T. (2006) Mitochondrial membrane potential and ischemic neuronal death. *Neuroscience Research,* 55, 234-243.

Jordan, B. A., Fernholz, B. D., Boussac, M., Xu, C., Grigorean, G., Ziff, E. B. & Neubert, T. A. (2004) Identification and verification of novel rodent postsynaptic density proteins. *Molecular and Cellular Proteomics,* 3, 857-871.

Kagedal, K., Johansson, U. & Ollinger, K. (2001) The lysosomal protease cathepsin D mediates apoptosis induced by oxidative stress. *FASEB Journal,* 15, 1592-1594.

Kharlamov, A., LaVerde, G. C., Nemoto, E. M., Jungreis, C. A., Yushmanov, V. E., Jones, S. C. & Boada, F. E. (2009) MAP2 immunostaining in thick sections for early ischemic stroke infarct volume in non-human primate brain. *Journal of Neuroscience Methods,* 182, 205-210.

Li, K. W., Hornshaw, M. P., Van Der Schors, R. C. et al. (2004) Proteomics analysis of rat brain postsynaptic density. Implications of the diverse protein functional groups for the integration of synaptic physiology. *Journal of Biological Chemistry,* 279, 987-1002.

Liu, C., Gao, Y., Barrett, J. & Hu, B. (2010) Autophagy and protein aggregation after brain ischemia. *Journal of Neurochemistry,* 115, 68-78.

MacManus, J. P., Graber, T., Luebbert, C., Preston, E., Rasquinha, I., Smith, B. & Webster, J. (2004) Translation-state analysis of gene expression in mouse brain after focal ischemia. *Journal of Cerebral Blood Flow and Metabolism,* 24, 657-667.

Malaspina, A., Kaushik, N. & de Belleroche, J. (2000) A 14-3-3 mRNA is up-regulated in amyotrophic lateral sclerosis spinal cord. *Journal of Neurochemistry,* 75, 2511-2520.

Martone, M. E., Jones, Y. Z., Young, S. J., Ellisman, M. H., Zivin, J. A. & Hu, B. R. (1999) Modification of postsynaptic densities after transient cerebral ischemia: a quantitative and three-dimensional ultrastructural study. *Journal of Neuroscience,* 19, 1988-1997.

Mattson, M. P. & Duan, W. (1999) "Apoptotic" biochemical cascades in synaptic compartments: roles in adaptive plasticity and neurodegenerative disorders. *Journal of Neuroscience Research,* 58, 152-166.

Mattson, M. P. & Gleichmann, M. (2005) The neuronal death protein par-4 mediates dopaminergic synaptic plasticity. *Molecular Interventions,* 5, 278-281.

Mattson, M. P., Keller, J. N. & Begley, J. G. (1998) Evidence for synaptic apoptosis. *Experimental Neurology,* 153, 35-48.

Morciano, M., Burre, J., Corvey, C., Karas, M., Zimmermann, H. & Volknandt, W. (2005) Immunoisolation of two synaptic vesicle pools from synaptosomes: a proteomics analysis. *Journal of Neurochemistry,* 95, 1732-1745.

Park, J. S., Bateman, M. C. & Goldberg, M. P. (1996) Rapid alterations in dendrite morphology during sublethal hypoxia or glutamate receptor activation. *Neurobiology of Disease,* 3, 215-227.

Passafaro, M., Nakagawa, T., Sala, C. & Sheng, M. (2003) Induction of dendritic spines by an extracellular domain of AMPA receptor subunit GluR2. *Nature,* 424, 677-681.

Pastuszko, A., Wilson, D. F. & Erecinska, M. (1982) Neurotransmitter metabolism in rat brain synaptosomes: effect of anoxia and pH. *Journal of Neurochemistry,* 38, 1657-1667.

Pedrioli, P. G., Eng, J. K., Hubley, R. et al. (2004) A common open representation of mass spectrometry data and its application to proteomics research. *Nature Biotechnology,* 22, 1459-1466.

Pekny, M. & Pekna, M. (2004) Astrocyte intermediate filaments in CNS pathologies and regeneration. *Journal of Pathology,* 204, 428-437.

Peng, J., Elias, J. E., Thoreen, C. C., Licklider, L. J. & Gygi, S. P. (2003) Evaluation of multidimensional chromatography coupled with tandem mass spectrometry (LC/LC-MS/MS) for large-scale protein analysis: the yeast proteome. *Journal of Proteome Research,* 2, 43-50.

Peng, J., Kim, M. J., Cheng, D., Duong, D. M., Gygi, S. P. & Sheng, M. (2004) Semiquantitative proteomic analysis of rat forebrain postsynaptic density fractions by mass spectrometry. *Journal of Biological Chemistry,* 279, 21003-21011.

Petrovski, G., Das, S., Juhasz, B., Kertesz, A., Tosaki, A. & Das, D. K. (2011) Cardioprotection by endoplasmic reticulum stress-induced autophagy. *Antioxidants & Redox Signaling,* 14, 2191-2200.

Phillips, G. R., Florens, L., Tanaka, H., Khaing, Z. Z., Fidler, L., Yates, J. R., 3rd & Colman, D. R. (2005) Proteomic comparison of two fractions derived from the transsynaptic scaffold. *Journal of Neuroscience Research,* 81, 762-775.

Rafalowska, U., Erecinska, M. & Wilson, D. F. (1980) The effect of acute hypoxia on synaptosomes from rat brain. *Journal of Neurochemistry,* 34, 1160-1165.

Sako, W., Morigaki, R., Kaji, R., Tooyama, I., Okita, S., Kitazato, K., Nagahiro, S., Graybiel, A. M. & Goto, S. (2011) Identification and localization of a neuron-specific isoform of TAF1 in rat brain: implications for neuropathology of DYT3 dystonia. *Neuroscience,* 189, 100-107.

Schrimpf, S. P., Meskenaite, V., Brunner, E., Rutishauser, D., Walther, P., Eng, J., Aebersold, R. & Sonderegger, P. (2005) Proteomic analysis of synaptosomes using isotope-coded affinity tags and mass spectrometry. *Proteomics,* 5, 2531-2541.

Stevens, S. M., Jr., Zharikova, A. D. & Prokai, L. (2003) Proteomic analysis of the synaptic plasma membrane fraction isolated from rat forebrain. *Brain Research. Molecular Brain Research,* 117, 116-128.

Sulkowski, G., Waskiewicz, J., Walski, M., Januszewski, S. & Rafalowska, U. (2002) Synaptosomal susceptibility on global ischaemia caused by cardiac arrest correlated with early and late times after recirculation in rats. *Resuscitation,* 52, 203-213.

Taylor, S. W., Fahy, E., Zhang, B. et al. (2003) Characterization of the human heart mitochondrial proteome. *Nature Biotechnology,* 21, 281-286.

Tsujimoto, Y. & Shimizu, S. (2007) Role of the mitochondrial membrane permeability transition in cell death. *Apoptosis,* 12, 835-840.

Vanderklish, P. W. & Bahr, B. A. (2000) The pathogenic activation of calpain: a marker and mediator of cellular toxicity and disease states. *International Journal of Experimental Pathology,* 81, 323-339.

Wang, B., Ling, S. & Lin, W. C. (2010) 14-3-3Tau regulates Beclin 1 and is required for autophagy. *PLoS ONE,* 5, e10409.

Witzmann, F. A., Arnold, R. J., Bai, F. et al. (2005) A proteomic survey of rat cerebral cortical synaptosomes. *Proteomics,* 5, 2177-2201.

Yamashima, T. & Oikawa, S. (2009) The role of lysosomal rupture in neuronal death. *Progress in Neurobiology,* 89, 343-358.

Zhang, S. & Murphy, T. H. (2007) Imaging the impact of cortical microcirculation on synaptic structure and sensory-evoked hemodynamic responses in vivo. *PLoS Biology,* 5, e119.

Zhao, H., Shimohata, T., Wang, J. Q., Sun, G., Schaal, D. W., Sapolsky, R. M. & Steinberg, G. K. (2005) Akt contributes to neuroprotection by hypothermia against cerebral ischemia in rats. *Journal of Neuroscience,* 25, 9794-9806.

6

Delayed Neuronal Death in Ischemic Stroke: Molecular Pathways

Victor Li, Xiaoying Bi, Paul Szelemej and Jiming Kong
University of Manitoba
Canada

1. Introduction

Ischemic stroke is caused by a loss of blood flow and deficiency in glucose and oxygen to the brain. The lack of sufficient glucose and oxygen results in varying degrees of tissue damage and cell death following stroke. Reperfusion of blood flow after ischemia often compounds tissue damage that is sustained during the initial drop in local blood availability.

The size and position of the affected region depends on which vessel is occluded. A complete loss of blood flow is rare, as rich networks of nearby blood vessels often compensate for reduced flow. The centre of the ischemic region, the core, is characterized by acute and mostly necrotic cell death resulting from severe anoxia and hypoglycemia. The region enveloping the core is known as the penumbra, which experiences a milder ischemic insult. The penumbra should be targeted for treatment strategies; it is usually much larger than the core and has a longer window of opportunity during which neurons can be prevented from dying. Many studies elucidate the molecular pathways of delayed neuronal death. This chapter presents the pathways and strategies that have been investigated to date.

2. Events in stroke

There are major differences in the physiology and biochemistry of cell death between the core and penumbra, which suggests that different mechanisms of cell death are at work in these two regions.

2.1 Core of ischemic infarct

During a stroke, the ischemic core suffers a drop in energy. ATP levels in the core fall to a level only 15% of typical basal values within one or two minutes (Katsura et al., 1993; Lipton, 1999; Lipton & Whittingham, 1982; Martin et al., 1994) and do not recover by much after reperfusion (Sun et al., 1995). The core rapidly loses ion transporter functions and undergoes anoxic depolarization (Balestrino, 1995). Homeostasis of potassium, calcium, and sodium ions is lost (Harris & Symon, 1984). After reperfusion, extracellular K^+ typically returns to control levels for six hours and then stays slightly elevated above normal (Gido et al., 1997). There is some restoration of K^+ transporter functions, despite widespread cell injury and cell death within the core. Other responses to ischemia-induced energy loss include reduction or a complete halting of protein synthesis due to translation initiation factor (IF) inactivation (White et al., 2000) and insufficient GTP for ribosomal function. Permanent absence of protein synthesis continuing beyond reperfusion results in necrotic cell death. Recovery of protein synthesis is necessary for cell survival. Necrosis in the core is accompanied by glutamate release and excitotoxic cell damage to neighbouring regions.

2.2 Penumbra of ischemic infarct

Blood flow within the penumbra can vary substantially, subjecting cells to a wide range of stresses. Ischemic injury within the penumbra is variable in whether it results in cell death and in which molecular mechanisms are involved. Many of these mechanisms induce cell death in a delayed manner in neurons, which allows them to be saved if some neuroprotection is provided. This delay allows for therapeutic treatment, since the majority of stroke patients present many hours after suffering a stroke.

Penumbral ischemia is milder than in the core; levels of ATP in the penumbra drop to an average of 50-70% of normal levels. Protein synthesis can be stalled following massive Ca^{2+} influx, which can inactivate eIF-2a by preventing activation of eIF-2 and guanine nucleotide exchange factor during the initiation of translation (Kumar et al., 2001). Protein synthesis resumes after reperfusion and has a role in determining the extent of delayed neuronal death.

2.3 Excitotoxicity

Penumbral cells are subject to excessive excitatory amino acid release from depolarized nearby cells in the ischemic core. Glutamate is the major excitatory neurotransmitter in the brain and the key mediator of intracellular communication, plasticity, growth and differentiation. The glutamate receptors implicated in excitotoxicity include the NMDA, AMPA, kainate, and other metabotropic glutamate receptors (Prass & Dirnagl, 1998). While present in synapses at micromolar concentrations, ischemia-induced depolarization causes a much larger release that triggers a chain reaction of depolarization and effects glutamate release in surrounding neurons (Paschen, 1996). The overstimulated neurons release Ca^{2+} into their cytosol, halting protein synthesis and activating cyclooxygenase-2 (COX-2), increased nitric oxide (NO) production, phospholipases, calpains, cathepsins, and calcineurin (Ferrer, 2006; White et al., 2000). Degradation of calpain substrates such as spectrin and eIF4G then follows (White et al., 2000), while cathepsin activation may increase lysosomal activity and lead to autophagic cell death (Yamashima et al., 1998). Membranes are degraded by hyperactivated phospholipases, which produce free arachidonic acid that is metabolized during reperfusion to produce peroxidative derivatives that then act as free radicals.

Excitotoxicity describes the damaging effects resulting from excessive excitatory neurotransmitter release. It is implicated in necrotic, apoptotic, and necroptotic cell death (Choi, 1996; Li et al., 2008).

2.4 Oxidative stress

Oxidative damage by free radical generation mediates cell damage in ischemia (Gilgun-Sherki et al., 2002). It is involved in excitotoxicity, apoptosis, autophagic cell death, and inflammation. Penumbral free radical levels increase during early ischemia, remain elevated, and then rise during reperfusion due to a variety of metabolic and inflammatory mechanisms (Beckman et al., 1990; Chambers et al., 1985; Clemens et al., 1997; Kuehl et al., 1980; Zhu et al., 2004b). Arachidonic acid metabolites are a source of oxidative stress following reperfusion. Mitochondrial dysfunction, COX-2 activation, endothelial and neural production of NO, and conversion of xanthine dehydrogenase to xanthine oxidase play significant roles in producing free radicals.

Oxidative stress can cause lipid peroxidation, sulfhydryl oxidation, proteolysis, and destruction of nuclear material. Excessive free radicals can activate p53, nuclear factor kappa-light-chain-enhancer of activated B cells (NF-κB), and activator protein-1, to drive their expression of pro-apoptotic genes. Free radicals and oxidative stress are involved in lysosomal dysfunction and autophagic cell death (Pivtoraiko et al., 2009). Free radicals can disrupt the electron transport chain in mitochondria, which results in autoxidation of flavoproteins and ubisemiquinone and an increase in superoxide generation (Zhu et al., 2004b).

2.5 Mitochondria-mediated death pathways

Neuronal mitochondria release cell-death factors and free radicals into the cytosol. Mitochondria have roles in apoptotic and necrosis-like cell death. ATP depletion, Ca^{2+} overload, and free radical damage causes the opening of mitochondrial permeability transition pores (Friberg & Wieloch, 2002) and releases cytochrome *c*, high temperature requirement protein A2 (HtrA2/Omi), second mitochondria-derived activator of caspases (Smac/DIABLO), apoptosis-inducing factor (AIF), and endonuclease G (EndoG).

The Bcl-2 family of proteins that regulate apoptosis includes both pro-apoptotic and anti-apoptotic proteins that counteract one another and regulate mitochondrial outer membrane permeability (MOMP) and release of mitochondrial apoptotic factors. After ischemic damage, Bcl-2 and Bcl-xL are inhibited, allowing Bax and Bak to act, which form channels in the mitochondria and release cytochrome *c*, HtrA2/Omi, and Smac/DIABLO and other cell-death-inducing factors.

2.6 Neurotrophins

Neurotrophins play a role in immediate protection of neurons and in long-term cellular remodeling and regeneration. Following ischemia, neurotrophic factors are upregulated (Ferrer et al., 1998; Takeda et al., 1993; Tsukahara et al., 1994), although local levels of brain-derived neurotrophic factor (BDNF) levels drop below baseline in vulnerable cell types (Kokaia et al., 1996). Other growth factors with neuroprotective effects include transforming growth factor-beta (TGF-β), acidic fibroblast growth factor (FGF1), and vascular endothelial growth factor (VEGF). Many mechanisms for the protective action of nerve growth factors that are induced or reduced post-ischemia have been proposed. FGF1 inhibits excitotoxicity by preventing or delaying the rise of Ca^{2+} during ischemia (Mitani et al., 1992). BDNF protects against excitotoxicity by preventing the decrease in protein kinase C that follows ischemia (Tremblay et al., 1999). The induction of BDNF is attributed to the reduction of free radicals (Mattson et al., 1995) and acts by upregulating antioxidant enzymes such as superoxide dismutases (SOD) and glutathione reductase. The function of BDNF depends on phosphorylating other cellular components (Dugan et al., 1997).

Maintenance of protein synthesis after ischemia is mediated by tyrosine kinase systems activated by neurotrophins or other growth factors. Lack of neurotrophic action in neurons results in a failure to restore protein synthesis (Hu & Wieloch, 1994). TGF-β may provide neuroprotection in ischemia by moderating transcription factors and cell-death pathways. TGF-β controls the activation of mitogen-activated protein kinases (MAPK) (Friguls et al., 2002) and inhibits Bad and caspase-3 to reduce cell death (Buisson et al., 2003; Zhu et al., 2002). These effects may be mediated by NF-κB (Zhu et al., 2004a).

VEGF promotes angiogenesis, vascular permeability, and endothelial proliferation. VEGF is implicated in neurogenesis (Storkebaum et al., 2004). VEGF is up-regulated between six and 24 hours after stroke in the penumbra (Marti et al., 2000; Plate et al., 1999). In the penumbra, VEGF modulates the PI3K/Akt/NF-κB signalling pathway and inhibits caspase-3 activity to reduce apoptosis (Sun & Guo, 2005).

2.7 Heat shock proteins

Heat shock proteins (Hsp) are involved in proper protein folding and are expressed following heat and oxidative stresses. During the first minutes of stroke, Hsp70 and Hsp90 mRNA expression rises and persists in the penumbra (Ikeda et al., 1994; Kawagoe et al., 1992; Kinouchi et al., 1993; Woodburn et al., 1993), with upregulated protein expression following a few hours later. Cell survival is positively correlated with Hsp70 production, since overexpression of Hsp70 protects against infarction in rats (Mestril et al., 1996). Lower or reduced expression of Hsp70 positively correlates with neuronal death.

Expression of Hsps inhibits the activation of the transcription factor NF-κB (Schell et al., 2005), which primarily serves a detrimental function in ischemia. Hsp70 inhibits apoptosis through interacting with key proteins in various cell-death pathways. Hsp70 prevents activation of caspase-8 and caspase-9 (Matsumori et al., 2006). Hsp70 protects cells after caspase-3 activation by blocking activation of phospholipase A-2 in the cell nucleus (Jaattela et al., 1998). Hsps may work by preserving proper protein conformation in neurons suffering ischemia (Lipton, 1999).

Ubiquitin decreases after ischemia. Expression then recovers except in vulnerable neurons destined to die (Deshpande et al., 1992; Magnusson & Wieloch, 1989). This phenomenon may be involved in cell damage, possibly by allowing the accumulation of denatured proteins (Lipton, 1999).

3. Modes of neuronal cell death

Mechanisms of cell death vary along a continuum between regulated, programmed cell death and unregulated, necrotic cell death. One on end of the spectrum, apoptotic cell death is tightly regulated and normally involved in tissue maintenance. Necrosis, at the opposite end of the spectrum, is unregulated and results from injury. Between these extremes are pathways with varying semblance to either necrosis or apoptosis, including necrosis-like cell death, necroptosis, and autophagic cell death.

3.1 Necrosis

Classical necrosis lacks regulation, order, and energy dependence. It is caused by physical or chemical insult. It is characterized by an acute loss of osmotic homeostasis and an early decline in plasma membrane integrity and ATP levels, resulting in burst cells and inflammation from the scattered cell contents. DNA cleavage occurs late in cell death through a mechanism dependent on serine proteases (Bicknell & Cohen, 1995; Dong et al.,

1997). DNA fragments are of random size. This form of necrotic cell death is present during a stroke; it is found within the ischemic core during severe acute ischemic damage.

3.2 Autophagy

Autophagy is a regulated catabolic process involving the degradation of a cell's own cytoplasmic macromolecules and organelles through digestion by the lysosomal system. Autophagy can be triggered by defective cell machinery. Through the formation of autophagolysosomes, a cell is capable of degrading the constituents, effectively recycling macronutrients and reducing the cell's metabolic requirements. The role of autophagy in cell homeostasis is undisputed. Autophagocytosis as a unique mechanism of programmed cell death is a controversial concept. There is evidence that autophagy is a separate mechanism of cell death and not merely an adaptive response to nutrient limitation (Cho & Toledo-Pereyra, 2008). It is unclear if the observed autophagic processes and mechanisms associated with cell death are the effectors of cell death or merely an overshoot of their initially beneficial intentions.

The autophagic cell death process is distinct from apoptosis and necrosis; it is characterized by autophagic degradation of cellular components prior to nuclear destruction (Bursch et al., 2000a; Schwartz et al., 1993). The most representative morphological feature is the formation of numerous autophagosomes in the cytosol with a condensed nucleus (Bursch et al., 2000b). Evidence suggests that autophagy contributes to the neuronal degeneration following cerebral ischemia. Autophagy occurs in both neonatal and adult mouse cortices and hippocampi after ischemic injury. Increased autophagosomal marker LC3-II levels are detected as early as 8 h after ischemia; more pronunciation occurs at 24 h and 72 h after hypoxic ischemia (Koike et al., 2008; Zhu et al., 2005). Damaged neurons show features of autophagic cell death, such as increased lysosomal cysteine proteinases, formation of cytoplasmic autophagic vacuoles, and the induction of GFP-LC3 immunofluorescence, during cerebral hypoxia or ischemia in adult mice (Adhami et al., 2006; Nitatori et al., 1995). Inhibition of autophagy provides neuroprotection in situations where most other pharmacological treatments are ineffective (Puyal & Clarke, 2009).

3.2.1 Autophagy pathways

A pathway for autophagous cell death has been proposed that relies on the runaway activation of beclin 1. Beclin 1 is a primary inducer of autophagy and the first identified mammalian autophagy gene product (Aita et al., 1999). Beclin 1 was originally isolated as a Bcl-2-interacting protein (Liang et al., 1999). Bcl-2 inhibits beclin 1 and beclin-1-dependent autophagy in yeast and mammalian cells. Beclin 1 mutants that cannot bind to Bcl-2 induce more autophagy (Pattingre et al., 2005). The pharmacological BH3 mimetic ABT-737 can inhibit the interaction between beclin 1 and Bcl-2 or Bcl-xL and also stimulate autophagy (Maiuri et al., 2007a; Maiuri et al., 2007b). Beclin 1 is regulated through binding with Bcl-2 proteins. Bcl-2 downregulation may result in excessive autophagy causing cell death. Autophagy regulation through Bcl-2 is attributed to its expression at the ER membrane, suggesting that signalling events originating from the ER are crucial for autophagy (Rodriguez et al., 2011). ER stress triggers autophagy; this is regulated by UPR stress sensors (Kouroku et al., 2007; Ogata et al., 2006). Stimuli that increase cytosolic calcium can activate ER stress and autophagy, which can be blocked by Bcl-2 (Hoyer-Hansen et al., 2007). ER and oxidative stresses, which are common in cerebral ischemia, are critical triggers of autophagy in neurons.

BH3-only proteins regulate autophagy under different settings, possibly by disrupting the interaction between beclin 1 and Bcl-2 or Bcl-xL via their BH3 domains (Bellot et al., 2009; Maiuri et al., 2007a). Prolonged expression or acute overexpression of BNIP3 beyond an autophagic survival threshold may result in autophagic cell death. Prolonged exposure to hypoxia of several apoptosis-competent cancer lines induces autophagy and cell death in a BNIP3-dependent manner. Beclin 1 liberation from Bcl-2 or Bcl-xL may be one of the mechanisms through which BH3-only members promote autophagy (Azad et al., 2008; Chinnadurai et al., 2008). BNIP3 may induce autophagy as a consequence of mitochondrial injury, as a loss of MPT induces autophagy (Elmore et al., 2001). Our lab has found a unique caspase-independent cell-death pathway that features the mitochondrial localization of BNIP3 followed by EndoG and AIF release from mitochondria and translocation into the nuclei, which results in cell death. Autophagy may play a part in this pathway by affecting mitochondrial stabilization or acting as a parallel cell-death-inducing pathway. Beclin 1 levels positively correlate with BNIP3 expression following ischemia. The increase in both proteins is accompanied by increased autophagic cell death that is inhibited by the autophagy inhibitor 3-methyladenine and by knockdown of BNIP3 with miRNA.

Autophagy and apoptosis can be triggered by upstream signals, often resulting in a mixed phenotype of both cell-death patterns. Neurons can switch between responses in a mutually exclusive manner. Both mechanisms are capable of inhibiting the other. Caspase inhibitors may arrest apoptosis but also promote autophagic cell death (Yu et al., 2004). Calpain-mediated cleavage of Beclin 1 can switch autophagy to apoptosis (Yousefi et al., 2006). Pathways linking the apoptotic and autophagic machineries have been deciphered at the molecular level (Maiuri et al., 2007c; Rubinsztein et al., 2005).

3.3 Apoptosis

Apoptosis is involved in cell development, differentiation, proliferation, homoeostasis, regulation, immune function, and removal of defective and harmful cells. In stroke, it is a mechanism of delayed neuronal death in response to ischemic injury. Key apoptotic proteins are activated and upregulated after cerebral ischemia, while inhibition of these proteins protects neurons from death (Chen et al., 1998).

Regulated apoptotic pathways activate cascades leading to cell suicide without the leakage of harmful cell contents. Main players in regulation include proteins from the Bcl-2 family, Smac/DIABLO (Du et al., 2000; Verhagen et al., 2000), HtrA2/Omi (Suzuki et al., 2001) and apoptotic protease-activating factor (Apaf-1) (Manfredi & Beal, 2000; Tatton & Olanow, 1999; Yuan & Yankner, 2000). Typical hallmarks of apoptosis include cell shrinkage and rounding, pyknosis and karyorhexis with DNA laddering on gel electrophoresis, membrane blebbing, and gradual disintegration of the cell into membrane-enclosed apoptotic bodies (Choi, 1996; Love, 2003; Zhang et al., 2004). Organelle structures, particularly mitochondria, are mostly preserved because apoptosis is an energy-consuming process (Friberg & Wieloch, 2002).

Coded proteins that are inactivated by covalent modifications or interactions with other anti-apoptotic regulatory molecules are necessary for pro-apoptotic signalling. Cell death stimuli are able to bring about cellular changes that remove the covalent modifications and block binding of anti-apoptotic regulators, thereby effecting apoptosis. In neurons, apoptosis can be carried out through a variety of discrete pathways, which can be categorized as either intrinsic or extrinsic. In neurons, intrinsic pathways can be triggered by intracellular damage that is caused by free radicals or excitotoxicity; extrinsic death pathways can be activated by tumour necrosis factors (TNF) or lack of neurotrophins and other growth factors. Once activated, both intrinsic and extrinsic pathways can trigger caspase-dependent or caspase-independent cell death.

3.3.1 Apoptotic pathways

The caspase family of proteases is the most common and best understood mediators of apoptosis. In humans, at least seven caspases are implicated in apoptosis, including the initiator caspases 2, 8, 9, and 10, and the executioner caspases 3, 6, and 7 (Kroemer & Martin, 2005). Activated initiator caspases are able to cleave themselves and downstream targets, causing a cascade of caspase activation culminating at the executioner caspases, which have cell structures as their substrates and directly induce apoptosis. Caspase-activated deoxyribonuclease (CAD) causes the characteristic laddered DNA fragmentation observed when its inhibitor, ICAD, is cleaved by executioner caspases (Liu et al., 1997; Liu et al., 1999).

Following cerebral ischemia, the caspase cascade can be initiated early on through cell-death receptors or by mitochondrially mediated pathways (Ashkenazi & Dixit, 1998). The two mechanisms are not necessarily mutually exclusive and can be activated sequentially depending upon cell type and insult stimuli.

The Fas receptor, a primary death receptor in ischemia-induced apoptosis (Ferrer & Planas, 2003), belongs to the TNF receptor (TNFR) family and is specific for the Fas ligand (FasL) expressed on T cells. Activation of the Fas receptor causes formation of the cell-death-inducing signalling complex (DISC), which activates caspase-8 through the Fas-associated death domain (FADD). Caspase-8 can then activate caspase-3 to bring about apoptosis or activate the mitochondrial death pathway by cleaving Bid, a promoter for mitochondrial apoptosis-induced channel (MAC) formation (Planas et al., 1997). TNFR1 is also a member of the TNFR family, which induces apoptosis through a similar mechanism (Stanger et al., 1995). The upstream activators of the TNFRs in stroke models are increased during inflammation and include FasL and TNF-α.

The mitochondrial pathway is activated by inducing MOMP through the formation of the MAC, which is thought to be an oligomerized product of the Bcl-2 proteins Bax and Bak (Dejean et al., 2010; Martinez-Caballero et al., 2009). Regulation of pore formation is carried out by the Bcl-2 family, which includes anti-apoptotic proteins Bcl-2 and Bcl-xL and pro-apoptotic proteins Bid (which is cleaved to become the active tBid), Bim, and Bad (Gross et al., 1999; Imazu et al., 1999; Susin et al., 1996; Yang et al., 1997). Upon formation, the MAC allows cytochrome *c* release to the cytoplasm, where it interacts with Apaf-1 and dATP to form apoptosomes that cleave and activate caspase-9 (Zou et al., 1997). Caspase-9 then activates executioner caspases 3, 6, and 7 to bring about apoptosis. Smac/DIABLO and HtrA2/Omi are also released from the mitochondria along with cytochrome *c* (Du et al., 2000; Suzuki et al., 2001; Verhagen et al., 2000). Both promote apoptosis by respectively removing inhibitor of apoptosis protein (IAP)'s and X-linked inhibitor of apoptosis protein (XIAP)'s inhibition of caspase-3 and caspase-9 (Suzuki et al., 2001). The action of Smac/DIABLO is inhibited by Bcl-2 and Bcl-xL, which gives some degree of control over apoptosis even after the activation of the MAC.

The mitochondrial permeability transition pore (mPTP) is activated by excess Ca^{2+} levels, loss of voltage between inner and outer mitochondrial membranes, and high levels of free radicals. It is regulated by Bcl-2 proteins and is capable of releasing cytochrome *c* to bring about caspase-dependent apoptosis. The mPTP is often associated with excitotoxicity, which provides the requisite levels of Ca^{2+} needed to induce the mPTP to open (Ichas & Mazat, 1998; Martin, 2011). The mPTP is associated with cytochrome *c* release and various reactive oxygen species (ROS). It is involved in oxidative-stress-mediated apoptosis (Baumgartner et al., 2009).

3.4 Necrosis-like cell death

Despite the prevalence of apoptosis in delayed neuronal death, there is another cell-death pathway capable of inducing cell death independently of caspase activation (Kim et al., 2005a; Kroemer & Martin, 2005; Lang-Rollin et al., 2003; Le et al., 2002; Lockshin & Zakeri, 2002). Because it is with features of necrosis, the caspase-independent cell death is also known as necrosis-like cell death (Vande Velde, et al. 2000). Preventing caspase activation by using broad caspase inhibitors such as zVAD-fmk or testing with caspase 3 or 9 knockouts provides only minor protection against cell death after brain ischemia (Himi et al., 1998; Kim et al., 2005b; Le et al., 2002). Dying neurons in the penumbra exhibit 50 kbp DNA fragments, which is atypical of the caspase-dependent chromatin fragmentation that usually results in fragments of 200-1000 bp (MacManus et al., 1997). These findings indicate that caspase-independent, or necrosis-like, cell-death pathways are probably involved in delayed neuronal death. AIF and EndoG may be important players in necrosis-like cell-death pathways (Cande et al., 2002; van Loo et al., 2001).

AIF is a mitochondrial protein localized in the inner mitochondrial membrane, where it is an oxidoreductase. Upon mitochondrial permeabilization, AIF is released into the cytoplasm and subsequently translocates into the nucleus, where it contributes to chromatin condensation and fragmentation (Krantic et al., 2007). The fragments produced are 50kbp in size, which is consistent with observations of caspase-independent cell death (Cao et al., 2003). Activation of the cell-death pathway ending in AIF is also independent of caspases, since the broad inhibitors zVAD-fmk and zDEVD-fmk do not provide neuroprotection. Inhibition of AIF or knockdown of AIF expression is able to protect against stroke-like conditions (Culmsee et al., 2005). Since AIF relies on passage through the MAC pore to cause cell death, the same regulators of the caspase-dependent mitochondrial pathway are applicable (Tsujimoto, 2003). Bcl-xL prevents AIF translocation to the nucleus (Cao et al., 2003), while tBid and Bax cause AIF efflux from the mitochondria (Cregan et al., 2002; van Loo et al., 2002). Since AIF is attached to the inner mitochondrial membrane, AIF is cleaved from the membrane before it can leave through mitochondrial pores (Donovan & Cotter, 2004). This step is not well-understood, though it is known to be caspase-independent and possibly carried out by tBid and Bax (Donovan & Cotter, 2004; Otera et al., 2005).

Endonuclease G (EndoG) is another well-established mediator of caspase-independent cell death (Li et al., 1997; van Loo et al., 2001). EndoG acts after transient cerebral ischemia (Lee et al., 2005) and oxygen-glucose deprivation (Tanaka et al., 2005), while working independently of caspase-activated DNase (Li et al., 2001; van Loo et al., 2001). Like AIF, EndoG is present in the mitochondrial inter-membrane space, localizes to the nucleus upon release, and causes cell death by cleaving chromatin into fragments. The Bcl-2 family moderates EndoG release from the mitochondria (Donovan & Cotter, 2004); tBid can cause

EndoG efflux. The pro-apoptotic protein BNIP3 causes caspase-independent cell death in hypoxia and stroke through the action of EndoG (Zhang et al., 2007b).

3.4.1 The BNIP3-activated and EndoG and AIF-mediated neuronal death pathway

BNIP3 is part of a unique subfamily of death-inducing mitochondrial proteins that includes BNIP3, NIX, BNIP3h and a Caenorhabditis elegans ortholog, ceBNIP3. Expression of BNIP3 can induce death of various cells (Chen et al., 1997), including neurons (Zhang et al., 2007a; Zhang et al., 2007b; Zhang et al., 2007c). Cell death mediated by BNIP3 is characterized through cell transfection studies by early permeabilization of the plasma membrane and damage to the mitochondria without release of cytochrome *c* or activation of caspases (Cizeau et al., 2000; Ray et al., 2000). BNIP3 triggers mPTP opening, decreases mitochondrial membrane potential, and increases generation of ROS once it localizes to the mitochondrial outer membrane (Vande Velde et al., 2000).

The BNIP3 protein has four domains: a PEST domain that targets BNIP3 for degradation, a putative Bcl-2 homology 3 (BH3) domain that is homologous to those on other members of the Bcl-2 family, a CD domain that is conserved from *C. elegans* to humans, and a C-terminal transmembrane domain that is necessary for its mitochondrial localization and for its cell-death-inducing activity (Chen et al., 1999; Farooq et al., 2001; Yasuda et al., 1998). The BH3 domain is often necessary for Bcl-2 proteins to mediate cell death. BNIP3 possesses a BH3 domain that is not necessary for its cell-death-inducing ability in vivo and in vitro (Cizeau et al., 2000; Ray et al., 2000). The mechanism may operate independently of interaction with the Bcl-2 family.

BNIP3 is not detectable in normal neurons but is inducible under hypoxia in a variety of cells and tissues (Bruick, 2000; Guo et al., 2001; Sowter et al., 2001). The BNIP3 promoter contains a functional HIF-1 response element (HRE) that is activated by either hypoxia or forced expression of HIF-1α (Bruick, 2000). HIF-1α accumulation and subsequent activation of BNIP3 is induced by oxidative stress (Zhang et al., 2007a).

HIF-1 is a basic helix-loop-helix PAS domain (BHLH-PAS) transcription factor that normally regulates homeostatic responses to hypoxia in cells (Greijer & van der Wall, 2004). HIF-1 is composed of HIF-1α and HIF-1β; HIF-1 requires heterodimerization of both to function. HIF-1β is constitutively expressed, while HIF-1α expression and stability is dependent on intracellular oxygen levels. Under hypoxia, HIF-1α stabilizes and binds to HIF-1β in order to form HIF-1, which activates genes with HREs in their promoters.

Our work shows that hypoxia increases both BNIP3 and HIF-1α levels in neurons and that knockdown of HIF-1α expression is able to protect cells from hypoxia-induced death (Z. Zhang et al., 2007). Delayed neuronal death is also reduced when cortical neuron cultures are given a dominant-negative form of HIF-1α (HIFdn) via a herpes amplicon (Halterman et al., 1999). Our proposed pathway and other major caspase-independent pathways are shown in figure 1.

4. Therapy

The root of ischemic damage can be traced to a loss of adequate oxygen and glucose due to interrupted blood flow. While this is a singular event responsible for most, if not all, subsequent neuronal death, it is unrealistic to design treatments that are able to restore blood flow in the few seconds to minutes before any damage occurs. Rather, treatment must focus on either prophylactic manipulations of these mechanisms or downstream pathways

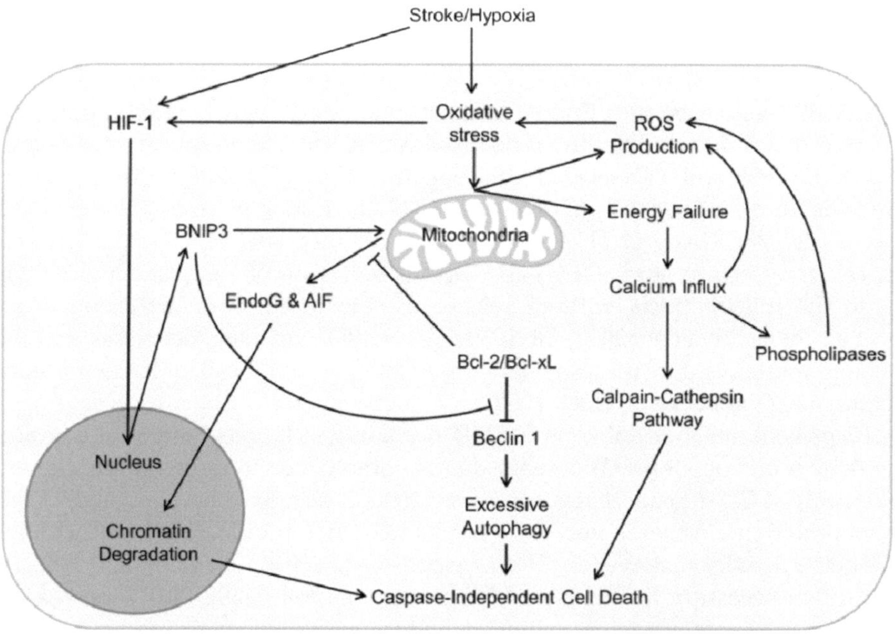

Fig. 1. Caspase-independent cell-death pathways. HIF-1 is induced directly by hypoxia or by oxidative stress and activates the expression of BNIP3 to cause the mitochondrial release of EndoG and AIF. Translocation of EndoG and AIF to the nucleus results in neuronal cell death without cytochrome c release and caspase activation. Bcl-2/Bcl-xL normally binds with beclin 1 to inhibit its activity. Sufficient BNIP3 displacement of Bcl-2/Bcl-xL from beclin 1 can cause runaway autophagy resulting in cell death. Immediate energy failure following stroke or hypoxia results in calcium disregulation and influx, triggering ROS production, phospholipase activity, and the calpain-cathepsin pathway. These processes can effect caspase-independent cell death.

that involve oxidative stress, energy depletion, ion deregulation, loss of protein synthesis, and activation of a host of protective and cell-death-inducing internal cell mechanisms. Due to the complex interactions that lead to delayed neuronal death in stroke, multi-approach strategies must be used. A comprehensive approach targeting as many pathways as possible would theoretically yield the best patient outcomes.

4.1 Antioxidants

Targeting a wide range of proteins and mechanisms involved in oxidative stress may provide beneficial therapeutic interventions for ischemia and reperfusion injury. Application of antioxidant compounds appears to be effective in combating oxidative stress in stroke (Huang et al., 2001). Antioxidant enzymes may protect against apoptosis after cerebral ischemia and reperfusion. Superoxide dismutase (SOD) has a protective role against focal cerebral ischemia. SOD-1 overexpression attenuates apoptotic cell death (Saito et al., 2004).

Melatonin is known for its neuroprotective free radical scavenging and antioxidant properties and may be a candidate for protecting against delayed neuronal death. Melatonin can readily cross the blood-brain barrier and effectively prevents neuronal loss in experimental models of ischemia and in various in vivo focal and global ischemia/reperfusion models (Letechipia-Vallejo et al., 2001; Sinha et al., 2001). Melatonin's protective mechanism may lie in its ability to bolster intracellular antioxidative mechanisms. Glutathione peroxidase activity is upregulated by melatonin, as are the gene expressions of Mn-SOD and Cu/Zn-SOD, while preventing the activation of the transcription factor NF-κB. Oxidative stress can activate several cell signalling cascades that may trigger further damage and cell-death programs. Targeting the messengers that mediate this crosstalk may prove as a viable strategy for preventing cell death. The mitogen-activated protein kinases (MAPKs) such as p38, ERK, and JNK/SAPK are important mediators of cell survival and death following ischemic injury; their activation can lead to cell death. Inhibition of their activity reduces cell damage and results in neuroprotection. Other immediate events downstream of oxidative stress, such as degradation of membranes and production of arachidonic acid by phospholipases, may be potential therapeutic targets in stroke.

4.2 Autophagy-related therapy

Blocking autophagy more than four hours after cerebral ischemia can be neuroprotective (Puyal & Clarke, 2009), despite controversy about autophagy's role as a protective or damaging mechanism. 3-methyladenine, injected intracerebroventricularly following stroke, reduces the volume of the lesion by almost half, even when given hours after a stroke has occurred. Knockdown of Atg7, the gene coding for beclin 1, also provides protection against hypoxia and ischemia (Koike et al., 2008; Nitatori et al., 1995). Other methods of downregulating beclin 1, and even BNIP3, should yield protection against autophagic cell death. Since there is the possibility that autophagy serves a mainly protective function in some neurons, too broad or unspecific an inhibition may exacerbate injury from stroke. More research needs to be done to determine the exact effects of blocking these autophagy inducers.

4.3 Hsp-related therapy

Hsp70 expression is related to a neuron's ability to survive an ischemic insult. During ischemia, Hsp expression depends on activation of NMDA receptors (Ahn et al., 2008; Lipton, 1999; Saleh et al., 2009). While this receptor is an attractive target for neuroprotection, it must be noted that NMDA receptor overstimulation may play a major role in excitotoxicity, since it mediates calcium influx. If treatment strategies are to be pursued, a balance must be established between the activation of Hsp70 expression and exacerbation of excitotoxic damage. A possible solution is to use melatonin, which is capable of inducing Hsp70 upregulation and has antioxidative effects. Gene therapy to induce the expression of Hsp72 is effective in mice and may also be an option once the technology becomes more mature.

Hsp-related therapy primarily relies on preconditioning. Hsps have protective effects only when they exist at sufficient levels in the cytoplasm. That is an unlikely scenario for a patient during a stroke, where no precondition has occurred, ischemic onset is quick and severe, and protein synthesis is halted or slowed. Most of the evidence for Hsp neuroprotection involves pretreatment to induce Hsp expression prior to the ischemic insult. Hsp-based treatment might find utility during reperfusion, if its expression can be induced rapidly and sufficiently and is shown to offer protection against this second wave of injury.

A recent study has implicated Hsp70 in blocking the release of AIF from the mitochondria. This may be an additional mechanism for preventing delayed neuronal death by inhibiting the activation of caspase-dependent cell-death pathways (Ruchalski et al., 2006).

4.4 Protective effects of exogenous growth factors

Neurotrophins, like Hsps, are exploitable as neuroprotective elements. Exogenous BDNF protects against delayed neuronal death in the rat (Beck et al., 1994; Tsukahara et al., 1994) after ischemia. Administration of VEGF is neuroprotective through inhibition of apoptosis (Hayashi et al., 1998; Jin et al., 2001; Manoonkitiwongsa et al., 2004). Gene therapy strategies for GDNF are also promising (Harvey et al., 2005; Shirakura et al., 2003; Tsai et al., 2000). Other neurotrophins are similarly able to exert protective actions by inhibiting death or triggering protective mechanisms. Neurotrophins suffer the drawback of being difficult to deliver. Many require administration before or immediately after an ischemic incident to be effective. Various methods have been devised to target neurotrophins to neurons in order to reduce delayed neuronal death.

Neurotrophins are difficult to localize to the neurons in a clinical setting. Most do not cross the blood-brain barrier, and large doses to overcome the minimal localization to brain neurons result in harmful side effects (Ferrer, 2006). The use of viral or ligand vectors to carry neurotrophins have had some success in ischemic models. Murine monoclonal antibody against rat transferrin receptors (OX26-SA) linked to a neurotrophin is capable of neuroprotection when injected into the carotid arteries, though treatment must be promptly administered after ischemia to observe any protective effects (Wu, 2005). Targeting also allows for lower doses to be used, which overcomes the obstacle of otherwise inducing side effects.

At least one study has found an increase in neuronal necrosis following BDNF pre-treatment in cell culture while reducing apoptosis in the same cells (Koh et al., 1995). The mechanism may be via the potentiation of NMDA-mediated Ca^{2+} influx, which can amplify excitotoxic effects. Another explanation may be that BDNF exacerbates free-radical-induced cell death (Gwag et al., 1995). A patient who has suffered a stroke would virtually never have received pre-treatment with neurotrophins, but the fact that neurotrophins could inadvertently exacerbate damage under certain conditions (Gwag et al., 1995) should be considered when designing neuroprotective strategies.

4.5 Caspase inhibitors

Caspases and their associated players in apoptosis may also be viable targets for preventing delayed neuronal death. Caspase inhibitors, such as the specific caspase-1 inhibitor Ac-WEHD-CHO, and broad capase inhibitors, such as z-VAD-fmk, protect against delayed neuronal death in CA-1 pyramidal cells (Hayashi et al., 2001). Injection of benzyloxycarbonyl-Asp-CH2-dichlorobenzene, a permanent inhibitor of caspases, also offers protection against delayed neuronal death by delaying chromatin condensation and DNA fragmentation (Himi et al., 1998). Administration of the broad inhibitors z-VAD-fmk and z-DEVD-fmk preserves neurological functions in addition to attenuating delayed death (Endres et al., 1998). Upregulation of the activity of intracellular caspase inhibitors is also an option. Induced overexpression of XIAP using viral vectors shows neuroprotective effects (Xu et al., 1999). UCF-101, an HtrA2/Omi inhibitor, prevents apoptosis by regulating Fas-mediated proteins in extrinsic apoptosis as well.

These caspase inhibitors can be a valuable tool to combat delayed neuronal death, despite many of them being unable to cross the blood brain barrier. Most studies involve the direct injection of the inhibitors into brain tissue or intraventricular space. Seeing as intrinsic caspase-dependent cell death depends on mitochondrial permeability, there is a chance that blocking caspase activation may allow caspase-independent death pathways to occur. As a result, inhibiting only caspases may allow a number of cells to die by alternative means. Caspase inhibitors alone do not help in preserving long-term potentiation and plasticity of neurons after ischemia (Gillardon et al., 1999). Theoretically, blocking as many of the cell death signalling pathways as possible may maximize neuroprotection.

A concern with the use of caspase inhibitors in therapy or inhibiting apoptosis in general is that it may increase the probability of developing cancer or autoimmune disorders. This risk must be balanced against the potential neuroprotective effects of directly inhibiting apoptosis. This risk may be minimized if the inhibitors are localized as much as possible to the infarct region.

4.6 AIF and EndoG

Recently, more therapeutic strategies have been targeted towards caspase-independent cell death that is mediated by AIF and EndoG. Reducing the levels of AIF in a cell by using neutralizing antibodies (Cregan et al., 2002), RNAi (Strosznajder & Gajkowska, 2006) or gene knockout (Klein et al., 2002) is strongly neuroprotective. Downregulation of EndoG activity has been explored. Our team has found that RNAi inhibition of BNIP3 reduces EndoG translocation and is neuroprotective against hypoxia-induced cell death (Zhang et al., 2007b). Other studies have found that mutant heterozygosity for EndoG in transgenic mice provides resistance to TNF-α-induced cell death (Zhang et al., 2003).

AIF and EndoG release can be inhibited by preventing mitochondrial outer membrane permeabilization (MOMP). Blocking MAC activation or preventing mitochondrial rupturing may be neuroprotective. Seeing as most stroke patients are treated for hours after a stroke occurs, when MOMP has already been induced, strategies centred on preventing mitochondrial release of death promoters are limited. Some benefit may still exist for those cases receiving prompt intervention, when treatment can prevent MOMP in affected but not yet compromised mitochondria. Preventing MOMP while simultaneously targeting downstream death effectors may prevent cell death (Galluzzi et al., 2009).

Hsp70 is capable of inhibiting AIF release from the mitochondria. This mechanism may be dependent on the C-terminal region of Hsp70 rather than its enzymatic activity (Sun et al., 2006). Hsp70 may be capable of inhibiting the nuclease functions of EndoG in an ATP-dependent manner as well (Kalinowska et al., 2005). Hsp70 may offer neuroprotection through a multitude of pathways.

MOMP inhibition by targeting upstream factors has achieved significant levels of neuroprotection in vivo and is another therapeutic possibility. For example, it has been found that inhibiting the family of MAPKs can protect against ischemic damage. Treating mice through inhibition of p53 by genetic (Morrison et al., 1996), pharmacological (Culmsee et al., 2001) means, or by using blockers of the JNK signalling pathway (Gao et al., 2005; Guan et al., 2006) has resulted in neuroprotection against ischemia and excitotoxicity, presumably in part by reducing mitochondrial permeability.

4.7 MOMP prevention by targeting Bcl-2 proteins

Regulating Bcl-2 proteins provides protection against delayed neuronal death by preserving mitochondrial integrity. The MAC pore is key in regulating mitochondrial permeability and is under the control of the Bcl-2 family of proteins. Inhibition or upregulation of select members by genetic or pharmacological means can modulate the downstream activation of caspase-dependent apoptosis and AIF- or EndoG-mediated necrosis-like cell death; and they have been investigated for treatment strategies.

Inhibiting the pro-apoptotic BH3-only Bcl-2 proteins prevents MOMP, providing protection against mitochondria-mediated cell death. Pharmacologically blocking Bid with 4-phenylsulfanyl-phenylamine derivatives prevents tBid-induced Smac release, AIF release, caspase-3 activation, and nuclear condensation (Culmsee & Plesnila, 2006; Culmsee et al., 2005). Knockouts of Bid (Plesnila et al., 2002; Plesnila et al., 2001) or Bax genes (Gibson et al., 2001; Tehranian et al., 2008) protect against ischemic cell death in stroke models as well.

Genetic means of boosting the effects of Bcl-2 antiapoptotic proteins provide neuroprotection. Transgenically upregulating the protective Bcl-2 gene provides protection in mice of neurons injured by ischemia (Martinou et al., 1994). A similar effect can be observed when human Bcl-2 is overexpressed with herpes simplex virus vectors (Linnik et al., 1995). Gene therapy using adeno-associated viruses carrying the Bcl-2 gene is also effective (Shimazaki et al., 2000). Human gene therapy, while powerful, is not yet mature, so it will take time for these approaches to be proven effective and integrated into a clinical setting. In the meantime, other methods of upregulating protective Bcl-2 members should be explored.

BDNF is capable of regulating cell-death pathways. BDNF is capable of counter-regulating Bax and Bcl-2 when administered intravenously after ischemia (Schabitz et al., 2000). Neuroprotection is achieved by conjugating the product of the bcl-x gene with the HIV-Tat PTD as a method of delivery (Asoh et al., 2002). The upregulation of Bcl-2 and downregulation of Bax is implicated as part of hypothermia's protective mechanism against ischemic damage. These and other methods for regulating the Bcl-2 family may prove clinically relevant and could be examined for extra neuroprotection when used in combination or with therapies targeting different cell death mechanisms.

4.8 Excitotoxicity and calcium-mediated damage prevention

Excitotoxic damage due to massive Ca^{2+} influx should be reduced to some extent by either preventing ion disturbance or targeting the resulting structural damage by calpains, free radical production, and caspase activation. Free radical production and caspase activation may demonstrate protective action for mild excitotoxic stress causing delayed neuronal death.

Neuroprotection by blocking glutamate release and reception has been attempted with some success. In experimental stroke models, glutamate blockade provides protection against cell death, but the results do not necessarily translate into human therapy. Blocking the release of glutamate and other excitatory amino acids through the use of various drugs has been unsuccessful in human trials. Too little is known about neuroprotection to rule out glutamate blockers entirely. It is possible that treatment in these trials occurred too late and was unable to block the excitotoxic chain reaction. If the drugs were administered within a couple hours of stroke, then the time conditions would be similar to those found in models used in studies successfully demonstrating neuroprotection (Babu & Ramanathan, 2011; Prass & Dirnagl, 1998).

Some potential therapeutic targets may alleviate calcium-induced neuronal damage. Calcium/calmodulin-dependent protein kinase kinase (CaM-KK) protects against delayed apoptosis following glutamate by activating Atk and CaM kinase IV (Yano et al., 2005), which both are anti-apoptotic players. Nimodipine (Mossakowski & Gadamski, 1990; Nuglisch et al., 1990), dantrolene (Wei & Perry, 1996), and the tetrapeptide Tyr-Val-Ala-Asp-chloromethyl ketone (Ac-YVAD-cmk) (Gray et al., 2001) are all able to block damage due to high cytosolic Ca^{2+} levels in a variety of stroke models and may be useful in preventing excitotoxic damage.

Energy depletion plays a large role in excitotoxicity. Methods that selectively inhibit poly (ADP-ribose) polymerase-1 (PARP-1) and PARP-2 offer neuroprotection (Chiarugi, 2005) by counteracting energy-consuming activities following ischemia and reducing the drop in high-energy molecules. Additional evidence implicates PARP in a pathway capable of inducing AIF release and activation (Niimura et al., 2006), which indicates that therapies targeting PARP may have a protective effect against AIF-mediated delayed neuronal death. Drugs that inhibit PHRP activation, such as PJ34 (Xu et al., 2010) or hepatocyte growth factor (Niimura et al., 2006), may be useful as part of multimodal early interventions.

5. Conclusions

Neuronal cell death following stroke occurs in necrosis, apoptosis and other alternative modes and is mediated through diverse molecular pathways. These pathways provide therapeutic targets for stroke management.

6. Acknowledgment

The authors would like to thank Ms. Jacqueline Hogue for her assistance in preparing the manuscript. This work was supported by grants from the Canadian Institutes of Health Research, Canadian Stroke Network and Manitoba Health Research Council (to J. Kong) and Shanghai Health Bureau Foundation (2008-2010,2008087 to X. Bi).

7. References

Adhami, F., Liao, G., Morozov, Y. M., Schloemer, A., Schmithorst, V. J., Lorenz, J. N., Dunn, R. S., Vorhees, C. V., Wills-Karp, M., Degen, J. L., Davis, R. J., Mizushima, N., Rakic, P., Dardzinski, B. J., Holland, S. K., Sharp, F. R. & Kuan, C. Y. (2006). Cerebral ischemia-hypoxia induces intravascular coagulation and autophagy. *Am J Pathol* 169, 566-83.

Ahn, J., Piri, N., Caprioli, J., Munemasa, Y., Kim, S. H. & Kwong, J. M. (2008). Expression of heat shock transcription factors and heat shock protein 72 in rat retina after intravitreal injection of low dose N-methyl-D-aspartate. *Neurosci Lett* 433, 11-6.

Aita, V. M., Liang, X. H., Murty, V. V., Pincus, D. L., Yu, W., Cayanis, E., Kalachikov, S., Gilliam, T. C. & Levine, B. (1999). Cloning and genomic organization of beclin 1, a candidate tumor suppressor gene on chromosome 17q21. *Genomics* 59, 59-65.

Ashkenazi, A. & Dixit, V. M. (1998). Death receptors: signaling and modulation. *Science* 281, 1305-8.

Asoh, S., Ohsawa, I., Mori, T., Katsura, K., Hiraide, T., Katayama, Y., Kimura, M., Ozaki, D., Yamagata, K. & Ohta, S. (2002). Protection against ischemic brain injury by protein therapeutics. *Proc Natl Acad Sci U S A* 99, 17107-12.

Azad, M. B., Chen, Y., Henson, E. S., Cizeau, J., McMillan-Ward, E., Israels, S. J. & Gibson, S. B. (2008). Hypoxia induces autophagic cell death in apoptosis-competent cells through a mechanism involving BNIP3. *Autophagy* 4, 195-204.

Babu, C. S. & Ramanathan, M. (2011). Post-ischemic administration of nimodipine following focal cerebral ischemic-reperfusion injury in rats alleviated excitotoxicity, neurobehavioural alterations and partially the bioenergetics. *Int J Dev Neurosci* 29, 93-105.

Balestrino M. (1995). Pathophysiology of anoxic depolarization: new findings and a working hypothesis. *J Neurosci Methods* 59, 99-103.

Baumgartner, H. K., Gerasimenko, J. V., Thorne, C., Ferdek, P., Pozzan, T., Tepikin, A. V., Petersen, O. H., Sutton, R., Watson, A. J. & Gerasimenko, O. V. (2009). Calcium elevation in mitochondria is the main Ca2+ requirement for mitochondrial permeability transition pore (mPTP) opening. *J Biol Chem* 284, 20796-803.

Beck, T., Lindholm, D., Castren, E. & Wree, A. (1994). Brain-derived neurotrophic factor protects against ischemic cell damage in rat hippocampus. *J Cereb Blood Flow Metab* 14, 689-92.

Beckman, J. S., Beckman, T. W., Chen, J., Marshall, P. A. & Freeman, B. A. (1990). Apparent hydroxyl radical production by peroxynitrite: implications for endothelial injury from nitric oxide and superoxide. *Proc Natl Acad Sci U S A* 87, 1620-4.

Bellot, G., Garcia-Medina, R., Gounon, P., Chiche, J., Roux, D., Pouyssegur, J. & Mazure, N. M. (2009). Hypoxia-induced autophagy is mediated through hypoxia-inducible factor induction of BNIP3 and BNIP3L via their BH3 domains. *Mol Cell Biol* 29, 2570-81.

Bicknell, G. R. & Cohen, G. M. (1995). Cleavage of DNA to large kilobase pair fragments occurs in some forms of necrosis as well as apoptosis. *Biochem Biophys Res Commun* 207, 40-7.

Bruick, R. K. (2000). Expression of the gene encoding the proapoptotic Nip3 protein is induced by hypoxia. *Proc Natl Acad Sci U S A* 97, 9082-7.

Buisson, A., Lesne, S., Docagne, F., Ali, C., Nicole, O., MacKenzie, E. T. & Vivien, D. (2003). Transforming growth factor-beta and ischemic brain injury. *Cell Mol Neurobiol* 23, 539-50.

Bursch, W., Ellinger, A., Gerner, C., Frohwein, U. & Schulte-Hermann, R. (2000a). Programmed cell death (PCD). Apoptosis, autophagic PCD, or others? *Ann N Y Acad Sci* 926, 1-12.

Bursch, W., Hochegger, K., Torok, L., Marian, B., Ellinger, A. & Hermann, R. S. (2000b). Autophagic and apoptotic types of programmed cell death exhibit different fates of cytoskeletal filaments. *J Cell Sci* 113 (Pt 7), 1189-98.

Cande, C., Cecconi, F., Dessen, P. & Kroemer, G. (2002). Apoptosis-inducing factor (AIF): key to the conserved caspase-independent pathways of cell death? *J Cell Sci* 115, 4727-34.

Cao, G., Clark, R. S., Pei, W., Yin, W., Zhang, F., Sun, F. Y., Graham, S. H. & Chen, J. (2003). Translocation of apoptosis-inducing factor in vulnerable neurons after transient cerebral ischemia and in neuronal cultures after oxygen-glucose deprivation. *J Cereb Blood Flow Metab* 23, 1137-50.

Chambers, D. E., Parks, D. A., Patterson, G., Roy, R., McCord, J. M., Yoshida, S., Parmley, L. F. & Downey, J. M. (1985). Xanthine oxidase as a source of free radical damage in myocardial ischemia. *J Mol Cell Cardiol* 17, 145-52.

Chen, G., Cizeau, J., Vande Velde, C., Park, J. H., Bozek, G., Bolton, J., Shi, L., Dubik, D. & Greenberg, A. (1999). Nix and Nip3 form a subfamily of pro-apoptotic mitochondrial proteins. *J Biol Chem* 274, 7-10.

Chen, G., Ray, R., Dubik, D., Shi, L., Cizeau, J., Bleackley, R. C., Saxena, S., Gietz, R. D. & Greenberg, A. H. (1997). The E1B 19K/Bcl-2-binding protein Nip3 is a dimeric mitochondrial protein that activates apoptosis. *J Exp Med* 186, 1975-83.

Chen, J., Nagayama, T., Jin, K., Stetler, R. A., Zhu, R. L., Graham, S. H. & Simon, R. P. (1998). Induction of caspase-3-like protease may mediate delayed neuronal death in the hippocampus after transient cerebral ischemia. *J Neurosci* 18, 4914-28.

Chiarugi, A. (2005). Poly(ADP-ribosyl)ation and stroke. *Pharmacol Res* 52, 15-24.

Chinnadurai, G., Vijayalingam, S. & Gibson, S. B. (2008). BNIP3 subfamily BH3-only proteins: mitochondrial stress sensors in normal and pathological functions. *Oncogene* 27 Suppl 1, S114-27.

Cho, B. B. & Toledo-Pereyra, L. H. (2008). Caspase-independent programmed cell death following ischemic stroke. *J Invest Surg* 21, 141-7.

Choi, D. W. (1996). Ischemia-induced neuronal apoptosis. *Curr Opin Neurobiol* 6, 667-72.

Cizeau, J., Ray, R., Chen, G., Gietz, R. D. & Greenberg, A. H. (2000). The C. elegans orthologue ceBNIP3 interacts with CED-9 and CED-3 but kills through a BH3- and caspase-independent mechanism. *Oncogene* 19, 5453-63.

Clemens, J. A., Stephenson, D. T., Dixon, E. P., Smalstig, E. B., Mincy, R. E., Rash, K. S. & Little, S. P. (1997). Global cerebral ischemia activates nuclear factor-kappa B prior to evidence of DNA fragmentation. *Brain Res Mol Brain Res* 48, 187-96.

Cregan, S. P., Fortin, A., MacLaurin, J. G., Callaghan, S. M., Cecconi, F., Yu, S. W., Dawson, T. M., Dawson, V. L., Park, D. S., Kroemer, G. & Slack, R. S. (2002). Apoptosis-inducing factor is involved in the regulation of caspase-independent neuronal cell death. *J Cell Biol* 158, 507-17.

Culmsee, C. & Plesnila, N. (2006). Targeting Bid to prevent programmed cell death in neurons. *Biochem Soc Trans* 34, 1334-40.

Culmsee, C., Zhu, C., Landshamer, S., Becattini, B., Wagner, E., Pellecchia, M., Blomgren, K. & Plesnila, N. (2005). Apoptosis-inducing factor triggered by poly(ADP-ribose) polymerase and Bid mediates neuronal cell death after oxygen-glucose deprivation and focal cerebral ischemia. *J Neurosci* 25, 10262-72.

Culmsee, C., Zhu, X., Yu, Q. S., Chan, S. L., Camandola, S., Guo, Z., Greig, N. H. & Mattson, M. P. (2001). A synthetic inhibitor of p53 protects neurons against death induced by ischemic and excitotoxic insults, and amyloid beta-peptide. *J Neurochem* 77, 220-8.

Dejean, L. M., Ryu, S. Y., Martinez-Caballero, S., Teijido, O., Peixoto, P. M. & Kinnally, K. W. (2010). MAC and Bcl-2 family proteins conspire in a deadly plot. *Biochim Biophys Acta* 1797, 1231-8.

Deshpande, J., Bergstedt, K., Linden, T., Kalimo, H. & Wieloch, T. (1992). Ultrastructural changes in the hippocampal CA1 region following transient cerebral ischemia: evidence against programmed cell death. *Exp Brain Res* 88, 91-105.

Dong, Z., Saikumar, P., Weinberg, J. M. & Venkatachalam, M. A. (1997). Internucleosomal DNA cleavage triggered by plasma membrane damage during necrotic cell death. Involvement of serine but not cysteine proteases. *Am J Pathol* 151, 1205-13.

Donovan, M. & Cotter, T. G. (2004). Control of mitochondrial integrity by Bcl-2 family members and caspase-independent cell death. *Biochim Biophys Acta* 1644, 133-47.

Du, C., Fang, M., Li, Y., Li, L. & Wang, X. (2000). Smac, a mitochondrial protein that promotes cytochrome c-dependent caspase activation by eliminating IAP inhibition. *Cell* 102, 33-42.

Dugan, L. L., Creedon, D. J., Johnson, E. M., Jr. & Holtzman, D. M. (1997). Rapid suppression of free radical formation by nerve growth factor involves the mitogen-activated protein kinase pathway. *Proc Natl Acad Sci U S A* 94, 4086-91.

Elmore, S. P., Qian, T., Grissom, S. F. & Lemasters, J. J. (2001). The mitochondrial permeability transition initiates autophagy in rat hepatocytes. *FASEB J* 15, 2286-7.

Endres, M., Namura, S., Shimizu-Sasamata, M., Waeber, C., Zhang, L., Gomez-Isla, T., Hyman, B. T. & Moskowitz, M. A. (1998). Attenuation of delayed neuronal death after mild focal ischemia in mice by inhibition of the caspase family. *J Cereb Blood Flow Metab* 18, 238-47.

Farooq, M., Kim, Y., Im, S., Chung, E., Hwang, S., Sohn, M., Kim, M. & Kim, J. (2001). Cloning of BNIP3h, a member of proapoptotic BNIP3 family genes. *Exp Mol Med* 33, 169-73.

Ferrer, I. (2006). Apoptosis: future targets for neuroprotective strategies. *Cerebrovascular diseases* 21 Suppl 2, 9-20.

Ferrer, I., Lopez, E., Pozas, E., Ballabriga, J. & Marti, E. (1998). Multiple neurotrophic signals converge in surviving CA1 neurons of the gerbil hippocampus following transient forebrain ischemia. *J Comp Neurol* 394, 416-30.

Ferrer, I. & Planas, A. M. (2003). Signaling of cell death and cell survival following focal cerebral ischemia: life and death struggle in the penumbra. *J Neuropathol Exp Neurol* 62, 329-39.

Friberg, H. & Wieloch, T. (2002). Mitochondrial permeability transition in acute neurodegeneration. *Biochimie* 84, 241-50.

Friguls, B., Petegnief, V., Justicia, C., Pallas, M. & Planas, A. M. (2002). Activation of ERK and Akt signaling in focal cerebral ischemia: modulation by TGF-alpha and involvement of NMDA receptor. *Neurobiol Dis* 11, 443-56.

Galluzzi, L., Morselli, E., Kepp, O. & Kroemer, G. (2009). Targeting post-mitochondrial effectors of apoptosis for neuroprotection. *Biochimica et biophysica acta* 1787, 402-13.

Gao, Y., Signore, A. P., Yin, W., Cao, G., Yin, X. M., Sun, F., Luo, Y., Graham, S. H. & Chen, J. (2005). Neuroprotection against focal ischemic brain injury by inhibition of c-Jun N-terminal kinase and attenuation of the mitochondrial apoptosis-signaling pathway. *J Cereb Blood Flow Metab* 25, 694-712.

Gibson, M. E., Han, B. H., Choi, J., Knudson, C. M., Korsmeyer, S. J., Parsadanian, M. & Holtzman, D. M. (2001). BAX contributes to apoptotic-like death following neonatal hypoxia-ischemia: evidence for distinct apoptosis pathways. *Mol Med* 7, 644-55.

Gido, G., Kristian, T. & Siesjo, B. K. (1997). Extracellular potassium in a neocortical core area after transient focal ischemia. *Stroke* 28, 206-10.

Gilgun-Sherki, Y., Rosenbaum, Z., Melamed, E. & Offen, D. (2002). Antioxidant therapy in acute central nervous system injury: current state. *Pharmacol Rev* 54, 271-84.

Gillardon, F., Kiprianova, I., Sandkuhler, J., Hossmann, K. A. & Spranger, M. (1999). Inhibition of caspases prevents cell death of hippocampal CA1 neurons, but not impairment of hippocampal long-term potentiation following global ischemia. *Neuroscience* 93, 1219-22.

Gray, J., Haran, M. M., Schneider, K., Vesce, S., Ray, A. M., Owen, D., White, I. R., Cutler, P. & Davis, J. B. (2001). Evidence that inhibition of cathepsin-B contributes to the neuroprotective properties of caspase inhibitor Tyr-Val-Ala-Asp-chloromethyl ketone. *J Biol Chem* 276, 32750-5.

Greijer, A. E. & van der Wall, E. (2004). The role of hypoxia inducible factor 1 (HIF-1) in hypoxia induced apoptosis. *J Clin Pathol* 57, 1009-14.

Gross, A., McDonnell, J. M. & Korsmeyer, S. J. (1999). BCL-2 family members and the mitochondria in apoptosis. *Genes Dev* 13, 1899-911.

Guan, Q. H., Pei, D. S., Zong, Y. Y., Xu, T. L. & Zhang, G. Y. (2006). Neuroprotection against ischemic brain injury by a small peptide inhibitor of c-Jun N-terminal kinase (JNK) via nuclear and non-nuclear pathways. *Neuroscience* 139, 609-27.

Guo, K., Searfoss, G., Krolikowski, D., Pagnoni, M., Franks, C., Clark, K., Yu, K. T., Jaye, M. & Ivashchenko, Y. (2001). Hypoxia induces the expression of the pro-apoptotic gene BNIP3. *Cell Death Differ* 8, 367-76.

Gwag, B. J., Koh, J. Y., Chen, M. M., Dugan, L. L., Behrens, M. M., Lobner, D. & Choi, D. W. (1995). BDNF or IGF-I potentiates free radical-mediated injury in cortical cell cultures. *Neuroreport* 7, 93-6.

Halterman, M. W., Miller, C. C. & Federoff, H. J. (1999). Hypoxia-inducible factor-1alpha mediates hypoxia-induced delayed neuronal death that involves p53. *J Neurosci* 19, 6818-24.

Harris, R. J. & Symon, L. (1984). Extracellular pH, potassium, and calcium activities in progressive ischaemia of rat cortex. *J Cereb Blood Flow Metab* 4, 178-86.

Harvey, B. K., Hoffer, B. J. & Wang, Y. (2005). Stroke and TGF-beta proteins: glial cell line-derived neurotrophic factor and bone morphogenetic protein. *Pharmacol Ther* 105, 113-25.

Hayashi, T., Abe, K. & Itoyama, Y. (1998). Reduction of ischemic damage by application of vascular endothelial growth factor in rat brain after transient ischemia. *J Cereb Blood Flow Metab* 18, 887-95.

Hayashi, Y., Jikihara, I., Yagi, T., Fukumura, M., Ohashi, Y., Ohta, Y., Takagi, H. & Maeda, M. (2001). Immunohistochemical investigation of caspase-1 and effect of caspase-1 inhibitor in delayed neuronal death after transient cerebral ischemia. *Brain Res* 893, 113-20.

Himi, T., Ishizaki, Y. & Murota, S. (1998). A caspase inhibitor blocks ischaemia-induced delayed neuronal death in the gerbil. *Eur J Neurosci* 10, 777-81.

Hoyer-Hansen, M., Bastholm, L., Szyniarowski, P., Campanella, M., Szabadkai, G., Farkas, T., Bianchi, K., Fehrenbacher, N., Elling, F., Rizzuto, R., Mathiasen, I. S. & Jaattela, M. (2007). Control of macroautophagy by calcium, calmodulin-dependent kinase kinase-beta, and Bcl-2. *Mol Cell* 25, 193-205.

Hu, B. R. & Wieloch, T. (1994). Tyrosine phosphorylation and activation of mitogen-activated protein kinase in the rat brain following transient cerebral ischemia. *J Neurochem* 62, 1357-67.

Huang, J., Agus, D. B., Winfree, C. J., Kiss, S., Mack, W. J., McTaggart, R. A., Choudhri, T. F., Kim, L. J., Mocco, J., Pinsky, D. J., Fox, W. D., Israel, R. J., Boyd, T. A., Golde, D. W. & Connolly, E. S., Jr. (2001). Dehydroascorbic acid, a blood-brain barrier transportable form of vitamin C, mediates potent cerebroprotection in experimental stroke. *Proc Natl Acad Sci U S A* 98, 11720-4.

Ichas, F. & Mazat, J. P. (1998). From calcium signaling to cell death: two conformations for the mitochondrial permeability transition pore. Switching from low- to high-conductance state. *Biochim Biophys Acta* 1366, 33-50.

Ikeda, J., Nakajima, T., Osborne, O. C., Mies, G. & Nowak, T. S., Jr. (1994). Coexpression of c-fos and hsp70 mRNAs in gerbil brain after ischemia: induction threshold, distribution and time course evaluated by in situ hybridization. *Brain Res Mol Brain Res* 26, 249-58.

Imazu, T., Shimizu, S., Tagami, S., Matsushima, M., Nakamura, Y., Miki, T., Okuyama, A. & Tsujimoto, Y. (1999). Bcl-2/E1B 19 kDa-interacting protein 3-like protein (Bnip3L) interacts with bcl-2/Bcl-xL and induces apoptosis by altering mitochondrial membrane permeability. *Oncogene* 18, 4523-9.

Jaattela, M., Wissing, D., Kokholm, K., Kallunki, T. & Egeblad, M. (1998). Hsp70 exerts its anti-apoptotic function downstream of caspase-3-like proteases. *EMBO J* 17, 6124-34.

Jin, K., Mao, X. O., Batteur, S. P., McEachron, E., Leahy, A. & Greenberg, D. A. (2001). Caspase-3 and the regulation of hypoxic neuronal death by vascular endothelial growth factor. *Neuroscience* 108, 351-8.

Kalinowska, M., Garncarz, W., Pietrowska, M., Garrard, W. T. & Widlak, P. (2005). Regulation of the human apoptotic DNase/RNase endonuclease G: involvement of Hsp70 and ATP. *Apoptosis* 10, 821-30.

Katsura, K., Rodriguez de Turco, E. B., Folbergrova, J., Bazan, N. G. & Siesjo, B. K. (1993). Coupling among energy failure, loss of ion homeostasis, and phospholipase A2 and C activation during ischemia. *J Neurochem* 61, 1677-84.

Kawagoe, J., Abe, K., Sato, S., Nagano, I., Nakamura, S. & Kogure, K. (1992). Distributions of heat shock protein-70 mRNAs and heat shock cognate protein-70 mRNAs after transient global ischemia in gerbil brain. *J Cereb Blood Flow Metab* 12, 794-801.

Kim, D. W., Eum, W. S., Jang, S. H., Kim, S. Y., Choi, H. S., Choi, S. H., An, J. J., Lee, S. H., Lee, K. S., Han, K., Kang, T. C., Won, M. H., Kang, J. H., Kwon, O. S., Cho, S. W., Kim, T. Y., Park, J. & Choi, S. Y. (2005a). Transduced Tat-SOD fusion protein protects against ischemic brain injury. *Mol Cells* 19, 88-96.

Kim, R., Emi, M. & Tanabe, K. (2005b). Caspase-dependent and -independent cell death pathways after DNA damage (Review). *Oncol Rep* 14, 595-9.

Kinouchi, H., Sharp, F. R., Koistinaho, J., Hicks, K., Kamii, H. & Chan, P. H. (1993). Induction of heat shock hsp70 mRNA and HSP70 kDa protein in neurons in the 'penumbra' following focal cerebral ischemia in the rat. *Brain Res* 619, 334-8.

Klein, J. A., Longo-Guess, C. M., Rossmann, M. P., Seburn, K. L., Hurd, R. E., Frankel, W. N., Bronson, R. T. & Ackerman, S. L. (2002). The harlequin mouse mutation downregulates apoptosis-inducing factor. *Nature* 419, 367-74.

Koh, J. Y., Gwag, B. J., Lobner, D. & Choi, D. W. (1995). Potentiated necrosis of cultured cortical neurons by neurotrophins. *Science* 268, 573-5.

Koike, M., Shibata, M., Tadakoshi, M., Gotoh, K., Komatsu, M., Waguri, S., Kawahara, N., Kuida, K., Nagata, S., Kominami, E., Tanaka, K. & Uchiyama, Y. (2008). Inhibition of autophagy prevents hippocampal pyramidal neuron death after hypoxic-ischemic injury. *Am J Pathol* 172, 454-69.

Kokaia, Z., Nawa, H., Uchino, H., Elmer, E., Kokaia, M., Carnahan, J., Smith, M. L., Siesjo, B. K. & Lindvall, O. (1996). Regional brain-derived neurotrophic factor mRNA and protein levels following transient forebrain ischemia in the rat. *Brain Res Mol Brain Res* 38, 139-44.

Kouroku, Y., Fujita, E., Tanida, I., Ueno, T., Isoai, A., Kumagai, H., Ogawa, S., Kaufman, R. J., Kominami, E. & Momoi, T. (2007). ER stress (PERK/eIF2alpha phosphorylation) mediates the polyglutamine-induced LC3 conversion, an essential step for autophagy formation. *Cell Death Differ* 14, 230-9.

Krantic, S., Mechawar, N., Reix, S. & Quirion, R. (2007). Apoptosis-inducing factor: a matter of neuron life and death. *Prog Neurobiol* 81, 179-96.

Kroemer, G. & Martin, S. J. (2005). Caspase-independent cell death. *Nat Med* 11, 725-30.

Kuehl, F. A., Jr., Humes, J. L., Ham, E. A., Egan, R. W. & Dougherty, H. W. (1980). Inflammation: the role of peroxidase-derived products. *Adv Prostaglandin Thromboxane Res* 6, 77-86.

Kumar, R., Azam, S., Sullivan, J. M., Owen, C., Cavener, D. R., Zhang, P., Ron, D., Harding, H. P., Chen, J. J., Han, A., White, B. C., Krause, G. S. & DeGracia, D. J. (2001). Brain ischemia and reperfusion activates the eukaryotic initiation factor 2alpha kinase, PERK. *J Neurochem* 77, 1418-21.

Lang-Rollin, I. C., Rideout, H. J., Noticewala, M. & Stefanis, L. (2003). Mechanisms of caspase-independent neuronal death: energy depletion and free radical generation. *J Neurosci* 23, 11015-25.

Le, D. A., Wu, Y., Huang, Z., Matsushita, K., Plesnila, N., Augustinack, J. C., Hyman, B. T., Yuan, J., Kuida, K., Flavell, R. A. & Moskowitz, M. A. (2002). Caspase activation and neuroprotection in caspase-3- deficient mice after in vivo cerebral ischemia and in vitro oxygen glucose deprivation. *Proc Natl Acad Sci U S A* 99, 15188-93.

Lee, B. I., Lee, D. J., Cho, K. J. & Kim, G. W. (2005). Early nuclear translocation of endonuclease G and subsequent DNA fragmentation after transient focal cerebral ischemia in mice. *Neurosci Lett* 386, 23-7.

Letechipia-Vallejo, G., Gonzalez-Burgos, I. & Cervantes, M. (2001). Neuroprotective effect of melatonin on brain damage induced by acute global cerebral ischemia in cats. *Arch Med Res* 32, 186-92.

Li, L. Y., Luo, X. & Wang, X. (2001). Endonuclease G is an apoptotic DNase when released from mitochondria. *Nature* 412, 95-9.

Li, P., Nijhawan, D., Budihardjo, I., Srinivasula, S. M., Ahmad, M., Alnemri, E. S. & Wang, X. (1997). Cytochrome c and dATP-dependent formation of Apaf-1/caspase-9 complex initiates an apoptotic protease cascade. *Cell* 91, 479-89.

Li, Y., Yang, X., Ma, C., Qiao, J. & Zhang, C. (2008). Necroptosis contributes to the NMDA-induced excitotoxicity in rat's cultured cortical neurons. *Neurosci Lett* 447, 120-3.

Liang, X. H., Jackson, S., Seaman, M., Brown, K., Kempkes, B., Hibshoosh, H. & Levine, B. (1999). Induction of autophagy and inhibition of tumorigenesis by beclin 1. *Nature* 402, 672-6.

Linnik, M. D., Zahos, P., Geschwind, M. D. & Federoff, H. J. (1995). Expression of bcl-2 from a defective herpes simplex virus-1 vector limits neuronal death in focal cerebral ischemia. *Stroke* 26, 1670-4; discussion 1675.

Lipton, P. (1999). Ischemic cell death in brain neurons. *Physiol Rev* 79, 1431-568.

Lipton, P. & Whittingham, T. S. (1982). Reduced ATP concentration as a basis for synaptic transmission failure during hypoxia in the in vitro guinea-pig hippocampus. *J Physiol* 325, 51-65.

Liu, X., Zou, H., Slaughter, C. & Wang, X. (1997). DFF, a heterodimeric protein that functions downstream of caspase-3 to trigger DNA fragmentation during apoptosis. *Cell* 89, 175-84.

Liu, X., Zou, H., Widlak, P., Garrard, W. & Wang, X. (1999). Activation of the apoptotic endonuclease DFF40 (caspase-activated DNase or nuclease). Oligomerization and direct interaction with histone H1. *J Biol Chem* 274, 13836-40.

Lockshin, R. A. & Zakeri, Z. (2002). Caspase-independent cell deaths. *Curr Opin Cell Biol* 14, 727-33.

Love, S. (2003). Apoptosis and brain ischaemia. *Prog Neuropsychopharmacol Biol Psychiatry* 27, 267-82.

MacManus, J. P., Rasquinha, I., Tuor, U. & Preston, E. (1997). Detection of higher-order 50- and 10-kbp DNA fragments before apoptotic internucleosomal cleavage after transient cerebral ischemia. *J Cereb Blood Flow Metab* 17, 376-87.

Magnusson, K. & Wieloch, T. (1989). Impairment of protein ubiquitination may cause delayed neuronal death. *Neurosci Lett* 96, 264-70.

Maiuri, M. C., Criollo, A., Tasdemir, E., Vicencio, J. M., Tajeddine, N., Hickman, J. A., Geneste, O. & Kroemer, G. (2007a). BH3-only proteins and BH3 mimetics induce autophagy by competitively disrupting the interaction between Beclin 1 and Bcl-2/Bcl-X(L). *Autophagy* 3, 374-6.

Maiuri, M. C., Le Toumelin, G., Criollo, A., Rain, J. C., Gautier, F., Juin, P., Tasdemir, E., Pierron, G., Troulinaki, K., Tavernarakis, N., Hickman, J. A., Geneste, O. & Kroemer, G. (2007b). Functional and physical interaction between Bcl-X(L) and a BH3-like domain in Beclin-1. *EMBO J* 26, 2527-39.

Maiuri, M. C., Zalckvar, E., Kimchi, A. & Kroemer, G. (2007c). Self-eating and self-killing: crosstalk between autophagy and apoptosis. *Nature reviews. Molecular cell biology* 8, 741-52.

Manfredi, G. & Beal, M. F. (2000). The role of mitochondria in the pathogenesis of neurodegenerative diseases. *Brain Pathol* 10, 462-72.

Manoonkitiwongsa, P. S., Schultz, R. L., McCreery, D. B., Whitter, E. F. & Lyden, P. D. (2004). Neuroprotection of ischemic brain by vascular endothelial growth factor is critically dependent on proper dosage and may be compromised by angiogenesis. *J Cereb Blood Flow Metab* 24, 693-702.

Marti, H. J., Bernaudin, M., Bellail, A., Schoch, H., Euler, M., Petit, E. & Risau, W. (2000). Hypoxia-induced vascular endothelial growth factor expression precedes neovascularization after cerebral ischemia. *Am J Pathol* 156, 965-76.

Martin, L. J. (2011). An approach to experimental synaptic pathology using green fluorescent protein-transgenic mice and gene knockout mice to show mitochondrial permeability transition pore-driven excitotoxicity in interneurons and motoneurons. *Toxicologic pathology* 39, 220-33.

Martin, R. L., Lloyd, H. G. & Cowan, A. I. (1994). The early events of oxygen and glucose deprivation: setting the scene for neuronal death? *Trends Neurosci* 17, 251-7.

Martinez-Caballero, S., Dejean, L. M., Kinnally, M. S., Oh, K. J., Mannella, C. A. & Kinnally, K. W. (2009). Assembly of the mitochondrial apoptosis-induced channel, MAC. *J Biol Chem* 284, 12235-45.

Martinou, J. C., Dubois-Dauphin, M., Staple, J. K., Rodriguez, I., Frankowski, H., Missotten, M., Albertini, P., Talabot, D., Catsicas, S., Pietra, C. & et al. (1994). Overexpression of BCL-2 in transgenic mice protects neurons from naturally occurring cell death and experimental ischemia. *Neuron* 13, 1017-30.

Matsumori, Y., Northington, F. J., Hong, S. M., Kayama, T., Sheldon, R. A., Vexler, Z. S., Ferriero, D. M., Weinstein, P. R. & Liu, J. (2006). Reduction of caspase-8 and -9 cleavage is associated with increased c-FLIP and increased binding of Apaf-1 and Hsp70 after neonatal hypoxic/ischemic injury in mice overexpressing Hsp70. *Stroke* 37, 507-12.

Mattson, M. P., Lovell, M. A., Furukawa, K. & Markesbery, W. R. (1995). Neurotrophic factors attenuate glutamate-induced accumulation of peroxides, elevation of intracellular Ca2+ concentration, and neurotoxicity and increase antioxidant enzyme activities in hippocampal neurons. *J Neurochem* 65, 1740-51.

Mestril, R., Giordano, F. J., Conde, A. G. & Dillmann, W. H. (1996). Adenovirus-mediated gene transfer of a heat shock protein 70 (hsp 70i) protects against simulated ischemia. *J Mol Cell Cardiol* 28, 2351-8.

Mitani, A., Oomura, Y., Yanase, H. & Kataoka, K. (1992). Acidic fibroblast growth factor delays in vitro ischemia-induced intracellular calcium elevation in gerbil hippocampal slices: a sign of neuroprotection. *Neurochem Int* 21, 337-41.

Morrison, R. S., Wenzel, H. J., Kinoshita, Y., Robbins, C. A., Donehower, L. A. & Schwartzkroin, P. A. (1996). Loss of the p53 tumor suppressor gene protects neurons from kainate-induced cell death. *J Neurosci* 16, 1337-45.

Mossakowski, M. J. & Gadamski, R. (1990). Nimodipine prevents delayed neuronal death of sector CA1 pyramidal cells in short-term forebrain ischemia in Mongolian gerbils. *Stroke* 21, IV120-2.

Niimura, M., Takagi, N., Takagi, K., Mizutani, R., Ishihara, N., Matsumoto, K., Funakoshi, H., Nakamura, T. & Takeo, S. (2006). Prevention of apoptosis-inducing factor translocation is a possible mechanism for protective effects of hepatocyte growth factor against neuronal cell death in the hippocampus after transient forebrain ischemia. *J Cereb Blood Flow Metab* 26, 1354-65.

Nitatori, T., Sato, N., Waguri, S., Karasawa, Y., Araki, H., Shibanai, K., Kominami, E. & Uchiyama, Y. (1995). Delayed neuronal death in the CA1 pyramidal cell layer of the gerbil hippocampus following transient ischemia is apoptosis. *J Neurosci* 15, 1001-11.

Nuglisch, J., Karkoutly, C., Mennel, H. D., Rossberg, C. & Krieglstein, J. (1990). Protective effect of nimodipine against ischemic neuronal damage in rat hippocampus without changing postischemic cerebral blood flow. *J Cereb Blood Flow Metab* 10, 654-9.

Ogata, M., Hino, S., Saito, A., Morikawa, K., Kondo, S., Kanemoto, S., Murakami, T., Taniguchi, M., Tanii, I., Yoshinaga, K., Shiosaka, S., Hammarback, J. A., Urano, F. &

Imaizumi, K. (2006). Autophagy is activated for cell survival after endoplasmic reticulum stress. *Mol Cell Biol* 26, 9220-31.

Otera, H., Ohsakaya, S., Nagaura, Z., Ishihara, N. & Mihara, K. (2005). Export of mitochondrial AIF in response to proapoptotic stimuli depends on processing at the intermembrane space. *EMBO J* 24, 1375-86.

Paschen, W. (1996). Glutamate excitotoxicity in transient global cerebral ischemia. *Acta Neurobiol Exp (Wars)* 56, 313-22.

Pattingre, S., Tassa, A., Qu, X., Garuti, R., Liang, X. H., Mizushima, N., Packer, M., Schneider, M. D. & Levine, B. (2005). Bcl-2 antiapoptotic proteins inhibit Beclin 1-dependent autophagy. *Cell* 122, 927-39.

Pivtoraiko, V. N., Stone, S. L., Roth, K. A. & Shacka, J. J. (2009). Oxidative stress and autophagy in the regulation of lysosome-dependent neuron death. *Antioxid Redox Signal* 11, 481-96.

Planas, A. M., Soriano, M. A., Estrada, A., Sanz, O., Martin, F. & Ferrer, I. (1997). The heat shock stress response after brain lesions: induction of 72 kDa heat shock protein (cell types involved, axonal transport, transcriptional regulation) and protein synthesis inhibition. *Prog Neurobiol* 51, 607-36.

Plate, K. H., Beck, H., Danner, S., Allegrini, P. R. & Wiessner, C. (1999). Cell type specific upregulation of vascular endothelial growth factor in an MCA-occlusion model of cerebral infarct. *J Neuropathol Exp Neurol* 58, 654-66.

Plesnila, N., Zinkel, S., Amin-Hanjani, S., Qiu, J., Korsmeyer, S. J. & Moskowitz, M. A. (2002). Function of BID -- a molecule of the bcl-2 family -- in ischemic cell death in the brain. *Eur Surg Res* 34, 37-41.

Plesnila, N., Zinkel, S., Le, D. A., Amin-Hanjani, S., Wu, Y., Qiu, J., Chiarugi, A., Thomas, S. S., Kohane, D. S., Korsmeyer, S. J. & Moskowitz, M. A. (2001). BID mediates neuronal cell death after oxygen/ glucose deprivation and focal cerebral ischemia. *Proc Natl Acad Sci U S A* 98, 15318-23.

Prass, K. & Dirnagl, U. (1998). Glutamate antagonists in therapy of stroke. *Restor Neurol Neurosci* 13, 3-10.

Puyal, J. & Clarke, P. G. (2009). Targeting autophagy to prevent neonatal stroke damage. *Autophagy* 5, 1060-1.

Ray, R., Chen, G., Vande Velde, C., Cizeau, J., Park, J. H., Reed, J. C., Gietz, R. D. & Greenberg, A. H. (2000). BNIP3 heterodimerizes with Bcl-2/Bcl-X(L) and induces cell death independent of a Bcl-2 homology 3 (BH3) domain at both mitochondrial and nonmitochondrial sites. *J Biol Chem* 275, 1439-48.

Rodriguez, D., Rojas-Rivera, D. & Hetz, C. (2011). Integrating stress signals at the endoplasmic reticulum: The BCL-2 protein family rheostat. *Biochim Biophys Acta* 1813, 564-74.

Rubinsztein, D. C., DiFiglia, M., Heintz, N., Nixon, R. A., Qin, Z. H., Ravikumar, B., Stefanis, L. & Tolkovsky, A. (2005). Autophagy and its possible roles in nervous system diseases, damage and repair. *Autophagy* 1, 11-22.

Ruchalski, K., Mao, H., Li, Z., Wang, Z., Gillers, S., Wang, Y., Mosser, D. D., Gabai, V., Schwartz, J. H. & Borkan, S. C. (2006). Distinct hsp70 domains mediate apoptosis-inducing factor release and nuclear accumulation. *J Biol Chem* 281, 7873-80.

Saito, A., Hayashi, T., Okuno, S., Nishi, T. & Chan, P. H. (2004). Modulation of the Omi/HtrA2 signaling pathway after transient focal cerebral ischemia in mouse brains that overexpress SOD1. *Brain Res Mol Brain Res* 127, 89-95.

Saleh, M. C., Connell, B. J. & Saleh, T. M. (2009). Ischemic tolerance following low dose NMDA involves modulation of cellular stress proteins. *Brain research* 1247, 212-20.

Schabitz, W. R., Sommer, C., Zoder, W., Kiessling, M., Schwaninger, M. & Schwab, S. (2000). Intravenous brain-derived neurotrophic factor reduces infarct size and counterregulates Bax and Bcl-2 expression after temporary focal cerebral ischemia. *Stroke* 31, 2212-7.

Schell, M. T., Spitzer, A. L., Johnson, J. A., Lee, D. & Harris, H. W. (2005). Heat shock inhibits NF-kB activation in a dose- and time-dependent manner. *J Surg Res* 129, 90-3.

Schwartz, L. M., Smith, S. W., Jones, M. E. & Osborne, B. A. (1993). Do all programmed cell deaths occur via apoptosis? *Proc Natl Acad Sci U S A* 90, 980-4.

Shimazaki, K., Urabe, M., Monahan, J., Ozawa, K. & Kawai, N. (2000). Adeno-associated virus vector-mediated bcl-2 gene transfer into post-ischemic gerbil brain in vivo: prospects for gene therapy of ischemia-induced neuronal death. *Gene Ther* 7, 1244-9.

Shirakura, M., Fukumura, M., Inoue, M., Fujikawa, S., Maeda, M., Watabe, K., Kyuwa, S., Yoshikawa, Y. & Hasegawa, M. (2003). Sendai virus vector-mediated gene transfer of glial cell line-derived neurotrophic factor prevents delayed neuronal death after transient global ischemia in gerbils. *Exp Anim* 52, 119-27.

Sinha, K., Degaonkar, M. N., Jagannathan, N. R. & Gupta, Y. K. (2001). Effect of melatonin on ischemia reperfusion injury induced by middle cerebral artery occlusion in rats. *Eur J Pharmacol* 428, 185-92.

Sowter, H. M., Ratcliffe, P. J., Watson, P., Greenberg, A. H. & Harris, A. L. (2001). HIF-1-dependent regulation of hypoxic induction of the cell death factors BNIP3 and NIX in human tumors. *Cancer Res* 61, 6669-73.

Stanger, B. Z., Leder, P., Lee, T. H., Kim, E. & Seed, B. (1995). RIP: a novel protein containing a death domain that interacts with Fas/APO-1 (CD95) in yeast and causes cell death. *Cell* 81, 513-23.

Storkebaum, E., Lambrechts, D. & Carmeliet, P. (2004). VEGF: once regarded as a specific angiogenic factor, now implicated in neuroprotection. *Bioessays* 26, 943-54.

Strosznajder, R. & Gajkowska, B. (2006). Effect of 3-aminobenzamide on Bcl-2, Bax and AIF localization in hippocampal neurons altered by ischemia-reperfusion injury. the immunocytochemical study. *Acta Neurobiol Exp (Wars)* 66, 15-22.

Sun, F. Y. & Guo, X. (2005). Molecular and cellular mechanisms of neuroprotection by vascular endothelial growth factor. *J Neurosci Res* 79, 180-4.

Sun, G. Y., Zhang, J. P., Lin, T. A., Lin, T. N., He, Y. Y. & Hsu, C. Y. (1995). Inositol trisphosphate, polyphosphoinositide turnover, and high-energy metabolites in focal cerebral ischemia and reperfusion. *Stroke* 26, 1893-900.

Sun, Y., Ouyang, Y. B., Xu, L., Chow, A. M., Anderson, R., Hecker, J. G. & Giffard, R. G. (2006). The carboxyl-terminal domain of inducible Hsp70 protects from ischemic injury in vivo and in vitro. *J Cereb Blood Flow Metab* 26, 937-50.

Susin, S. A., Zamzami, N., Castedo, M., Hirsch, T., Marchetti, P., Macho, A., Daugas, E., Geuskens, M. & Kroemer, G. (1996). Bcl-2 inhibits the mitochondrial release of an apoptogenic protease. *J Exp Med* 184, 1331-41.

Suzuki, Y., Imai, Y., Nakayama, H., Takahashi, K., Takio, K. & Takahashi, R. (2001). A serine protease, HtrA2, is released from the mitochondria and interacts with XIAP, inducing cell death. *Mol Cell* 8, 613-21.

Takeda, A., Onodera, H., Sugimoto, A., Kogure, K., Obinata, M. & Shibahara, S. (1993). Coordinated expression of messenger RNAs for nerve growth factor, brain-derived neurotrophic factor and neurotrophin-3 in the rat hippocampus following transient forebrain ischemia. *Neuroscience* 55, 23-31.

Tanaka, S., Takehashi, M., Iida, S., Kitajima, T., Kamanaka, Y., Stedeford, T., Banasik, M. & Ueda, K. (2005). Mitochondrial impairment induced by poly(ADP-ribose) polymerase-1 activation in cortical neurons after oxygen and glucose deprivation. *J Neurochem* 95, 179-90.

Tatton, W. G. & Olanow, C. W. (1999). Apoptosis in neurodegenerative diseases: the role of mitochondria. *Biochim Biophys Acta* 1410, 195-213.

Tehranian, R., Rose, M. E., Vagni, V., Pickrell, A. M., Griffith, R. P., Liu, H., Clark, R. S., Dixon, C. E., Kochanek, P. M. & Graham, S. H. (2008). Disruption of Bax protein prevents neuronal cell death but produces cognitive impairment in mice following traumatic brain injury. *J Neurotrauma* 25, 755-67.

Tremblay, R., Hewitt, K., Lesiuk, H., Mealing, G., Morley, P. & Durkin, J. P. (1999). Evidence that brain-derived neurotrophic factor neuroprotection is linked to its ability to reverse the NMDA-induced inactivation of protein kinase C in cortical neurons. *J Neurochem* 72, 102-11.

Tsai, T. H., Chen, S. L., Chiang, Y. H., Lin, S. Z., Ma, H. I., Kuo, S. W. & Tsao, Y. P. (2000). Recombinant adeno-associated virus vector expressing glial cell line-derived neurotrophic factor reduces ischemia-induced damage. *Exp Neurol* 166, 266-75.

Tsujimoto, Y. (2003). Cell death regulation by the Bcl-2 protein family in the mitochondria. *J Cell Physiol* 195, 158-67.

Tsukahara, T., Yonekawa, Y., Tanaka, K., Ohara, O., Wantanabe, S., Kimura, T., Nishijima, T. & Taniguchi, T. (1994). The role of brain-derived neurotrophic factor in transient forebrain ischemia in the rat brain. *Neurosurgery* 34, 323-31; discussion 331.

van Loo, G., Saelens, X., Matthijssens, F., Schotte, P., Beyaert, R., Declercq, W. & Vandenabeele, P. (2002). Caspases are not localized in mitochondria during life or death. *Cell Death Differ* 9, 1207-11.

van Loo, G., Schotte, P., van Gurp, M., Demol, H., Hoorelbeke, B., Gevaert, K., Rodriguez, I., Ruiz-Carrillo, A., Vandekerckhove, J., Declercq, W., Beyaert, R. & Vandenabeele, P. (2001). Endonuclease G: a mitochondrial protein released in apoptosis and involved in caspase-independent DNA degradation. *Cell Death Differ* 8, 1136-42.

Vande Velde, C., Cizeau, J., Dubik, D., Alimonti, J., Brown, T., Israels, S., Hakem, R. & Greenberg, A. H. (2000). BNIP3 and genetic control of necrosis-like cell death through the mitochondrial permeability transition pore. *Mol Cell Biol* 20, 5454-68.

Verhagen, A. M., Ekert, P. G., Pakusch, M., Silke, J., Connolly, L. M., Reid, G. E., Moritz, R. L., Simpson, R. J. & Vaux, D. L. (2000). Identification of DIABLO, a mammalian protein that promotes apoptosis by binding to and antagonizing IAP proteins. *Cell* 102, 43-53.

Wei, H. & Perry, D. C. (1996). Dantrolene is cytoprotective in two models of neuronal cell death. *J Neurochem* 67, 2390-8.

White, B. C., Sullivan, J. M., DeGracia, D. J., O'Neil, B. J., Neumar, R. W., Grossman, L. I., Rafols, J. A. & Krause, G. S. (2000). Brain ischemia and reperfusion: molecular mechanisms of neuronal injury. *J Neurol Sci* 179, 1-33.

Woodburn, V. L., Hayward, N. J., Poat, J. A., Woodruff, G. N. & Hughes, J. (1993). The effect of dizocilpine and enadoline on immediate early gene expression in the gerbil global ischaemia model. *Neuropharmacology* 32, 1047-59.

Wu, D. (2005). Neuroprotection in experimental stroke with targeted neurotrophins. *NeuroRx* 2, 120-8.

Xu, D., Bureau, Y., McIntyre, D. C., Nicholson, D. W., Liston, P., Zhu, Y., Fong, W. G., Crocker, S. J., Korneluk, R. G. & Robertson, G. S. (1999). Attenuation of ischemia-induced cellular and behavioral deficits by X chromosome-linked inhibitor of apoptosis protein overexpression in the rat hippocampus. *J Neurosci* 19, 5026-33.

Xu, X., Chua, K. W., Chua, C. C., Liu, C. F., Hamdy, R. C. & Chua, B. H. (2010). Synergistic protective effects of humanin and necrostatin-1 on hypoxia and ischemia/reperfusion injury. *Brain Res* 1355, 189-94.

Yamashima, T., Kohda, Y., Tsuchiya, K., Ueno, T., Yamashita, J., Yoshioka, T. & Kominami, E. (1998). Inhibition of ischaemic hippocampal neuronal death in primates with cathepsin B inhibitor CA-074: a novel strategy for neuroprotection based on 'calpain-cathepsin hypothesis'. *Eur J Neurosci* 10, 1723-33.

Yang, J., Liu, X., Bhalla, K., Kim, C. N., Ibrado, A. M., Cai, J., Peng, T. I., Jones, D. P. & Wang, X. (1997). Prevention of apoptosis by Bcl-2: release of cytochrome c from mitochondria blocked. *Science* 275, 1129-32.

Yano, S., Morioka, M., Kuratsu, J. & Fukunaga, K. (2005). Functional proteins involved in regulation of intracellular Ca(2+) for drug development: role of calcium/calmodulin-dependent protein kinases in ischemic neuronal death. *J Pharmacol Sci* 97, 351-4.

Yasuda, M., D'Sa-Eipper, C., Gong, X. L. & Chinnadurai, G. (1998). Regulation of apoptosis by a Caenorhabditis elegans BNIP3 homolog. *Oncogene* 17, 2525-30.

Yousefi, S., Perozzo, R., Schmid, I., Ziemiecki, A., Schaffner, T., Scapozza, L., Brunner, T. & Simon, H. U. (2006). Calpain-mediated cleavage of Atg5 switches autophagy to apoptosis. *Nat Cell Biol* 8, 1124-32.

Yu, L., Alva, A., Su, H., Dutt, P., Freundt, E., Welsh, S., Baehrecke, E. H. & Lenardo, M. J. (2004). Regulation of an ATG7-beclin 1 program of autophagic cell death by caspase-8. *Science* 304, 1500-2.

Yuan, J. & Yankner, B. A. (2000). Apoptosis in the nervous system. *Nature* 407, 802-9.

Zhang, F., Yin, W. & Chen, J. (2004). Apoptosis in cerebral ischemia: executional and regulatory signaling mechanisms. *Neurol Res* 26, 835-45.

Zhang, J., Dong, M., Li, L., Fan, Y., Pathre, P., Dong, J., Lou, D., Wells, J. M., Olivares-Villagomez, D., Van Kaer, L., Wang, X. & Xu, M. (2003). Endonuclease G is required for early embryogenesis and normal apoptosis in mice. *Proc Natl Acad Sci U S A* 100, 15782-7.

Zhang, S., Zhang, Z., Sandhu, G., Ma, X., Yang, X., Geiger, J. D. & Kong, J. (2007a). Evidence of oxidative stress-induced BNIP3 expression in amyloid beta neurotoxicity. *Brain Res* 1138, 221-30.

Zhang, Z., Yang, X., Zhang, S., Ma, X. & Kong, J. (2007b). BNIP3 upregulation and EndoG translocation in delayed neuronal death in stroke and in hypoxia. *Stroke* 38, 1606-13.

Zhang, Z. F., Yang, X. F., Zhang, S., Ma, X. & Kong, J. (2007c). The proapoptotic protein BNIP3 plays a role in the delayed neuron death in stroke. *Stroke* 38, 548-548.

Zhu, C., Wang, X., Xu, F., Bahr, B. A., Shibata, M., Uchiyama, Y., Hagberg, H. & Blomgren, K. (2005). The influence of age on apoptotic and other mechanisms of cell death after cerebral hypoxia-ischemia. *Cell Death Differ* 12, 162-76.

Zhu, Y., Culmsee, C., Klumpp, S. & Krieglstein, J. (2004a). Neuroprotection by transforming growth factor-beta1 involves activation of nuclear factor-kappaB through phosphatidylinositol-3-OH kinase/Akt and mitogen-activated protein kinase-extracellular-signal regulated kinase1,2 signaling pathways. *Neuroscience* 123, 897-906.

Zhu, Y., Yang, G. Y., Ahlemeyer, B., Pang, L., Che, X. M., Culmsee, C., Klumpp, S. & Krieglstein, J. (2002). Transforming growth factor-beta 1 increases bad phosphorylation and protects neurons against damage. *J Neurosci* 22, 3898-909.

Zhu, Y. Z., Huang, S. H., Tan, B. K., Sun, J., Whiteman, M. & Zhu, Y. C. (2004b). Antioxidants in Chinese herbal medicines: a biochemical perspective. *Nat Prod Rep* 21, 478-89.

Zou, H., Henzel, W. J., Liu, X., Lutschg, A. & Wang, X. (1997). Apaf-1, a human protein homologous to C. elegans CED-4, participates in cytochrome c-dependent activation of caspase-3. *Cell* 90, 405-13.

7

The Matrix Metalloproteinases and Cerebral Ischemia

Wan Yang and Guangqin Li
Department of Neurology, the First Affiliated Hospital, Chongqing Medical University
China

1. Introduction

Matrix metalloproteinases(MMPs) are a family of zinc-containing endopeptidases which can degrade extracellular matrix (ECM) components at physiological PH. Thirty members of MMPs have been found so far [1]. They are widely distributed in plants,vertebrates and invertebrates cells.In human body, MMPs are mainly produced by vascular smooth muscle cells, monocytes, endothelial cells and so on. MMPs are synthesized as latent enzymes (zymogens) that are secreted or membrane-associated and must be proteolytically processed to their active form. Additionally, MMPs can be inhibited by endogenous inhibitors (e.g. TIMPs, tissue inhibitors of metalloproteinases).

1.1 Construction and function of matrix metalloproteinases

1.1.1 Construction of MMPs

MMP members have similar structures. They are usually composed of six structural domains with different functions.

1.2 The signal peptide and propeptide domain

Human MMPs(except MMP14) have a signal peptide sequence. The role of the signal peptide is to guide the post-translation substrate to the cytoplasm endoplasmic reticulum. Propeptide domain contains the conserved sequence of Pro-Arg-Cys-Gly-Val/Asn-Pro-Asp(PRCGV/NPD) which is responsible for maintaining the stability of plasminogen. When the propeptide domain is cut off by the exogenous enzymes, MMPs plasminogen can be activated.

1.3 The catalysis domain

There are two zinc ion binding domains and at least one calcium binding domain in the catalysis domain. Of the 2 zinc ion binding domains, one is in the activation center which is responsible for the catalytic process of MMPs. The other one is the structural zinc ion domain. In the catalysis domain, both gelatinase A and B have a insertion sequence of 175 residues. This insertion sequence is the type-fibronectin binding domain. Studies suggest that this domain may be responsible for the integration between gelatinase and its substrate.

1.4 The hinge domain and hemopexin binding domain

The hinge domain is located between the catalysis and the hemopexin binding domian and is linked with the terminal amino acid residues of the hemopexin binding domain by the disulfide bond. The hemopexin domain contains four duplicate sequences which has the weak homology with hemopexin and vitronectin. This domain is considered to be relevant to most MMPs' substrate specificity and also plays an important role in the integration between MMPs and tissue inhibitors of metalloproteinases (TIMPs).

1.5 The transmembrane domain

This domain exists in the carboxyl terminal of the Membrane-type MMPs(MT-MMPs) and can fix MT-MMPs to the cell membrane.
MMP members have different characteristics based on the six structural domains.

2. Function of matrix metalloproteinases

MMPs are the essential enzymes that may play a role in the degradation of ECM in the connective tissue. They can degrade almost all components of ECM and play an important role in various physiological and pathological processes in human body. Under physiological conditions, MMPs participate in the process of tissue demodeling such as wound healing, bone resorption, pregnancy, childbirth and breast atrophy. Normal physiological process depends on the control and coordination between MMPs and TIMPs. When infection or other stimulation occurs, the expression and activation of MMP are out of control, which may lead to the excessive degradation of ECM.
MMPs family can be divided into the following six categories based on the strucuture of their substrate, sequence simlilarity and characteristics of structural domain.

2.1 Collagenases

MMP-1, MMP-8,MMP-13 and MMP-18 are included. The main feature of these enzymes is to resolve collagen types I, II, III. Collagenase can also resolve some ECM components and other non-extracellular matrix molecules.

2.2 Gelatinases

Gelatinase A(MMP-2) and gelatinase B(MMP-9) are included. They are secreted or membrane-associated and must be proteolytically processed to their active form. MMP-2 can digest gelatin, collagen types IV, V, VIII, X laminin, elastin and fibronectin. The molecular weight of MMP-9 is 92KD which is the largest one. MMP-9 can be synthesized by various cells, such as astrocytes, vascular endothelial cells, microglias, neutrophils and macrophages. MMP-9 is mainly affected by the regulation of plasminogen activator and its subsrates inclucde gelatinase, collagen types IV, V and elastin[2]. Researches have shown that MMP-2 and MMP-9 may play a role in angiogenesis[3], atherosclerosis[4,5] and ischemic brain injury[6].

2.3 Stromelysins

Stromelysin-1(MMP-3) and stromelysin-2(MMP-10) have the same substrate specificity. However, the proteolytic efficiency of MMP-3 is higher than that of MMP-10. In addition to digesting extracellular matrix components, MMP-3 can also activate some pro-MMPs (e.g.

It is extremely important for pro-MMP-1 to produce MMP-1). MMP-11 is also called stromelysin-3,but it is often classified to other types because of its different structural sequence and substrate specificity.

2.4 Matrilysins

The structure of matrilysins lacks hemopexin domain. Matrilysin-1(MMP-7) and matrilysin-2(MMP-26) are included. In addition to degrading ECM, MMP-7 can process cell surface factors, such as pro TNF-α and E-cadherin. The matrilysin-2 (MMP-26) can also digest many ECM components.

2.5 Membrane-type MMPs(MT-MMPs)

There are six types of MT-MMPs, four types of MT-MMPs are type I transmembrane protein(MMP-14,-15, -16,-24), the other two types are GPI-ankyrin(MMP-17,-25). In addition to MT4-MMP, all other MT-MMPs can activate pro MMP-2. These enzymes can also digest some ECM components. MT1-MMP(MMP-14) has the activity to degrade collagen types I, II, III. MT5-MMP(MMP-24)
is mainly expressed in the cerebellum. MT6-MMP(MMP-25) is almost exclusively expressed in peripheral blood leucocytes, the original astrocytomas and the glioblastomas. However, it is not expressed in the meningiomas.

MT-MMPs have the following characteristics:

a. Binding with cell membrane and provide the focus area for the decomposition and degradation of extracellular matrix protein;
b. In the process of migration to the cell membrane, MT-MMPs are responsible for the cell activation of pro convertase pathway. Therefore, different from other types of MMPs, MT-MMPs have the proteolytic activity once it is inserted into the cell membrane.
c. MT-MMPs have the substrate recognition sites of other types of MMPs and participate in an important pathway to activate other types of MMPs. It has been proved that MT1-MMP participates in the hydrolysis of MMP-2 and MMP-13.

2.6 Other types of MMPs

There are at least seven types of MMPs which are not mentioned in the prevous text. MMP-12 is mainly expressed in macrophages and may take part in the migration of macrophages. MMP-12 can digest elastin and some other proteins. MMP-19 is identified through the liver c-DNA cloning and exists as T-cell antigens in the rheumatoid arthritis patients. Enamelysin (MMP-20) is mainly expressed in newly formed enamel and can digest amelogenin. The function of MMP-22 is not clear. MMP-23 is mainly expressed in the regeneration tissue and Epilysin (MMP-28) is mainly expressed in keratinocytes[7].

3. Influence factors to the activation of matrix metalloproteinases

The activation of MMPs is adjusted by three parts: gene transcription, zymogen activation and endogenous inhibitors.

3.1 Gene transcription

The genetic study has confirmed that there is promotor polymorphisms in MMP-1, -3, -9, -12 which affects the expression of MMPs gene[8].The expression of MMPs mRNA is affected by

a variety of chemical factors, such as ECM components, carcinogens, oncogene, neural hormones, cytokines and corticosteroids. For example, TNF-α affects the expression of MMPs gene by affecting the multi-cell system transcription factors (the latter is combined with the specific response elements in the MMPs gene enhancer);Tissue-type plasminogen activator (tPA) and urokinase can induce the expression of MMP-9[9,10]. The signal transduction mechanism of MMPs' activation remains to be elucidated. Previous studies suggest that MAPK pathway may be relevant to MMPs gene expression, transcription factor (AP-1 and NF-KB) is closely relevant to activation of MMPs [10]. The signal transduction mechanisms in different types of cells or for different types of MMPs may be different.
Mengshol et al[11] have showed that p38, JNK and NF-KB are essential for IL-1 to induce cartilage cells to produce MMP-13. For the production of MMP-1, p38 is still essential while JNK and NF-KB are not essential. Studies have also shown that some factors such as glucocorticoid and TGF-β, can inhibit MMP gene expression at the genetic level.

3.2 Zymogen activation

After translation and modification, the vast majority of MMPs mRNA is secreted to ECM in the form of zymogen. And it will be activated after hydrolysis of the propeptide domain. The activation mechanism found now includes stepwise activation, activation by MT-MMP, and cell activation. The initial activation of MMP is often associated with plasmin parenzyme, elastase, kallikrein. Among them, plasmin is considered to be the most powerful physiological activator in human body. In addition, SH-reagent (iodoacetic acid, HOCL, oxidized glutathione), denaturant (urea, SDS, NaSCN) and heat treatment have the ability to hydrolyze propeptide domain.

3.3 Endogenous inhibitors

The proteolytic activity of MMP is inhibited by non-specific and specific inhibitors. Non-specific inhibitors include α 2-macroglobulin,α 1-antiprotease and BB-94(batimistat). Specific inhibitors are the tissue inhibitors of metalloproteinases(TIMPs). TIMPs, which are the coding proteins of multi-gene family, are the natural inhibitors of MMPs. The expression of TIMPs is regulated during development and tissue remodeling. To date, a total of four types of TIMPs have been found in vertebrates. They form the high affinity complexes with activated MMPs at the molar ratio of 1:1 and inhibit the degradation of ECM by blocking the catalysis domain of MMPs. TIMP-1 inhibits the activity of most MMPs, except for MT1-MMP and MMP-2; TIMP-2 inhibits majority of MMPs except MMP-9. In addition, TIMP-2 can form the complexes with MT1-MMP in the cell membrane which may have the regulation to activate the proteolytic activity of MMP-2; TIMP-3 inhibits MMP-1, -2, -3, -9, -13; TIMP-4 inhibits MMP-1, -3, -7, -9 and is highly expressed in human heart. Corresponding to MMPs, TIMPs play a negative role in the regulation of the ECM metabolism. They can prevent the activation of MMPs, inhibit the function and affect the extent of protein breakdown and duration of injury[12]. In some excessive matrix degradation diseases, the imbalance between MMPs and TIMPs leads to a net increase in overall activity of MMPs[13].
Although TIMPs play an important role in preventing excessive matrix degradation caused by MMPs, recent research shows that TIMP-1 and TIMP-2 are the multifunctional proteins with different biological functions. It has been reported that TIMP-1 and TIMP-2 demonstrate growth factor-like activity and inhibit the angiogenesis;while TIMP-3 is associated with apoptosis[7].

TIMPs inhibit the MMPs activity by two steps. In the stage of zymogen activation, TIMP-2 can form a stable complex with pro MMP-2,as well as TIMP-1 and pro MMP-9. Therefore, they can impede the zymogen self-activation of pro MMP-1. In the stage of activated MMPs, both TIMP-1 and TIMP-2 can directly form a tight 1:1 complex with the activated MMPs and inhibit their activity. Naturally, the TIMP-MMP complexes may also be activated under certain conditions.

4. Role of matrix metalloproteinase in cerebral ischemia

In recent years, there is growing research interest on MMPs in central nervous system. In the normal central nervous system, MMP-2 and MMP-9 have been found in perivascular cells, brain vascular endothelial cells, astrocytes and microglias. The microglias in cultured rat can secrete MMP-9 once they are activated. Human hippocampal pyramidal cells can also synthesize MMP-9. It is reported that MMP-9 mRNA can be expressed in the developing mouse embryo brain, suggesting that MMP-9 is related to neurodevelopment. Studies also show that MMP-2 is related to the regeneration of axons. A growing number of scholars believe that MMPs plays an important role in the pathologic processes of central nervous system diseases[5].

4.1 MMPs and pathogenesis of stroke

Atherosclerosis is one of the underlying vascular risk factors for developing cerebrovascular disease. It is reported that the gelatinase of MMPs plays a key role in the process of intimal injury and the formation of atherosclerotic lesions. The endothelial cells covered on the plaque have the activity to express MMP-2 and MMP-9. The over-expression of MMPs can dissolve collagens and significantly change the proportion of plaque composition which leads to the relative increase in lipid content and increases the plaque instability. Then the plaque cap thinningzs and splits, eventually leading to the occurrence of cerebral ischemia disease[14,15]. Studies have shown that MMP-8 and MMP-1, MMP-12 might play a decisive role in maintaining the stability of atherosclerotic plaques[16]. The rupture of atherosclerotic plaque partially depends on the activity and content of MMP-9[17]. Another study reported that the focal increase of MMP-9 activity was an early warning of acute plaque rupture.

4.2 MMPs and ischemic brain injury

In the normal state, cerebral vascular endothelial cells can not express or only express a small amount of MMP-9[18]. By the animal experiments, Fukuda[19] confirmed that ischemic brain tissue could produce some active proteases and these proteases led to the rapid and significant degradation of microvessels. Another studies suggested that cerebral ischemia and reperfusion could induce the expression of MMPs. Especially, the activity of MMP-2 and MMP-9 would increase, which was related to cerebral microvascular permeability, blood-brain barrier (BBB) permeability, BBB damage, inflammatory cell invasion and cerebral edema[6,12,13,20]. Gidday et al[21] showed that MMP-9 in ischemic brain tissue played a pro-inflammatory role which helped neutrophil leukocytes migrate from the blood circulation into the tissue. At first, MMP-9 caused BBB damage, then MMP-9 contributed to the proteolysis of microvascular basement membrane and eventually led to neurological damage. The possible mechanism may be the following: In the ischemic brain tissue, MMP-9 is mainly expressed in vascular endothelial cells, the increased MMP-9 may act on the tight junctions and basement membrane among the BBB endothelial cells which leads to the BBB damage,increase of permeability and vasogenic brain edema. The worst is the occurrence of herniation[22]. In addition, the degradation of vascular basement membrane makes neutrophil leukocytes exudated to the brain tissue. MMP-2 and MMP-9 expressed by macrophages may contribute to their entry into the ischemic lesions and promote the wound healing after focal stroke [13]. However, MMP-9 expressed by neutrophil leukocytes may also contribute to the ischemic damage of brain. Zalewska et al[23] proposed that activated MMP-9 may act on a certain link of the cell apoptosis cascade in the hippocampus CAI area after transient ischemic brain. Previous experimental studies also showed that MMP-9 could degrade the myelin basic protein of brain white matter and lead to the damage after ischemic brain[24]. Early studies have showed that injecting MMP-2 to the rat brain can contribute to the opening of BBB. MMP-2 and MMP-9 destroy the capillary tight junctions and basement membrane by protein hydrolysis after brain ischemia, thus leading to vasogenic brain edema. In 1996, Rosenberg et al[25] monitored of the expression of MMP-9 in rats with first onset cerebral infarction. They found the upregulated expression of MMP-9 4 hours after the occlusion of middle cerebral artery,. Within 12 hours and 24 hours, the expression of MMP-9 in the infarction site significantly increased which was consistent with the peak of the vasogenic brain edema, suggesting that MMP-9 played an important role in secondary brain damage and vasogenic edema. Montaner' et al[26] also showed that the activity of MMP-9 abnormally increased in the early stage of stroke and pro-inflammatory response, while the activity of MMP-2 appeared in the repair phase of vascular regeneration. Autopsy results showed that one week after infarction, MMP-9 was expressed in neutrophils, and one week later the macrophages expressing matrilysin and MMP-2 were observed. Montaner et al also found that the level of plasma MMP-2 was higher in the patients with previous history of stroke. The above results suggested that MMP-9 plays an important role in secondary brain damage and vasogenic brain edema,while MMP-2 is involved in tissue repair and nerve regeneration.

Previous studies also suggested that MMP-9 may also related to the hemorrhage translation after tPA or urokinase thrombolysis[24].

4.3 MMPs and cerebral ischemia reperfusion

Animal model studies showed that 3 hours and 48 hours of reperfusion occurred after cerebral ischemia, BBB was opened and the opening reached to the peak in the 48th hour; The first opening was related to the increased level of MMP-2 while the second opening occurred in the stage when the level of MMP-9 was significantly higher; the content of MMP-2 reached to the peak 5 days after reperfusion and the repair process began at the same time; the content of TIMP-1 significantly increased in the 48th hour while that of TIMP-2 increased to the maximum on day 5[12]. These results suggested that reperfusion may affect MMPs and TIMPs, while MMPs and TIMPs promoted the reperfusion injury by complex ways. When the synthetic inhibitors of MMPs (BB-1101) was applicated to inhibit MMPs, both the BBB's first opening and cerebral edema after reperfusion were prevented, suggesting that BBB's opening and brain edema after reperfusion were related to MMPs.

5. Effect of inhibiting matrix metalloproteinase on cerebral ischemia

Matrix metalloproteinase inhibitors have been used to treat cancer metastasis. Currently, many MMP inhibitors are also used in experimental models of neurological diseases[6], such as bacterial meningitis, cerebral infarction and experimental allergic meningitis. Studies have shown that the content of MMPs increased after cerebral ischemia and reperfusion, exogenous inhibitors could reduce the ischemic and reperfusion injury[12,13]. Thus, MMPs may become a new potential target for stroke therapy and matrix metalloproteinase inhibitors can be used for treatment of cerebrovascular diseases[2].

5.1 Matrix metalloproteinase inhibitors and cerebral ischemia

Previous studies have showed that the activated leukocytes could increase the reperfusion injury in the central nervous system. So, the drugs which can inhibit the leukocyte adhesion (including the intracellular adherence factor antibodies) have a neuroprotective effect. Matrix metalloproteinase inhibitors can combine with the divalent cation in vitro, inhibit the leukocytes function, and reduce the reperfusion injury.

Lee' et al[3] have shown that MMP inhibitors could inhibit the MMP-9 production in brain after stimulated and parenchymal angiogenesis.Horstmann[27] found that MMP-1 not only had the direct proteolytic capacity, but also played a role in the activation cascade of MMPs. It could crack collagen types I, II, III and be involved in the activation of MMP-2, MMP-9. Non-specific matrix metalloproteinase inhibitors are clustered in atherosclerosis tissues and inhibit the activity of MMP-9 in the carotid artery plaques, thereby stabilizing the easily broken atherosclerotic plaques. Matrix metalloproteinase inhibitors can also reduce the incidence of acute plaque rupture by reducing MMP-9 activity. The content of TIMPs is significantly higher in cerebral ischemia-reperfusion. They combine with the corresponding MMPs and prevent the activation of MMPs. They inhibit the function of MMPs, stabilize the ECM, significantly reduce the blood-brain barrier damage and the brain edema after ischemia[12].

5.2 Matrix metalloproteinase inhibitors and therapies for cerebral ischemia

Previous studies suggested that MMP-9 monoclonal antibody may significantly reduce the infarction volume in a rat model of ischemia[13]. Clinical studies have also confirmed that MMP-9 is related to the total infarction volume. It is reported that matrix metalloproteinase inhibitors and MMPs neutralizing antibodies can reduce the vasogenic brain edema and infarction volume[26]. In addition, MMPs inhibitors are also effective in preventing atherosclerosis and the ischemic brain damage.

rt-PA and urokinase are effective drugs for acute ischemic stroke. However, the clinical application of thrombolytics is limited by the narrow therapeutic time window and the complication of bleeding after thrombolysis. But if we combine rt-PA or urokinase with the MMP inhibitors (BB-94 or doxycycline)in thrombolysis treatment, the incidence of hemorrhage and the amount of hemorrhage after thrombolysis may be decreased and the thrombolytic time window will be prolonged[28,29]. This is because that if MMPs inhibitors are used before the application of rt-PA or urokinase, MMP-2, MMP-3 and MMP-9 (which have the potential damage for BBB) would be inhibited. BBB would be closed and the integrity of blood vessels would be maintained, thus might increase the safety of the thrombolytic therapy[6,30].

6. Conclusion

MMPs may play an important role in the brain ischemia and reperfusion by degrading the ECM and destroying the blood -brain barrier which can lead to the vasogenic brain edema and secondary brain injury. The matrix metalloproteinase inhibitors and MMPs neutralizing antibodies can reduce the vasogenic brain edema and infarction volume. In addition, MMPs inhibitors are also effective in preventing atherosclerosis and the ischemic brain damage. Thus, MMPs may become a new potential target for stroke therapy and matrix metalloproteinase inhibitors can be used for the treatment of cerebrovascular diseases.

7. References

[1] Sheppeck JE 2nd, Tebben A, Gilmore JL, et al.A molecular modeling analysis of novel non-hydroxamate inhibitors of TAGE.Bioorg Med Chem Leit,2007,17:1408-1412.
[2] Hashimoto T, Wen G, Lawton MT, et al. Abnormal expression of matrix metalloproteinases and tissue inhibitors of metalloproteinases in brain arteriovenous malformations. Stroke,2003,34:925-931.
[3] Lee CZ, Xu B, Hashimoto T, er al. Doxycycline suppresses cerebral matrix metalloproteinase-9 and angiogenesis induced by focal hyperstimulation of vascular endothelial growth factor in a mouse model.Stroke,2004,35:1715-1719.
[4] Newby AC.Dual Role of Matrix Metalloproteinases(Matrixins) in Intimal Thickening and Atherosclerotic Plaque Rupture.Physiol Rev,2005,85:1-31.
[5] Axiso B, Loftus I, Ross Naylor A. Prospective, randomized, double-blind trial investigating the effect of Doxycycline on matrix metalloproteinase expression within delayed carotid plaques(J).Stroke,2002,33:2858-2865.
[6] Pfefferkorn T, Rosenberg GA. Closure of the blood-brain barrier by matrix metalloproteinase inhibition reduces rtPA-mediated mortality in cerebral ischemia with delayed reperfusion.Stroke,2003,34:2025-2030.
[7] Visse R, Nagase H. Matrix metalloproteinases and tissue inhibitors of metalloproteinases: structure, function and biochemistry.Cire Res,2003,92:827-839.
[8] Ye S. Polymorphism in matrix metalloproteinase gene promoters:implication in regulation of gene expression and susceptibility of various diseases.Matrix Biol,2000,19:623-629.
[9] LI Jie,LI Guang-qin,JIANG Guo-hui.Effects of rt-PA and urokinase on expression of MMP-9 and blood-brain barrier permeability in thrombolytic therapy.Chin J Contemp Neurol Neurosurg,2009,9:445-449.
[10] ZHANG Shu-tang,LI Guangqin.The effect of urokinase on the expression of MMP-9 in human endothelial cell and its mechanism.Journal of Chongqing Medical University,2009,34:269-272.
[11] Mengshol JA, Vincenti MP, Coon CI, et al. Interleukin-1 induction of collagenase3 (matrix metelloproteinase 13) gene expression in chondrocytes requires p38,c-Jun N-terminal kinase,and nuclear factor kappaB: differential regulation of collagenase 1 and collagenase 3.Arthritis Rheum,2000,43:801-811.
[12] Rosenberg GA, Estrada EY, Dencoff JE. Matrix metalloproteinases and TIMPs are associated with blood-brain barrier opening after reperfusion in rat brain. Stroke,1998,29:2189-2195.

[13] Romanic AM, White RF, Arleth AJ, er al. Matrix metalloproteinases expression increases after cerebral focal ischemia in rats: inhibition of matrix metalloproteinase-9 reduces infarct size. Stroke,1998,29:1020-1030.
[14] Morgan AR, Rerkasem K, Gallagher PJ, et al. Differences in matrix metalloproteinase-1 and matrix metalloproteinase-12 transcript levels among carotid atherosclerotic plaques with different histopathological characteristics. Stroke,2004,35:1310-1315.
[15] Fatar M, Stroick M, Griebe M, er al. Matrix metalloproteinases in cerebrovascular diseases. Cerebrovasc Dis,2005,20:141-148.
[16] Molloy KJ, Thompson MM, Jones JL, et al. Unstable carotid plaques exhibit raised matrix metalloproteinase-8 activity. Circulation,2004,110:337-343.
[17] Heo JH, Kim SH, Lee KY, et al. Increase in plasma matrix metalloproteinase-9 in acute stroke patients with thrombolysis failure. Stroke,2003,34:e48-50.
[18] Guzener ML, Gveric D, Strand C, et al. The expression of tissue-type plasminogen activator,matrix metalloproteinases and endogenous inhibitors in the central nervous system in multiple sclerosis: comparision of stages in lesion evulution.J Neuopathol Exp Neurol,1996,55:1194.
[19] Fukuda S, Fini CA, Mabuchi T, et al. Focal cerebral ischemia induces active proteases that degrade microvascular matrix(J). Stroke,2004,35(4):998-1004.
[20] Gasche Y, Fujimura M, Morita-Fujimura Y, et al. Early appearance of activated matrix metalloproteinase-9 after focal cerebral ischemia in mice: a possible role in blood-brain barrier dysfunction. J Cereb Blood Flow Metab,1999,19:1020-1028.
[21] Giddy JM, Gasche YG, Copin JC, et al. Leukocyte derived matrix metalloproteinase-9 mediates blood-brain barrier breakdown and is proinflammatory following transient focal cerebral ischemia. Am J Physiol Heart Circ Physiol,2005,289:H558-H568.
[22] Eldrup N, Gronholdt ML, Sillesen H, et al. Elevated matrix metalloproteinase-9 associated with stroke or cardiovascular death in patients with carotid stenosis. Circulation,2006,114:1847-1854.
[23] Zalewska T, Ziemka-Nalecz M, Sarnowska A, et al. Involvement of MMPs in delayed neuronal death after global ischmia. Acta Neurobiol Expe,2002,62:53-61.
[24] LI Jie,LI Guang-qin.Effects of urokinase thrombolysis on matrix metalloproteinase-9, blood-brain barrier permeability and intracerebral hemorrhage in a rat modal of middle cerebral artery thromboembolism.Int J Cerebrovasc Dis,2009,17:668-672.
[25] Rosenberg GA, Navratil M, Borane F, et al. Proteolytic cascade enzymes increase in focal cerebral ischemia in rat. J Cereb Blood Flow Metab,1996,16:360-366.
[26] Montaner J, Alvarez-Sabin J, Molina C, et al. Matrix metalloproteinase expression after human cardioembolic stroke: temporal profile and relation to neurological impairment. Stroke,2001,32:1759-1766.
[27] Horstmann S, Kalb P, Koziol J, et al. Profiles of matrix metalloproteinases: their inhibitors, and Jaminin in stroke patients: infulence of different therapies. Stroke,2003,34:2165-2170.
[28] Lapchak PA,Chapman DF,Zivin JA. Metalloproteinase inhibition reduces thrombolytic (tissue plasminogen activator)-induced hemorrhage after thromboembolic stroke.Stroke,2000,31:3034-3040

[29] JIANG Guo-hui,LI Guang-qin,LI Jie.Inhibtion of matrix metalloproteinase-9 can prolonging urokinase thrombolytic time window after embolic stroke in rats.Journal of Brain and Nervous Diseases,2009,17:354-358
[30] Montaner J, Molina CA, Monasterio J, et al. Matrix metalloproteinase-9 pretreatment level predicts intracranial hemorrhagic complications after thrombolysis in human stroke. Circulation,2003,107:598-603.

8

Folate Deficiency Enhances Delayed Neuronal Death in the Hippocampus After Transient Cerebral Ischemia

Jun Hyun Yoo
Department of Family Medicine, Samsung Medical Center, Samsung Biomedical Research Institute, Sungkyunkwan University School of Medicine, Seoul, Republic of Korea

1. Introduction

Transient cerebral ischemia, in which the brain is temporarily deprived of nutrients and oxygen, results in delayed degeneration of vulnerable neurons within the CA1 region of the hippocampus. The pathophysiology of cerebral ischemic disease is a complex series of cellular biochemical process that involves intracellular ATP depletion, excitotoxicity, oxidative stress, microvascular injury, hypercoagulable hemostatic activation, post-ischemic inflammation and final cell death of neuronal, glial, and endothelial cells (Brouns et al, 2009; Jin et al, 2010).

Folate is an essential micronutrient as a methyl donor for the DNA nucleotides synthesis and cytosine methylation for the control of gene expression. Clinically, folate deficiency is linked to megaloblastic anemia and atherothrobotic vascular disease. On the biochemical basis, folate deficiency increases nuclear DNA damage via uracil misincorporation and which induces chromosome breaks (Blount et al, 1997; Fenech, 2010). A metabolic consequence of folate deficiency is the accumulation of intermediate metabolite, homocysteine. Dietary folate deficiency has been shown to decrease mitochondrial folate concentration and mitochondrial DNA content and increase mitochondrial DNA deletion in brain, leading to leakage of ROS and increase of oxidative stress (Chang et al, 2007; Ho et al, 2003; Crott et al, 2005). Electron microscopic finding showed mitochondrial degeneration in the endothelium and perivascular fibrosis in microvascular wall in the rat brain (Kim et al, 2002).

Homocysteine is a toxic amino acid to neuronal and vascular endothelial cells. Numerous epidemiological studies have recognized the association of folate deficiency and hyperhomocysteinemia with increased risk of vascular disease and ischemic stroke (Yoo et al, 1998, 2000, Kang et al, 1992). Hyperhomocysteinemia produces complex alterations in the blood vessels including oxidative stress, endothelial dysfunction and inflammatory response via the activation of transcription factor such as nuclear factor-kB (NF-kB) or activiator protein-1(AP-1). Homocysteiene upregulate E-selectin, P-selectin, ICAM-1, V-CAM-1, MCP-1 via activation of NF-kB, and AP-1 (Hwang et al, 2008; Woo et al, 2008).

No study has yet evaluated the morphological characteristics of the folate-deficient hippocampus after transient forebrain ischemia. This study examined the delayed neuronal death and morphologic changes in the hippocampal CA1 region after transient forebrain ischemia in a gerbil model.

2. Materials and methods

2.1 Experimental animals, diets, measurements of body weight and serum homocysteine level

For a detailed description of the present experimental method is referred to the published article (Hwang IK et al, 2008). The animals were fed with the respective diet *ad libitum* for 3 months. After 3 months on the folate deficient-diets (FAD), blood was taken for analysis of homocysteine levels. Homocysteine levels in serum samples were quantified with the use of an high performance liquid chromatography(Yoo et al, 1998).

2.2 Induction of transient forebrain ischemia and tissue processing for histology

After 3 months of folate deficient-diet, animals were anesthetized with isoflurane in 33% oxygen and 67% nitrous oxide. Bilateral common carotid arteries were isolated and occluded using non-traumatic aneurysm clips. After 5 min of occlusion, the aneurysm clips were removed from the common carotid arteries. The body temperature under free-regulating or normothermic (37 ± 0.5°C) conditions was monitored with a rectal temperature probe and maintained during and after the surgery until the complete recovery from anesthesia. Thereafter, animals were kept on the thermal incubator to maintain the body temperature of animals until the euthanasia. Sham-operated animals served as controls: these sham-operated animals were subjected to the same surgical procedures except no occlusion of common carotid artery.

For the tissue preparation, sham- and ischemia-operated animals were anesthetized and perfused transcardially with 0.1 M phosphate-buffered saline (pH 7.4) followed by 4% paraformaldehyde in 0.1 M phosphate-buffer (pH 7.4). The brains were removed and post-fixed in the same fixative for 6 hours. The brain tissues were cryoprotected by infiltration with 30% sucrose overnight.

2.3 Examination of neuronal damage: Cresyl violet staining

The sections in the hippocampal CA1 region were mounted on gelatin-coated microscopy slides. Cresyl violet acetate (Sigma) was dissolved at 1.0% (*w/v*) in distilled water, and glacial acetic acid was added to this solution. The sections were stained and dehydrated by immersing in serial ethanol baths, and they were then mounted with Canada balsam (Kanto Chemical, Tokyo, Japan). All animals (n=7 at each time) were sampled according to the time lines to evaluate the evolving histopathologic changes (3 hour, 12 hour, 1 day, 2day, 3day, 4day after reperfusion).

2.4 Examination of neuronal damage: NeuN immunohistochemistry

The sections in the hippocampal CA1 region were sequentially treated with 0.3% hydrogen peroxide in PBS for 30 min and 10% goat serum in 0.05 M PBS for 30 min. The sections were next incubated with diluted mouse anti-NeuN (diluted 1:1,000, Chemicon International, Temecula, CA) overnight at room temperature. Thereafter the tissues were exposed to biotinylated goat anti-mouse IgG and streptavidin peroxidase complex (Vector, Burlingame, CA). And they were visualized with 3,3′-diaminobenzidine in 0.1 M Tris-HCl buffer and mounted on the gelatin-coated slides. After dehydration the sections were mounted in Canada Balsam (Kanto Chemical).

2.5 Examination of neuronal apoptosis: TUNEL staining

The sections in the hippocampal CA1 region were stained using terminal deoxynucleotidyl transferase dUTP-biotin nick-end-labeling (TUNEL) staining. The sections were washed in 0.1 M PBS (pH 7.4) for 30 min before being incubated in blocking solution (3% H_2O_2 in 0.01 M PBS) at room temperature for 20 min, and were then washed in PBS for 5 min and treated with permeabilization solution (0.1% Triton X-100 in 0.1% sodium citrate) at 4°C for 2 min. Next, the sections were washed 3 times, and then incubated in TUNEL reaction mixture according to kit instructions (Roche Molecular Biochemicals, Mannheim, Germany). The TUNEL reaction mixture was prepared with a 1:2 dilution of the enzyme solution. The sections were washed 3 times with PBS (10 min per wash) before being incubated in converter-POD (Roche Molecular Biochemicals) at 37°C for 30 min and treated with DAB-substrate solution for 1.5-2 min. After washing the sections 3 times, the sections were counterstained with methyl green, dehydrated and coverslipped with Canada Balsam (Kanto Chemical).

2.6 Examination of neuronal damage: Fluoro-Jade B (F-J B) histofluorescence staining

According to the experiment of Candelario-Jalil et al (2003), the sections were first immersed in a solution containing 1% sodium hydroxide in 80% alcohol, and followed in 70% alcohol. They were then transferred to a solution of 0.06% potassium permanganate, and transferred to a 0.0004% F-J B (Histochem, Jefferson, AR) staining solution. After washing, the sections were placed on a slide warmer (approximately 50°C), and then examined using an epifluorescent microscope (Carl Zeiss, Göttingen, Germany) with blue (450-490 nm) excitation light and a barrier filter (Schmued and Hopkins, 2000).

2.7 Immunohistochemistry for 8-hydroxy-2'-deoxyguanosine (8-OHdG)

At designated times (30 min, 3 h, 6 h, 12 h, 24 h, 2 days, 3 days and 4 days) after the surgery, sham- and ischemia-operated animals (n = 7 at each time point) were used for this experiment. To obtain the exact data in this study, tissues of sham-operated and operated animals were processed under the same conditions. The sections were sequentially treated with 0.3% hydrogen peroxide in PBS for 30 min, 150 μM/ml RNase A for 1 h at 37°C, 50 mM sodium hydroxide in 40% ethanol for 10 min. The sections were incubated with mouse anti-8-OHdG antiserum (1:100) (Bail et al., 1996; Won et al., 1999, 2001) in PBS containing 0.3% Triton X-100 and 2% normal goat serum overnight at room temperature. After washing 3 times for 10 min with PBS, the sections were incubated sequentially, in goat anti-mouse IgG and Vectastain (Vector), diluted 1:200 in the same solution as the primary antiserum. Between incubations, the tissues were washed with PBS 3 times for 10 min each. The sections were visualized using 3,3'-diaminobenzidine tetrachloride (Sigma) in 0.1 M Tris-buffer and mounted on gelatin-coated slides.

2.8 Platelet endothelial cell adhesion molecule-1 (PECAM-1) staining

Immunohistochemistry for PECAM-1 (final mediator of neutrophil transendothelial migration) was conducted according to the method by Hwang et al (2005b). In brief, the sections were sequentially treated with 0.3% hydrogen peroxide (H_2O_2) in PBS and 10%

normal horse serum in 0.05 M PBS. The sections were next incubated with diluted mouse anti-PECAM-1 antibody (diluted 1:1000, Santa Cruz Biotechnology, Santa Cruz, CA) overnight. Thereafter, the tissues were exposed to biotinylated horse anti-mouse IgG and streptavidin–peroxidase complex (Vector). The sections were visualized with DAB in 0.1 M Tris-HCl buffer and mounted on the gelatin-coated slides.

2.9 Immunohistochemistry for glial fibrillary acidic protein (GFAP) and ionized calcium-binding adapter molecule 1 (Iba-1)

In order to examine the degree of reactive gliosis in the CA1 region in the CD- and FAD-treated groups after ischemia/reperfusion, we carried out immunohistochemical staining with rabbit anti-GFAP (diluted 1:1,000, Chemicon) for astrocytes and rabbit anti-Iba-1 (diluted 1:500, Wako, Osaka, Japan) for microglia according to the above mentioned-method (see the NeuN immunohistochemistry). The tissues were exposed to biotinylated goat anti-rabbit IgG (diluted 1:200; Vector) and streptavidin peroxidase complex (diluted 1:200; Vector). And they were visualized with DAB in 0.1 M Tris-HCl buffer and mounted on the gelatin-coated slides. After dehydration the sections were mounted in Canada Balsam (Kanto Chemical).

2.10 Quantification of data

All measurements were performed in order to ensure objectivity in blind conditions, by two observers for each experiment, carrying out the measures of control and experimental samples under the same conditions.

The number of survived pyramidal cells in the stratum pyramidale within the CA1 region was counted using an AxioM1 light microscope (Carl Zeiss) photomicroscope at a magnification of 400×. Histologic analysis was performed by a blinded observer and the average of the right and left survived cell numbers (neurons per 1 mm liner length) in a single section of the dorsal hippocampal CA1 region was calculated as reported by Kirino group (1986). Five sections of cresyl violet/NeuN and TUNEL/F-J B staining from each animal were used for counting.

Fifteen sections from a animal were randomly selected from the corresponding areas of the hippocampus in order to quantitatively analyze 8-OHdG, GFAP, Iba-1 and PECAM-1 immunoreactivity in the hippocampal CA1 region. The mid-point areas of the hippocampal CA1 region were measured on the monitor at a magnification of 25-50×. Images of all 8-OHdG, GFAP, Iba-1 and PECAM-1 immunoreactive structures taken from 3 layers (strata oriens, pyramidale and radiatum in the hippocampus proper, and molecular, granule cell and polymorphic layers in the dentate gyrus) were obtained through light microscope (Carl Zeiss, Germany). The staining intensity of all 8-OHdG, GFAP, Iba-1 and PECAM-1 immunoreactive structures was evaluated on the basis of a optical density (OD).

3. Results

3.1 Folate deficient change of body weight and serum concentration of homocysteine

Folate deficiency rendered the FAD-(folate deficient-diet) group susceptible to ischemia/reperfusion. After 3 months on the folate deficient-diets, serum levels of homocysteine were determined and found to be 5- to 8-fold higher in gerbils subjected to FAD compared to CD-(control diet) group. The body weight gain during the first diet month was significantly lower in the FAD group than in the CD group, this was consistent throughtout the 3 months of observation.

3.2 Neuronal damage

Cresyl violet and NeuN stainings show the positive pyramidal neurons on the first day. The cell densities decreased over the time after ischemia/reperfusion. Two days after ischemia/reperfusion, neurodegeneration were found in the neurons in the FAD-group (Figs. 1F, 1N), when no significant changes were seen in the CD-group (Figs. 1B, 1J). In FAD-group, CA1 pyramidal neurons showed cytoplasmic shrinkage and chromatic condensation. Starting from day three after ischemia/reperfusion, pyramidal neurons in FAD-group showed delayed neuronal death, which became morphologically similar to that of day four in CD-group (Figs. 1D, 1G, 1K and 1O).

Delayed neuronal death in the CA1 region was identified using TUNEL or F-J B staining. CA1 pyramidal neurons in the CD- and FAD-groups 1 day after ischemia/reperfusion did not show TUNEL or F-J B staining (Figs. 2B, 2F, 2J, 2N). Two days after ischemia/reperfusion, pyramidal neurons in the FAD-group showed TUNEL or F-J B staining representing neurodegeneration (Figs. 2G, 2O). Four days after ischemia/reperfusion, pyramidal neurons in the CD-group showed TUNEL or F-J B staining (Figs. 2D, 2L), but TUNEL or F-J B stained pyramidal neurons decreased in FAD-group (Figs. 2H, 2P). These shows that folate deficiency enhances delayed neuronal death in the hippocampus after transient cerebral ischemia

3.3 Change in 8-hydroxy-deoxyguanosine immunoreactivity

In this study, we found a significant difference in 8- hydroxy-deoxyguanosine immunoreactivity between the CD- and FAD-groups after ischemia/reperfusion (Figs. 3, 4). In both the sham-operated groups, very weak 8- hydroxy-deoxyguanosine immunoreactivity was detected in the CA1 region (Figs. 3A, 3E). The oxidative change in both groups began to increase at 30 min after ischemia/reperfusion, which the peak changes were noted at 12 hour after ischemia/reperfusion (Figs. 3C, 3G, Fig 4). At 12 hour after ischemia, 8- hydroxy-deoxyguanosine immunoreactivity in FAD-group was much higher than that in CD-group (Fig. 4). Thereafter, it decreased with time (Figs. 3D and 4). Four days after ischemic insult, 8-OHdG immunoreactivity in both groups was lower than that in the sham-operated groups (Fig. 4).

3.4 Change in PECAM-1 immunoreactivity

PECAM-1 immunoreactivity in microvessels in the hippocampal CA1 region changed after ischemia/reperfusion (Figs. 5, 6). In the CD- and FAD-fed-sham-operated groups, microvessels showed weak PECAM-1 immunoreactivity (Fig. 5A, 5B), and this immunoreactivity increased with time after ischemic insult in both of these groups (Figs. 5C-5H, Fig 6). PECAM-1 immunoreactivity in CA1 in both groups increased significantly 3 days after ischemia/reperfusion (Figs. 5G, 5H, Fig 6) and PECAM-1 immunoreactivity in FAD-group was much higher than that in CD-group (Fig. 6).

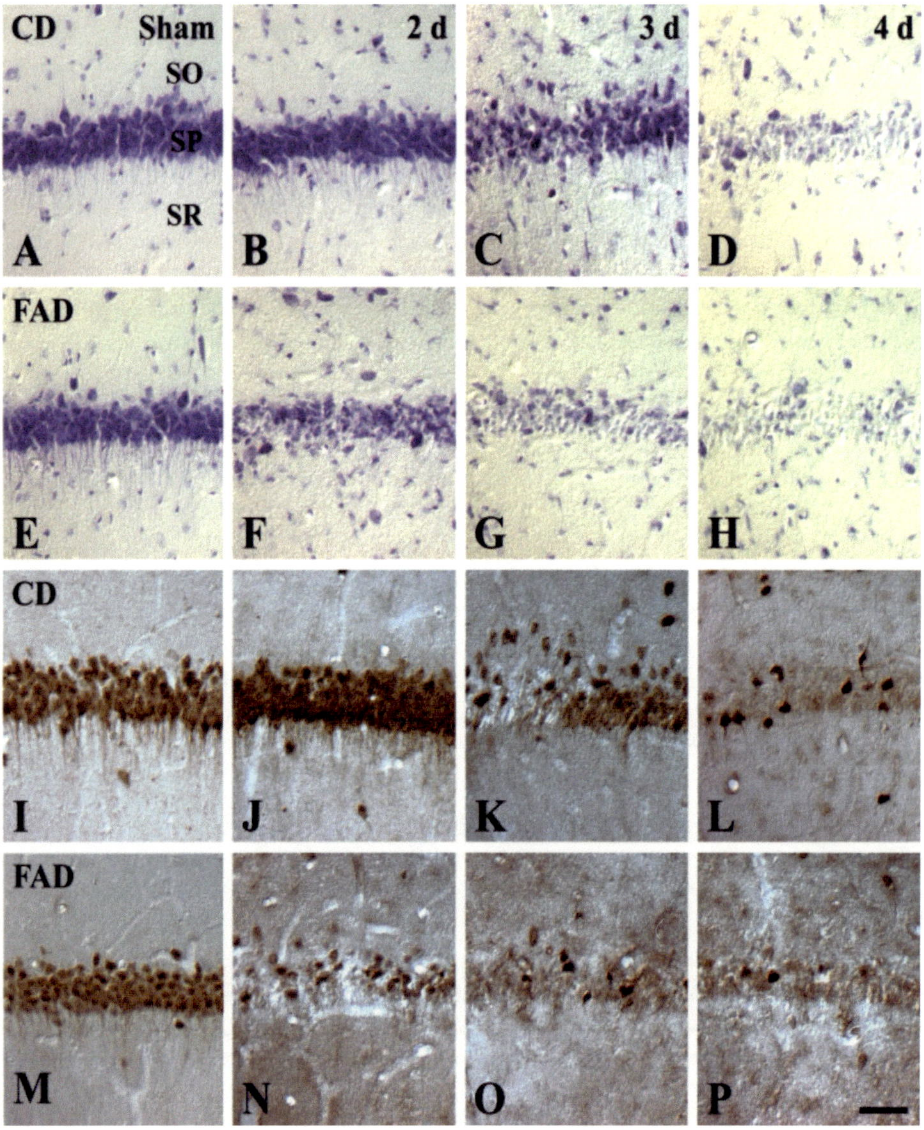

Fig. 1. Cresyl violet (CV) and NeuN staining of the CA1 region in sham-operated (A,E,I,M) and ischemia-operated groups 2 days (B,F,J,N), 3 days (C,G,K,O) and 4 days (D,H,L,P) after ischemia/reperfusion and feeding with a folic acid-deficient or control diet. Two days after ischemia/reperfusion, CV- or NeuN-positive pyramidal neurons in the folate-deficient diet-treated group show cytoplasmic shrinkage and chromatic condensation. Three days after ischemia/reperfusion, CV- or NeuN-positive pyramidal neurons in the folate-deficient diet-treated group show "delayed neuronal death" like that in the control diet-treated group 4 days after ischemia/reperfusion. SO, stratum oriens; SP, stratum pyramidale; SR,stratum radiatum.

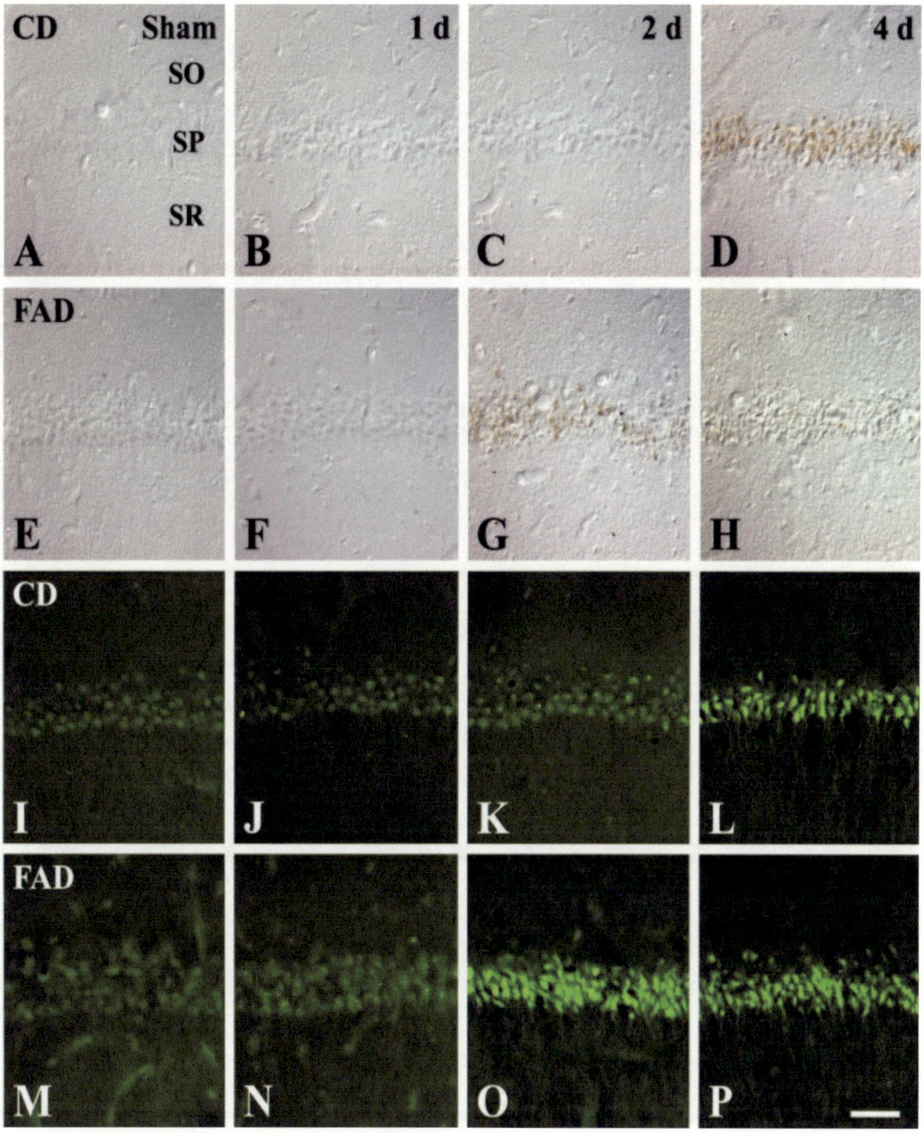

Fig. 2. TUNEL and Fluoro-Jade B (F-JB) staining of the CA1 region in the sham-operated (A,E,I,M) and ischemia-operated groups 1 days (B,F,J,N), 2 days (C,G,K,O), and 4 days (D,H,L,P) after ischemia/reperfusion and feeding with a folic acid-deficient or control diet. Two days after ischemia/reperfusion, TUNEL- or F-JBpositive pyramidal neurons are observed in stratum pyramidale (SP) of the folate-deficient diet-treated group. Four days after ischemia-reperfusion, TUNEL or F-JB reaction decreases in pyramidal neurons in the SP of the folate-deficient diet-treated group. SO, stratum oriens; SR, stratum radiatum.

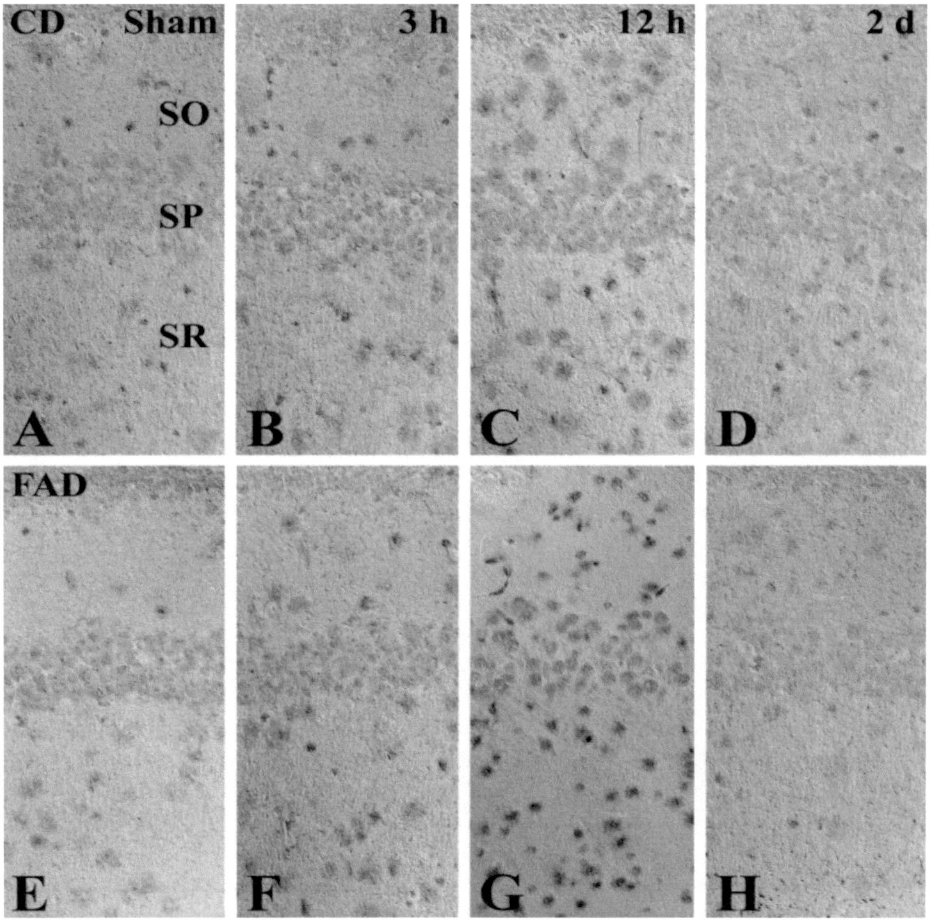

Fig. 3. Immunohistochemistry for 8-hydroxy-deoxyguanosine in the CA1 region in the control diet- and folate deficient diet-sham(A,E) and ischemia-operated groups at 3 hr (B,F), 12 hr (C,G), and 2 days (D,H) after ischemia/reperfusion. At 12 hr after ischemic insult, 8- hydroxy-deoxyguanosine immunoreactivity in both groups is highest in CA1 (C,G), showing more dense immunoreactivity in folate-deficient diet- than in the control diet-group. Two days after ischemia/reperfusion, 8- hydroxy-deoxyguanosine immunoreactivity in folate-deficient diet-group is much lower than that in control diet-group (D,H). SP, stratum pyramidale; SO, stratum oriens; SR, stratum radiatum.

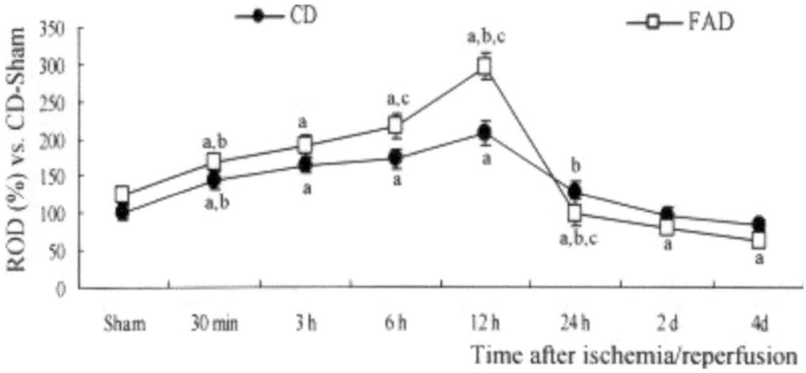

Fig. 4. Relative optical density (ROD) as percentage of 8-hydroxy-deoxyguanosine immunoreactivity in the CA1 region after transient ischemia (n= 5-7 per group; aP < 0.05 significantly different from the control diet- or folate-deficient diet-fed sham-operated group, bP < 0.05 significantly different from the control diet- or folate-deficient diet-treated preadjacent group, cP < 0.05 between the control diet- and the folate deficient diet-groups). Bars indicate means ± SEM.

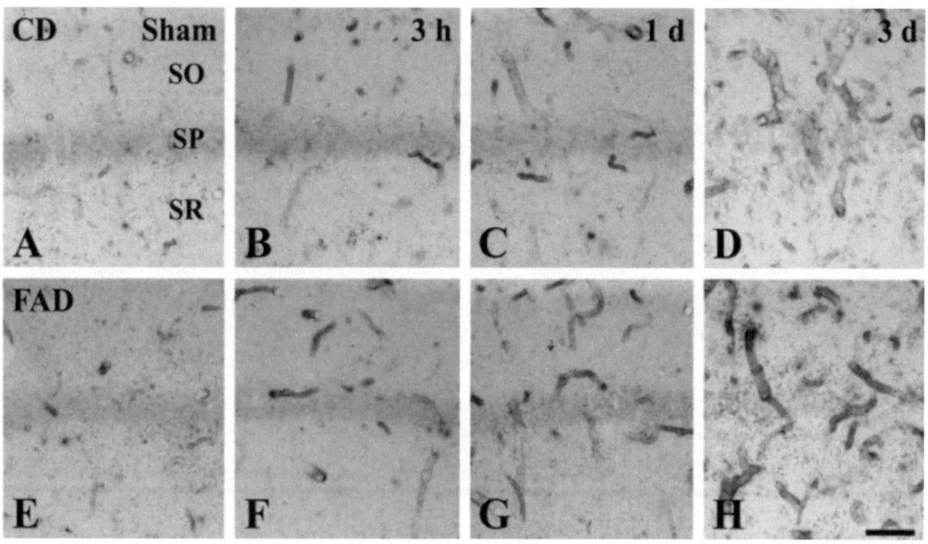

Fig. 5. Immunohistochemistry for platelet endothelial cell adhesion molecule-1 (PECAM-1) in the CA1 region in sham-operated (A,E) and in ischemia-operated groups at 3 hr (B,F), 1 day (C,G), and 3 days (D,H) after ischemia/reperfusion in control diet- and folate-deficient diet-groups. In control diet-(A) and folate-deficient diet -sham-operated (E) groups, weak PECAM-1 immunoreactivity is detected in microvessels. Three days after ischemia /reperfusion, PECAM-1 immunoreactivity in both groups increased significantly (G,H); the immunoreactivity in folate deficient diet-group is higher than that in control diet-group. SP, stratum pyramidale; SO, stratum oriens; SR, stratum radiatum.

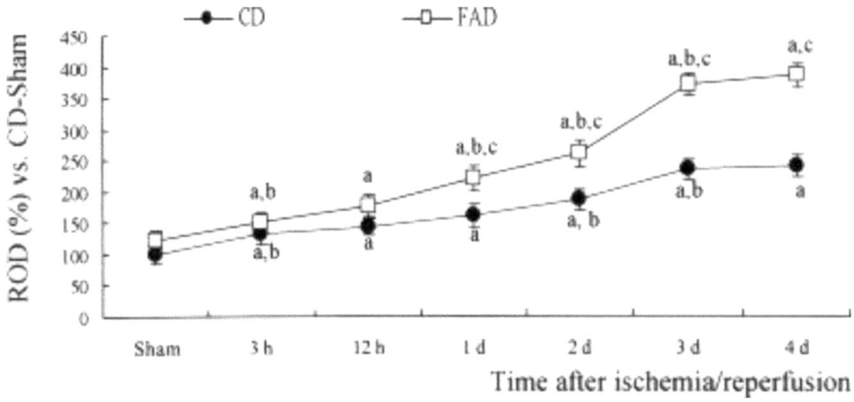

Fig. 6. Relative optical density (ROD) as percentage of PECAM-1 immunoreactivity in the CA1 region after transient ischemia (n 5 7 per group; aP < 0.05 significantly different from the control diet- or folate deficient diet treated sham-operated group, bP < 0.05 significantly different from the CD- or folate-deficient diet-treated preadjacent group, cP < 0.05 between the control diet- and the folate-deficient diet-treated groups). Bars indicate means ± SEM.

3.5 Reactive gliosis

Significant morphological changes were observed in glial cells in the CA1 region in the CD- and FAD-groups after ischemia/reperfusion. This change began 2 days after ischemia/reperfusion (Figs. 7).

Astrocytes. In the FAD-sham-operated group, weak GFAP immunoreactivity was detected in the CA1 region as in the CD-group (Fig. 7A, 7E). GFAP immunoreactive astrocytes had thin processes. Two days after ischemia/reperfusion, many astrocytes showed morphological changes in both groups (Fig. 7B, 7F), although at this time many more astrocytes in the FAD-treated group showed hypertrophied processes. Three days after ischemia/reperfusion, GFAP immunoreactive astrocytes in the FAD-treated group showed punctuated cytoplasm, whereas in the CD-group the cytoplasm of GFAP immunoreactive astrocytes was hypertrophied (Fig. 7C, 7G). Four days after ischemia/reperfusion, the processes of GFAP-immunoreactive astrocytes became hypertrophied, and the number and immunoreactivity in GFAP-immunoreactive astrocytes in the FAD-group were higher in the CD-group (Figs. 7D, 7H).

Microglia. Iba-1 immunoreactivity in the FAD-sham-operated group was similar to that in the CD-sham-operated group (Figs. 7I, 7M). Microglia in the CD-group were activated 2 days after ischemia/reperfusion, and many activated microglia in the FAD-group had aggregated to the stratum pyramidale, in which pyramidal neurons showed delayed neuronal death (Fig. 7J, 7N). Three days after ischemia/reperfusion, Iba-1 immunoreactive microglia in the FAD-group were concentrated in the stratum pyramidale of the CA1 region (Fig. 7O), whereas in the CD-group Iba-1 immunoreactive microglia were dispersed in CA1 (Fig. 7K). Four days after ischemia/reperfusion, microgliosis in the FAD-group was severer than in the CD-group (Figs. 7L, 7P).

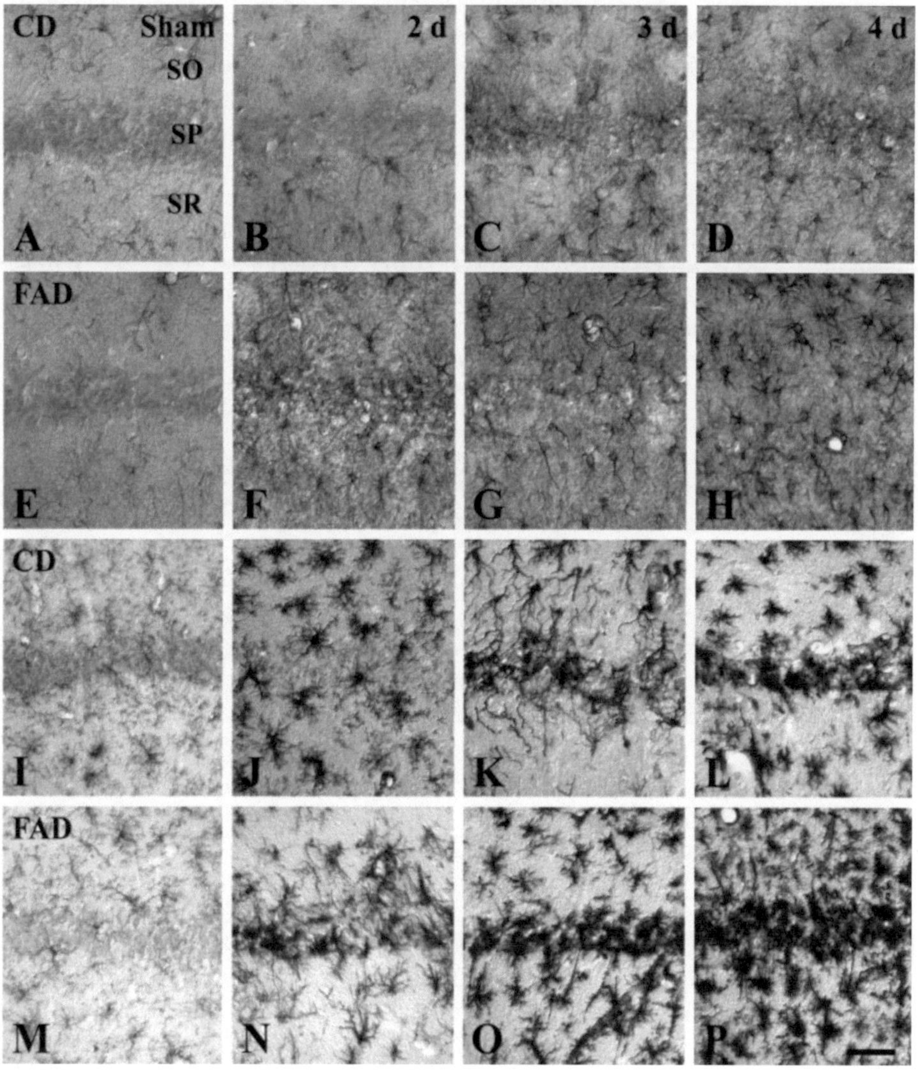

Fig. 7. Immunohistochemistry for GFAP representing astrocytes and Iba-1 representing microglia in the CA1 region in sham-operated (A,E,I,M) and ischemia-operated groups 2 days (B,F,J,N), 3 days (C,G,K,O), and 4 days (D,H,L,P) after ischemia/reperfusion and feeding with folate-deficient diet or control diet. GFAP immunoreactivity-punctuated astrocytes in folate-deficient diet-group are detected 3 days after ischemia/reperfusion, whereas, in control diet-group, they are detected 4 days after ischemia/reperfusion. An increase of Iba-1-immunoreactive microglia is noted 3 days after ischemia/reperfusion in the stratum pyramidale of folate-deficient diet -group, whereas, in control diet-group, Iba-1-immunoreactive microglia is markedly increased 4 days after ischemia/reperfusion.

4. Discussion

Folate deficiency is common condition, especially in geriatric population which is caused by environmental and genetic factor. The genetic variant of methylenetetrahydrofolate reductase is very common (10-15%). Moderate hyperhomocysteinemia (15-30 μmol/L) is very common condition which is linked to increased risk of artherothrombotic vascular disease (Yoo et al). Low dietary intake of folic acid is associated with increased homocysteine levels and an increased risk of heart disease and stroke (Giles et al., 1995; hankey GJ et al, 2001). Homocysteine has direct effects on the endothelium (Wall et al,1980; Kamath et al., 2006; Lominadze et al., 2006) and astrocytes (Kranich et al., 1998), which are mediate signaling between endothelium and neurons (Nedergaard et al., 2003). In addition, the treatment of folic acid with vitamin B_{12} and B_6 improves the blood-brain barrier function in human (Lehmann et al., 2003). Among the hypoxic brain damage, most sensitive are the pyramidal neurons in the CA1 region of the hippocampus. In experimental animal, transient forebrain ischemia, which temporarily deprives the brain of glucose as well as oxygen, results in the insidious delayed degeneration of specific vulnerable neurons within the CA1 region of the hippocampus (Kirino, 1982; Pulsinelli et al., 1982).

In FAD-group, cresyl violet or NeuN positive neurons began to decrease day 2 after ischemia/reperfusion, while in CD-group, cresyl violet or NeuN positive neurons began to decrease day 3 after ischemia/reperfusion. Delayed neuronal death of CA1 pyramidal neurons in the CD-groups occurred day 4 after ischemia/reperfusion, whereas in the FAD-group, delayed neuronal death in CA1 pyramidal neurons occurred day 3 after ischemia/reperfusion. In addition, CA1 pyramidal neurons in the FAD-group showed TUNEL or F-J B staining representing neurodegeneration day 2 after ischemia/reperfusion. This is the first report that neuronal damage in the ischemic CA1 region is accelerated by folate deficiency.

4.1 Excitotoxicity of homocysteine

Homocysteine is easily carried into neuronal cells via a specific membrane transporter, leading to high intracellular homocysteine concentrations (Grieve et al., 1992). It has been shown that homocysteine and its metabolic derivatives activate both group I metabotropic glutamate receptors (mGluR) (Dalton et al, 1997) and NMDA receptors (Pullan et al., 1987), suggesting the role of homocysteine-induced excitotoxicity. Homocysteine can play as an endogenous glutamate receptor agonist (Lipton et al, 1997; Do et al, 1986; Ito et al, 1991) by activating on N-methyl-D-aspartate(NMDA) receptor subtype. The oxidative product of homocysteine, homocysteic acid, can functions as an excitatory neurotransmitter by activating NMDA receptor (Olney et al, 1987) The neurotoxicity of homocysteic acid in the brain can be partially abrogated by using a NMDA antagonist, suggesting a role for agonistic function (Olney et al, 1987; Kim et al, 1987).

Depending on glycine concentration, homocysteine showed dual response. In the condition of low glycine, homocysteine acts as a antagonist of the glycine site of the NMDA receptor, resulting in neuroprotective function. However, in the situation of high glycine levels after brain ischemia, homocysteine can bind and activate NMDA receptor, leading to excitotoxic damage (Lipton et al, 1997). These actions suggest that folate deficiency accompanied by hyperhomocysteinemia may contribute to the early brain damage after ischemia.

In addition, homocysteine has been reported to induce an extra-cellular signal regulated kinase in the hippocampus(Robert et al, 2005). Homocysteine also activates group I metabotropic glutamate receptors (mGluRl), leading to activation of protein kinase C and increased intracellular IP_3 formation, increasing the intracellular calcium ion, especially in endoplasmic reticulum (Dalton et al, 1997).

4.2 Homocysteine and apoptosis pathway

Homocysteine-induced ROS generation enhances the activation of NF-kB (Chern et al., 2001). NF-kB is one of the transcriptional factors that can be controlled by the cellular redox status. NF-kB plays a role in the control of oxidative stress-mediated apoptosis. In the oxidative conditions, neuronal cell death derives from excessive calcium influx and ROS leading to excitotoxicity. In a transient middle cerebral artery occlusion experiment, increased DNA binding was detected after reperfusion following 2 hour ischemia (Schneider et al., 1999), suggesting the activation of NF-kB. Increased transcriptional activity of NF-kB has been identified in mouse models of both permanent and transient cerebral ischemia using kB-dependent β-globin reporter gene assay (Schneider et al., 1999). NF-kB target genes include proinflammatory cytokines shown to be expressed in cerebral ischemia. TNF, IL-6, inducible nitric oxide synthase, intercellular adhesion molecule 1 (ICAM-1), and matrix metallopeptidase (MMP) 9 are major players in the post-ischemic inflammation of brain (Wang et al., 2007; Gilmore, 2008). IL-1 is another possible inducer of NF-kB activity in the ischemic brain (Kunz et al., 2008). Both IL-1α and IL-1β are rapidly induced in cerebral ischemia (Allan et al., 2005).

4.3 Hyperhomocysteinemia and hypercoagulable state of blood

The mechanism by which hyperhomocysteinemia can cause the hypercoagulable state of blood and an increased risk of thrombosis has poorly established. There have been growing evidences from the various aspects. In vitro study of cultured cells showed a toxic effect of homocysteine on endothelial cell viability (Wall, 1980). Cultured endothelial cells under high concentration of homocysteine were not viable with copper that led to the oxidation of homocysteine, concomitant with hydrogen peroxide generation (Starkebaum and Harlan, 1986). Homocysteine inhibited the synthesis of prostacyclin, a potent inhibitor of platelets in cultured cells (Wang,1993). In vitro studies have shown that high concentration of homocysteine promote blood clotting cascade. Homocysteine activated factor V on cultured endothelial cells (Rodgers and Kane, 1986) and inhibited protein C activation in cultured endothelial cells (Rodgers, 1990). At concentrations greater than 5mmol/L, homocysteine inhibited thrombomodulin surface expression (thrombomodulin promote activation of the anticoagulant protein C and inhibit procoagulant activity of thrombin) (Lentz , 1991). Homocysteine blocked tissue-type plasminogen activiator in endothelial cells (Hajjar, 1993). Homocysteine increased platelet adhesion (Blann, 1992), and induced tissue factor (Fryer, 1993), and suppressed anticoagulant, heparan sulfate expression (Nishinaga, 1993). It has been documented that homocysteine level as low as 8 micromol/L increased affinity of lipoprotein(a) for plasmin modified fibrin surfaces, inhibiting plasminogen activation (Harpel, 1992). In vivo studies showed an abnormally increased biosynthesis of thromboxane A2 in patients with CBS deficiency (Di Minno, 1993), and endothelial dysfunction (Lentz, 1996). It have been reported that impaired regulation of endothelium-de-rived relaxing factor & nitrogen oxides (Stamler, 1993) and oxidation of low-density lipoprotein in vitro (Pathasarathy, 1987). Folate deficiency may contribute the development of atherothrombogenic condition. In the rat model, dietary folate deficiency, a major cause

of hyperhomocysteinemia, was associated with 20-fold enhanced macrophage-derived tissue factor activity and increased ADP- and thrombin-induced platelet aggregation (Durand et al, 1996). In vitro endothelial cell study, cell treated with homocysteine showed a significant decrease in glutathione peroxidase transcription and activity, suggesting the impairment of endothelial ability to detoxify oxidative stress and leading to attenuation of bioavailable nitric oxide, a potent anti-thrombotic factor (Upchurch, 1997)
Recent oligo-array technology data validated by real time reverse transcriptase-polymerase chain reaction showed the changed gene expression in animal fed folate deficient diet, suffering from hyperhomocystinemia. Folate deficiency upregulate integrin beta-3, Rap1b, glycoprotein V, platelet-endothelial cell adhesion molecule-1(PECAM-1) and von Willebrand factor, leading to platelet activation and aggregation. In addition, upregulation of coagulation factor XIIIa, plasminogen activator inhibitor-1, and down regulation of tissue-type plasminogen activator were observed (Ebbesen LS et al, 2006).

4.4 Oxidative stress and neurotoxicity in hyperhomocysteinemia and folate deficiency

The highly reactive sulfhydryl group in the homocysteine is readily oxidized to generate reactive oxygen species (Starkebaum and Harlan, 1986), suggesting that homocysteine can cause cell injury through a mechanism involving oxidative damage. The oxidative stress has been noted that hyperhomocysteinemia and folate deficiency induces or potentiates the toxic effects on the neuronal cells in vivo or in vitro. In early study, Wall et al.(1980) showed homocysteine oxidation is related to hydrogen peroxide generation. In human neuroblastoma cells cultured in folate-deprived media, oxidative stress played a role for homocysteine toxicity in neuronal cells (Ho et al, 2003). The cytotoxicity of homocysteine was compromised by antioxidants including N-acetyl cysteine, vitamin E or C (Reis et al, 2002; Wyse et al, 2002). Antoxidants vitamin including vitamin E or C prevented memory dysfunction induced by homocysteine administration in the rats (Reis et al, 2002) and the reduction of Na-K ATPase activity caused by hyperhomocyeteinemia in rats(Wyse et al, 2002). Folate deficiency decreased the proliferating cells in the dentate gyrus of adult mice hippocampus (Kruman et al, 2005). Folate deprivation led to pronounced hyperhomocysteinemia and reactive oxygen species. Folate deficient condition increased amyloid-beta-induced apoptosis, while high level of folate supplementation abrogated the reactive oxygen species generation by amyloid-beta(Ho et al, 2003). Folate deprivation in neuroblastoma cells showed an increased immunoreactivity of phospho-tau (Ho et al, 2003).
In apolipoprotein E-deficient mice, iron challenge increased oxidative stress in folate deprived animals, but not in vitamin E. Oxidative damage can be mitigated by folate supplementation by reducing intracellular superoxide generation or scavenging hydrogen peroxide. (Shea and Rogers, 2002). In primary culture of rat cerebellar granular cells, homocysteine neurotoxicity was partially prevented by NMDA receptor antagonist. Homocysteine-induced neuronal death was effectively blocked by the combination of catalase and superoxide dismutase or catalase alone. These findings support that the homocysteine-induced neurotoxicity is based on the oxidative stress and excitotoxicity(Kim and Pae, 1996).
A number of evidence supports the roles of DNA damage and apoptosis in the pathogenesis of several neurodegenerative disorders, including cerebral ischemia (Liu et al., 1996; Won et al., 1999, 2001; Bazan, 2005). In the present study, 8-hydroxy-deoxyguanosine immunoreactivity in the CA1 region in FAD-group increased in advance of that in CD-group, and its peak level was noted at 12 hour after ischemia/reperfusion, which was more

pronounced in FAD-group. This result indicates that CA1 neurons in folate deficient condition are more vulnerable to ischemic DNA damage.

Endres et al. (2005) reported that cerebral lesion volumes after ischemia and 72-hour reperfusion were significantly increased by 2.1-fold in folic acid-deficient 129/SV wild-type mice versus controls on a normal diet, and this could not be explained by obvious differences in physiological parameters. They also reported that abasic sites, a marker of oxidative DNA damage, are significantly increased in DNA from the ischemic brains of folate-deficient 129/SV wild-type mice at early time points after MCA occlusion than control mice (Endres et al., 2005). These are supported by those of previous studies which found that folate deficiency in humans induces extensive chromosome damage, fragile site expression, micronucleus formation, and increased uracil levels in bone marrow cell DNA (Blount et al., 1997; Crott et al., 2001). The misincorporation of uracil appears to be a key event in the neurotoxicity associated with folate deficiency, because the pretreatment of culture medium with thymidine and hypoxanthine (precursors of purines) reduces neuronal cell death induced by methyl donor deficiency (Blount et al., 1997). Folate deficiency could cause the misincorporation of uracil into the DNA of proliferating cells caused by the impairment of deoxynucleoside triphosphate pools (Pogribny et al., 1997; Mol et al., 1999). In addition, homocysteine is rapidly taken up by neurons via a specific membrane transporter. Increased levels of homocysteine in cell nuclei may induce DNA strand breaks by disturbing the DNA methylation cycle (Blount et al., 1997) or may promote DNA damage accumulation in neurons by impairing DNA repair (Kruman et al., 2002).

4.5 Folate deficiency and platelet endothelial cell adhesion molecule-1

Adhesion and trans-endothelial migration of leucocytes play a significant roles in the pathophysiologic events in brain inflammation after stroke. Platelet endothelial cell adhesion molecule-1 (PECAM-1, CD31) is a 130-kDa protein member of the immunoglobulin gene superfamily, which is expressed on the surface of platelets, monocytes, neutrophils, selected T cell subsets and on endothelial cell intercellular junctions (Newman, 1997). Expression levels of PECAM-1 differ in the type of organ tissues. It is highly expressed in kidney, lung, and trachea, while its level is at lower in brain, heart and liver. But, fibroblasts, epithelial cells, muscle, nonvascular cells or red blood cells do not express it.(Newman, 1997; Wang, 2003).

Muller et al. (1993) showed for the first time that monocytes or neutrophils treated with the specific antibodies for PECAM-1 blocked transmigration across the endothelial monolayer in vitro assay. Blocking endothelial cell junctional PECAM-1 also inhibited leukocyte transmigration, indicating that PECAM-1 molecules on both the endothelial cell as well as the leukocyte side contributed to the transmigration process. Most of PECAM in endothelium is distributed in the intercellular junctions, and 15% is on the exposed apical surface. Qing et al(2001) found that anti-PECAM-1 antibody or PECAM-Ig chimeric molecule injection blocked the T cell trafficking into the CNS in TCR transgenic mice during inflammation. Rosenblum et al.(1994) demonstrated that anti-CD31 mAb injection before the damage of endothelium in pial arteriole of mouse doubled the platelet aggregation time. Vaporciyan et al. (1993) also showed that antibody to human PECAM-1 could block in vivo accumulation of rat neutrophils into the peritoneal cavity and the alveolar compartment of the lung. These results suggest that PECAM-1 plays a key role in the transendothelial migration of leukocytes in the process of inflammation. Gumina et al.(1996) showed that antibodies to PECAM-1 reduce myocardial infarct size in both rat. and Murohara et al(1996) showed blockade of platelet endothelial cell adhesion molecule-1 protects against myocardial ischemia and reperfusion injury in cats.

Brain ischaemia eventually enhances local inflammatory reaction. Accumulated leucocytes adhere to endothelium, probably leading to the microvasculature occlusion (Schmid-Schonbein, 1987; del Zoppo et al, 1991). Hwang et al. (2005b) demonstrated that transient ischaemia in gerbils results in a significant increase of PECAM-1 immunoreactivity in the hippocampus. PECAM-1 expression was particularly prominent in the vulnerable neurons of the hippoccampal CA1 region. PECAM-1 immunoreactivity was significantly increased by 4 days after ischaema. In addition, serum sPECAM-1 levels in ischemic group were higher than those of sham group. Zaremba and Losy (2002). reported that sPECAM-1 increases significantly in serum and in CSF in patients within 24 h after ischaemic stroke, compared with control group. In addition, serum and CSF sPECAM-1 levels within 24 h after ischaemic stroke correlated to volume of early brain CT hypodense areas, indicating the cerebral hypoperfusion. This suggests that PECAM-1 may be involved in inflammatory response mediated extent of early ischaemic brain damage. Also, sPECAM-1 levels within 24 h and at second week after ischaemic stroke correlated positively with neurological stroke severity, and with the degree of functional disability within 24 h of stroke and at second week after the incident. Therefore, initial sPECAM-1 might be of predictive value for the short-term outcome of stroke (Zaremba and Losy, 2002b).

O'Brien et al(2003) demonstrated that PECAM-1 mediates neutrophil migration through IL-1 beta stimulated endothelial cells. It has shown that hyperhomocysteinemia at moderate level activates human monocyte and induces cytokine expression including tumor necrosis alpha, IL-1 beta, IL-6, IL-8, and IL-12 (Su et al, 2005). In this experiment, PECAM-1 immunoreactivity in the CA1 region was higher in folate deficient group than in the controls. This result suggests that folate deficiency and elevated homocysteine can enhance inflammatory response in post ischemic condition through NF-kB activation. Increased gliosis in folate deficient group may be due to elevations of PECAM-1 immunoreactivity and of its protein level in vessels, inducing the transmigration of lymphocytes and neutrophils (Michiels et al., 1998; Dangerfield et al., 2002; Hwang et al., 2005b).

In summary, folate deficiency was found to induce early and significant neuronal death and gliosis in CA1 with concomitant oxidative DNA damage. These findings suggest that folate deficiency accelerate the pathological neuronal loss and inflammation that are activated after the onset of transient cerebral mild ischemia.

5. Acknowledgements

The author wish to thank Hwang IK, Yoo KY, Suh HW, Kim YS, Kwon DY, Kwon YG, and Won MH for excellent technical work. This work was supported by BioFoods Project in Korea Biotechnology Research Plan under the Ministry of Science and Technology of the Korea Government; Contract grant number: M10510120004-05N1012-00411; MRC program of MOST/KOSEF; R13-2005-022-01002-0; Samsung Biomedical Research Institute; CA5-220-1.

6. References

Allan SM, Tyrrell PJ, Rothwell NJ. (2005). Interleukin-1 and neuronal injury. Nat Rev Immunol 5:629-640.

Baik SC, Youn HS, Chung MH, Lee WK, Cho MJ, Ko GH, Park CK, Kasai H, Rhee KH. (1996). Increased oxidative DNA damage in Helicobacter pylori-infected human gastric mucosa. Cancer Res 56: 1279-1282.

Bazan NG. (2005). Lipid signaling in neural plasticity, brain repair, and neuroprotection. Mol Neurobiol 32:89-103.

Blann AD: Endothelial cell damage and homocysteine. (1992). Atherosclerosis 94:89.

Bleich S, Degner D, Sperling W, Bönsch D, Thürauf N, Kornhuber J. (2004). Homocysteine as a neurotoxin in chronic alcoholism. Prog Neuropsychopharmacol Biol Psychiatry 28(3):453-64.

Blount BC, Mack MM, Wehr CM, MacGregor JT, Hiatt RA, Wang G, Wickramasinghe SN, Everson RB, Ames BN. (1997). Folate deficiency causes uracil misincorporation into human DNA and chromosome breakage: implications for cancer and neuronal damage. Proc Natl Acad Sci USA 94: 3290-3295.

Brouns R, De Deyn PP. (2009). The complexity of neurobiological processes in acute ischemic stroke. Clin Neurol Neurosurg 111(6):483-95.

Candelario-Jalil E, Alvarez D, Merino N, León OS. (2003). Delayed treatment with nimesulide reduces measures of oxidative stress following global ischemic brain injury in gerbils. Neurosci Res 47: 245-253.

Chang CM, Yu CC, Lu HT, Chou YF, Huang RF. (2007). Folate deprivation promotes mitochondrial oxidative decay: DNA large deletions, cytochrome c oxidase dysfunction, membrane depolarization and superoxide overproduction in rat liver. Br J Nutr 97(5):855-63.

Chern, C.L., Huang, R.F., Chen, Y.H., Cheng, J.T., Liu, T.Z., (2001). Folate deficiency-induced oxidative stress and apoptosis are mediated via homocysteine-dependent overproduction of hydrogen peroxide and enhanced activation of NF-kappa B in human Hep G2 cells. Biomed. Pharmacother 55, 434-442.

Crott JW, Mashiyama ST, Ames BN, Fenech MF. (2001). Methylenetetrahydrofolate reductase C677T polymorphism does not alter folic acid deficiency-induced uracil incorporation into primary human lymphocyte DNA in vitro. Carcinogenesis 22: 1019-1025.

Dalton, M.L., Gadson Jr., P.F., Wrenn, R.W., Rosenquist, T.H., (1997). Homocysteine signal cascade: production of phospholipids, activation of protein kinase C, and the induction of c-fos and c-myb in smooth muscle cells. FASEB J 11, 703-711.

Dangerfield J, Larbi KY, Huang MT, Dewar A, Nourshargh S.(2002). PECAM-1 (CD31) homophilic interaction up-regulates $\alpha6\beta1$ on transmigrated neutrophils in vivo and plays a functional role in the ability of $\alpha6$ integrins to mediate leukocyte migration through the perivascular basement membrane. J Exp Med 196: 1201-1211.

del Zoppo GJ, Schmid-Scho¨ nbein GW, Mori E, Copeland BR, Chang CM. (1991). Polymorphonuclear leukocytes occlude capillaries following middle cerebral artery occlusion and reperfusion in baboons. Stroke 22: 1276–1283.

Di Minno G Davi'G, Margaglione M, Cirillo F, Grandone E, Ciabattoni E, Catalano I, Strisciuglio P, Andria G, Patrono C, Mancini M. (1993). Abnormally high thromboxane biosynthesis in homozygous homocystinuria. Evidence for platelet involvement and Probucol-sensitive mechanism. J Clin Invest 92:1400.

Do, K.Q., Herrling, P.L., Streit, P., Turski, W.A. and Cuenod, M. (1986). In vitro release and electrophysiological effects in situ of homocysteic acid, an endogenous N-methyl-(D)-aspartic acid agonist, in the mammalian striatum. J. Neurosci 6, 2226-2234.

Durand P, Prost M, Blache D. (1996). Prothrombotic effects of folic acid deficienct diet in rat platelets and macrophages related to elevated homocysteine and decreased n-3 polyunsaturated fatty acids. Atherosclerosis 121:231-243.

Endres M, Ahmadi M, Kruman I, Biniszkiewicz D, Meisel A, Gertz K. (2005). Folate deficiency increases postischemic brain injury. Stroke 36: 321-325.

Ebbesen LS, Olesen SH, Kruhoffer M, Ingerslev J, Orntoft TF. (2006). Folate deficiency induced hyperhomocysteinemia changes the expression of thrombosis-related genes. Blood Coagul Fibrinolysis 17:293-301.

Fenech M. (2010). Folate, DNA damage and the aging brain. Mech Ageing Dev 131(4):236-41.

Fryer RH, Wilson BD, Gubler DB, Fitzgerald LA, Fodgers GM. (1993). Homocysteine, a risk factor for premature vascular disease and thrombosis, induces tissue factor activity in endothelial cells. Arterioscler Thromb 13:1327.

Giles WH, Kittner SJ, Anda RF, Croft JB, Casper ML. (1995). Serum folate and risk for ischemic stroke. First national health and nutrition examination survey epidemiologic follow-up study. Stroke 26: 1166-1170.

Gilmore TD. (2008). Rel/NF-xB transcription factors. www.nf-kb.org.

Grieve, A., Butcher, S.P., Griffiths, R., (1992). Synaptosomal plasma membrane transport of excitatory sulphur amino acid transmitter candidates: kinetic characterization and analysis of carrier specificity. J. Neurosci. Res 32, 60-68.

Gumina, R.J., J.E. Schultz, Z. Yao, D. Kenny, D.C. Warltier, P.J. Newman, and G.J. Gross. (1996). Antibody to platelet/endothelial cell adhesion molecule-1 reduces myocardial infarct size in a rat model of ischemia-reperfusion injury. *Circulation* 15;94(12):3327-33.

Hajjar KA. (1993). Homocysteine-induced modulation of tissue plasminogen activator binding to its endothelial cell membrane receptor. *J Clin Invest* 91:2873

Hankey GJ, Eikelboom JW. (2001). Homocysteine and stroke. Curr Opin Neurol 14:95-102

Harpel PC, Chang VT, Borth W. (1992). Homocysteine and other sulfhydryl compounds enhance the binding of lipoprotein(a) to fibrin: A potential biochemical link between thrombosis, atherogenesis and sulfhydryl compounds metabolism. Proc Natl Acad Sci USA 89:10193

Ho.,P.I., Ashline, D., Dhitavat, S., Ortiz, D., Collins, S.C., Shea, T.B. and Rogers, E. (2003). Folate deprivation induces neurodegeneration: roles of oxidative stress and increased homocysteine. Neurobiol. Dis. 14, 32-42.

Hwang IK, Eum WS, Yoo KY, Cho JH, Kim DW, Choi SH, Kang TC, Kwon OS, Kang JH, Choi SY, Won MH. (2005a). Copper chaperone for Cu,Zn-SOD supplement potentiates the Cu,Zn-SOD function of neuroprotective effects against ischemic neuronal damage in the gerbil hippocampus. Free Radic Biol Med 39: 392-402.

Hwang IK, Kim DW, Yoo KY, Jung BK, Song JH, Jung JY, Choi SY, Kang TC, Lee JY, Kwon YG, Won MH. (2005b). Ischemia-induced changes of platelet endothelial cell adhesion molecule-1 in the hippocampal CA1 region in gerbils. Brain Res 1048: 251-257.

Hwang IK, Yoo KY, Li H, Lee BH, Suh HW, Kwon YG, Won MH. (2007). Aquaporin 9 changes in pyramidal cells before and is expressed in astrocytes after delayed neuronal death in the ischemic hippocampal CA1 region of the gerbil. J Neurosci Res 85: 2470-2479.

Hwang IK, Yoo K-Y, Suh H-W, Kim YS, Kwon DY, Kwon Y-G, Yoo J-H, Won M-H. (2008). Folic Acid deficiency increases delayed neuronal death, DNA damage, platelet endothelial cell adhesion molecule-1 immunoreactivity, and gliosis in the hippocampus after transient cerebral ischemia. J Neurosci Res 86:2003-2015.

Hwang SY, Woo CW, Au-Yeung KK, Siow YL, Zhu TY, O K. (2008). Homocysteine stimulates monocyte chemoattractant protein-1 expression in the kidney via nuclear factor-kappaB activation. Am J Physiol Renal Physiol. 294(1):F236-44.

Ito, S., Provini, L. and Cherubini, E. (1991). L-homocysteic acid mediates synaptic excitation at NMDA receptors in the hippocampus. Neurosci. Lett. 124, 157-161

Jin R, Yang G, Li G. (2010). Inflammatory mechanisms in ischemic stroke: role of inflammatory cells. J Leukoc Biol. 87(5):779-89.

Kamath AF, Chauhan AK, Kisucka J, Dole VS, Loscalzo J, Handy DE, Wagner DD. (2006). Elevated levels of homocysteine compromise blood-brain barrier integrity in mice. Blood 107: 591-593.

Kang SS, Wong PW. (1996) Genetic and nongenetic factors for moderate hyperhomocyst(e)inemia. Atherosclerosis. 119(2):135-8.

Kang SS, Wong PW, Malinow MR. (1992) Hyperhomocyst(e)inemia as a risk factor for occlusive vascular disease. Annu Rev Nutr. 12:279-298.

Kanwar YS, Manaligod JR, Wong PW. (1976). Morphologic studies in a patient with homocystinuria due to 5,10-methylenetetrahydrofolate reductase deficiency. Pediatr Res 10:598-609.

Kim, J.P., Koh, J.Y. and Choi, D.W. (1987). L-homocysteate is a potent neurotoxin on cultured cortical neurons. Brain Res 437, 103-110.

Kim, W.K., Pae, Y.S. (1996). Involvement of N-methyl-D-aspartate receptor and free radical in homocysteine-mediated toxicity on rat cerebellar granule cells. Neurosci. Lett. 216, 117-120.

Kirino T, Tamura A, Sano K. (1986). A reversible type of neuronal injury following ischemia in the gerbil hippocampus. Stroke 17: 455-459.

Kirino T. (1982). Delayed neuronal death in the gerbil hippocampus following ischemia. Brain Res 239: 57-69.

Kranich O, Dringen R, Sandberg M, Hamprecht B. (1998). Utilization of cysteine and cysteine precursors for the synthesis of glutathione in astroglial cultures: preference for cysteine. Glia 22: 11-18.

Kruman II, Culmsee C, Chan SL, Kruman Y, Guo Z, Penix L, Mattson MP. (2000). Homocysteine elicits a DNA damage response in neurons that promotes apoptosis and hypersensitivity to excitotoxicity. J Neurosci 20: 6920-6926.

Kruman II, Kumaravel TS, Lohani A, Pedersen WA, Cutler RG, Kruman Y, Haughey N, Lee J, Evans M, Mattson MP. (2002). Folic acid deficiency and homocysteine impair DNA repair in hippocampal neurons and sensitize them to amyloid toxicity in experimental models of Alzheimer's disease. J Neurosci 22: 1752-1762.

Kunz A, Abe T, Hochrainer K, Shimamura M, Anrather J, Racchumi G, Zhou P, ladecola C. (2008). Nuclear factor-kappaB activation and postischemic inflammation are suppressed in CD36-null mice after middle cerebral artery occlusion. J Neurosci 28:1649-1658.

Lehmann M, Regland B, Blennow K, Gottfries CG. (2003). Vitamin B_{12}-B_6-folate treatment improves blood-brain barrier function in patients with hyperhomocysteinaemia and mild cognitive impairment. Dement Geriatr Cogn Disord 16: 145-150.

Lentz SR, Sadler JE. (1991). Inhibition of thrombomodulin surface expression and protein C activation by the thrombogenic agent homocysteine. J Clin Invest 88:1906

Lentz RS, Sobey CG, Pigeors, DJ, Bhopatkar MY, Faraci FM, Faraci FM, Malinow MR, Heistad DD. (1991). Vascular dysfunction in monkeys with diet-induced hyperhomocyst(e)inemia. J Clin Invest 98:24

Lipton SA, Kim WK, Choi YB, Kumar S, D'Emilia DM, Rayudu PV, Arnelle DR, Stamler JS. (1997). Neurotoxicity associated with dual actions of homocysteine at the *N*-methyl-*D*-aspartate receptor. Proc Natl Acad Sci U S A 94: 5923-5928.

Liu PK, Hsu CY, Dizdaroglu M, Floyd RA, Kow YW, Karakaya A, Rabow LE, Cui JK. (1996). Damage, repair, and mutagenesis in nuclear genes after mouse forebrain ischemia-reperfusion. J Neurosci 16: 6795-6806.

Lominadze D, Roberts AM, Tyagi N, Moshal KS, Tyagi SC. (2006). Homocysteine causes cerebrovascular leakage in mice. Am J Physiol Heart Circ Physiol 290: H1206-H1213.

Michiels C, Arnould T, Remacle J. (1998). Role of PECAM-1 in the adherence of PMN to hypoxic endothelial cells. Cell Adhes Commun 5: 367-374.

Mol CD, Parikh SS, Putnam CD, Lo TP, Tainer JA. (1999). DNA repair mechanisms for the recognition and removal of damaged DNA bases. Annu Rev Biophys Biomol Struct 28: 101-128.

Muller, W.A., S.A. Weigl, X. Deng, and D.M. Phillips. (1993). PECAM-1 is required for transendothelial migration of leukocytes. *J. Exp. Med* 178:449-460.

Murohara, T., J.A. Delyani, S.M. Albelda, and A.M. Lefer. (1996). Blockade of platelet endothelial cell adhesion molecule-1 protects against myocardial ischemia and reperfusion injury in cats. *J. Immunol.* 156:3550–3557

Nedergaard M, Ransom B, Goldman SA. 2003. New roles for astrocytes: redefining the functional architecture of the brain. Trends Neurosci 26: 523-530.

Newman PJ. (1997). The Biology of PECAM-1. Journal of Clinical Investigation 99: 3-8.

Nishinaga M, Ozawa T, Shimada K. (1993). Homocysteine, a thrombogenic agent, suppresses anticoagulant heparin sulfate expression in cultured porcine aortic endothelial cells. J Clin Invest 92:1381

O'Brien CD, Lim P, Sun J, Albelda SM. (2003). PECAM-1-dependent neutrophil transmigration is independent of monolayer PECAM-1 signaling or localization. Blood. 101:2816 -2825.

Olney, J.W., Price, M.T., Salles, K.S., Labruyere, J., Ryerson, R., Mahan, K., Frierdich, GG. And Samson, L.(1987). L-homocysteic acid: an endogenous excitotoxic ligand of the NMDA receptor. Brain Res. Bull. 19, 597-602.

Pathasarathy S. (1987). Oxidation of low-density lipoprotein by thiol compounds leads to its recognition by the acetyl LDL receptor. Biochim Biophys Acta 917:337

Pogribny IP, Muskhelishvili L, Miller BJ, James SJ. (1997). Presence and consequence of uracil in preneoplastic DNA from folate/methyl-deficient rats. Carcinogenesis 18: 2071-2076.

Pullan, L. M., Olney, J.W., Price, M.T., Compton, R.P., Hood, W.F., Michel, J., Monahan, J.B. (1987). Excitatory amino acid receptor potency and subclass specificity of sulfur-containing amino acids. J. Neurochem. 49, 1301-1307

Pulsinelli WA, Brierley JB, Plum F. (1982). Temporal profile of neuronal damage in a model of transient forebrain ischemia. Ann Neurol 11: 491-498.

Qing Z, Sandor M, Radvany Z et al. (2001). Inhibition of antigen-specific T cell trafficking into the central nervous system via blocking PECAM1/CD31 molecule. Journal of Neuropathology and Experimental Neurology 60:798-807.

Reis, E.A., Zugno, A.I., Franzon, R., Tagliari, B., Matte, C., Lammers, M.L., Netto, C.A. and Wyse, A.T. (2002). Preteatment with vitamins E and C prevent the impairment of memory caused by homocysteine administration in rats. Metab. Brain Dis. 17, 211-217.

Robert, K., Pages, C., Ledru, A., Delabar, J., Caboche, J. and Janel, N. (2005). Regulation of extracellular signal-regulated kinase by homocysteine in hippocampus. Neuroscience 133,925-935.

Rodgers GM, Kane WH. (1986). Activation of endogenous factor V by a homocysteine-induced vascular endothelial cell activator. J Clin Invest 77:1909

Rodgers GM, Conn MT. (1990). Homocysteine, an atherogenic stimulus, reduces protein C activation by arterial and venous endothelial cells. Blood 75:895

Rosenblum WI, Murata S, Nelson GH, Werner PK, Ranken R, Harmon RC. (1994). Anti-CD31 delays platelet adhesion/aggregation at sites of endothelial injury in mouse cerebral arterioles. American Journal of Pathology 145: 33-36.

Saposnik G. (2011) The role of vitamin B in stroke prevention: a journey from observational studies to clinical trials and critique of the VITAmins TO Prevent Stroke (VITATOPS). Stroke. 42(3):838-42.

Schmid-Schonbein GW. (1987). Capillary plugging by granulocytes and the no-reflow phenomenon in the microcirculation. Federation Proceedings 46: 2379–2401.

Schmued LC, Hopkins K.J. (2000). Fluoro-Jade B: a high affinity fluorescent marker for the localization of neuronal degeneration. Brain Res 874: 123-130.

Schneider A, Martin-Villalba A, Weih F, Vogel J, Wirth T, Schwaninger M. (1999). NF-$_k$B is activated and promotes cell death in focal cerebral ischemia. Nat Med 5:554-559.

Shea, T.B., Rogers, E. (2002). Folate quenches oxidative damage in brains of aploipoprotein E-deficient mice: augmentation by vitamin E. Brain Res Mol Brain Res. 108:1-6.

Stamler JS, Osborne JA, Jaraki M, Rabbini LE, Mullins M, Singel D, Loscalzo J. (1993). Adverse vascular effects of homocysteine are modulated by endothelium-derived relaxing factor and related oxides of nitrogen. J Clin Invest 91:308

Starkebaum G, Harlan JM. (1986). Endothelial cell injury die to dopper-catalyzed hydrogen peroxide generation form homocysteine. J Clin Invest 77:1370

Starkebaum G, Harlan JM. (1986). Endothelial cell injury die to dopper-catalyzed hydrogen peroxide generation form homocysteine. J Clim Invest 77:1370

Su SJ, Huang LW, Pai LS, Liu HW, Chang KL. (2005). Homocysteine at pathophysiologic concentrations activates human monocyte and induces cytokine expression and inhibits macrophage migration inhibitory factor expression. Nutrition 21:994-1002.

Upchurch, G.R., Welch, G.N., Fabian, A.J., Freedman, J.E., Johnson, J.E., Keaney, J.F. Jr, Loscalzo, J. (1997). Homocysteine decreases bioavail-able nitric oxide by a mechanism involving glutathione peroxidase. J. Biol, Chem. 272, 17012-17017.

Vaporciyan AA, DeLisser HM, Yan HC et al. (1993). Involvement of platelet-endothelial cell adhesion molecule-1 in neutrophil recruitment in vivo. Science 262: 1580-1582.

Wall RT, Harlan JM, Harker LA, Striker GE. (1980). Homocysteine-induced endothelial cell injury in vitro: A model for the study of vascular injury. Thromb Res 18:113

Wang J, Dudman NPB, Wilcken DE. (1993). Effects of homocys-teine and related compounds on prostacyclin production by cultured human vascular endothelial cells. Thromb Haemost 6:1047

Wang Q, Tang XN, Yenari MA. (2007). The inflammatory response in stroke. J Neuroimmunol 184:53-68.

Wang Q, Sun AY, Simonyi A, Jensen MD, Shelat PB, Rottinghaus GE, MacDonald RS, Miller DK, Lubahn DE, Weisman GA, Sun GY. (2005). Neuroprotective mechanisms of curcumin against cerebral ischemia-induced neuronal apoptosis and behavioral deficits. J Neurosci Res 82:138-148.

Wang Y, Su X, Sorenson CM, Sheibani N. (2003). Tissue-specific distributions of alternatively spliced human PECAM-1 isoforms. American Journal of Physiology. Heart and Circulatory Physiology 284: H1008-H1017.

Won MH, Kang TC, Jeon GS, Lee JC, Kim DY, Choi EM, Lee KH, Choi CD, Chung MH, Cho SS. (1999). Immunohistochemical detection of oxidative DNA damage induced by ischemia-reperfusion insults in gerbil hippocampus in vivo. Brain Res 836: 70-78.

Won MH, Kang TC, Park SK, Jeon GS, Kim Y, Seo JH, Choi E, Chung MH, Cho SS. (2001). The alterations of *N*-methyl-*D*-aspartate receptor expressions and oxidative DNA damage in the CA1 area at the early time after ischemia-reperfusion insult. Neurosci Lett 301: 139-142.

Woo CW, Siow YL, O K. (2008). Homocysteine induces monocyte chemoattractant protein-1 expression in hepatocytes mediated via activator protein-1 activation. J Biol Chem 283(3):1282-92

Wyse, A.T., Zugno, A.I., Streck, E. L., Matte, C., Calcagnotto, T., Wannmacher, C.M. and Wajner, M. (2002). Inhibition of Na (+), K(+)-ATPase activity in hippocampus of rats subjected to acute administration of homocysteine is prevented by vitamins E and C treatment. Neurochem. Res 27, 1685-1689.

Yoo JH, Chung CS, Kang SS. (1998). Relation of plasma homocyst(e)ine to cerebral infarction and cerebral atherosclerosis. Stroke 29: 2478-2483.

Yoo JH, Park JE, Hong KP, Lee SH, Kim DK, Lee WR, Park SC. (1999). Moderate hyperhomocyst(e)inemia is associated with the presence of coronary artery disease and the severity of coronary atherosclerosis in Koreans. Thromb Res 94: 45-52.

Yoo JH, Park SC. (2000). Low plasma folate in combination with the 677 C to T methylenetetrahydrofolate reductase polymorphism is associated with increased risk of coronary artery disease in Koreans. Thromb Res 97: 77-84.

Yoo JH, Choi GD, Kang SS. (2000). Pathogenicity of thermolabile methylenetetrahydrofolate reductase for vascular dementia. Arterioscler Thromb Vasc Biol 20:1921-1925.

Yoo JH, Lee SC. (2001). Elevated levels of plasma homocyst(e)ine and asymmetric dimethylarginine in elderly patients with stroke. Atherosclerosis 158:425-430.

Zaremba J, Losy J. (2002). sPECAM-1 in serum and CSF of acute ischaemic stroke patients. Acta Neurologica Scandinavica 106: 292–298.

Zaremba J, Losy J. (2002). Soluble platelet endothelial cell adhesion molecule-1 in ischaemic stroke patients is related to the extent of early brain damage. Central-European Journal of Immunology 27: 90–96.

9

Glial Cells, Inflammation and Heat Shock Proteins in Cerebral Ischemia

Vivianne L. Tawfik, Robin E. White and Rona Giffard
Department of Anesthesia, Stanford University School of Medicine, Stanford, CA USA

1. Introduction

Each year approximately 795,000 people in the United States suffer a new or recurrent stroke and it is the third leading cause of death after heart disease and cancer (Lloyd-Jones et al., 2010). The estimated cost of stroke was $73.7 billion nationwide in 2010, the majority of which was related to payments for inpatient care and rehabilitation for significant morbidity (hemiparesis, aphasia and loss of independence). Stroke is broadly divided into two categories: ischemic and hemorrhagic. The former is related to too little blood supplied to the brain, secondary to thrombus or embolus, and the latter results from excess blood escaping into the cranial cavity. Ischemic brain injury represents conditions including focal ischemia, with subsequent loss of blood flow and nutrients to one area of the brain, and global ischemia, as seen in cardiopulmonary arrest and resuscitation which, when brief, results specifically in neuronal death in the CA1 region of the hippocampus (Pulsinelli, 1985). In either case, decreased cerebral blood flow initiates a cascade of ATP depletion, ion gradient disruption, excessive glutamate release, formation of reactive oxygen species and increased lactic acidosis that leads to neuronal death (Doyle et al., 2008). To date, the only FDA-approved treatment for focal ischemic stroke is recombinant tissue plasminogen activator which aims to restore blood flow by recanalization of the occluded vessel (The National Institute of Neurological Disorders and Stroke rt-PA Stroke Study Group, 1995). In global ischemia, multiple clinical trials have demonstrated that therapeutic hypothermia increases survival and improves neurologic outcome (Bernard et al., 2002; Sahota and Savitz, 2011; The Hypothermia after Cardiac Arrest Study Group, 2002). Though the exact mechanisms remain unclear, effects on several different pathways have been observed. In spite of this one treatment modality, survival to hospital discharge after cardiac arrest and attempted resuscitation remains a dismal 5-18% depending on the cause and rapidity of the response (de Vreede-Swagemakers et al., 1997; Eckstein et al., 2005).

To date, more than one hundred potential pharmacological strategies for stroke have failed to show improved outcome in phase III trials. As such, the role of central nervous system glial cells has recently come under scrutiny as work focused on neurons alone has failed to reverse neuronal death in ischemic areas of the brain. Glial cells (microglia, astrocytes and oligodendrocytes) constitute over 70% of the total cell population in the CNS and are active contributors to neuromodulatory, neurotrophic and neuroimmune events in the brain and spinal cord (Pellerin, 2005; Reichenbach and Wolburg, 2005). Once thought of merely as neuronal support cells, astrocytes and microglia, in their physiologic role, dynamically control synaptic function and neuronal activity by performing a variety of crucial functions. Microglia, the intrinsic macrophages of the CNS, provide immune surveillance against invading pathogens or nervous system insults (Aloisi, 2001) while astrocytes regulate synaptic glutamate levels, contribute to the blood-brain-barrier and supply neuronal growth factors (Liberto et al., 2004). Given their complex involvement in normal CNS function, glial cells must be considered in any strategy focused on neuronal preservation after ischemic injury.

Heat shock proteins (HSP) are a phylogenetically conserved group of chaperones that assist in ATP-dependent protein folding, translocation across membranes, suppression of protein aggregation, presentation of substrates for degradation and modulate a host of other intracellular processes (Hartl, 1996). The 70 kDa heat shock protein family (HSP70) is the most extensively studied group of chaperones and consists of at least twelve constitutive and inducible proteins which aid in a coordinated response to cellular stressors. The most important members include: the constitutively expressed primarily cytosolic Hsc70/Hsp73, the heat inducible cytosolic form Hsp70/72, the glucose regulated mitochondrial protein Grp75/mortalin/mtHsp70 and the endoplasmic reticulum glucose regulated protein Grp78/BiP. The HSP70s are structurally comprised of a 44 kDa amino-terminal ATPase domain, 18 kDa carboxyl-terminal substrate-binding domain and a more variable 10 kDa segment that terminates in the highly conserved EEVD sequence that regulates intramolecular interactions and ATPase activity (Freeman et al., 1995). Our laboratory has demonstrated that the carboxyl-terminal domain of Hsp72 is sufficient to protect astrocytes from oxygen-glucose deprivation and decrease infarct volume after transient middle cerebral artery occlusion (MCAO) (Sun et al., 2006b).

Extensive work using overexpression and knockout of HSP70 family members has highlighted integral cytoprotective, anti-apoptotic and immune regulatory roles for these proteins. Induction of Hsp70/72 by heat stress or targeted overexpression in multiple experimental disease models including stroke (Rajdev et al., 2000), sepsis (Ryan et al., 1992), renal injury (Jo et al., 2006) and acute lung injury (Villar et al., 1994) demonstrated decreased organ injury and enhanced survival. Lee et al. (2001) showed that while *hsp70.1* knockout mice have a normal baseline phenotype; cerebral infarct volume was 30% larger and mortality was higher than in wild type littermates after focal ischemia. In addition, using a combined *hsp70.1/3* knockout (the two genes are separated by only 8kb on chromosome 17 and show 99% homology), Lee et al. (2004) later determined that cytochrome *c* release into the cytosol and levels of activated caspase-3 were increased after MCAO suggesting that Hsp 70/72 plays a role in preventing initiation of apoptosis after injury. The *hsp70.1/3* knockout also exhibited an enhanced inflammatory response to cecal perforation and ligation (an animal model of acute respiratory distress syndrome/sepsis) as evidenced by increased NF-κB activation, TNF-α and IL-6 expression and lung injury highlighting a role in controlling immune function in injury states (Singleton and Wischmeyer, 2006). In this same model, Weiss et al. (2002) demonstrated that targeted overexpression of Hsp70 in rat lung significantly attenuated interstitial and alveolar edema, protein exudation and dramatically decreased neutrophil accumulation leading to improvement of acute respiratory distress syndrome.

Overall, this chapter seeks to review the importance of astrocytes and microglia in the post-ischemic inflammatory response and the role of heat shock proteins in modulating inflammation and outcome after cerebral ischemia.

2. Microglia: Immune cells of the CNS

Microglia are monocyte-derived CNS tissue macrophages that are phenotypically adapted to the neural environment. As such, they are characterized by minimal phagocytic activity and low expression of the macrophage-specific antigen, CD45 (Kreutzberg, 1996) which may be used to differentiate resident microglia from infiltrating macrophages (Babcock et al., 2003). Microglia constitutively and inducibly express a variety of immune-related receptors on their surface including cytokine, chemokine, prostaglandin, pattern recognition and complement receptors (Aloisi, 2001). In addition, microglia can function as antigen presenting cells, and through CD40 on their membranes can form an "immunological synapse" with CD40L-expressing T-cells recruited centrally (Gerritse et al., 1996). As a result, microglia can respond to diverse stresses by performing innate immune functions such as phagocytosis, and can release potentially beneficial factors such as glial-derived neurotrophic factor (GDNF).

Microglia can release a host of factors to protect the CNS; however, when activated after ischemia by necrotic cell debris and other substances, they can produce free radicals, proinflammatory cytokines (IL-1β, TNFα, IL-6 and interferon-γ), reactive oxygen species, matrix metalloproteinases and glutamate in an aberrant fashion (Lucin and Wyss-Coray, 2009; Yenari et al., 2010). Such compounds are instrumental in the subsequent activation of astrocytes (see below), induction of cell adhesion molecules and T-lymphocyte recruitment into the CNS following various injuries (Liu and Hong, 2003; Sweitzer et al., 2002). Several studies have been performed testing inhibition of microglial activation as a strategy to protect neurons following ischemic injury. Transgenic mice lacking the pattern recognition receptor TLR4 (Hyakkoku et al., 2010), mice overexpressing the anti-inflammatory cytokine IL-10 (De Bilbao et al., 2009) and treatment with a neutralizing antibody against TNF-alpha (Barone et al., 1997), all resulted in suppressed microglial activation and significantly decreased infarct size following focal cerebral ischemia. Taken together, these studies suggest that inhibition of the post-ischemia inflammatory response is a viable option for stroke treatment. Although microglia quickly respond to ischemia by producing proinflammatory cytokines (Yenari et al., 2010), proliferating (Denes et al., 2007) and exhibiting an altered cell morphology (Tanaka et al., 2003), only a small percentage (1-8%) of the microglia in the corpus callosum and lesion penumbra, and no microglia in the lesion core, express Hsp72 early after focal ischemia (Soriano et al., 1994). This indicates that a robust increase in Hsp72 protein expression is not a normal aspect of the post-ischemic microglial phenotype.

Interestingly, the majority of inflammatory mediators produced by microglia after stroke are produced by NFκB pathway activation (Yenari et al., 2010). Hsp72 has been implicated in modulation of inflammation by suppressing NFκB through multiple interactions. Previous work has shown that Hsp72 directly binds to the NFκB:IκB complex, thus preventing IκB phosphorylation and subsequent NFκB activation (Feinstein et al., 1996; Zheng et al., 2008). Ran et al. (2004) further demonstrated that Hsp72 binds directly to IκB kinase-γ (IKK-γ), an essential regulatory component of the IKK complex, blocking activation of IκB and release of

NFκB. Mice overexpressing Hsp72 have decreased infarcts compared to their wild-type counterparts, along with attenuated microglial activation and TNF-α production (Rajdev et al., 2000; Zheng et al., 2008). Microglia isolated from these mice showed decreased toxicity towards cultured astrocytes, accompanied by decreased NFκB signaling. Thus, the use of heat shock proteins to inhibit NFκB signaling in microglia may be an effective treatment for stroke by inhibiting a plethora of downstream factors that ultimately lead to further glial cell activation and neuronal cell death.

3. Astrocytes: Multiple roles in physiology & pathophysiology

Historically, astrocytes were considered to be passive elements in the CNS and neurotransmitter receptor expression was believed to be solely a characteristic of neurons. To the contrary, astrocytes express a variety of receptors on their surface, including metabotropic glutamate receptors, GABA receptors, adenosine receptors and the mu, delta and kappa opioid receptors, among others (Kettenmann and Steinhauser, 2005). In addition, these cells express a variety of ion channels on their surface, including Ca^{2+} channels. These are important because astrocytes are thought to function as part of a syncytia linked by connexins in order to transfer information in the form of ATP and Ca^{2+} (Kielian, 2008). In a model of ischemia, Cotrina et al. (1998) demonstrated that gap junctions remain open after oxygen-glucose deprivation (OGD) and may contribute to infarct evolution through direct astrocytic intercellular communication.

Astrocytes derive from the neuroectoderm and express a series of "marker antigens" during development such as the cytoskeletal protein vimentin and nestin (Eliasson et al., 1999) and the fatty acid binding protein brain lipid binding protein (Schmid et al., 2006). Once they reach their adult phenotype, other proteins are expressed including Aldh1L1 and glial fibrillary acidic protein (GFAP) (Cahoy et al., 2008). This intermediate filament is commonly considered to be astrocyte-specific, though it may also be found on reactive choroid plexus epithelium cells and neuronal precursor cells (Reichenbach and Wolburg, 2005) and there are also astrocyte populations that are GFAP negative (Kimelberg, 2004). GFAP functions as a structural protein and enhancement of GFAP remains the mainstay for demonstrating astrocytic reactivity in the CNS (Eng et al., 2000), however, it is important to note that only 15% of the total astrocyte cell volume is labeled with GFAP (Bushong et al., 2002). Remarkably, GFAP knockout mice do not exhibit an altered phenotype at baseline; however, after trauma, astrocyte hypertrophy is suppressed, scar formation is less organized and healing is slowed (Pekny et al., 1995; Pekny and Pekna, 2004). In further work using a lesion model of the entorhinal cortex, Wilhelmsson et al. (2004) demonstrated that double $GFAP^{-/-}$ $Vim^{-/-}$ mice display increased neuronal loss in the dentate gyrus at day 4 post-injury but enhanced synaptic regeneration at day 10. These data suggest a two-part response of reactive astrocytes to CNS injury: beneficial for neuronal survival in the initial post-injury period and detrimental to CNS regeneration in the recovery phase (Pekny and Nilsson, 2005).

3.1 Role in the blood-brain barrier

Astrocytes play an integral role in the structure of the blood-brain barrier (BBB), which limits the entry of circulating elements into the nervous system. Though recent data suggests that pericytes, not astrocytes, are required for the formation of the BBB during development (Daneman et al., 2010), ablation of astrocytes in the process of CNS restoration leads to failure of blood-brain barrier repair, an enhanced infiltration of leukocytes and subsequent excitotoxic neuronal death (Bush et al., 1999). In addition, astrocytes have been postulated to mediate functional hyperemia, the coupling of neuronal activity with increased cerebral blood flow, via changes in intracellular calcium in astrocytic endfeet leading to release of vasoactive substances (cyclooxygenase, adenosine) and modulation of adjacent arterioles (Iadecola and Nedergaard, 2007; Takano et al., 2006). It is estimated that 56% of rat cortical synapses are ensheathed by astrocyte domains (Chao et al., 2002) and an individual astrocyte occupies an exclusive, non-overlapping territory; each interfacing with the vasculature and thousands of synapses suggesting a complex process of synaptic integration (Bushong et al., 2004). Indeed, mice lacking GFAP exhibit increased infarct following ischemia, possibly due to blood-brain barrier and cerebral blood flow dysfunction (Nawashiro et al., 2000). The implication is that following ischemia, astrocytes are poised to influence penumbral blood flow and provision of neuronal nutrients in a coordinated fashion.

3.2 Astrocytes and ischemic injury

While it was established over a hundred years ago that neurons of the CA1 region of the hippocampus are selectively vulnerable to forebrain ischemia (Pulsinelli, 1985); evidence for injury to astrocytes has been more recent (Petito et al., 1998). The two main types of astrocytes found in the CNS are protoplasmic astrocytes found in the gray matter and fibrous astrocytes found in the white matter. This is important because astrocytes isolated from different brain regions exhibit varying sensitivity to oxygen-glucose deprivation (OGD) with striatal cells most vulnerable followed by hippocampal and cortical astrocytes (Xu et al., 2001). *In vivo*, using the middle cerebral artery occlusion (MCAO) model of focal ischemia, Lukaszevicz et al. (2002) demonstrated selective degeneration of protoplasmic cortical astrocytes with associated breakdown of the blood brain barrier. Yu et al. (1989) first demonstrated that cultured astrocytes are sensitive to hypoxia, exhibiting swelling and 80% suppression of glutamate uptake after 12-24 hours of oxygen deprivation. Using in situ hybridization and immunohistochemistry, Liu et al. (1999) demonstrated an early decline in mRNA and protein for GFAP in the ischemic core after middle cerebral artery occlusion (MCAO) with a corresponding increase in astrocyte markers in the penumbra, both of which temporally preceded neuronal death. In agreement, Zhao et al. (2003) showed early loss of GFAP after traumatic brain injury. Early *in vitro* work determined that co-culture of neurons with astrocytes protected them from OGD; specifically, when cultured alone and exposed to 4 hour of OGD only 5% of neurons survived compared to 75% survival in mixed cultures (Vibulsreth et al., 1987). Neurons co-cultured with astrocytes have also been shown to survive exposure to 100-fold higher concentrations of glutamate (Rosenberg and Aizenman, 1989). Taken together, these studies suggest that therapeutics aimed at maintaining astrocyte viability and function may protect neurons from ischemic injury.

3.3 Astrocytes as regulators of synaptic glutamate

Another key function of astrocytes is the control of extracellular glutamate homeostasis through sodium-dependent uptake via the excitatory amino acid transporters (EAATs) (Danbolt, 2001). The glutamate-aspartate transporter (GLAST/EAAT1) and the glutamate transporter-1 (GLT-1/EAAT2) are primarily localized in astrocytes. GLT-1 is the most studied astrocyte transporter and is suggested to be responsible for over 90% of synaptic glutamate clearance (Tanaka et al., 1997). Dysregulation of synaptic glutamate clearance by these transporters has been implicated in many disease processes (Gegelashvili and Schousboe, 1997; Maragakis and Rothstein, 2001; Rothstein et al., 1996). For example, glutamate levels have been shown to increase 50 times from baseline after ischemia and glutamate efflux from astrocytes has been suggested to occur by reversal of glutamate transport (Mitani et al., 1994; Seki et al., 1999). Transient MCAO leads to downregulation of GLT-1 which precedes neuronal death and antisense knockdown of GLT-1 exacerbates neuronal death in the same model (Rao et al., 2001a; Rao et al., 2001b; Rao et al., 2000). Furthermore, using pre-treatment with ceftriaxone, a known inducer of GLT-1, Chu et al. (2007) demonstrated a dose-dependent decrease in infarct volume and levels of the proinflammatory cytokine TNFα after MCAO. In addition, work from our laboratory showed that upregulation of GLT-1 in astrocytes using ceftriaxone decreases CA1 neuronal cell death in a global ischemia model (Ouyang et al., 2007). Complete knock-out of GLT-1 results in spontaneous seizures, selective death of CA1 neurons and 20% survival of animals at 12 weeks (Tanaka et al., 1997) and mice lacking GLT-1 display enhanced neuronal death after brief ischemia compared to wild type controls (Mitani and Tanaka, 2003). These findings underline the importance of exquisite regulation of synaptic glutamate by astrocytes in maintaining neuronal integrity.

4. Heat shock proteins affect astrocyte regulation of ischemia

4.1 A role for Hsp72 in ischemia

Our laboratory has been particularly interested in the role of astrocytic heat shock proteins as regulators of ischemic injury. Initial studies demonstrated induction of Hsp72 in cultured astrocytes exposed to heat shock or OGD (Bergeron et al., 1996) and further work confirmed that Hsp72 overexpression in astrocytes exposed to glucose deprivation (Xu and Giffard, 1997) or oxygen-glucose deprivation (Papadopoulos et al., 1996) was cytoprotective. Interestingly, overexpression of Hsp72 in astrocytes was shown to protect co-cultured neurons from ischemic injury (Xu et al., 1999); highlighting the integral role of astrocytes in neuronal homeostasis and survival. As discussed above, we have also demonstrated that the carboxyl-terminal domain of Hsp72 is sufficient to protect astrocytes from oxygen-glucose deprivation by suppressing protein aggregation and further decreases infarct volume after transient middle cerebral artery occlusion (MCAO) (Sun et al., 2006b). Astrocytes in the CA1 region of the brain, which is particularly sensitive to forebrain ischemia, lose glutamate transporter expression and activity prior to the death of CA1 neurons (Chen et al., 2005; Ouyang et al., 2007; Yeh et al., 2005). We have shown that astrocyte-targeted overexpression of Hsp72 not only protects CA1 neurons from transient forebrain ischemia, but also preserves GLT-1 immunoreactivity in the region (Xu et al., 2010) suggesting a possible mechanism for the observed protection.

4.2 Hsp72 as a regulator of apoptosis

Multiple studies have highlighted a neuroprotective role of Hsp72 overexpression in models of ischemia (Hoehn et al., 2001; Rajdev et al., 2000; van der Weerd et al., 2005). The mechanism was initially attributed to the known chaperone functions of Hsp72 including maintaining correct protein folding and inhibiting aggregation, however, a body of work has now emerged that indicates a direct role for Hsp72 in regulation of cell death by apoptosis and potentially even necrosis (Giffard and Yenari, 2004). Mitochondria are central to both cell death pathways; severe ischemia renders mitochondria unable to produce ATP and in less extreme stress conditions, mitochondria may increase production of reactive oxygen species (ROS), lose membrane potential and undergo changes in respiratory function (Dugan and Kim-Han, 2004). Ischemia can activate mitochondrial cytochrome *c* which translocates to the cytosol where it interacts with Apaf1 to form the apoptosome and activate caspase 9, initiating a cascade leading to DNA fragmentation (Chan, 2004; Leist and Jaattela, 2001). We have shown that overexpression of Hsp72 in cultured astrocytes subjected to glucose deprivation leads to decreased formation of ROS, stabilization of the mitochondrial membrane potential and prevention of increases in state IV respiration suggesting decreased cytochrome *c* release and activation of apoptosis (Ouyang et al., 2006). Furthermore, in the MCAO model of ischemia, we have shown that transfection of Hsp72 leads to inhibition of apoptosis-inducing factor (AIF) translocation to the nucleus thereby blocking caspase-independent apoptosis (Sun et al., 2006b). This is supported by previous work by Ravagnan et al. (2001) demonstrating that Hsp72 protects Apaf -/- cells against death via an interaction with AIF. For a comprehensive review of the role of Hsp72 in cell death please see Giffard et al. (2008).

4.3 Mitochondrial protection and mortalin/mitochondrial Hsp70

Mitochondrial dysfunction leading to a loss of ATP production impairs many of the energy-demanding neuroprotective functions of astrocytes after ischemic injury including ion homeostasis and neurotransmitter turnover (Bambrick et al., 2004). Mortalin forms part of the mitochondrial protein import machinery by binding a translocase in the inner membrane to form an ATP-dependent motor (Voos et al., 1999) and while it is not heat inducible it has been shown to increase after a variety of other stressors including glucose deprivation, oxidative stress and focal cerebral ischemia (Hadari et al., 1997; Lee, 2001; Massa et al., 1995).

Using LXSN-mortalin-transduced astrocytes, our laboratory has shown that overexpression of mortalin produces mitochondrial protection after glucose deprivation (Voloboueva et al., 2008). Specifically, we found decreased hydroethidine fluorescence (an indicator of the accumulation of reactive oxygen species (ROS)) and preserved mitochondrial membrane potential as measured by tetramethyl rhodamine staining (TMRE), a dye whose sequestration by mitochondria depends on the mitochondrial membrane potential, in astrocytes expressing increased levels of mortalin. In addition, mortalin overexpression preserved ATP levels in astrocytes subjected to oxygen-glucose deprivation and enhanced cell survival. In a more clinically relevant model of stroke, middle cerebral artery occlusion (MCAO), we further investigated the role of mortalin in mitochondrial protection. Rats overexpressing mortalin in astrocytes and neurons by direct intraventricular injection of a DNA plasmid encoding mortalin were subjected to MCAO and found to have a reduction in infarct area, decreased ROS and lipid oxidation compared to vector-transfected controls. Similar to our *in vitro* data we showed that mortalin overexpression reduced the ischemia-induced depletion of ATP and maintained electron transport chain complex IV activity (Xu et al., 2009).

To investigate the specific role of astrocytic mitochondrial inhibition in ischemia we treated astrocyte cultures with the Krebs cycle inhibitor, fluorocitrate (Voloboueva et al., 2007).

After glucose deprivation, astrocytes treated with fluorocitrate showed depletion of ATP, cell death and suppressed glutamate uptake within 3 hours. In addition, we demonstrated that inhibition of astrocytic mitochondria increased cell death in co-cultured neurons and enhanced changes in mitochondrial membrane potential in astrocytes suggesting a two-way crosstalk between these cells after injury related to energy supply and demand (Voloboueva et al., 2007).

4.4 The role of Grp78/BiP in calcium handling

The endoplasmic reticulum (ER) controls several cellular processes including protein synthesis, folding and trafficking. Under conditions of physiologic stress, including ischemia, that perturb ER Ca^{2+} homeostasis and therefore ER protein folding, the concerted actions of multiple pathways that influence protein synthesis and folding are activated; this is termed the unfolded protein response (UPR). Grp78/BiP is an ER chaperone protein involved in protein folding, suppression of apoptosis and regulation of the UPR. It is strongly induced as part of the UPR and translocates to mitochondria and other compartments after stress where it is postulated to mediate ER-mitochondria crosstalk (Sun et al., 2006a). Several prior studies also supported a role for Grp78/BiP in protection from ischemia-induced cell death using BIX, a Grp78 inducer, prior to transient global forebrain ischemia in gerbils (Oida et al., 2008) and focal ischemia in mice (Kudo et al., 2007). Work from our laboratory further showed that overexpression of Grp78/BiP protected cultured astrocytes from OGD, suppressed the GD-induced increase in mitochondrial Ca^{2+} and preserved mitochondrial function (Ouyang et al., 2011).

5. Conclusion

The processes leading to neuronal death following ischemia are complex and involve the integrated action of multiple pathways in a variety of cells types. Data from our laboratory, among others, has highlighted a role for dysfunction of astrocytes and microglia in the pathophysiology of cerebral ischemia. Currently, the most promising areas for intervention are ischemia-induced inflammation and oxidative stress with several drugs in clinical trials at this time aimed at suppressing cytokine release and reactive oxygen species, respectively. For example, the microglial inhibitor minocycline, which affects the release of inflammatory mediators from activated microglia is in Phase IV trials (Yenari et al., 2006), and epoetin alfa, which may be downregulated in astrocytes after ischemic injury is in Phase II/III trials (Zhao and Rempe, 2010). In this chapter we have reviewed several key functions of glial cells including control of inflammation, apoptosis and synaptic glutamate clearance as well as modulation of blood flow and mitochondrial protection (see Figure 1) that may be therapeutically targeted to protect neurons from injury. As the roles of glial cells and heat shock proteins in normal function and cerebral ischemia continue to be elucidated novel neuroprotective strategies may be developed in the future.

Astrocytes are well poised to respond to changes in blood flow by release of vasodilators such as cyclooxygenase (COX) and adenosine. In the case of ischemia from thrombus or embolus, the decrease in oxygen and glucose delivery can initiate a stress response in astrocytes including changes in morphology, increase in intermediate filaments such as GFAP (not shown), decreases in glutamate transporters and activation of mitochondrial cell death pathways. Heat shock proteins have been shown to modulate several of these pathways to inhibit astrocyte dysfunction leading to neuronal death. Microglia play an important role in the inflammatory cascade following ischemia. Activation of NFκB leads to the production of pro-inflammatory cytokines which can exacerbate damage to neurons. Heat shock proteins may also have a role in inhibiting the activation of NFκB, by direct interaction and stabilization of the IκB:NFκB complex or by inhibition of IKK preventing phosphorylation of degradation of IκB.

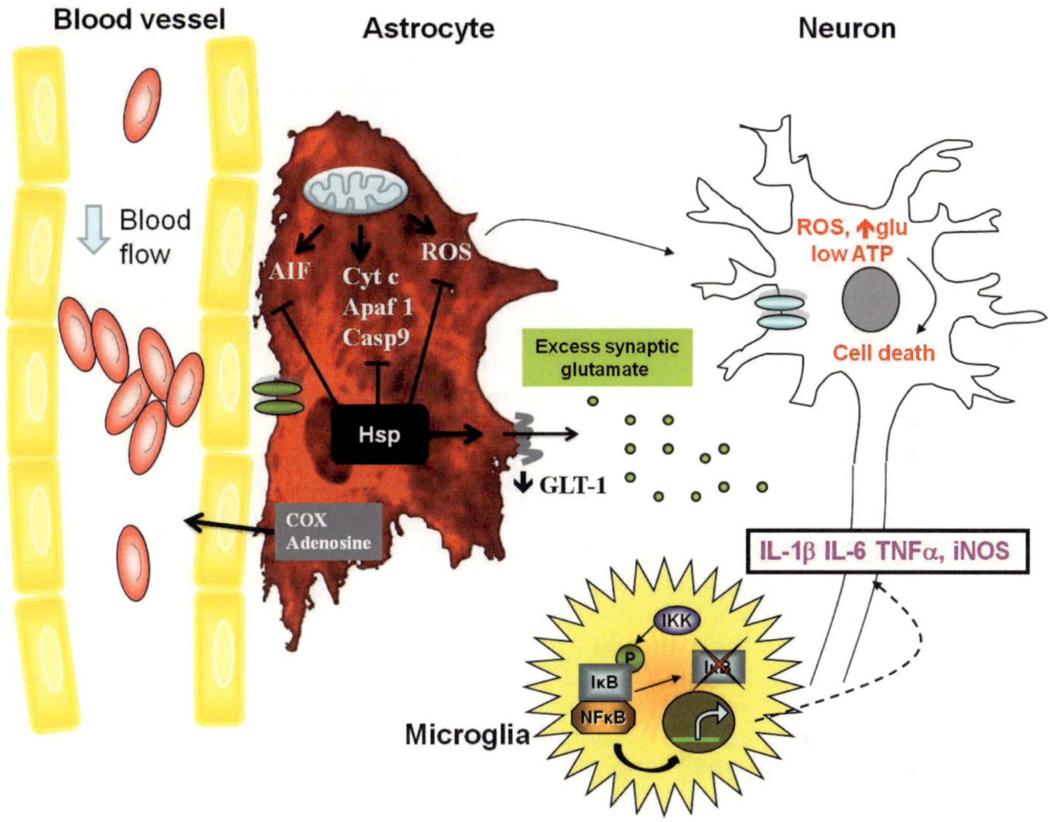

Fig. 1. Glial involvement in neuronal death from ischemia.

6. Acknowledgment

This work was supported in part by NIH grants NS053898 and GM49831 to RGG and T32 GM089626 to REW.

7. References

Aloisi, F. (2001). Immune function of microglia. *Glia,* Vol. 36, No. 2, pp. 165-179

Babcock, A. A., Kuziel, W. A., Rivest, S.& Owens, T. (2003). Chemokine expression by glial cells directs leukocytes to sites of axonal injury in the CNS. *J Neurosci,* Vol. 23, No. 21, pp. 7922-7930

Bambrick, L., Kristian, T.& Fiskum, G. (2004). Astrocyte mitochondrial mechanisms of ischemic brain injury and neuroprotection. *Neurochem Res,* Vol. 29, No. 3, pp. 601-608

Barone, F. C., Arvin, B., White, R. F., Miller, A., Webb, C. L., Willette, R. N., Lysko, P. G.& Feuerstein, G. Z. (1997). Tumor Necrosis Factor-α : A Mediator of Focal Ischemic Brain Injury. *Stroke,* Vol. 28, No. 6, pp. 1233-1244

Bergeron, M., Mivechi, N. F., Giaccia, A. J.& Giffard, R. G. (1996). Mechanism of heat shock protein 72 induction in primary cultured astrocytes after oxygen-glucose deprivation. *Neurol Res,* Vol. 18, No. 1, pp. 64-72

Bernard, S. A., Gray, T. W., Buist, M. D., Jones, B. M., Silvester, W., Gutteridge, G.& Smith, K. (2002). Treatment of Comatose Survivors of Out-of-Hospital Cardiac Arrest with Induced Hypothermia. *New England Journal of Medicine,* Vol. 346, No. 8, pp. 557-563

Bush, T. G., Puvanachandra, N., Horner, C. H., Polito, A., Ostenfeld, T., Svendsen, C. N., Mucke, L., Johnson, M. H.& Sofroniew, M. V. (1999). Leukocyte infiltration, neuronal degeneration, and neurite outgrowth after ablation of scar-forming, reactive astrocytes in adult transgenic mice. *Neuron,* Vol. 23, No. 2, pp. 297-308

Bushong, E. A., Martone, M. E.& Ellisman, M. H. (2004). Maturation of astrocyte morphology and the establishment of astrocyte domains during postnatal hippocampal development. *Int J Dev Neurosci,* Vol. 22, No. 2, pp. 73-86

Bushong, E. A., Martone, M. E., Jones, Y. Z.& Ellisman, M. H. (2002). Protoplasmic astrocytes in CA1 stratum radiatum occupy separate anatomical domains. *J Neurosci,* Vol. 22, No. 1, pp. 183-192

Cahoy, J. D., Emery, B., Kaushal, A., Foo, L. C., Zamanian, J. L., Christopherson, K. S., Xing, Y., Lubischer, J. L., Krieg, P. A., Krupenko, S. A., Thompson, W. J.& Barres, B. A. (2008). A Transcriptome Database for Astrocytes, Neurons, and Oligodendrocytes: A New Resource for Understanding Brain Development and Function. *The Journal of Neuroscience,* Vol. 28, No. 1, pp. 264-278

Chan, P. H. (2004). Mitochondria and neuronal death/survival signaling pathways in cerebral ischemia. *Neurochem Res,* Vol. 29, No. 11, pp. 1943-1949

Chao, T. I., Rickmann, M.& Wolff, J. R. (2002). The synapse-astrocyte boundary: an anatomical basis for an integrative role of glial in synaptic transmission. In: *The Tripartite Synapse: glia in synaptic transmission,* A. Volterra, P. Magistretti and P. Haydon, Eds, Oxford University Press, Oxford, pp. 3-23.

Chen, J. C., Hsu-Chou, H., Lu, J. L., Chiang, Y. C., Huang, H. M., Wang, H. L., Wu, T., Liao, J. J.& Yeh, T. S. (2005). Down-regulation of the glial glutamate transporter GLT-1 in rat hippocampus and striatum and its modulation by a group III metabotropic glutamate receptor antagonist following transient global forebrain ischemia. *Neuropharmacology,* Vol. 49, No. 5, pp. 703-714

Chu, K., Lee, S. T., Sinn, D. I., Ko, S. Y., Kim, E. H., Kim, J. M., Kim, S. J., Park, D. K., Jung, K. H., Song, E. C., Lee, S. K., Kim, M.& Roh, J. K. (2007). Pharmacological Induction of Ischemic Tolerance by Glutamate Transporter-1 (EAAT2) Upregulation. *Stroke,* Vol. 38, No. 1, pp. 177-182

Cotrina, M. L., Kang, J., Lin, J. H., Bueno, E., Hansen, T. W., He, L., Liu, Y.& Nedergaard, M. (1998). Astrocytic gap junctions remain open during ischemic conditions. *J Neurosci,* Vol. 18, No. 7, pp. 2520-2537

Danbolt, N. C. (2001). Glutamate uptake. *Prog Neurobiol,* Vol. 65, No. 1, pp. 1-105

Daneman, R., Zhou, L., Kebede, A. A.& Barres, B. A. (2010). Pericytes are required for blood-brain barrier integrity during embryogenesis. *Nature,* Vol. 468, No. 7323, pp. 562-566

De Bilbao, F., Arsenijevic, D., Moll, T., Garcia-Gabay, I., Vallet, P., Langhans, W.& Giannakopoulos, P. (2009). In vivo over-expression of interleukin-10 increases resistance to focal brain ischemia in mice. *Journal of Neurochemistry,* Vol. 110, No. 1, pp. 12-22

de Vreede-Swagemakers, J. J., Gorgels, A. P., Dubois-Arbouw, W. I., van Ree, J. W., Daemen, M. J., Houben, L. G.& Wellens, H. J. (1997). Out-of-hospital cardiac arrest in the 1990's: a population-based study in the Maastricht area on incidence, characteristics and survival. *J Am Coll Cardiol,* Vol. 30, No. 6, pp. 1500-1505

Denes, A., Vidyasagar, R., Feng, J., Narvainen, J., McColl, B. W., Kauppinen, R. A.& Allan, S. M. (2007). Proliferating resident microglia after focal cerebral ischaemia in mice. *J Cereb Blood Flow Metab,* Vol. 27, No. 12, pp. 1941-1953

Doyle, K. P., Simon, R. P.& Stenzel-Poore, M. P. (2008). Mechanisms of ischemic brain damage. *Neuropharmacology,* Vol. 55, No. 3, pp. 310-318

Dugan, L. L.& Kim-Han, J. S. (2004). Astrocyte mitochondria in in vitro models of ischemia. *J Bioenerg Biomembr,* Vol. 36, No. 4, pp. 317-321

Eckstein, M., Stratton, S. J.& Chan, L. S. (2005). Cardiac Arrest Resuscitation Evaluation in Los Angeles: CARE-LA. *Ann Emerg Med,* Vol. 45, No. 5, pp. 504-509

Eliasson, C., Sahlgren, C., Berthold, C. H., Stakeberg, J., Celis, J. E., Betsholtz, C., Eriksson, J. E.& Pekny, M. (1999). Intermediate filament protein partnership in astrocytes. *J Biol Chem,* Vol. 274, No. 34, pp. 23996-24006

Eng, L. F., Ghirnikar, R. S.& Lee, Y. L. (2000). Glial fibrillary acidic protein: GFAP-thirty-one years (1969-2000). *Neurochem Res,* Vol. 25, No. 9-10, pp. 1439-1451

Feinstein, D. L., Galea, E., Aquino, D. A., Li, G. C., Xu, H.& Reis, D. J. (1996). Heat Shock Protein 70 Suppresses Astroglial-inducible Nitric-oxide Synthase Expression by Decreasing NFκB Activation. *Journal of Biological Chemistry,* Vol. 271, No. 30, pp. 17724-17732

Freeman, B. C., Myers, M. P., Schumacher, R.& Morimoto, R. I. (1995). Identification of a regulatory motif in Hsp70 that affects ATPase activity, substrate binding and interaction with HDJ-1. *EMBO J,* Vol. 14, No. 10, pp. 2281-2292

Gegelashvili, G.& Schousboe, A. (1997). High affinity glutamate transporters: regulation of expression and activity. *Mol Pharmacol,* Vol. 52, No. 1, pp. 6-15

Gerritse, K., Laman, J. D., Noelle, R. J., Aruffo, A., Ledbetter, J. A., Boersma, W. J.& Claassen, E. (1996). CD40-CD40 ligand interactions in experimental allergic encephalomyelitis and multiple sclerosis. *Proc Natl Acad Sci U S A,* Vol. 93, No. 6, pp. 2499-2504

Giffard, R. G., Han, R. Q., Emery, J. F., Duan, M.& Pittet, J. F. (2008). Regulation of apoptotic and inflammatory cell signaling in cerebral ischemia: the complex roles of heat shock protein 70. *Anesthesiology,* Vol. 109, No. 2, pp. 339-348

Giffard, R. G.& Yenari, M. A. (2004). Many mechanisms for hsp70 protection from cerebral ischemia. *J Neurosurg Anesthesiol,* Vol. 16, No. 1, pp. 53-61

Hadari, Y. R., Haring, H. U.& Zick, Y. (1997). p75, a member of the heat shock protein family, undergoes tyrosine phosphorylation in response to oxidative stress. *J Biol Chem,* Vol. 272, No. 1, pp. 657-662

Hartl, F. U. (1996). Molecular chaperones in cellular protein folding. *Nature,* Vol. 381, No. 6583, pp. 571-579

Hoehn, B., Ringer, T. M., Xu, L., Giffard, R. G., Sapolsky, R. M., Steinberg, G. K.& Yenari, M. A. (2001). Overexpression of HSP72 after induction of experimental stroke protects neurons from ischemic damage. *J Cereb Blood Flow Metab,* Vol. 21, No. 11, pp. 1303-1309

Hyakkoku, K., Hamanaka, J., Tsuruma, K., Shimazawa, M., Tanaka, H., Uematsu, S., Akira, S., Inagaki, N., Nagai, H.& Hara, H. (2010). Toll-like receptor 4 (TLR4), but not TLR3 or TLR9, knock-out mice have neuroprotective effects against focal cerebral ischemia. *Neuroscience,* Vol. 171, No. 1, pp. 258-267

Iadecola, C.& Nedergaard, M. (2007). Glial regulation of the cerebral microvasculature. *Nat Neurosci,* Vol. 10, No. 11, pp. 1369-1376

Jo, S. K., Ko, G. J., Boo, C. S., Cho, W. Y.& Kim, H. K. (2006). Heat preconditioning attenuates renal injury in ischemic ARF in rats: role of heat-shock protein 70 on NF-kappaB-mediated inflammation and on tubular cell injury. *J Am Soc Nephrol,* Vol. 17, No. 11, pp. 3082-3092

Kettenmann, H.& Steinhauser, C. (2005). Receptors for neurotransmitters and hormones. In: *Neuroglia,* H. Kettenmann and B. R. Ransom, Eds, Oxford University Press, Oxford, pp. 131-145.

Kielian, T. (2008). Glial connexins and gap junctions in CNS inflammation and disease. *Journal of Neurochemistry,* Vol. 106, No. 3, pp. 1000-1016

Kimelberg, H. K. (2004). The problem of astrocyte identity. *Neurochem Int,* Vol. 45, No. 2-3, pp. 191-202

Kreutzberg, G. W. (1996). Microglia: a sensor for pathological events in the CNS. *Trends Neurosci,* Vol. 19, No. 8, pp. 312-318

Kudo, T., Kanemoto, S., Hara, H., Morimoto, N., Morihara, T., Kimura, R., Tabira, T., Imaizumi, K.& Takeda, M. (2007). A molecular chaperone inducer protects neurons from ER stress. *Cell Death Differ,* Vol. 15, No. 2, pp. 364-375

Lee, A. S. (2001). The glucose-regulated proteins: stress induction and clinical applications. *Trends Biochem Sci,* Vol. 26, No. 8, pp. 504-510

Lee, S. H., Kim, M., Yoon, B. W., Kim, Y. J., Ma, S. J., Roh, J. K., Lee, J. S.& Seo, J. S. (2001). Targeted hsp70.1 disruption increases infarction volume after focal cerebral ischemia in mice. *Stroke,* Vol. 32, No. 12, pp. 2905-2912

Lee, S. H., Kwon, H. M., Kim, Y. J., Lee, K. M., Kim, M.& Yoon, B. W. (2004). Effects of hsp70.1 gene knockout on the mitochondrial apoptotic pathway after focal cerebral ischemia. *Stroke,* Vol. 35, No. 9, pp. 2195-2199

Leist, M.& Jaattela, M. (2001). Four deaths and a funeral: from caspases to alternative mechanisms. *Nat Rev Mol Cell Biol,* Vol. 2, No. 8, pp. 589-598

Liberto, C. M., Albrecht, P. J., Herx, L. M., Yong, V. W.& Levison, S. W. (2004). Pro-regenerative properties of cytokine-activated astrocytes. *J Neurochem,* Vol. 89, No. 5, pp. 1092-1100

Liu, B.& Hong, J. S. (2003). Role of microglia in inflammation-mediated neurodegenerative diseases: mechanisms and strategies for therapeutic intervention. *J Pharmacol Exp Ther,* Vol. 304, No. 1, pp. 1-7

Liu, D., Smith, C. L., Barone, F. C., Ellison, J. A., Lysko, P. G., Li, K.& Simpson, I. A. (1999). Astrocytic demise precedes delayed neuronal death in focal ischemic rat brain. *Brain Res Mol Brain Res,* Vol. 68, No. 1-2, pp. 29-41

Lloyd-Jones, D., Adams, R. J., Brown, T. M., Carnethon, M., Dai, S., De Simone, G., Ferguson, T. B., Ford, E., Furie, K., Gillespie, C., Go, A., Greenlund, K., Haase, N., Hailpern, S., Ho, P. M., Howard, V., Kissela, B., Kittner, S., Lackland, D., Lisabeth,

L., Marelli, A., McDermott, M. M., Meigs, J., Mozaffarian, D., Mussolino, M., Nichol, G., Roger, V. L., Rosamond, W., Sacco, R., Sorlie, P., Thom, T., Wasserthiel-Smoller, S., Wong, N. D.& Wylie-Rosett, J. (2010). Heart disease and stroke statistics--2010 update: a report from the American Heart Association. *Circulation,* Vol. 121, No. 7, pp. e46-e215

Lucin, K. M.& Wyss-Coray, T. (2009). Immune Activation in Brain Aging and Neurodegeneration: Too Much or Too Little? *Neuron,* Vol. 64, No. 1, pp. 110-122

Lukaszevicz, A. C., Sampaio, N., Guegan, C., Benchoua, A., Couriaud, C., Chevalier, E., Sola, B., Lacombe, P.& Onteniente, B. (2002). High sensitivity of protoplasmic cortical astroglia to focal ischemia. *J Cereb Blood Flow Metab,* Vol. 22, No. 3, pp. 289-298

Maragakis, N. J.& Rothstein, J. D. (2001). Glutamate transporters in neurologic disease. *Arch Neurol,* Vol. 58, No. 3, pp. 365-370

Massa, S. M., Longo, F. M., Zuo, J., Wang, S., Chen, J.& Sharp, F. R. (1995). Cloning of rat grp75, an hsp70-family member, and its expression in normal and ischemic brain. *J Neurosci Res,* Vol. 40, No. 6, pp. 807-819

Mitani, A., Andou, Y., Matsuda, S., Arai, T., Sakanaka, M.& Kataoka, K. (1994). Origin of ischemia-induced glutamate efflux in the CA1 field of the gerbil hippocampus: an in vivo brain microdialysis study. *J Neurochem,* Vol. 63, No. 6, pp. 2152-2164

Mitani, A.& Tanaka, K. (2003). Functional Changes of Glial Glutamate Transporter GLT-1 during Ischemia: An In Vivo Study in the Hippocampal CA1 of Normal Mice and Mutant Mice Lacking GLT-1. *The Journal of Neuroscience,* Vol. 23, No. 18, pp. 7176-7182

Nawashiro, H., Brenner, M., Fukui, S., Shima, K.& Hallenbeck, J. M. (2000). High susceptibility to cerebral ischemia in GFAP-null mice. *J Cereb Blood Flow Metab,* Vol. 20, No. 7, pp. 1040-1044

Oida, Y., Izuta, H., Oyagi, A., Shimazawa, M., Kudo, T., Imaizumi, K.& Hara, H. (2008). Induction of BiP, an ER-resident protein, prevents the neuronal death induced by transient forebrain ischemia in gerbil. *Brain Research,* Vol. 1208, No. 217-224

Ouyang, Y. B., Voloboueva, L. A., Xu, L. J.& Giffard, R. G. (2007). Selective dysfunction of hippocampal CA1 astrocytes contributes to delayed neuronal damage after transient forebrain ischemia. *J Neurosci,* Vol. 27, No. 16, pp. 4253-4260

Ouyang, Y. B., Xu, L. J., Emery, J. F., Lee, A. S.& Giffard, R. G. (2011). Overexpressing GRP78 influences Ca2+ handling and function of mitochondria in astrocytes after ischemia-like stress. *Mitochondrion,* Vol. 11, No. 2, pp. 279-286

Ouyang, Y. B., Xu, L. J., Sun, Y. J.& Giffard, R. G. (2006). Overexpression of inducible heat shock protein 70 and its mutants in astrocytes is associated with maintenance of mitochondrial physiology during glucose deprivation stress. *Cell Stress Chaperones,* Vol. 11, No. 2, pp. 180-186

Papadopoulos, M. C., Sun, X. Y., Cao, J., Mivechi, N. F.& Giffard, R. G. (1996). Over-expression of HSP-70 protects astrocytes from combined oxygen-glucose deprivation. *Neuroreport,* Vol. 7, No. 2, pp. 429-432

Pekny, M., Leveen, P., Pekna, M., Eliasson, C., Berthold, C. H., Westermark, B.& Betsholtz, C. (1995). Mice lacking glial fibrillary acidic protein display astrocytes devoid of intermediate filaments but develop and reproduce normally. *EMBO J,* Vol. 14, No. 8, pp. 1590-1598

Pekny, M.& Nilsson, M. (2005). Astrocyte activation and reactive gliosis. *Glia,* Vol. 50, No. 4, pp. 427-434

Pekny, M.& Pekna, M. (2004). Astrocyte intermediate filaments in CNS pathologies and regeneration. *J Pathol,* Vol. 204, No. 4, pp. 428-437

Pellerin, L. (2005). How astrocytes feed hungry neurons. *Mol Neurobiol,* Vol. 32, No. 1, pp. 59-72

Petito, C. K., Olarte, J. P., Roberts, B., Nowak, T. S., Jr.& Pulsinelli, W. A. (1998). Selective glial vulnerability following transient global ischemia in rat brain. *J Neuropathol Exp Neurol,* Vol. 57, No. 3, pp. 231-238

Pulsinelli, W. A. (1985). Selective Neuronal Vulnerability: Morphological and Molecular Characteristics. In: *Progress in Brain Research,* K. A. H. B. K. S. K. Kogure and F. A. Welsh, Eds, Vol. Volume 63, Elsevier, pp. 29-37.

Rajdev, S., Hara, K., Kokubo, Y., Mestril, R., Dillmann, W., Weinstein, P. R.& Sharp, F. R. (2000). Mice overexpressing rat heat shock protein 70 are protected against cerebral infarction. *Ann Neurol,* Vol. 47, No. 6, pp. 782-791

Ran, R., Lu, A., Zhang, L., Tang, Y., Zhu, H., Xu, H., Feng, Y., Han, C., Zhou, G., Rigby, A. C.& Sharp, F. R. (2004). Hsp70 promotes TNF-mediated apoptosis by binding IKKγ and impairing NF-κB survival signaling. *Genes & Development,* Vol. 18, No. 12, pp. 1466-1481

Rao, V. L., Bowen, K. K.& Dempsey, R. J. (2001a). Transient focal cerebral ischemia down-regulates glutamate transporters GLT-1 and EAAC1 expression in rat brain. *Neurochem Res,* Vol. 26, No. 5, pp. 497-502

Rao, V. L., Dogan, A., Todd, K. G., Bowen, K. K., Kim, B. T., Rothstein, J. D.& Dempsey, R. J. (2001b). Antisense knockdown of the glial glutamate transporter GLT-1, but not the neuronal glutamate transporter EAAC1, exacerbates transient focal cerebral ischemia-induced neuronal damage in rat brain. *J Neurosci,* Vol. 21, No. 6, pp. 1876-1883

Rao, V. L. R., Rao, A. M., Dogan, A., Bowen, K. K., Hatcher, J., Rothstein, J. D.& Dempsey, R. J. (2000). Glial glutamate transporter GLT-1 down-regulation precedes delayed neuronal death in gerbil hippocampus following transient global cerebral ischemia. *Neurochem Int,* Vol. 36, No. 6, pp. 531-537

Ravagnan, L., Gurbuxani, S., Susin, S. A., Maisse, C., Daugas, E., Zamzami, N., Mak, T., Jaattela, M., Penninger, J. M., Garrido, C.& Kroemer, G. (2001). Heat-shock protein 70 antagonizes apoptosis-inducing factor. *Nat Cell Biol,* Vol. 3, No. 9, pp. 839-843

Reichenbach, A.& Wolburg, H. (2005). Astrocytes and ependymal glia. In: *Neuroglia,* H. Kettenmann and B. R. Ransom, Eds, Oxford University Press, Oxford, pp. 19-35.

Rosenberg, P. A.& Aizenman, E. (1989). Hundred-fold increase in neuronal vulnerability to glutamate toxicity in astrocyte-poor cultures of rat cerebral cortex. *Neurosci Lett,* Vol. 103, No. 2, pp. 162-168

Rothstein, J. D., Dykes-Hoberg, M., Pardo, C. A., Bristol, L. A., Jin, L., Kuncl, R. W., Kanai, Y., Hediger, M. A., Wang, Y., Schielke, J. P.& Welty, D. F. (1996). Knockout of glutamate transporters reveals a major role for astroglial transport in excitotoxicity and clearance of glutamate. *Neuron,* Vol. 16, No. 3, pp. 675-686

Ryan, A. J., Flanagan, S. W., Moseley, P. L.& Gisolfi, C. V. (1992). Acute heat stress protects rats against endotoxin shock. *J Appl Physiol,* Vol. 73, No. 4, pp. 1517-1522

Sahota, P.& Savitz, S. I. (2011). Investigational Therapies for Ischemic Stroke: Neuroprotection and Neurorecovery. *Neurotherapeutics,* Vol. 8, No. 3, pp. 434-451

Schmid, R. S., Yokota, Y.& Anton, E. S. (2006). Generation and characterization of brain lipid-binding protein promoter-based transgenic mouse models for the study of radial glia. *Glia,* Vol. 53, No. 4, pp. 345-351

Seki, Y., Feustel, P. J., Keller, R. W., Jr., Tranmer, B. I.& Kimelberg, H. K. (1999). Inhibition of ischemia-induced glutamate release in rat striatum by dihydrokinate and an anion channel blocker. *Stroke,* Vol. 30, No. 2, pp. 433-440

Singleton, K. D.& Wischmeyer, P. E. (2006). Effects of HSP70.1/3 gene knockout on acute respiratory distress syndrome and the inflammatory response following sepsis. *American Journal of Physiology - Lung Cellular and Molecular Physiology,* Vol. 290, No. 5, pp. L956-L961

Soriano, M. A., Planas, A. M., Rodríguez-Farré, E.& Ferrer, I. (1994). Early 72-kDa heat shock protein induction in microglial cells following focal ischemia in the rat brain. *Neuroscience Letters,* Vol. 182, No. 2, pp. 205-207

Sun, F.-C., Wei, S., Li, C.-W., Chang, Y.-S., Chao, C.-C.& Lai, Y.-K. (2006a). Localization of GRP78 to mitochondria under the unfolded protein response. *Biochem J,* Vol. 396, No. 1, pp. 31-39

Sun, Y., Ouyang, Y. B., Xu, L., Chow, A. M., Anderson, R., Hecker, J. G.& Giffard, R. G. (2006b). The carboxyl-terminal domain of inducible Hsp70 protects from ischemic injury in vivo and in vitro. *J Cereb Blood Flow Metab,* Vol. 26, No. 7, pp. 937-950

Sweitzer, S. M., Hickey, W. F., Rutkowski, M. D., Pahl, J. L.& DeLeo, J. A. (2002). Focal peripheral nerve injury induces leukocyte trafficking into the central nervous system: potential relationship to neuropathic pain. *Pain,* Vol. 100, No. 1-2, pp. 163-170

Takano, T., Tian, G. F., Peng, W., Lou, N., Libionka, W., Han, X.& Nedergaard, M. (2006). Astrocyte-mediated control of cerebral blood flow. *Nat Neurosci,* Vol. 9, No. 2, pp. 260-267

Tanaka, K., Watase, K., Manabe, T., Yamada, K., Watanabe, M., Takahashi, K., Iwama, H., Nishikawa, T., Ichihara, N., Kikuchi, T., Okuyama, S., Kawashima, N., Hori, S., Takimoto, M.& Wada, K. (1997). Epilepsy and exacerbation of brain injury in mice lacking the glutamate transporter GLT-1. *Science,* Vol. 276, No. 5319, pp. 1699-1702

Tanaka, R., Komine-Kobayashi, M., Mochizuki, H., Yamada, M., Furuya, T., Migita, M., Shimada, T., Mizuno, Y.& Urabe, T. (2003). Migration of enhanced green fluorescent protein expressing bone marrow-derived microglia/macrophage into the mouse brain following permanent focal ischemia. *Neuroscience,* Vol. 117, No. 3, pp. 531-539

The Hypothermia after Cardiac Arrest Study Group. (2002). Mild Therapeutic Hypothermia to Improve the Neurologic Outcome after Cardiac Arrest. *New England Journal of Medicine,* Vol. 346, No. 8, pp. 549-556

The National Institute of Neurological Disorders and Stroke rt-PA Stroke Study Group. (1995). Tissue Plasminogen Activator for Acute Ischemic Stroke. *New England Journal of Medicine,* Vol. 333, No. 24, pp. 1581-1588

van der Weerd, L., Lythgoe, M. F., Badin, R. A., Valentim, L. M., Akbar, M. T., de Belleroche, J. S., Latchman, D. S.& Gadian, D. G. (2005). Neuroprotective effects of HSP70 overexpression after cerebral ischaemia--An MRI study. *Experimental Neurology,* Vol. 195, No. 1, pp. 257-266

Vibulsreth, S., Hefti, F., Ginsberg, M. D., Dietrich, W. D.& Busto, R. (1987). Astrocytes protect cultured neurons from degeneration induced by anoxia. *Brain Research,* Vol. 422, No. 2, pp. 303-311

Villar, J., Ribeiro, S. P., Mullen, J. B., Kuliszewski, M., Post, M.& Slutsky, A. S. (1994). Induction of the heat shock response reduces mortality rate and organ damage in a sepsis-induced acute lung injury model. *Crit Care Med,* Vol. 22, No. 6, pp. 914-921

Voloboueva, L. A., Duan, M., Ouyang, Y., Emery, J. F., Stoy, C.& Giffard, R. G. (2008). Overexpression of mitochondrial Hsp70/Hsp75 protects astrocytes against ischemic injury in vitro. *J Cereb Blood Flow Metab,* Vol. 28, No. 5, pp. 1009-1016

Voloboueva, L. A., Suh, S. W., Swanson, R. A.& Giffard, R. G. (2007). Inhibition of mitochondrial function in astrocytes: implications for neuroprotection. *J Neurochem,* Vol. 102, No. 4, pp. 1383-1394

Voos, W., Martin, H., Krimmer, T.& Pfanner, N. (1999). Mechanisms of protein translocation into mitochondria. *Biochim Biophys Acta,* Vol. 1422, No. 3, pp. 235-254

Weiss, Y. G., Maloyan, A., Tazelaar, J., Raj, N.& Deutschman, C. S. (2002). Adenoviral transfer of HSP-70 into pulmonary epithelium ameliorates experimental acute respiratory distress syndrome. *The Journal of Clinical Investigation,* Vol. 110, No. 6, pp. 801-806

Wilhelmsson, U., Li, L., Pekna, M., Berthold, C. H., Blom, S., Eliasson, C., Renner, O., Bushong, E., Ellisman, M., Morgan, T. E.& Pekny, M. (2004). Absence of glial fibrillary acidic protein and vimentin prevents hypertrophy of astrocytic processes and improves post-traumatic regeneration. *J Neurosci,* Vol. 24, No. 21, pp. 5016-5021

Xu, L., Emery, J. F., Ouyang, Y. B., Voloboueva, L. A.& Giffard, R. G. (2010). Astrocyte targeted overexpression of Hsp72 or SOD2 reduces neuronal vulnerability to forebrain ischemia. *Glia,* Vol. 58, No. 9, pp. 1042-1049

Xu, L.& Giffard, R. G. (1997). HSP70 protects murine astrocytes from glucose deprivation injury. *Neurosci Lett,* Vol. 224, No. 1, pp. 9-12

Xu, L., Lee, J. E.& Giffard, R. G. (1999). Overexpression of bcl-2, bcl-XL or hsp70 in murine cortical astrocytes reduces injury of co-cultured neurons. *Neurosci Lett,* Vol. 277, No. 3, pp. 193-197

Xu, L., Sapolsky, R. M.& Giffard, R. G. (2001). Differential sensitivity of murine astrocytes and neurons from different brain regions to injury. *Exp Neurol,* Vol. 169, No. 2, pp. 416-424

Xu, L., Voloboueva, L. A., Ouyang, Y., Emery, J. F.& Giffard, R. G. (2009). Overexpression of mitochondrial Hsp70/Hsp75 in rat brain protects mitochondria, reduces oxidative stress, and protects from focal ischemia. *J Cereb Blood Flow Metab,* Vol. 29, No. 2, pp. 365-374

Yeh, T. H., Hwang, H. M., Chen, J. J., Wu, T., Li, A. H.& Wang, H. L. (2005). Glutamate transporter function of rat hippocampal astrocytes is impaired following the global ischemia. *Neurobiol Dis,* Vol. 18, No. 3, pp. 476-483

Yenari, M. A., Kauppinen, T. M.& Swanson, R. A. (2010). Microglial activation in stroke: therapeutic targets. *Neurotherapeutics,* Vol. 7, No. 4, pp. 378-391

Yenari, M. A., Xu, L., Tang, X. N., Qiao, Y.& Giffard, R. G. (2006). Microglia potentiate damage to blood-brain barrier constituents: improvement by minocycline in vivo and in vitro. *Stroke,* Vol. 37, No. 4, pp. 1087-1093

Yu, A. C., Gregory, G. A.& Chan, P. H. (1989). Hypoxia-induced dysfunctions and injury of astrocytes in primary cell cultures. *J Cereb Blood Flow Metab,* Vol. 9, No. 1, pp. 20-28

Zhao, X., Ahram, A., Berman, R. F., Muizelaar, J. P.& Lyeth, B. G. (2003). Early loss of astrocytes after experimental traumatic brain injury. *Glia,* Vol. 44, No. 2, pp. 140-152

Zhao, Y.& Rempe, D. A. (2010). Targeting astrocytes for stroke therapy. *Neurotherapeutics,* Vol. 7, No. 4, pp. 439-451

Zheng, Z., Kim, J. Y., Ma, H., Lee, J. E.& Yenari, M. A. (2008). Anti-inflammatory effects of the 70 kDa heat shock protein in experimental stroke. *J Cereb Blood Flow Metab,* Vol. 28, No. 1, pp. 53-63

10

Role of Creatine Kinase – Hexokinase Complex in the Migration of Adenine Nucleotides in Mitochondrial Dysfunction

Elena Erlykina and Tatiana Sergeeva
Nizhny Novgorod State Medical Academy
Russian Federation

1. Introduction

Creatine phosphokinase (CK) (ATP: creatine phosphotransferase, EC 2.7.3.2.) is found in a variety of cells with high and fluctuating energy requirements. It catalyses the reversible transfer of the high-energy-N-phosphoryl group from phosphocreatine to ADP. Creatine kinase connects sites of energy production with sites of energy consumption (Dolder et. al., 2001; Focant et al., 1970; Grossmann et al., 1985; Lipskaya et al., 1989; Walzel et al., 2002; Wyss, 2000).

There are know to be three cytosolic and two mitochondrial isoforms of CK. The more basic mitochondrial creatine kinase $MiCK_b$ is accumulated in mitochondria of cardiac muscle and skeletal muscle. The more acidic mitochondrial creatine kinase $MiCK_a$ was found in the brain (Eppenberger-Eberhardt et al., 1991; Fridman, Roberts, 1994).

Creatine kinase can exist in two interconvertible forms: dimer and octamer (Eriksson et al., 1998; Shen et al., 2002). Creatine kinase binds to the outer leaflet of the entire inner mitochondrial membrane and is specifically enriched in the so-called contact sites where inner and outer membranes are in close proximity (Boero et al., 2003; Chen et al, 1994; Lin et al., al., 1996; Wang et al., 2005).

A change in the octamer/dimer ratio may influence on the association behavior of mitochondrial creatine kinase in general and thus modulate mitochondrial energy flux (Brdiczka, 2003; Dolder et al., 2001; Schnyder et al., 1995).

Mitochondrial creatine kinase forms the functional microcompartment together with the mitochondrial porin (voltage-dependent anion channel) in the outer membrane and as well as the transmembrane protein adenine nucleotide translocase in the inner membrane (Fritz-Wolf et al., 1996; Kaldis, Wallimann, 1994; Schnyder et al., 1988).

Hexokinase (HK) (ATP:D-hexokinase-6-phosphotransferase, EC 2.7.11) is the enzyme with variable cellular localization (Mulichak et al., 1998; Xie & Wilson, 1990).

The type I isoenzyme of mammalian hexokinase is ubiquitously expressed in mammalian tissues but is found particularly at high levels in the brain where it plays an important role in regulating the rate of cerebral glucose metabolism (Schwab & Wilson, 1989; Wilson, 1985). The major portion of the hexokinase activity in the brain is associated with mitochondria. About 85% of hexokinase is bound to the outer mitochondrial membrane, forming the specific complex with porin (Magnani et al., 1982; Redker et al., 1972; Wilson, 1995). This physical proximity provides the basis for functional interaction between glucose phosphorylation by hexokinase and mitochondrial ATP production by oxidative phosphorylation with resulting coordination of the glycolytic and oxidative phases of glucose metabolism (Aleshin, 1998; Rosano et al., 1999). The outer mitochondrial membrane protein - porin, which forms the transmembrane channel, is responsible for specific interaction with hexokinase (Aflalo & Azoulay, 1998; Linden et al., 1982; Schlattner et al., 2001; Vyssokikh & Brdiczka, 2003).

The preferential mitochondrial localization of hexokinase in rat brain provides a predominant access to ATP, generated in mitochondria. The ADP produced by hexokinase activity is known to control both membrane potential and reactive oxygen species generation (Rose & Warms, 1967; Smith and Wilson, 1991; Viitanen et al., 1984; Wilson, 1980).

Thus both enzymes - creatine kinase and hexokinase - play an important role in dynamic compartmentation of adenine nucleotides.

Mitochondrial creatine kinase is a key enzyme of oxidative cellular energy metabolism in the brain (Bessman, 1981; Guo et al., 2003; Hemmer et al., 1994; Levin et al., 1990; Takagi et al., 2001; Wallimann et. al., 1992; Wallimnann et al., 1998). Hexokinase is an enzyme involved in the first step of glycolysis. Mitochondrial creatine kinase - hexokinase complex takes part in transport of adenine nucleotides from mitochondria to cytoplasm. Functioning of this complex depends on interaction of enzymes with the mitochondrial membrane and the oligomeric state of mitochondrial creatine kinase.

Mitochondrial dysfunction is one of the main reasons of the pathological changes in cerebral ischemia (Clostre, 2001; Delivoria-Papadopoulos et al., 2007; Fiscum, 2000; Kuznetsov, Margreiter, 2009; Mattson, Liu, 2002; Sas et al., 2007; Siesjo, 1999).

Stroke is a leading cause of disability and death in many countries. Understanding the molecular mechanisms of ischemic injury helps to find the novel therapeutic strategies for stroke. 80% of human strokes are ischemic in origin (Levine et al., 1992; Sappey-Marinier et al., 2002; Ueda et al., 2000).

Thus experimental models of cerebral ischemia have been developed in an attempt to closely mimic the changes that occur during and after human ischemic stroke. Changes in the amount and activity of enzyme proteins are critical factors in regulating intracellular metabolism under ischemic conditions (Cherubini et al., 2000; Dos Santos et al., 2004; Maulik et al., 1999; Rauchova et al., 2002).

According to modern data, membrane-associated enzyme in contrast to soluble enzyme has other catalytic properties (Beutner et al., 1998; da-Silva et al., 2004; Dolder et al., 2001; Kellershohn & Ricard, 1994; Linden et al., 1982; Lyubarev, 1997; Ovadi & Srere, 2000). The reverse adsorption on the mitochondrial membrane is controlled by ions and metabolites thus broadening the regulatory possibility of the cells under hypoxic conditions.

2. Materials and methods

Animals

Experiments were performed on male outbred albino rats weighing 150-180 g.

Cerebral ischemia was produced by bilateral ligation of the common carotid arteries. The animals were anesthetized with nembutal (30 mg/kg intraperitoneally). The brain tissue was examined 30 minutes (acute ischemia), 1.5, 4, 18 hours after surgical impairment of cerebral hemodynamics.

The animals were divided into two groups due to their physiological state after acute ischemia (severe and moderate). The severity of ischemia was estimated according to the behavior of rats, the respiratory rate and survival one. In acute severe ischemia the rats after ligation of the common carotid arteries were in severe state: they were passive, in lateral recumbent position, with agonal breathing (20-30 times per minute with respiratory arrest). In acute moderate ischemia the state of animals was satisfactory: they were active, moved in a cage, the respiratory rate was 50-70 times per minute. Due to the increase in the severity of general physiological state of rats in case of long-term ischemia we could not divide the animals into two groups; they were included into one group.

Preparation of brain tissue

The mitochondrial fraction of the brain was isolated by differential centrifugation (Fonyo, Somogy, 1960; Dizhe et al., 2003). The brain tissue was homogenized at 4 ^{0}C in a medium containing 0.32 M sucrose, 10 mM tris-HCl , 1 mM EDTA, pH 7,4. The total tissue homogenate was centrifuge at 2000 g for 10 minutes. The resulting supernatant was collected and centrifuged further at 12 500g for 15 minutes. The pellet containing mitochondria was resuspended in 0.32 M sucrose and centrifuged at 16 500g for 15 minutes. The fraction enriched mitochondria was collected and washed by 0.32 M sucrose.
The mitochondria were then swollen by incubation in distilled water (at a protein concentration of 1 mg) for 30 minutes, followed by centrifugation at 20 000g for 30 minutes. The resulting supernatant was collected for further analysis. The pellet containing mitochondrial membranes was resuspended in 0.32 M sucrose with 0.25 M dithiothreitol, pH 7.4.

Enzyme assay

Creatine kinase activity was measured by the pH-stat method using ADP and creatine phosphate as substrates (Kuby, Noltman, 1962). The velocity of the creatine kinase reaction is estimated by the change in pH. The reaction mixture (3 ml) contained (final concentration): 0.25 M sucrose, 2.5 mM tris-HC1, 12 mM $MgCl_2$, 10 mM KC1, 0.25 mM dithiothreitol, 5 mM creatine phosphate, 2 mM ADP. The reaction was started by addition of 100 µg protein. Then the mixture was titrated by addition of 10 µl 0.1 N HCl.
Creatine kinase activity is expressed as 1 unit corresponds to 1 µg-equ H^+/ min per 1 mg of protein.
Hexokinase activity was measured spectrophotometrically (Felgner, Wilson 1976). The reaction mixture (3 ml) contained (final concentration): 50 mM tris-HC1, pH 8.0, 2 mM glucose, 2 mM ATP, 5 mM $MgCl_2$, 0,25 mM NADP, 0.4 IU/min glucose-6-phosphate dehydrogenase. The reaction was started by addition of 100 µg protein.
Hexokinase activity is expressed as follows: 1 unit corresponds to 1 nmol of NADP transformed/min per 1 mg of protein.

Solubilization of creatine kinase

Mitochondria were resuspended in the proper (0.1M KCl; K-Na phosphate buffer 0.1-1.75 M, 0.5% (v/v) Triton X-100; 0.1% deoxycholate Na) solubilizing solution and incubated for 30 minutes. The samples were centrifuged at 4^{0}C and 20 000g, 60 minutes. Percentage of solubilization was determined as the difference of the activity before and after solubilization of the enzyme.

Solubilization of hexokinase

Mitochondria were resuspended at a protein concentration of 0.5-1 mg/ml in 0.1M tris-HCl pH 6.6, 0.1 M KCl or 0.5% (v/v) Triton X-100. After incubation for 30 minutes on ice, with occasional mixing, the samples were centrifuged at 4ºC and 20 000g for 30 minutes. Percentage of solubilization was determined as the difference of the activity before and after solubilization of the enzyme.

According to Wilson (2003) there are 2 types of binding sites for hexokinase on brain mitochondria. Hexokinase is readily solubilized from Type A sites by glucose-6-phosphate while hexokinase bound to Type B sites remains bound even in the presence of glucose-6-phosphate.

Mitochondria were resuspended in 2 mM glucose-6-phosphate; tris-HCl buffer, pH 8 and incubated for 30 minutes at the room temperature, and centrifuged 100 000g for 15 minutes. Aliquots of supernatant contain hexokinase Type A.

The sediment of mitochondria which contained hexokinase type B was resuspended again in 0,32 M sucrose, 0.5% (v/v) Triton X-100, 0.1M tris-HCl, pH 8. After incubation for 5 minutes on ice the samples were centrifuged at 20 000g for 10 minutes. The sediment was resuspended again in 0.32M sucrose, 0.1M KCl, 1% (v/v) Triton X-100, 0.1M tris-HCl, pH 8. After incubation for 20 minutes on ice the samples were centrifuged at 20 000g for 10 minutes. The aliquots of supernatant contained hexokinase Type B.

Dissociation of creatine kinase

Mitochondrial creatine kinase was dissociated by incubation of the total mitochondrial fraction and mitochondrial membrane pellet with substrates for the transition-state analogue complex ($MgCl_2$, ADP, KNO_3, and creatine) at 4 ºC for 2 hours (Lipskaya et al., 1989).

The free radical oxidation intensity assay

The intensity of the free radical oxidation (FRO) was estimated by the method of H_2O_2, Fe^{2+}-induced chemiluminescence on a BChL-07 biochemiluminometer. This method is based on the catalytic decomposition of hydrogen peroxide by ions of metal with variable valency (bivalent iron) (the Phenton reaction). The reaction mixture contained: 0,05 mM Fe_2SO_4, a phosphate buffer and a mitochondrial fraction. The reaction was started by addition of 2 % solution of hydrogen peroxide. Proceeding process of free radical oxidation was registered within 30 seconds. It is the time of the greatest information about its intensity. The ideal curve of the process is presented in figure 1.

The following parameters are the most informative for the estimation of the chemiluminescence intensity: the total luminescence yield (S, enables to estimate a balance between lipid peroxidation and antioxidants), maximum flash amplitude (Imax, shows a potential ability of the biological sample to free radical oxidation), and K index characterizing antioxidant potential were used as integral parameters of chemiluminescence (Kuzmina et al., 2009).

The protein concentration assay

Protein concentration was measured by the method of Bredford (Bredford & Spector, 1978).

Statistical analysis

The data are expressed as mean and standard error of the mean (SEM). The results were analyzed by means of Primer of Biostatistics 4.03 (Glantz, 2005). The significance of differences between the samples was evaluated by Student's test. The level of significance was set at $p<0.05$.

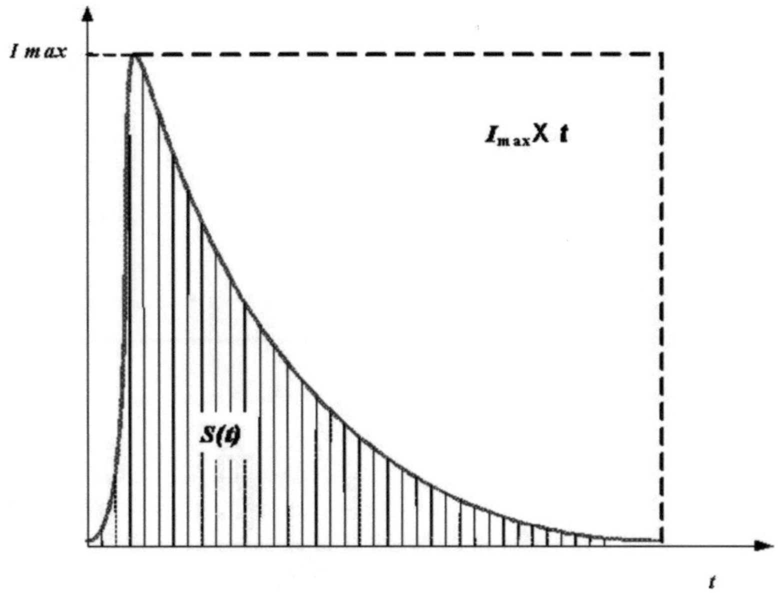

Fig. 1. The kinetic curve of the development of an induced chemiluminescence signal.

3. Results

Two forms of creatine kinase and hexokinase - membrane and soluble - were found in the brain.

The activity of membrane-associated creatine kinase equals to half of the enzyme activity in mitochondria. In contrast hexokinase activity is concentrated on the outer surface of the mitochondrial membrane (Table 1).

Form of the enzyme	Creatine kinase, U/ mg*min.	Hexokinase, U/ mg*min.
Membrane-associated	1.40±0.07 n=23	11.56±0.19 n=12
Soluble	1.78±0.10 n=19	1.53±0.04 n=12

Table 1. The distribution of creatine kinase and hexokinase activity between membrane-associated and soluble forms of the enzymes

Catalytic and kinetic properties of mitochondrial creatine kinase and hexokinase were shown to depend on the interaction with the membrane.

Different solubilizing agents (electrolyte, detergent and the endogenous metabolite glucose-6-phosphate) were used to analyze the character of interaction of hexokinase with the mitochondrial membrane.

All these agents solubilized only a third of the hexokinase activity, and only the sequence of action of electrolyte, detergent and glucose-6-phosphate removed the enzyme from the mitochondrial membrane (Fig. 2). Thus it shows the lability of protein-protein interaction and the possibility of its regulation under the certain pathological conditions.

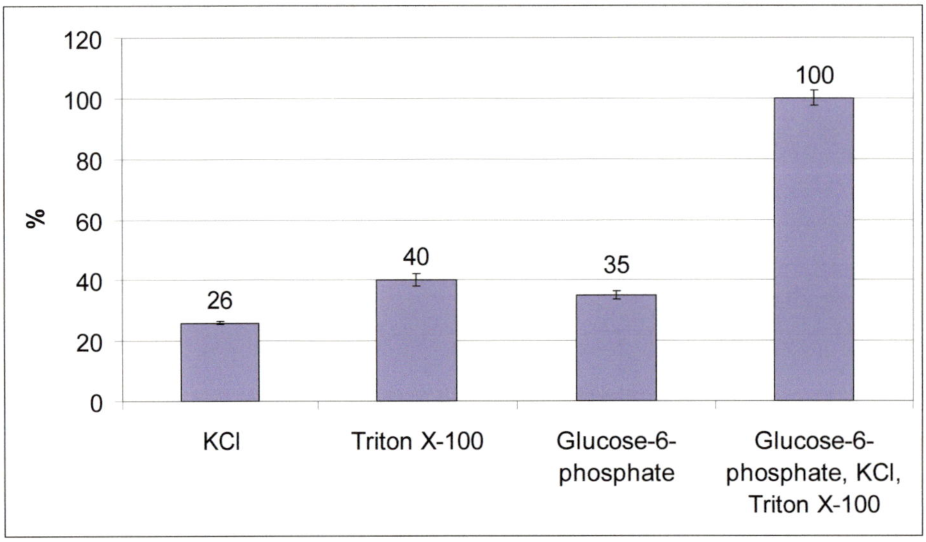

Fig. 2. Solubilization (%) of hexokinase from mitochondrial membranes of intact rats.

Creatine kinase can not dissociate from the mitochondrial membrane even in the presence of the simultaneous action of electrolyte and detergent (Fig. 3).

So the brain creatine kinase exists in different molecular forms: the first - soluble, which is located in the intermembrane space, the second is associated, which is loosely bound to the inner mitochondrial membrane and under the certain solubilizing agents can remove into the intermembrane space, the third form (about 18%) is tightly bound with the membrane.

In mitochondria from intact animals, mitochondrial creatine kinase presents as a mixture of two oligomeric forms (dimer and octamer; 65 and 35%, respectively). We consider that the tightly bound creatine kinase to exist mainly in the contact sites in the octamer form.

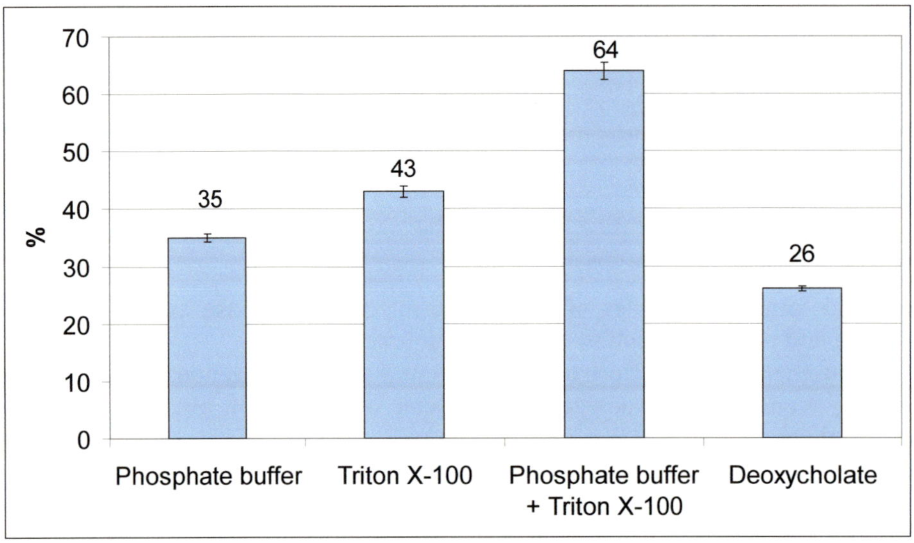

Fig. 3. Solubilization (%) of creatine kinase from mitochondrial membranes of intact rats.

Rebinding of both phosphokinases with the membrane changes their catalytic properties. Binding of hexokinase with the membrane increases the velocity of the reaction in 3 fold, but the kinetic behavior is not changed (Fig. 4).

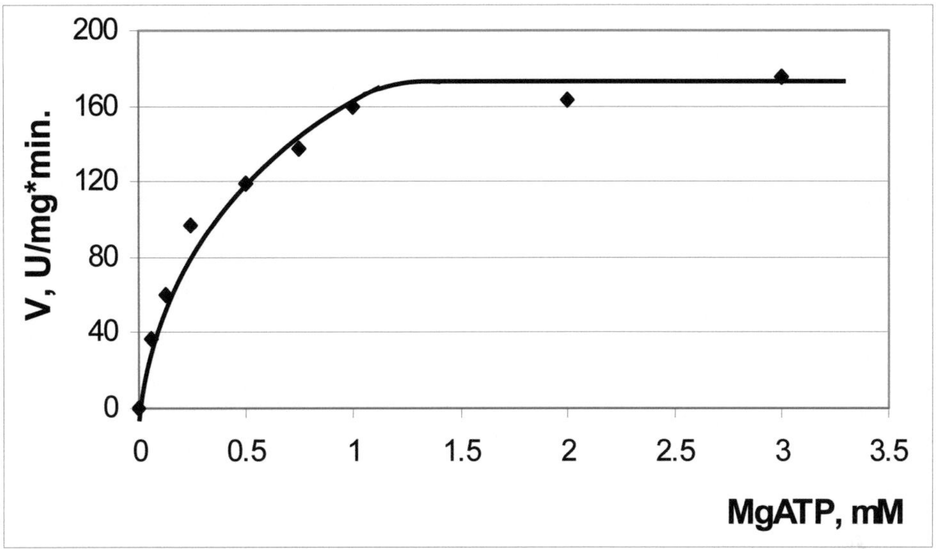

Fig. 4. Dependence of V_0 on concentration of MgATP of membrane-associated hexokinase of intact rats.

Creatine kinase has different types of kinetic behavior (Fig. 5-7). We consider that the membrane associated form of the enzyme binds by ionic interaction with the membrane and the character of the curve reveals the classical kinetic behavior (Fig. 6). The tightly bound

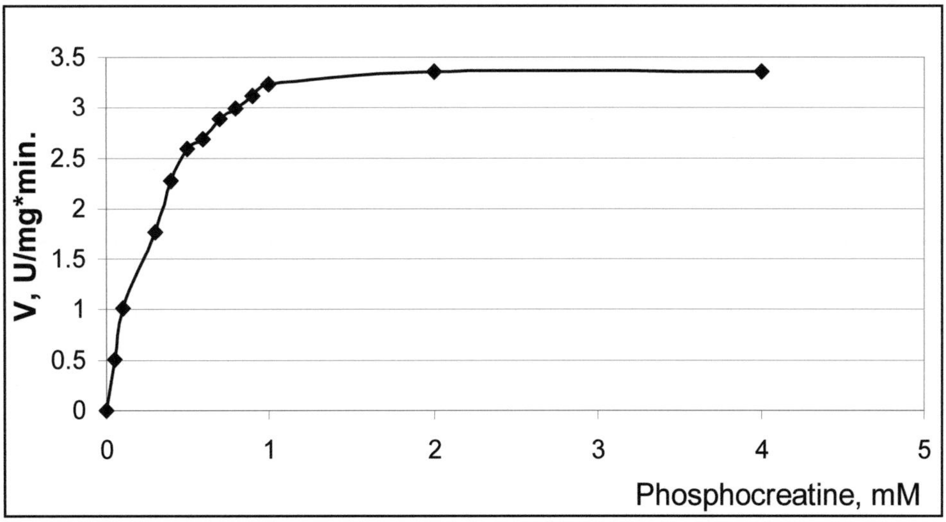

Fig. 5. Kinetic of creatine kinase reaction in total mitochondrial fraction of intact rats.

form of membrane enzyme has the abnormal kinetic behavior due to ionic and hydrophobic interaction (Fig. 7). These data discribe the role of specific microenvironment in the modification of the enzyme properties.

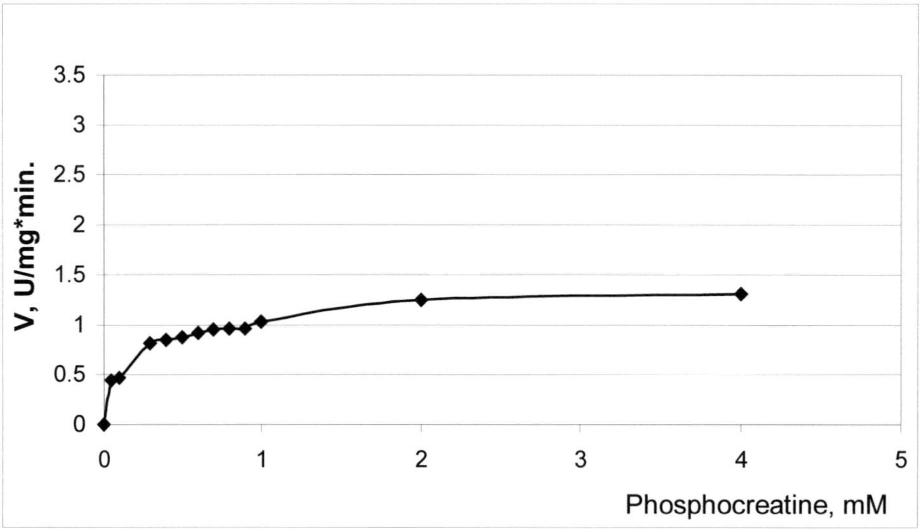

Fig. 6. Kinetic of creatine kinase reaction on mitochondrial membrane of intact rats.

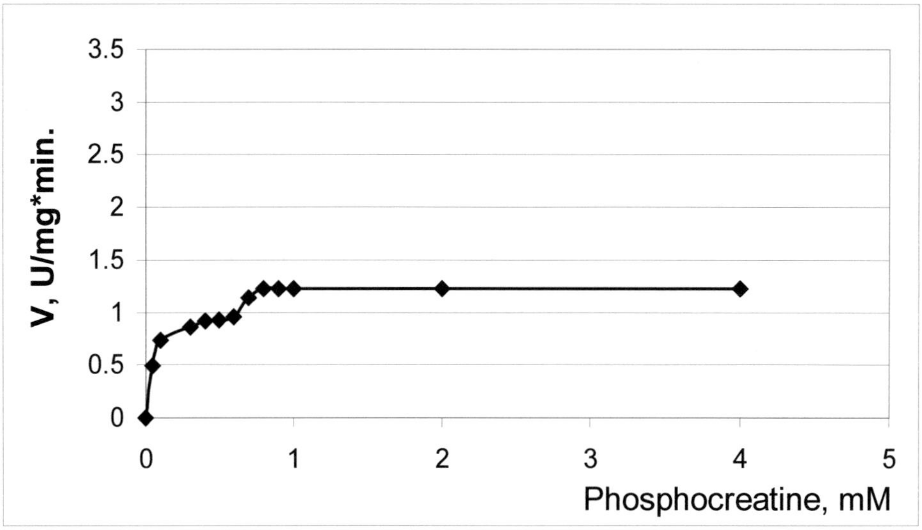

Fig. 7. Kinetic of creatine kinase reaction on mitochondrial membrane after solubilization by phosphate buffer of intact rats.

Thus the catalytic properties depend on the binding with the membrane and this process is controlled by the endogenous metabolites and the functional state of mitochondria.
All forms of hypoxia and ischemia are accompanied by activation of free radical oxidation (Ayer, Zhang, 2008; da-Silva et al., 2004; Kuznetsov, Margreiter, 2009; Meyer et al., 2006;

Wang et al., 2005). As a result of this activation the properties of the mitochondrial membrane-associated enzymes are changed in acute ischemia.

Severe ischemia reduced the binding of the investigated enzymes with the membrane (Fig. 8, 9). The activity of the enzymes decreased 2 fold for creatine kinase and 3 fold for hexokinase. Glucose-6-phosphate and the products of membrane degradation inhibited hexokinase activity in cerebral ischemia (Ishibashi, 1999; Wilson et al., 2000).

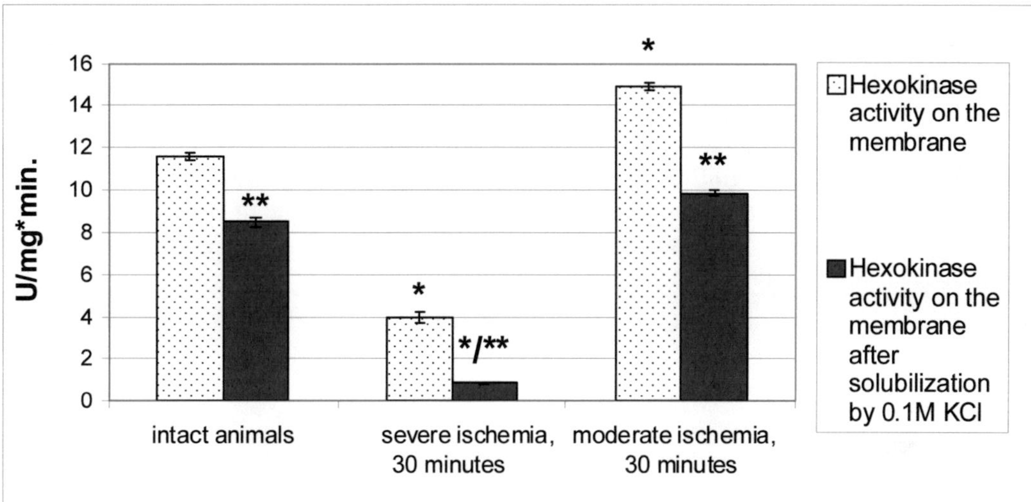

Fig. 8. Membrane associated hexokinase activity on the membrane before and after solubilization by 0.1M KCl of intact rats and in 30 minutes ischemia.

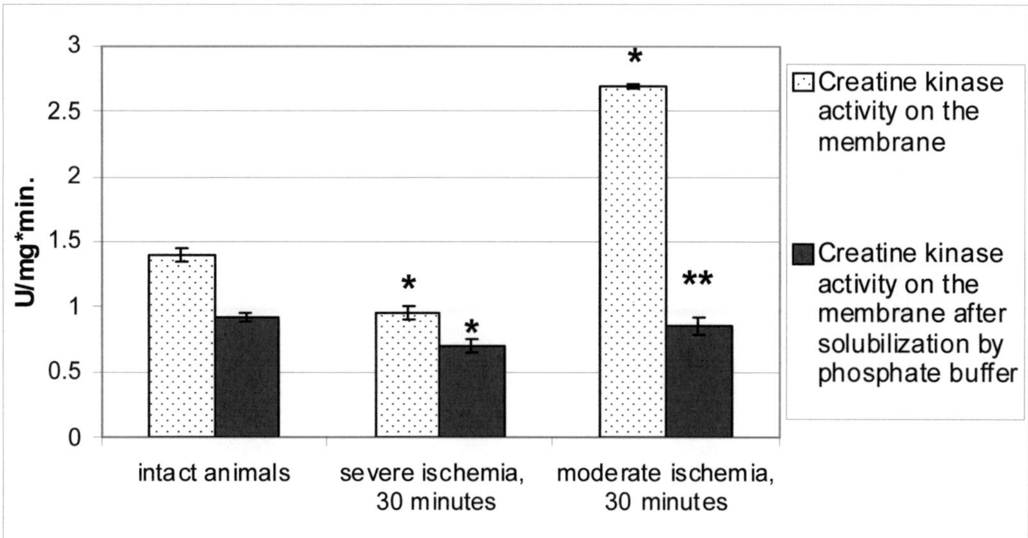

Fig. 9. Creatine kinase activity on the membrane of intact rats and in 30 minutes ischemia before and after solubilization by phosphate buffer.

The bar diagrams display average activities with error bars representing the standard deviation. *$p<0.05$ versus intact animals. ** $p<0.05$ versus initial hexokinase activity on the membrane within the same group.
The bar diagrams display average activities with error bars representing the standard deviation. $p<0.05$ versus intact animals. ** $p<0.05$ versus initial creatine kinase activity on the membrane within the same group.
In the second group (moderate ischemia) the activity of hexokinase was increased by 29% and by 92% for creatine kinase in comparison with intact animals. After the solubilization of the hexokinase by 0.1 M KCl the enzyme lost 38% of the initial activity. The effect of solubilization for membrane- bound creatine kinase was 69% instead of 35% for the intact rats.
The study of behavior of creatine kinase revealed the modification of its properties in acute ischemia. They differed significantly from those of the intact rats. It is connected with the realization of interconvertible transformation of oligomeric subunits of creatine kinase. This changing in kinetic behavior provides the higher sensitivity of the enzyme to the changes in substrate concentration (Fig. 10-13).

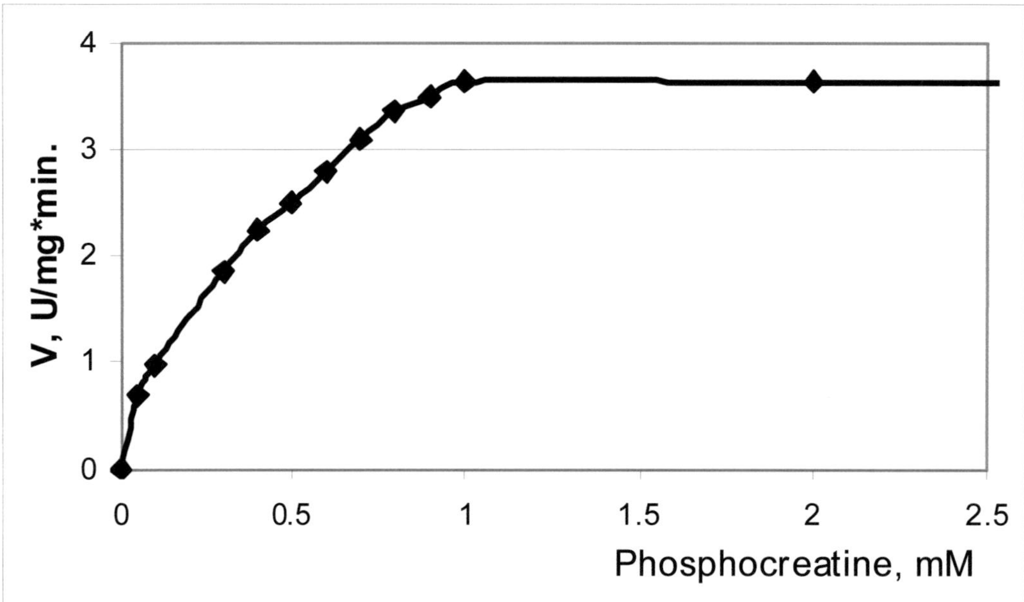

Fig. 10. Dependence of V_0 on concentration of phosphocreatine in total mitochondrial fraction in moderate ischemia

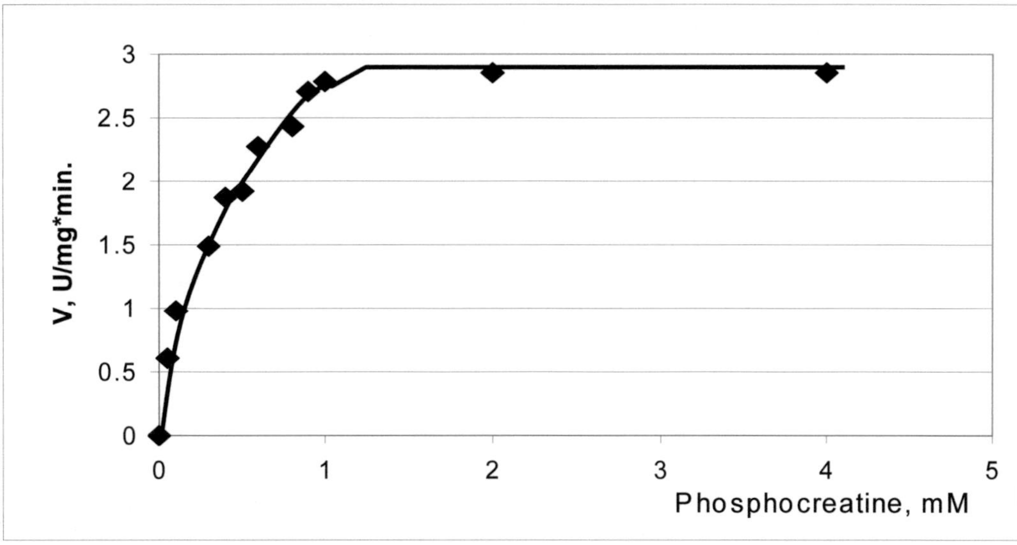

Fig. 11. Dependence of V_0 on concentration of phosphocreatine in fraction of mitochondrial membranes in moderate ischemia

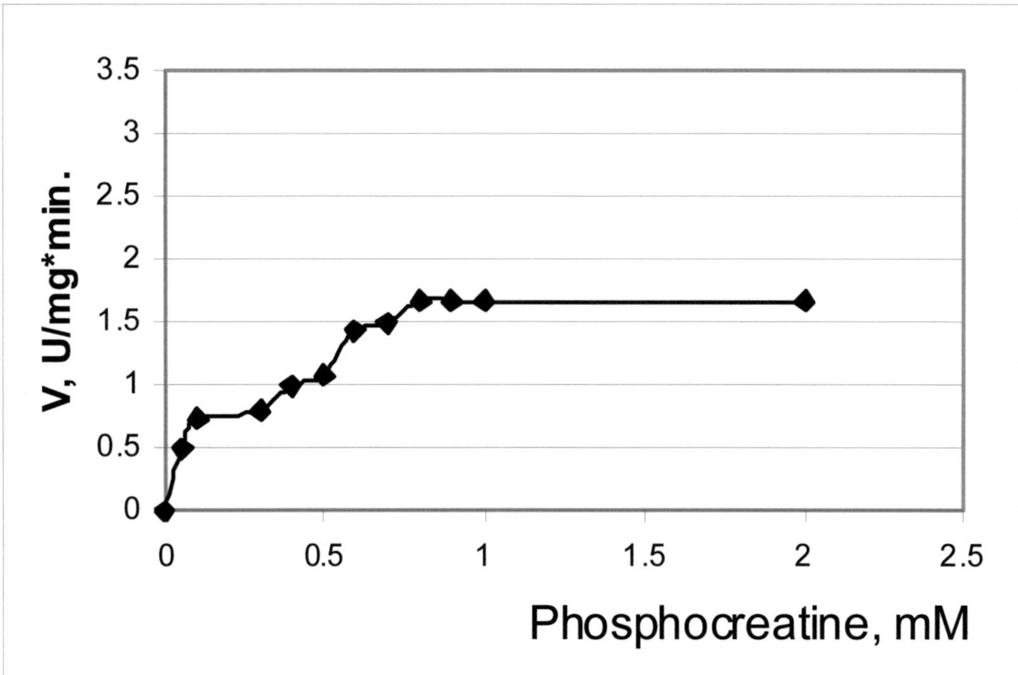

Fig. 12. Dependence of V_0 on concentration of phosphocreatine in total mitochondrial fraction in severe ischemia.

The study of the creatine kinase reaction in the group of animals after severe ischemia showed the abnormal kinetic behavior of the enzyme, the appearance of the intermediate plateau at the low concentration (0.3-0.4 mM) of creatine phosphate, the V_0 decreased 1.4-2 fold in comparison with intact rats.

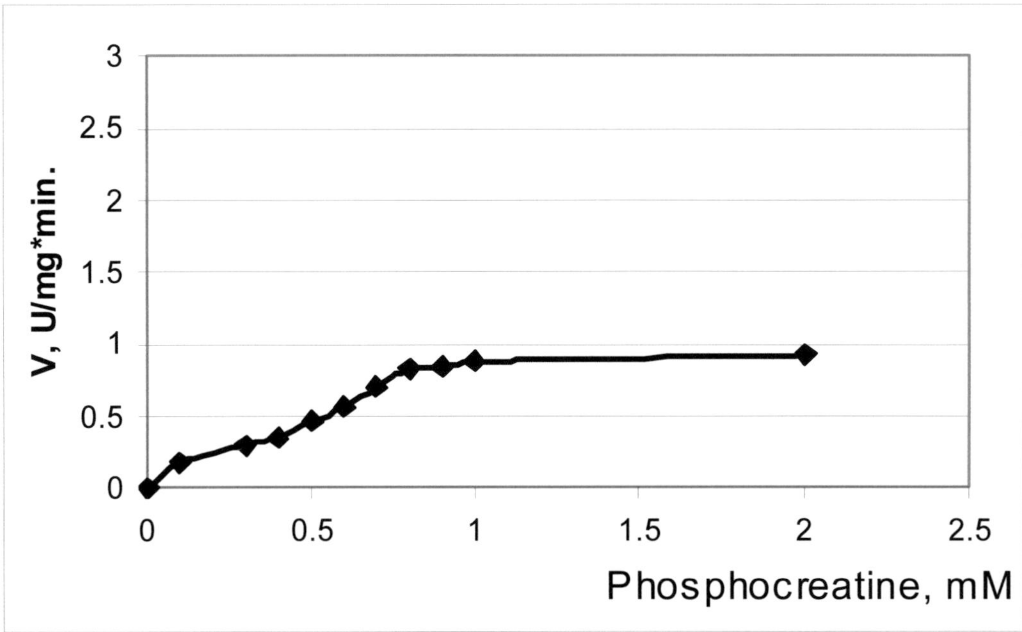

Fig. 13. Dependence of V_0 on concentration of phosphocreatine in fraction of mitochondrial membranes in severe ischemia.

The reversibility of these alterations has been shown during the increasing of duration of ischemia.

Increasing of the duration of cerebral ischemia to 4 and 18 hours was accompanied by changes in activity distribution for hexokinase. The activity of hexokinase progressively increased. The level of activity of the enzyme under these conditions was higher than in acute ischemia. However, the level of hexokinase activity in animals during long-term ischemia remained lower than in intact specimens (Fig. 14).

The bar diagrams display average activities with error bars representing the standard deviation. *$p<0.05$ versus intact animals. ** $p<0.05$ versus severe ischemia (30 minutes).

An increase in duration of cerebral ischemia influenced on the adsorption properties of hexokinase. Solubilization of hexokinase by 0.1 KCl was accompanied by decrease in the activity of the enzyme by 78% in acute cerebral ischemia. The percentage of solubilizing enzyme was 37% in 1.5 hours ischemia. It was by 11% higher than in intact specimens. The percentage of solubilizing enzyme was 30% and 27% in 4 hours and 18 hours ischemia, respectively. It did not differ from that in intact animals.

Therefore increase in the duration of cerebral ischemia was followed by an increase in the resistance of membrane structures. These changes were manifested in reduction of hexokinase desorption from the mitochondrial membrane.

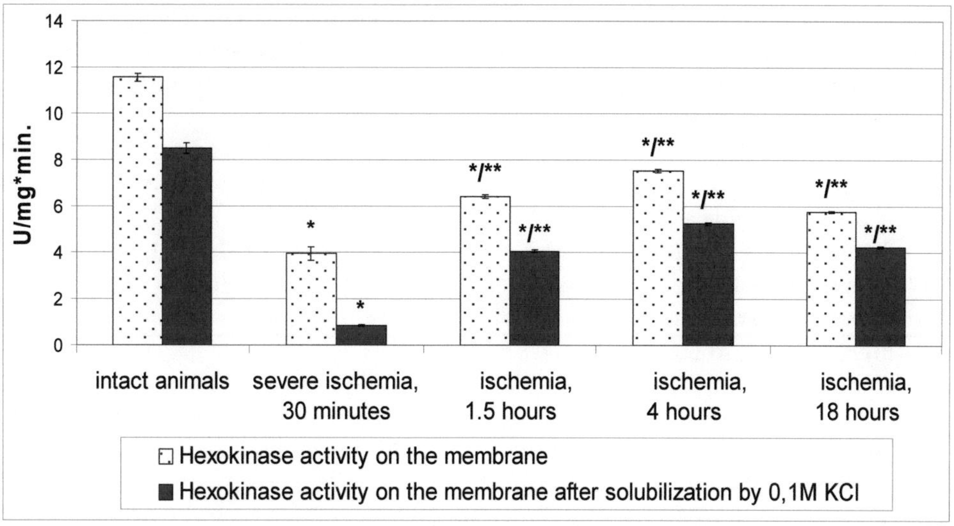

Fig. 14. The activity of membrane-bound hexokinase before and after solubilization by 0.1M KCl in cerebral ischemia

The cerebral ischemia causes the imbalance between reactive oxygen species production and the level of antioxidant defense, which leads to oxidative stress. Neuronal membranes contain a considerable amount of unsaturated lipids. The low level of activity of antioxidant enzymes and formation of free radicals in neurochemical reactions provide conditions for lipid oxidation and induce enzyme modification. To evaluate the state of membranes, the intensity of free radical oxidation and antioxidant properties of the brain tissue were estimated in various periods of ischemia (Table 2).

Experimental groups	Imax, mV	S, imp.*30 sec.	K=1/S
Intact animals	1.02±0.03 n=8	10.64±0.34 n=8	0.094
Ischemia, 30 minutes	1.89±0.07* n=7	17.22±0.98* n=7	0.058
Ischemia, 1.5 hours	1.52±0.04* n=7	15.18±0.91* n=7	0.066
Ischemia, 4 hours	1.47±0.05* n=8	14.55±0.03* n=8	0.068
Ischemia, 18 hours	1.08±0.11 n=8	12.63±0.79* n=8	0.079

*$p<0.05$ versus intact animals

Table 2. The intensity of free radical oxidation and the activity of antioxidant system in the brain.

Various characteristics of chemiluminescence (maximum flash amplitude and total yield of slow flash) in the mitochondrial fraction were elevated during various periods of cerebral ischemia. These changes reflect activation of free radical processes in the brain. Total yield of slow flash was 1.6-fold and 1.4-fold higher than in the intact animals in 30 min and 1.5 hours ischemia.

Parameters of free radical oxidation (Imax and S) remained practically unchanged by 4 hours ischemia. The increase in the duration of cerebral ischemia to 18 hours was accompanied by a decrease in the intensity of free radical oxidation. Parameter Imax did not differ from the corresponding parameter in intact animals.

Acute ischemia was not only followed by damage of the cell membrane structures and activation of free radical oxidation, but also induced the antioxidant system (Dziennis et al., 2008; Lai et al., 2003; Perez-Pinzon et al., 2005; Suzuki et al., 1997).

The K index serves as a criterion for the antioxidant potential of the cell. The level of the antioxidant activity of the brain tissue was elevated after ischemia for 1.5 and 4 hours. The conclusion was derived from the decrease in this index. By 18 hours ischemia, the K index did not differ from that in intact animals.

These data indicate that the prooxidant/antioxidant ratio returns to normal with increasing in the duration of cerebral circulatory disorder. The observed changes are probably related to activation of defense protein synthesis, which increases the resistance of membrane structures to the adverse effect of ischemia.

The kinetic curve for hexokinase was shown to have hyperbola form in various periods of ischemia except for 1.5 hours ischemia (Fig. 15). MgATP did not inhibit hexokinase when increasing the duration of ischemia. By 18 hours, the Km (0.13 mM) is 2-fold lower than in intact animals (0.26 mM) and is 5-fold lower than in 30 minutes ischemia (0.7 mM).

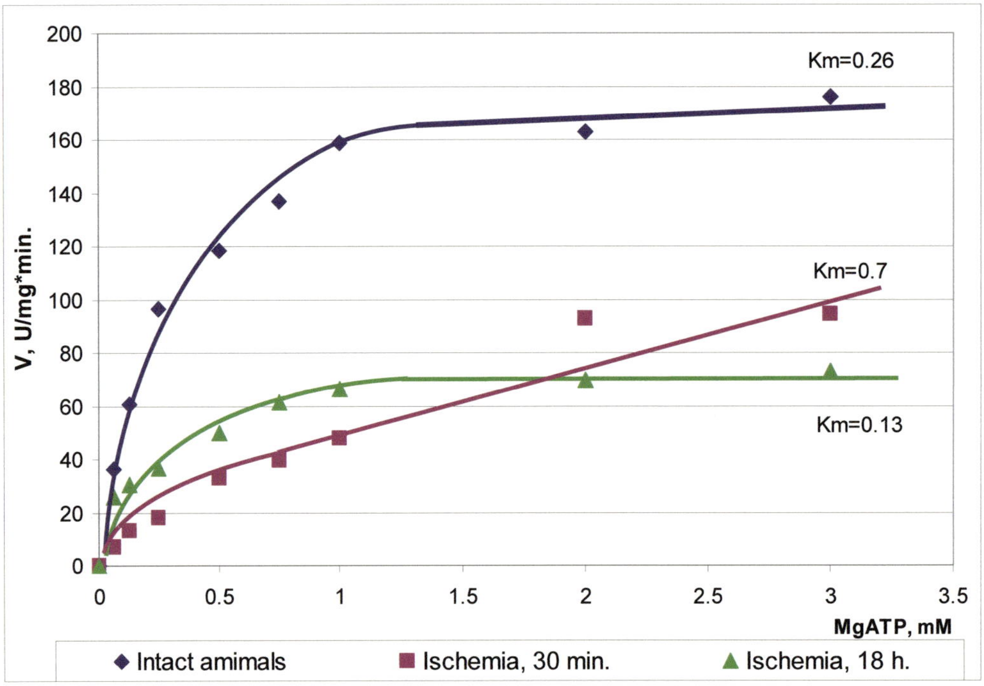

Fig. 15. Kinetic of the hexokinase reaction.

The major problem in the involvement of cell structures in the regulation of enzyme activity is the dependence of enzyme properties on the association of this enzyme with the membrane under conditions of functional changes in the organism.

Mitochondrial creatine kinase is associated with mitochondrial membranes due to the forces of electrostatic and hydrophobic interaction. Cerebral ischemia was followed by changes in the activity of associated and tightly-bound mitochondrial creatine kinase (Fig. 16).
The activity of associated mitochondrial creatine kinase increased in comparison with intact animals in 1.5 hours ischemia. However the activity of tightly-bound creatine kinase did not change. The activity of tightly-bound mitochondrial creatine kinase increased and the ratio between two forms of mitochondrial creatine kinase restored in 4 hours ischemia. By 18 hours, the percentage of tightly-bound form of the enzyme reached 90%.

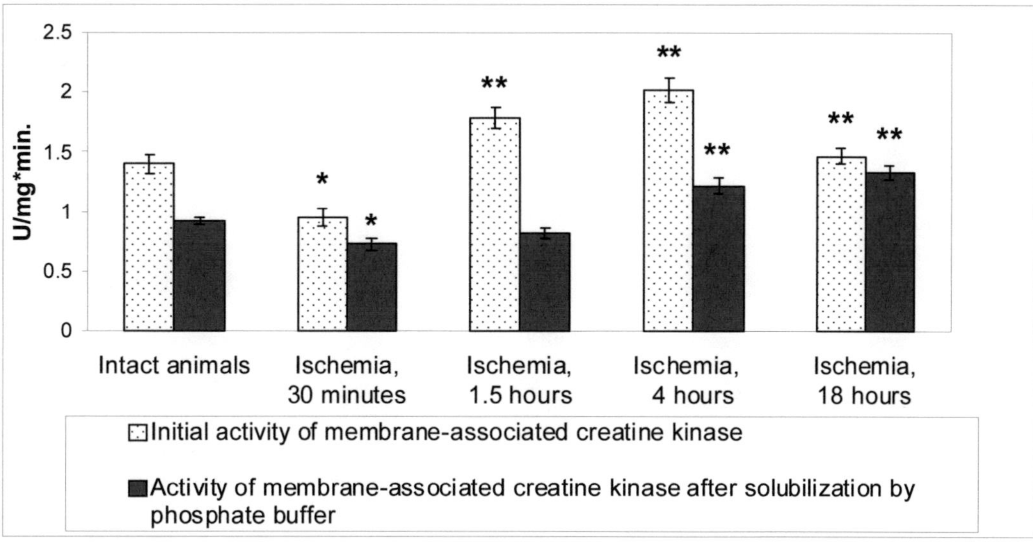

Fig. 16. The activity of membrane-associated creatine kinase before and after solubilization by phosphate buffer in cerebral ischemia.

The bar diagrams display average activities with error bars representing the standard deviation. *$p<0.05$ versus intact animals. ** $p<0.05$ versus severe ischemia (30 minutes).
Cerebral ischemia was shown to change the kinetic properties of mitochondrial creatine kinase (Fig. 17). Mitochondrial creatine kinase showed abnormal kinetic with the appearance of intermediate plateau. By 18 hours, the kinetic curve acquired a hyperbola form.
In mitochondria, mitochondrial creatine kinase is presented by two oligomeric forms (dimer and octamer). They are characterized by dynamic equilibrium (Lipskaya et al., 1989). The transition-state analogue complex of mitochondrial creatine kinase was induced to evaluate the ratio between oligomeric forms of this enzyme under conditions of cerebral circulatory disorders.
Cerebral ischemia changes the dimer/octamer ratio. This ratio is shifted toward the formation of dimers after 30-min ischemia (79%). Phospholipids serve as the structural elements of membranes that are bound to mitochondrial creatine kinase. Membrane binding properties of mitochondrial creatine kinase depend strongly on the protein dimer/octamer ratio and degree of lipid oxidation. Activation of free radical oxidation during acute ischemia is probably followed by partial dissociation of octamers to dimers. Increasing of the duration of ischemia to 18 hours was followed by an increase in the octamer ratio (53%).

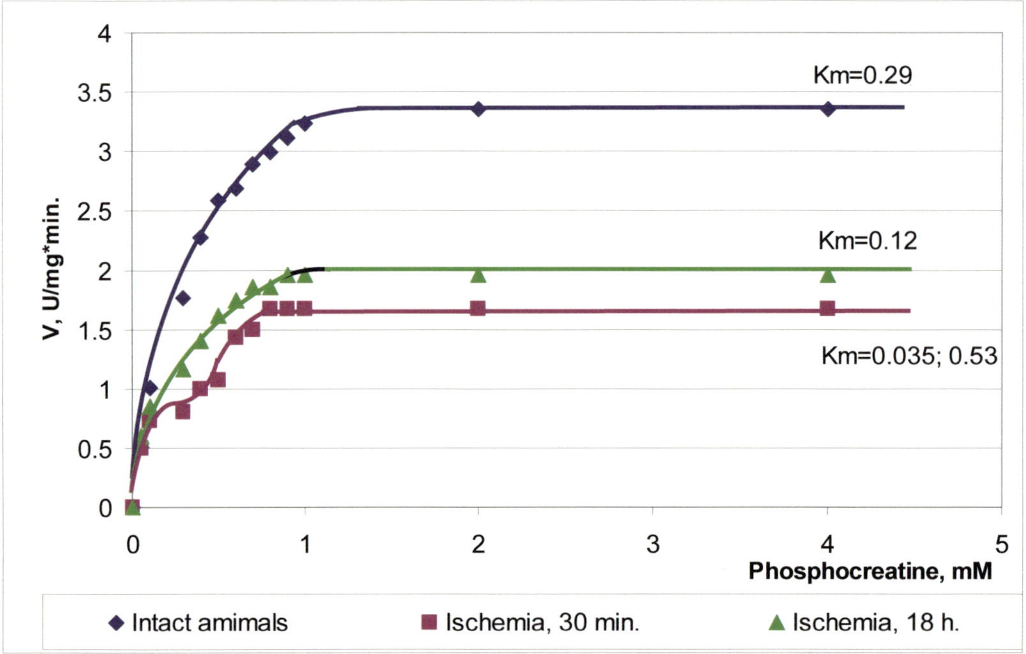

Fig. 17. Kinetic of the membrane-bound creatine kinase reaction

Published data suggest that octameric mitochondrial creatine kinase contributes to the appearance and strengthening of contact sites, which increases the efficiency of energy formation in brain mitochondria, consolidates the membrane structure, and determines the resistance of membranes to the adverse effect of hypoxia (Gross, Wallimann, 1995; Koufen et al., 1999; Lenz et al., 2007; Meyer et al., 2006). The existence of two oligomeric forms of this enzyme probably maintains the near-equilibrium state of reaction in a wide range of physiological conditions.

4. Conclusion

The results indicate that catalytic properties of mitochondrial creatine kinase and hexokinase depend on the functional interaction with mitochondrial membranes.

Acute ischemia impairs enzyme interaction with the mitochondrial membrane. Increasing in the duration of ischemia is not only followed by injury and dysfunction, but also activates the defense systems in the nervous tissue. It is manifested in the decrease in the intensity of free radical oxidation, increase in the percentage of tightly-bound mitochondrial creatine kinase, changes in kinetic properties of the enzyme and change in the dimer/octamer ratio toward the formation of octamer for the mitochondrial creatine kinase. These changes stabilize the mitochondrial creatine kinase complex. In contrast, increase in the duration of ischemia is accompanied by the decrease in the hexokinase activity on the membrane in spite the fact that it becomes higher than in acute 30 min ischemia, but the percentage of solubilizing enzyme does not differ from that in intact animals.

Therefore, the long-term ischemia leads to stabilization of the functional interaction between hexokinase and creatine kinase complex with the mitochondrial membranes at a new level, providing the adequate energy supply of the nervous cells due to the new adaptive conditions.

5. References

Aflalo, C. & Azoulay, H. (1998). Association of rat brain hexokinase to yeast mitochondria: effect of environmental factors and the source of porin. *J. Bioenerg. Biomembr.*, Vol. 30, pp. 245-255.

Aleshin, A.E.; Fromm, H.J. & Honzatko, R.B. (1998). Multiple crystal form of hexokinase I: new insights regarding conformational dynamics, subunit interactions, and membrane association. *FEBS Lett*, Vol. 434, pp. 42-46.

Bessman, S.P. & Carpenter, C.L. (1985). The creatine-creatine phosphate energy shuttle. *Annu. Rev. Biochem.*, Vol. 54, pp. 831-862.

Beutner, G.; Ruck, A., Riede, B. & Brdiczka, D. (1998). Complexes between porin, hexokinase, mitochondrial creatine kinase and adenylate translocator display properties of the permeability transition pore. Implication for regulation of permeability transition by the kinases. *Biochem. Biophys. Acta*, Vol. 1368, pp. 7-18.

Boero, J.; Qin, W., Cheg, J., Woolsey, T.A., Strauss, A.W. & Rhuchua, Z. (2003). Restricted neuronal expression of ubiquitous mitochondrial creatine kinase; changing patterns in development and with increased activity. *Mol. Cell Biochem*, Vol. 244, No 102, pp. 69-76.

Brdiczka, D. (1994). Function of the outer mitochondrial compartment in regulation of energy metabolism. *Biochem. Biophys. Acta*, Vol. 1187, No 2, pp. 264-269.

Bredford, T. & Spector, T. (1978). Refinement of the coomassie blue method of protein quantitation. A simple and linear spectrophotometric assay for less than or equal to 0.5 to 50 microgram of protein. *Anal. Biochem*, Vol. 86, No 1, pp. 142-146.

Chen, L.; Roberts, R. & Friedman, D.L. (1995). Expression of brain-type creatine kinase and ubiquitous mitochondrial creatine kinase in the fetal rat brain: evidence for a nuclear energy shuttle. *J. Comp. Neurol.*, Vol. 363, No 3, pp. 389-401.

Cherubini, A.; Ruggiero, C., Polidori, M.C. & Mecocci P. (2005). Potential markers of oxidative stress in stroke. *Free Radic. Biol. Med.*, Vol. 39, No 7, pp. 841-852.

Clostre, F. (2001). Mitochondria: recent pathophysiological discoveries and new therapeutic perspectives. *Ann. Pharm. Fr.*, Vol. 59, No 1, pp. 3-21.

da-Silva, W.S.; Gomez-Puyou, A., de Gomez-Puyou, M.T., Moreno-Sanchez, R., De Felice, F.G., de Meis, L., Oliveira, M.F. & Galina, A. (2004). Mitochondrial bound hexokinase activity as a preventive antioxidant defense: steady-state ADP formation as a regulatory mechanism of membrane potential and reactive oxygen species generation in mitochondria. *J. Biol. Chem.*, Vol. 279, No 38, pp. 39846-39855.

Delivoria-Papadopoulos, M.; Gorn M., Ashraf, Q.M. & Mishra, O.P. (2007). ATP and cytochrome c-dependent activation of caspase-9 during hypoxia in the cerebral cortex of newborn piglets. *Neurosci. Lett.*, Vol. 429, No 2-3, pp. 115-119.

Dizhe, G. P.; Eshchenko, N.D., Dizhe, A.A. & Krasovskaya, I.E. (2003). *Introduction to the Technique of Biochemical Assay* [in Russian], St. Petersburg, p. 86.

Dolder, M., Wendt, S. & Wallimann, T. (2001). Mitochondrial creatine kinase in contact sites: interaction with porine and adenine nucleotide translocase, role in permeability transition and sensivity to oxidative damage. *Biol. Signals Recept.*, Vol. 10, No 1-2, pp. 93-111.

Dos Santos, P.; Laclau, M.N., Boudina, S. & Garlid, K.D. (2004). Alteration of the bioenergetics systems of the cell in acute chronic myocardial ischemia. *Mol. Cell Biochem.*, Vol. 256-257, No 1-2, pp. 157-166.

Eppenberger-Eberhardt, M.; Riesinger, I., Messerli, M. et al. (1991). Adult rat cardiomyocytes cultured in creatine-deficient medium display large mitochondria with paracrystalline inclutions, enriched for creatine kinase. *J. Cell Biol.*, Vol. 113, pp. 289-302.

Eriksson, O.; Fontaine, E. & Bernandi, P. (1998). Chemical modification of arginines by 2,3-butanedione and phenylglyoxal causes closure of the mitochondrial permeability transition pore. *Biol. Chem.*, Vol. 273, pp. 12669-12674.

Felgner, P.L. & Wilson, J.E.(1976) Purification of nonbindable and membrane bindable mitochondrial hexokinase from rat brain. *Biochem. Biophys. Res. Communs.*, Vol. 68, No 2, pp. 592-597.

Fiscum, G. (2000) Mitochondrial participation in ischemic and traumatic neural cell death. J. *Neurotrauma*, Vol. 17, No 10, pp. 843-855.

Focant, T. (1970). Isolement et proprietes de la creatine-kinase de muscle lisse de boeuf. *FEBS Lett.*, Vol. 10, pp. 57-61.

Fonyo, A. & Somogyi, J. (1960). The phosphorylation of adenosinediphosphate and glucose in isolated brain mitochondria at different osmatic concentrations. *Acta physiol. Acad. Sci., Hung.*, Vol. 8, No 3, pp. 191.

Fridman, D.L & Roberts, R. (1994). Compartmentation of brain type creatine kinase and ubiquitous mitochondrial creatine kinase in neurons; evidence for a creatine phosphate shuttle in adult rat brain. *J. Comp. Neurol*, Vol. 343, No 3, pp. 500-511.

Fritz-Wolf, K. ; Schnyder, T. , Wallimann, T. & Kabsch, W (1996). Structure of mitochondrial creatine kinase. *J. Nature*, Vol. 381, No 6580, pp. 341-345.

Glantz, S.A. (2005). *Primer of Biostatistics*, 6th ed., McGraw-Hill Medical Publishing, p. 500.

Gross, M. & Wallimann, T. (1995). Dimer-dimer interactions in octameric mitochondrial creatine kinase. *Biochemistry*, Vol. 34, No 20, pp. 6660-6667.

Grossman, S. & Mixon, D. (1985). Further Characterization of the reassembly of creatine kinase and effect of substrate. *Arch. Biochem. Biophys.*, Vol. 236, pp. 797.

Guo, Z.; Wang, Z. & Wang, X. (2003). Studies on the stability of creatine kinase isoenzymes. *Biochem Cell Biol.*, Vol.81, No 1, pp. .9-16.

Hemmer, W.; Zanolla, E., Furter-Graves, E.M., Eppenberger, H.M. & Wallimann, T. (1994). Creatine kinase isozymes in chicken cerebellum: specific localization of brain-type creatine kinase in Bergmann glial cells and muscle-type creatine kinase in Purkinje neurons. *Eur. J. Neurosci*, Vol. 6, No 4, pp. 538-549.

Ishibashi, S. (1999). Cooperation of membrane proteins and cytosolic proteins in metabolic regulation – involvement of binding of hexokinase to mitochondria in regulation of glucose metabolism and association and complex formation between membrane proteins and cytosolic proteins in regulation of active oxygen production. *Yakugaku Zasshi*, Vol. 119, No 1, pp. 16-35.

Kaldis, P.; Wallimann T. (1995). Functional differences between dimeric and octameric mitochondrial creatine kinase. *Biochem. J.*, Vol. 308, pp. 623-627.

Kellershohn, N. & Ricard, J. (1994). Coordination of catalytic activities within enzyme complex. *Eur. J. Biochem.*, Vol. 220, No 2, pp. 955-961.

Koufen, P. et al. (1999). Free radical-induced inactivation of creatine kinase: influence on the octameric and dimeric states of the mitochondrial enzyme (Mi_b-CK). *Biochem. J.*, Vol. 344, pp. 413-417.

Kuby, S.A.; Noda, L. & Lardy, H.A. (1954). Adenosinetriphosphate-creatine transphosphorylase. I. Isolation of the crystalline enzyme from rabbit muscle. *J. Biol. Chem.*, Vol. 209, No 1, pp. 191-201.

Kuzmina, E.I. et al. (2009). The evaluation of antioxidant action of medications on modeling systems in vitro. *Revista de Ozonoterapia*, Vol. 3, suppl., No 1, pp. 67-68.

Kuznetsov, A.V.; Margreiter, R. (2009). Heterogeneity of mitochondria and mitochondrial function within cells as another level of mitochondrial complexity. *Int. J. Mol. Sci*, Vol. 10, No 4, pp. 1911-1929.

Lai, J.C.; White, B.K., Buerstatte, C.R.б Haddad G.G., Novotny, E.J. Jr. & Behar, K.L. (2003). Chronic hypoxia in development selectively alters the activities of key enzymes of glucose oxidative metabolism in brain regions. *Neurochem. Res.*, Vol. 28, No 6, pp. 933-940.

Lenz, H.; Schmidt, M., Welge, V., Kueper, T., Schlattner, U., Wallimann, T., Elsässer, H.P., Wittern, K.P., Wenck, H., Staeb, F. & Blatt, T. (2007). Inhibition of cytosolic and mitochondrial creatine kinase by siRNA in HaCaT - and HeLaS3-cells affects cell viability and mitochondrial morphology. *Mol. Cell. Biochem.*, Vol. 306, pp. 153-162.

Levin, R.M.; Longhurst, P.A., Levin, S.S., Haugaard, N. & Wein, A.J. (1990). Creatine kinase activity of urinary bladder and skeletal muscle from control and streptozotocin-diabetic rats. *Mol. Cell Biochem.*, Vol. 97, No 2, pp. 153-159.

Levine, S.R. et al. Human focal cerebral ischemia: evaluation of brain pH and energy metabolism with P-31 NMR spectroscopy. *Radiology*, Vol. 185, No 2, pp. 537-544.

Lin, L.; Perrymann, M.B., Friedman, D., Roberts, R. & Ma, T.S. (1994). Determination of the catalytic site of creatine kinase by site-directed mutagenesis. *Biochim Biophys Acta*, Vol. 1206, No 1, pp. 97-104.

Linden, M.; Gellerfors, P. & Nelson, B.D. (1982). Pore protein and the hexokinase- binding protein from the outer membrane of rat liver mitochondria are identical. *FEBS Lett*, Vol. 141, pp. 189-192.

Lipskaya, T.Yu.; Trofimova, M.E. & Moiseeva, N.S. (1989). Kinetic properties of the octameric and dimeric forms of mitochondrial creatine kinase and physiological role of the enzyme. *Biochem. Int.*, Vol. 19, No 3, pp. 603-613.

Lyubarev, A.E. (1977). Origin of biochemical organization. *Biosystems*, Vol. 42, No 2-3, pp. 103-110.

Magnani, M.; Serafini, G., Stocche, V., Bossù, M. & Dachà, M. Solubilization, purification and properties of rabbit brain hexokinase. *Arch. Biochem. and Biophys.*, Vol. 216, No 2, pp. 449-454.

Mattson, M.P.; Liu, D. (2002). Energetics and oxidative stress in synaptic plasticity and neurodegenerative disorders. *Neuromolecular Med*, Vol. 2, No 2, pp. 215-231.

Maulik, N.; Goswani, S., Galang, N. & Das, D.K. (1999). Differential regulation of Bcl-2, AP-1 and NF-kappaB on cardiomyocyte apoptosis during myocardial ischemic stress adaptation. *FEBS Lett.*, Vol. 443, No 3, pp. 331-336.

Meyer, L.E.; Machado, L.B., Santiago, A.P., da-Silva, W.S., De Felice, F.G., Holub, O., Oliveira, M.F. & Galina, A. (2006). Mitochondrial creatine kinase activity prevents reactive oxygen species generation. Antioxidant role of mitochondrial kinase-dependent ADP re-cycling activity. *The journal of biological chemistry*, Vol. 281, No 49, pp. 37361-37371.

Mulichak, A.M.; Wilson, J.E., Padmanabhan, K. & Garavito, R.M. (1998). The structure of mammalian hexokinase I. *Nat. Struct. Biol.*, Vol. 5, pp. 555-560.

Ovadi, J. & Srere, P.A. (2000). Macromolecular compartmentation and channeling. *Intl. Rev. Cytol.*, Vol. 192, pp. 255-280.

Perez-Pinzon, M.A.; Dave, K.R. & Raval, A.P. (2005). Role of reactive oxygen species and protein kinase C in ischemic tolerance in the brain. *Antioxid. Redox Signal*, Vol. 7, No 9-10, pp. 1150-1157.

Rauchova, H.; Kaudelova, J., Drahota, Z. & Mourek J. (2002). Hypoxia-induced lipid peroxidation in rat brain and protective effect of carnitine and phosphocreatine. *Neurochem. Res.*, Vol. 27, No 9, pp. 899-904.

Redker, V.D. & Kenkare, V.W. (1972). Bovine brain mitochondrial hexokinase. Solubilization, purification and role of sulphydryl residues. *J. Biol. Chem.*, Vol. 247, pp. 1576-1584.

Rosano, C. E.; Sabini, M. Rizzi, M., Deriu, D., Murshudov, G., Bianchi, M., Serafini, G., Magnani, M. & Bolognesi, M. (1999). Binding of non-catalytic ATP to human hexokinase I highlights the structural components for enzyme-membrane association control. *Structure*, Vol. 7, No 11, pp. 1427-1437.

Rose, I. & Warms, J.V.B. (1967). Mitocondrial hexokinase. Release. Rebinding, and location. *J. Biol. Chem.*, Vol. 242, pp. 1635-1645.

Sappey-Marinier, D.; Hubesch, B., Matson, G.B. & Weiner, M.W. (2002). Decreased phosphorus metabolite concentrations and alkalosis in chronic cerebral infarction. *Radiology*, Vol. 182, pp. 29-34.

Sas, K.; Robotka, H., Toldi, J. & Vécsei, L. (2007). Mitochondria, metabolic disturbances, oxidative stress and the kynurenine system, with focus on neurodegenerative disorders. *J. Neurol. Sci*, Vol. 257, No 1-2, pp. 221-239.

Schlattner, U.; Dolder, M., Wallimann, N. & Tokarska-Schlattner, M. (2001). Mitochondrial creatine kinase and mitochondrial outer membrane porin show a direct interaction that is modulated by calcium. *J. Biol. Chem.*, Vol. 276, No 51, pp. 48027-48030.

Schnyder, T.; Engel, A., Lustig, A. & Wallimann, T. (1988). Native mitochondrial creatine kinase forms octameric structures. II. Characterization of dimers and octamers by ultracentrifugation, direct mass measurements by scanning transmission electron microscopy, and image analysis of single mitochondrial creatine kinase octamers. *J. Biol. Chem*, Vol. 263, No 32, pp. 16954-16962.

Schnyder, T.; Tittmann, P., Winkler, H., Gross, H. & Wallimann, T. (1995). Localization of reactive cysteine residues by maleidoyl undecagold in the mitochondrial creatine kinase octamer. *J. Struct. Biol*, Vol. 114, No 3, pp. 209-217.

Schwab, D.A & Wilson, J.E. (1989). Complete amino acid sequence of rat brain hexokinase, deduced from the cloned cDNA, and proposed structure of a mammalian hexokinase. *Biochem.*, Vol. 86, pp. 2563-2567.

Shen, W.; Willis, D., Zhang, Y., Schlattner, U., Wallimann, T. & Molloy, G.R. (1978). Expression of creatine kinase isozyme genes during postnatal development of rat brain cerebellum: Evidence for transcriptional regulation. *Biochem. J.*, Vol. 367, No 2, pp. 369-380.

Siesjo, B.K. Brain energy metabolism / B.K. Siesjo. - Ed. J.Wiley and Sons, 1978. - 607p.

Smith, A.D. & Wilson, J.E. (1991). Disposition of mitochondrially bound hexokinase at the membrane surface, deduced from reactivity with monoclonal anti bodies recognizing epitopes of defined location. *Arch. Biochem. Biophys.*, Vol. 287, pp. 359-366.

Suzuki, Y.J.; Forman, H.J. & Sevanian, A. Oxidants as stimulators of signal transduction. *Free Radic. Biol. Med.*, Vol. 22, No 1-2, pp. 269-285.

Takagi, Y.; Yasuhara, T. & Gomi K. (2001). Creatine kinase and its isozymes. *Rinsho Byori*, Suppl. 116, pp. 52-61.

Ueda, M.; Muramatsu, H., Kamiya, T., Muramatsu, A., Mori, T., Terashi, A. & Katayama, Y. (2000). Pyruvate dehydrogenase activity and energy metabolite level following bilateral common carotid artery occlusion in rat brain. *Life Sci*, Vol. 67, No 7, pp. 821-826.

Viitanen, P.V.; Geiger, P.J., Erickson-Viitanen, S. & Bessman, S.P. (1984). Evidence for functional hexokinase compartmentation in rat skeletal muscle mitochondria. *J. Biol. Chem.*, Vol. 259, No 15, pp. 9679-9686.

Vyssokikh, M. & Brdiczka, D. (2003). The Function of complexes between the outer mitochondrial membrane pore (VDAC) and the adenine nucleotide translocase in regulation of energy metabolism and apoptosis. *Acta Biochimica Polonica*, Vol. 50, No 2, pp. 389-404.

Wallimann, T. et al. (1992). Intracellular compartmentation, structure and function of creatine kinase isoenzymes in tissues with high and fluctuating energy demands: the "phosphocreatine circuit" for cellular energy homeostasis. *Biochem. J.*, Vol. 281, pp. 21-40.

Wallimann, T. et al. (1998). Some new aspects of creatine kinase (CK): compartmentation, structure, function and regulation for cellular and mitochondrial bioenergetics and physiology. *Biofactors*, Vol. 8, No 3-4, pp. 229-234.

Walzel, B.; Speer,O., Zanolla, E., et al. (2002). Novel mitochondrial creatine transport activity: implications for intracellular creatine compartments and bioenergetics. *J. Biol. Chem.*, Vol. 277, pp. 37503-375511.

Wang, P.F.; Flynn, A.J., McLeish, M.J. & Kenyon, G.L. (2005). Loop movement and catalysis in creatine kinase. *IUBMB Life*, Vol. 57, No 4-5, pp. 355-362.

Wilson, J.E. (1980). Brain hexokinase, the prototype ambiquitous enzyme. *Curr. Top. Cell. Regul.*, Vol. 16., pp. 2-54.

Wilson, J.E. (1985). Regulation of mammalian hexokinase activity Regul. *Carbohydr. Metab.*, No 1, pp. 45-85.

Wilson, J.E. (1995). Hexokinases. *Rev. Physiol. Biochem. Pharmacol.*, Vol. 126, pp. 65-198.

Wilson, J.E. (2003). Isozymes of mammalian hexokinase: structure, subcellular localization and metabolic function. *The J. Exp. Biol.,* Vol. 206, pp. 2049-2057.

Wyss, M. & Kaddurah-Daouk, R. (2000). Creatine and creatinine metabolism. *Physiol. Rev.,* Vol. 80, pp. 1107-1213.

Xie, G. & Wilson, J.E. (1990). Tetrameric structure of mitochondrially bound rat brain hexokinase: a crosslinking study. *Arch. Biochem. Biophys.,* Vol. 276, No 1, pp. 285-293.

11

Diabetes-Mediated Exacerbation of Neuronal Damage and Inflammation After Cerebral Ischemia in Rat: Protective Effects of Water-Soluble Extract from Culture Medium of *Ganoderma lucidum* Mycelia

Naohiro Iwata[1], Mari Okazaki[1,*], Rika Nakano[1], Chisato Kasahara[1], Shinya Kamiuchi[1], Fumiko Suzuki[2], Hiroshi Iizuka[2], Hirokazu Matsuzaki[1] and Yasuhide Hibino[1]

[1]*Department of Immunobiochemistry, Josai University Graduate School of Pharmaceutical Sciences, Saitama,*
[2]*Noda Shokukinkogyo Co., Ltd.*
Japan

1. Introduction

Diabetes mellitus is a metabolic disorder, suffered by hundreds of millions of people throughout the world, which is characterized by hyperglycemia resulting from insufficiency of insulin secretion and/or action (Wild et al., 2004). Complications associated with diabetes affecting vessels, eyes, kidney, and peripheral nerves reduce the QOL of diabetic patients. Also, diabetes is widely recognized as a major risk factor for atherosclerotic disease such as acute brain ischemia. Indeed, diabetic patients have a higher risk of stroke compared with non-diabetic patients (Baynes 1991; Stephens et al., 2009). Additionally, they are more likely to have a poor prognosis and increased mortality after stroke (Biller et al., 1993; Vinik et al., 2002). Previous studies have demonstrated that the diabetic state increases oxidative stress in the brain and aggravates cerebral ischemic injury in both type I (Li et al., 2004; Saito et al., 2005; Rizk et al., 2005) and type II diabetic animal models (Anabela et al., 2006; Tureyen et al., 2011). In addition to neuronal damage attributed to hypoxia and ATP depletion caused by vascular obstruction in ischemic core region, cerebral injury caused by subsequent reperfusion is also involved in the pathophysiology of transient ischemia (Doyle et al., 2008; Nakka et al., 2008; Wang et al., 2010). During reperfusion, the production of reactive oxygen species (ROS) and reactive nitrogen species (RNS) is enhanced by abrupt re-oxygenation (Cuzzocrea et al., 2001; Saito et al., 2005). Besides direct injurious effects to the cell membrane, proteins and DNA by

* Corresponding Author

oxidation, ROS and RNS activate the pro-apoptotic pathway including the activation of caspase family proteases leading to DNA fragmentation in the neuronal cells of the ischemic penumbral region (Sugawara et al., 2007; Nakka et al., 2008). Hyperglycemia is assumed to be a major factor responsible for excessive generation of ROS. In the diabetic state, "glucose toxicity" caused by augmentation of the intracellular glucose oxidation process and non-enzymatic glycation of protein molecules leads to over production of ROS (Baynes, 1991; Giacco et al., 2010). Moreover, experimental transient hyperglycemia caused by intravenous infusion of glucose has been shown to increase ROS production and exacerbate brain injury after ischemia and subsequent reperfusion in rats (Tsuruta et al., 2010).

In addition to apoptotic cell death, inflammatory neurodegeneration is a crucial process contributing to cerebral damage after ischemia and reperfusion (Brown et al., 2010). ROS has been shown to activate nuclear factor-κB (NF-κB), which enhances transcription of the genes encoding pro-inflammatory cytokines and cell adhesion molecules, leading to neuroinflammatory responses (Saeed et al., 2007). Activation of the transcription factor NF-κB by ROS in microglia and astrocytes leads to an increase in the expression of cyclooxygenase-2 (COX-2), inducible nitric oxide synthase (iNOS) and pro-inflammatory cytokines including TNF-α, IL-1β and IL-6, which accelerate inflammatory responses and promote neuronal cell death in the ischemic region (Brown et al., 2010). Gene expression of IL-1β and IL-6 is much higher in type2-diabetic mice as compared with normoglycemic control mice (Tureyen et al., 2011). These pro-inflammatory cytokines and inflammatory mediators have been indicated to induce further inflammatory responses involving extravasation of neutrophils, macrophages/microglia through the expression of intracellular adhesion molecule 1 (ICAM-1) in endothelial cells (Wang et al., 2002; Chrissobolis et al., 2011). Myeloperoxidase (MPO) expressing in neutrophils and macrophages/ microglia, which has often been used as a histopathological marker for inflammation, generates ROS such as hypochloride and super oxide anion radical ($O_2^{-}\cdot$) and leads to further tissue damage (Breckwoldt et al., 2008). Thus, enhanced oxidative stress and inflammatory responses induced by hyperglycemia may substantially contribute to the exacerbation of cerebral injury caused by transient ischemia and subsequent reperfusion in the diabetic state.

Ganoderma lucidum (*G. lucidum*), a very popular medicinal fungus, has long been known for its beneficial effects on human health and longevity in Asian countries. Its fruiting bodies and cultured mycelia are used to treat chronic hepatopathy (Shi et al., 2008), hypertension (Kabir et al., 1988), hyperglycemia (Zhang et al., 2004), and tumor (Lu et al., 2003; Kubo et al., 2005). The pharmacological activities of *G. lucidum* constituents responsible for many of its health benefits, such as antioxidant (Zhu et al., 1999), anticancer (Lu et al., 2003; Kubo et al., 2005), anti-inflammatory (Akihisa et al., 2007), and immunomodulatory activities (Lai et al., 2010) have been elucidated. The water-soluble extract from culture medium of *G. lucidum* mycelia (MAK), a commercially available nutritional supplement, is a freeze-dried powder of a hot-water extract prepared from a solid culture medium composed of bagasse and defatted-rice bran overgrown with *G. lucidum* mycelia by cultivation for about 3.5 months. In a previous study, we demonstrated that the orally administered MAK attenuated oxidative stress and relieved exacerbation of cerebral injury induced by middle cerebral artery occlusion and reperfusion (MCAO/Re) in streptozotocin (STZ)-induced diabetic rats (Iwata et al., 2008). However, the mechanism of its cerebroprotective effect still remains unclear. Thus, we evaluated the effects of chronic oral pretreatment of MAK on the production of $O_2^{-}\cdot$ and apoptosis in STZ-rat brain after MCAO/Re. Furthermore, to clarify whether MAK suppresses inflammatory responses induced by the transient ischemia and reperfusion, we examined the effects of MAK on the expression profile of TNF-α, IL-1β, iNOS, COX-2, ICAM-1 and MPO in the brain during reperfusion.

2. Materials and methods

2.1 Experimental diabetic animals

Male Sprague Dawley rats (4-week old, weight 120-140 g; Tokyo Exp. Animal Co., Ltd., Tokyo, Japan) were purchased and housed in a temperature-controlled environment (23 ± 0.5°C) with a cycle of 12 hrs light and 12 hrs dark. The rats were given a standard rodent chow and water *ad libitum*. Animal care and the surgical procedure were performed in accordance with guidelines approved by the National Institutes of Health and the Josai University Animal Investigation Committee. A diabetic state was induced in the rats (diabetic group) by a single injection of STZ (60 mg/kg, i.p.) dissolved in 0.1 mM sodium citrate (pH 4.5), while the rats of the non-diabetic group were injected with buffer only (Iwata et al., 2008). Seven days after the STZ-injection, the plasma glucose level was determined using a glucose analyzer (Ascensia, Bayer Medical Co., Ltd., Land Nordrhein-Westfalen, Germany). Diabetes was defined by a blood glucose level greater than 300 mg/dl. Then, the diabetic and non-diabetic groups were divided into two groups respectively and were housed for an additional 6 weeks until stroke was induced by MCAO. MAK (1 g/kg; MAK group) or distilled water (control group) was administrated orally once daily for the last 2 weeks.

2.2 Middle cerebral artery occlusion and reperfusion

Focal cerebral ischemia was induced by MCAO with a standard intraluminal filament technique as previously described (Iwata et al., 2010). The animals were anesthetized with 4% halothane and maintained with 1.5% halothane and 30% oxygen under spontaneous respiration. After a midline incision at the neck, the right common carotid artery was exfoliated under an operating microscope. All branches of the external carotid artery were isolated and ligated. The tip of the 4-0 surgical nylon monofilament rounded by flame heating was inserted up through the internal carotid artery. When a small resistance was felt, insertion was stopped. The distance from bifurcation of the common carotid artery to the tip of the suture was approximately 20 mm in all rats. Cerebral blood flow was detected by laser Doppler Flowmetry (ATBF-LC1, Unique Medical Co., LTD., Tokyo) and about 50% reduction of its baseline associated with MCAO was ascertained in the rats. Rectal temperature was maintained at 37°C with a heat lamp and a heating pad during the operation. After 2 hrs of occlusion, the filament was withdrawn to allow for reperfusion. Then, the animals were permitted to recover from the anesthesia at room temperature. The rats were reperfused for 3 or 24 hrs before they were killed. The sham operation with the same manipulation without introduction of the monofilament was also performed in the 4 rats of the non-diabetic and diabetic groups, respectively.

2.3 Neurological evaluation

Post-ischemic neurological deficits were evaluated after 3 or 24 hrs of reperfusion on a 5-point scale as described as follows: grade 0:no deficit, grade 1:failure to extend right forepaw fully, grade 2:spontaneous circling or walking to contralateral side, grade 3:walking only when stimulated, grade 4:unresponsive to stimulation and a depressed level of consciousness, grade 5:death (Iwata et al., 2008; Vinik et al., 2002). Animals that did not show neurological deficits were excluded from the study.

2.4 Infarct and edema assessment

After 3 or 24 hrs of reperfusion, the animals were deeply anesthetized with diethyl ether and decapitated. The brain was removed and cut into four 2-mm coronal sections using a rat brain matrix, and stained with 2% 2,3,5-triphenyltetrazolium chloride (TTC; Wako Pure Chemicals) at 37°C for 15 min. The coronal slices were fixed in 10% formaldehyde for photography (Iwata et al., 2008; Vinik et al., 2002). Then, infarct areas were determined by using the image analysis system (Scion Image 1.62), and were added to obtain the infarct volumes per brain. Corrected infarct volume (%) = [left hemisphere volume - (right hemisphere volume - the infarct volume)] / left hemisphere volume × 100. Edema in the ischemic hemisphere was also calculated: edema (%) = (right hemisphere volume - the infarct volume) / left hemisphere volume.

2.5 Detection of $O_2^{-}\cdot$ generation in brain

Detection of intracellular $O_2^{-}\cdot$ generation in the penumbral region of the cortex following MCAO/Re was performed by staining freshly frozen brain sections (8 μm thick) with the fluorescent probe dihydroethidium (DHE). The brain sections were immediately incubated with DHE (10 μmol/l, Sigma) in phosphate-buffered saline for 30 min at 37°C (Muranyi et al., 2006). To determine the fluorescent intensity of oxidized DHE, three microscopic fields at the penumbral cortex regions of each hemisphere were captured using a confocal laser-scanning microscope at excitation of 510 nm and emission of 580 nm. Fluorescence intensity of the oxidized DHE was quantified using imaging software (FV10-ASW 1.7, OLYMPUS Co. Ltd., Tokyo, Japan).

2.6 TUNEL staining

Apoptosis in the brain tissues was measured using the Apoptosis in situ Detection Kit Wako (Wako, Laboratories, Osaka, Japan), which is based on the TUNEL (Terminal deoxynucleotidyl Transferase (TdT)-mediated dUTP nick end labeling) procedure, that is the addition of fluorescein-dUTP to 3′-terminals of apoptotically fragmented DNA with TdT followed by immunochemical detection using anti-fluorescein antibody conjugated with horseradish peroxidase (POD) and DAB (3-3′-diaminobenzidine tetrachloride) as a substrate. Coronal brain sections (8 μm thick) were used for the assay. The slides were lightly counterstained with hematoxylin and observed under a microscope (BX51W1, OLYMPUS). Quantification of TUNEL positive cells was achieved by cell counting in areas of the penumbral cortex affected by ischemia. Three randomly chosen visual fields were counted in each region by an investigator without knowledge of the experimental conditions. The percentage of apoptotic cells was calculated by the apoptotic index, i.e. dividing the number of positive-staining nuclei by the total number of nuclei (Li et al., 2004).

2.7 Real-time PCR analysis

The temporal gene expression patterns of pro-inflammatory cytokines (IL-1β and TNF-α) and inflammatory mediators (COX-2, iNOS and ICAM-1) were evaluated by quantitative real-time PCR analysis as described earlier (Liu et al. 2007). The rats subjected to MCAO were killed at 3 or 24 hrs of reperfusion, and the total RNA sample was obtained from the ischemic penumbral cortex of each rat. Total RNA was extracted with RNeasy Mini Kit (QIAGEN, Hilden, Germany) according to the manufacturer's instructions. Total RNA (0.5 μg) from each sample was reverse-transcribed with oligo dT and random hexamer primers using reverse transcriptase (PrimeScript™ RT Enzyme Mix I, Takara RNA PCR Kit, Takara Biomedicals, Shiga, Japan). Real-time PCR was performed with 10 ng of cDNA and a pair of gene specific primers (Takara Biomedicals) added to the SYBR Premix EX *Taq* (Takara Biomedicals) and subjected to PCR amplification in the iCycler iQ Real-Time Detection System (Bio-Rad Laboratories, Inc., Hercules, CA, USA) (1 cycle at 95°C for 10 sec, and 50 cycles at 95°C for 5 sec and 60°C for 34 sec). The expression of β-actin was used to normalize cDNA levels. The PCR products were analyzed by a melting curve to ascertain the specificity of amplification. Data were normalized to β-actin and were expressed as mean ± SD relative to the sham-operated non-diabetic group.

2.8 Immunohistochemistry

Immunostaining was performed as previously described (Faraco et al., 2007). Briefly, rats were sacrificed at the indicated time points and transcardially perfused with cold saline. Brains were fixed with 4% phosphate-buffered paraformaldehyde. Coronal brain sections (8 μm thick) were incubated sequentially with 3% hydrogen peroxide for 40 min at room temperature to inhibit endogenous peroxidase, followed by incubation with blocking buffer (100% block ace; Dainippon Sumitomo Pharma Co. Ltd., Osaka, Japan) for 2 hrs. Slides were incubated with polyclonal rabbit anti-IL-1β antibody (1:300, Santa Cruz Biotechnology, CA, USA), polyclonal rabbit anti-TNF-α antibody (1:200; Rabbit mAb, Hycult Biotech, PB Uden, The Netherlands), polyclonal rabbit anti-COX-2 antibody (1:200, Cayman Chemical, Michigan, USA), polyclonal rabbit anti-iNOS antibody (1:200, Santa Cruz), monoclonal mouse anti-RECA-1 (1:200, Abcam Biotechnology, Cambridge, UK), polyclonal rabbit anti-Cleaved caspase-3 (1:100, Cell Signalling Technology, Danvers, MA, USA), and monoclonal mouse anti-MPO (1:100, Hycult Biotech) in 0.01 mol/l phosphate-buffered saline overnight at 4°C. After washing with PBS, these were correspondingly incubated with Cy3- and FITC-conjugated secondary antibodies (1:200, Chemicon, California, USA) for 2 hrs at room temperature. Finally, sections were incubated with the nuclear stain TO-PRO-3 (1:10000, Invitrogen, California, USA) in phosphate-buffered saline for 10 min at room temperature with gentle agitation, washed and mounted using 70% glycerol mounting medium. Immunofluorescence was visualized using a Laser Scanning Confocal Microscope (FluoView FV1000, OLYMPUS). Fluorescence intensity was quantified using imaging software (FV10-ASW 1.7, OLYMPUS).

2.9 Western blotting

The cytosolic and nuclear extracts were prepared by the method of Meldrum (Meldrum et al., 1997; Aragno et al., 2005). Briefly, the penumbral cortex was homogenized at 10% (w/v) in a polytron homogenizer (Kinematica AG, Switzerland) using a homogenization buffer (20 mM HEPES (pH 7.9), 1 mM $MgCl_2$, 0.5 mM EDTA, 1% Nonidet P-40, 1 mM

EGTA, 1 mM dithiothreitol, 0.5 mM phenylmethylsulfonyl fluoride, 4 μg/ml pepstatin A, and 4 μg/ml leupeptin). Homogenates were centrifuged at 1,000×g for 5 min at 4°C. Supernatants were removed and centrifuged at 105,000×g at 4°C for 40 min to obtain the cytosolic fraction. The pelleted nuclei were resuspended in extraction buffer (20 mM HEPES (pH 7.9), 1.5 mM $MgCl_2$, 300 mM NaCl, 0.2 mM EDTA, 20% glycerol, 1 mM EGTA, 1 mM dithiothreitol, 0.5 mM phenylmethylsulfonyl fluoride, 4 μg/ml pepstatin A, and 4 μg/ml leupeptin). The suspensions were incubated on ice for 30 min for high-salt extraction followed by centrifugation at 15,000×g for 20 min at 4°C. The samples were stored at -80℃ until used. Brain tissues were homogenized in the SDS sample buffer (125 mM Tris (pH 6.8), 4% SDS, 10% sucrose, 0.01% bromophenol blue, and 10% 2-mercaptoethanol) and boiled for 1 min. Protein concentration was quantified by using the Bradford method (Protein Assay Reagent Kit, Bio-Rad Laboratories). The samples (40 μg) were separated by SDS-polyacrylamide gel electrophoresis, transferred onto a nitrocellulose membrane (Amersham Biosciences, Buckinghamshire, England) through a semidry-type blotting (Bio-Rad) method, blocked by 5% nonfat dry milk in PBS with Tween-20 (PBS-T) (137 mM NaCl, 8.10 mM Na_2HPO_4, 2.68 mM KCl, 1.47 mM KH_2PO_4, 0.1% Tween-20), and incubated with appropriate antibodies as described below. The filters were incubated with each primary antibody overnight at 4°C, with the corresponding horseradish peroxidase (HRP)-conjugated secondary antibody for 1 hr at room temperature in 5% nonfat dry milk/PBS-T. Finally, the target molecules were visualized through an enhanced chemiluminescence western blotting detection system (Amersham Biosciences) on the X-ray film (Amersham Biosciences). The following primary and secondary antibodies used in this study were NF-κB (rabbit, 1:2,000 Santa Cruz) and β-actin (mouse, 1:10,000, Sigma), anti-rabbit IgG HRP antibody (1:5,000, Amersham Biosciences), and anti-mouse IgG HRP antibody (1:10,000, Amersham Biosciences).

2.10 Statistical analysis

Statistical analysis was performed with a two-way ANOVA followed by post hoc Tukey's multiple-comparison test. Neurological deficit scores were analyzed by the Kruskal-Wallis test followed by the Mann-Whitney *U* test. In all cases a *P*-value of <0.05 was regarded as statistically significant.

3. Results

3.1 Physiological characteristic parameter

The control diabetic group had typical characteristics of type 1 diabetes such as a decrease in the body weight (296.6 ± 33.3 g) and hyperglycemia (535.4 ± 104.0 mg/dl) compared with the control non-diabetic group (340.0 ± 22.4 g, 119.8 ± 17.1 mg/dl), which were similar to previous reports (Iwata et al., 2008; 2010). Chronic treatment of MAK for 2 weeks showed a slight but significant decrease in blood glucose of the diabetic rats (404.4 ± 109.2 mg/dl, $P<0.01$), whereas MAK had little effect on the body weight (266.6 ± 33.3 g).

3.2 Infarct volume and neurological deficits after transient MCAO with reperfusion

Figure 1 shows the effects of MAK on the brain infarction by MCAO/Re in the non-diabetic and diabetic groups. Representative coronal brain sections stained by TTC after MCAO/Re showing viable (red) and dead (white) tissues are in (A). In the sham operated animals, there was no apparent damage in any brain region. The infarct area in the control non-diabetic rats after 24 hrs of reperfusion extended to the corpus striatum and cortex, whereas only a small striatal infarct was observed after 3 hrs of reperfusion. In the control diabetic group, brain injury induced by MCAO/Re was remarkably exacerbated. The cerebral infarct was produced within 3 hrs of reperfusion and the infarct region was extended to a large part of the left striatum and cortex in the diabetic rats. In contrast, the ischemic damage in the MAK-pretreated non-diabetic and diabetic animal brain was smaller as compared to those of the respective controls. Quantitative determination of infarct volume (B) indicated that the cerebral infarct volume was increased and associated with reperfusion time, which was markedly accelerated in the control diabetic group. The infarct volume evaluated at 3 hrs after reperfusion in the control diabetic group was significantly increased about 5-fold as compared with the non-diabetic group. Brain edema also tended to be exacerbated by diabetes, whereas no significant difference was detected between the non-diabetic and diabetic groups (data not shown). Consistent with the result of brain infarct volume, neurological deficits were exacerbated by reperfusion and diabetes (Fig. 2). MAK-pretreated diabetic rats showed significant alleviation in the neurological deficits compared to the control diabetic rats.

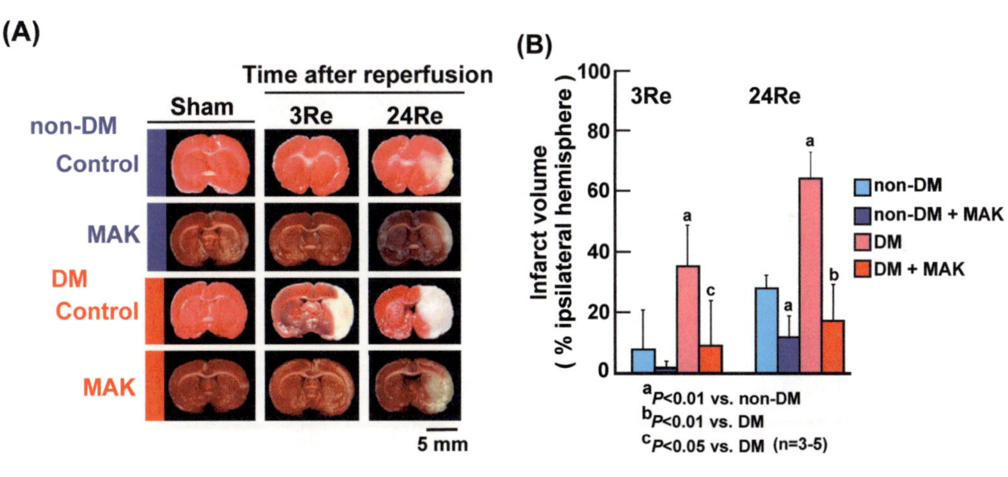

Fig. 1. Effects of MAK on infarction induced by MCAO/Re in non-diabetic (DM) and DM rat brains.

Representative coronal brain section photographs of the DM and non-DM rats stained by TTC at 3 or 24 hrs of reperfusion after 2 hrs MCAO (A). Infarct volume in ischemic hemispheres of the DM and non-DM groups after MCAO/Re by TTC staining (B).

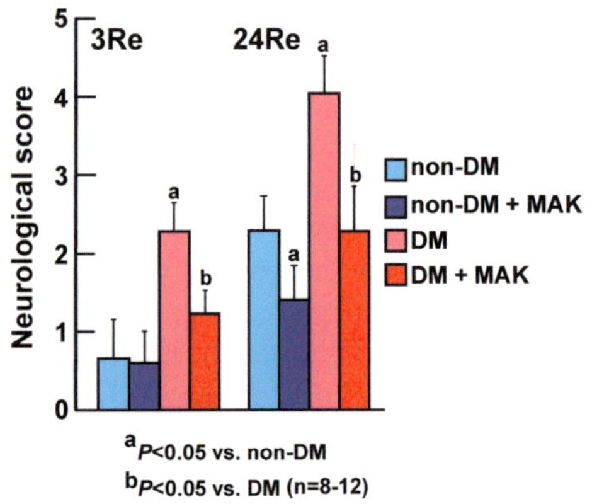

Neurological evaluation

grade 0 :	no deficit
grade 1 :	failure to extend right forepaw fully
grade 2 :	spontaneous circling or walking to contralateral side
grade 3 :	walking only when stimulated
grade 4 :	unresponsive to stimulation and a depressed level of consciousness
grade 5 :	death

Fig. 2. Effects of MAK on neurological deficits induced by MCAO/Re in non-DM and DM rats.

Post-ischemic neurological deficits were evaluated at 3 or 24 hrs of reperfusion after 2 hrs of MCAO by a 5-point scale as described in the table.

3.3 $O_2^-\cdot$ generation after transient MCAO with reperfusion

Intracellular $O_2^-\cdot$ generation in the ischemic penumbral region of the cortex induced by MCAO/Re was detected using the fluorescent probe DHE (Fig. 3). $O_2^-\cdot$ generation was increased by diabetes and MCAO/Re. No fluorescence of DHE was detected in the cortex of sham operated non-diabetic rats, whereas DHE fluorescence was present in the cortex of sham-operated diabetic rats. MCAO and subsequent following 24 hrs of reperfusion induced DHE fluorescence in the ischemic region of both the non-diabetic and diabetic cortex, which was remarkably augmented in the diabetic brain. Pretreatment of MAK reduced the $O_2^-\cdot$ generation in the cortex enhanced by MCAO/Re and diabetes.

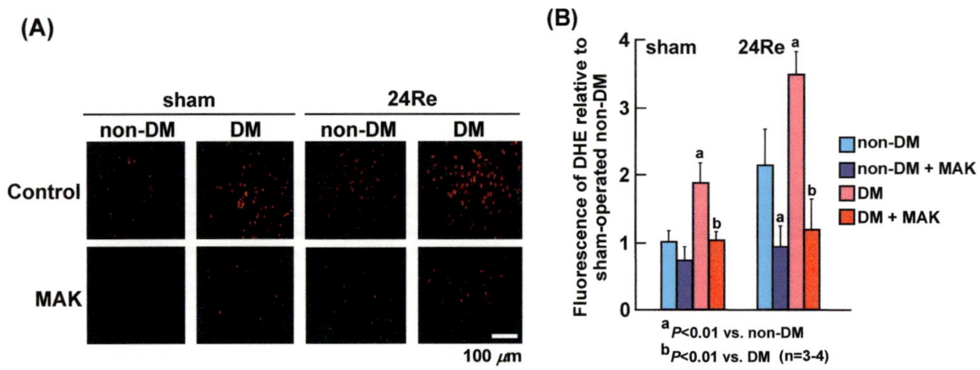

Fig. 3. Effects of MAK on production of superoxide after MCAO/Re in non-DM and DM rat brains.

Representative photographs of superoxide production detected by DHE staining in the cortex coronal sections of the non-DM and DM rats (A). Quantitative analysis of DHE fluorescence intensity in the cortex (B).

3.4 Apoptosis after transient MCAO with reperfusion

Representative histological images of TUNEL staining and cleaved caspase-3 activity in the control non-diabetic, MAK-pretreated non-diabetic, control diabetic and MAK-pretreated diabetic groups subjected to MCAO and 3 or 24 of hrs reperfusion are observed in Figs. 4 and 5. TUNEL staining of the ischemic penumbral region of the cortex was performed to determine nucleosomal DNA fragmentation accompanied by apoptotic cell death. In sham-operated non-diabetic and diabetic rats without MCAO/Re, no TUNEL positive cells were detected in the brain sections. TUNEL positive cells were increased in both the control non-diabetic and diabetic rats especially by MCAO and 3 hrs of reperfusion, which was remarkably suppressed by the pretreatment of MAK. The activation level of caspase-3, which directly activates DNase in the apoptotic final process was determined by immunostaining for cleaved caspase-3 in the ischemic penumbral cortex of non-diabetic and diabetic rats. Similar to the result of TUNEL staining, the number of cells expressing cleaved caspase-3, an activated form of this enzyme, was remarkably increased by MCAO/Re in the control diabetic group as compared with the control non-diabetic group. Pretreatment of MAK significantly inhibited the caspase-3 activation induced by MCAO/Re in these groups.

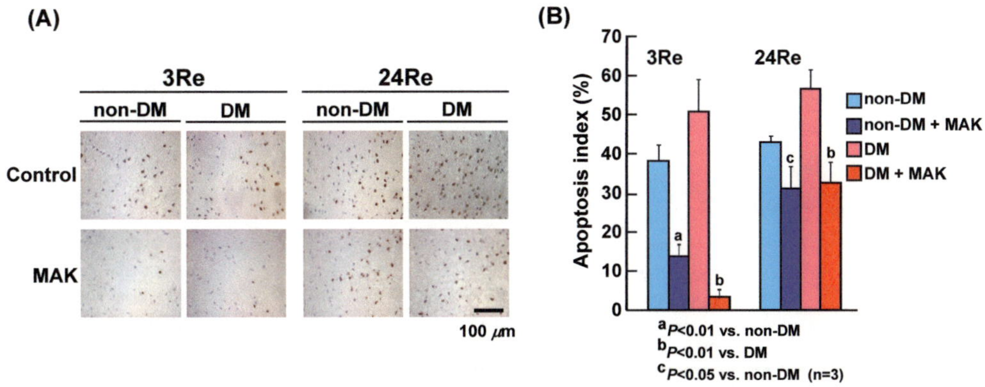

Fig. 4. Effects of MAK on neuronal apoptosis induced by MCAO/Re in non-DM and DM rat brains.

Representative photographs of apoptotic cells detected by TUNEL staining in the cortex coronal sections of non-DM and DM rats (A). Quantitative analysis of TUNEL-positive cells index in the cortex (B).

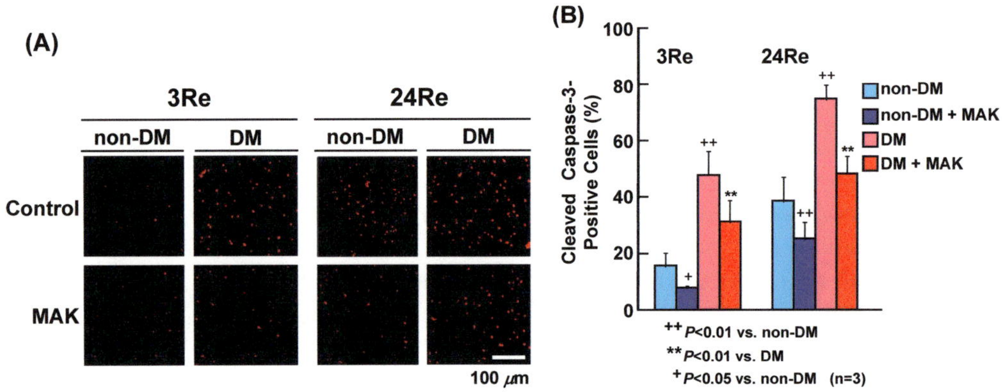

Fig. 5. Effects of MAK on cleaved caspase-3 after MCAO/Re in non-DM and DM rat brains. Representative photographs of cleaved caspase-3 staining in the cortex coronal sections of non-DM and DM rats (A). Quantitative analysis of cleaved caspase-3 positive cells fluorescence intensity in the cortex (B).

3.5 Expression of IL1-β and TNF-α in the cortex

Figure 6 shows the effects of MAK on the expression of mRNA of IL-1β (A) and TNF-α (B) in the non-diabetic and diabetic rat penumbral cortex after MCAO/Re. The control diabetic group had a 5.6-fold increase in the level of basal expression of IL-1β mRNA as compared with the control non-diabetic group. MCAO/Re increased the expression level of IL-1β mRNA in the ischemic cortex of both groups, which was remarkably accelerated and augmented by diabetes. The expression level of IL-1β mRNA in the control diabetic group reached maximum in an early period of reperfusion and at 3 hrs of reperfusion was about 10-fold higher than that of the control non-diabetic rats, which was significantly suppressed by pretreatment of MAK. Also, the control diabetic group had an increased level of the basal

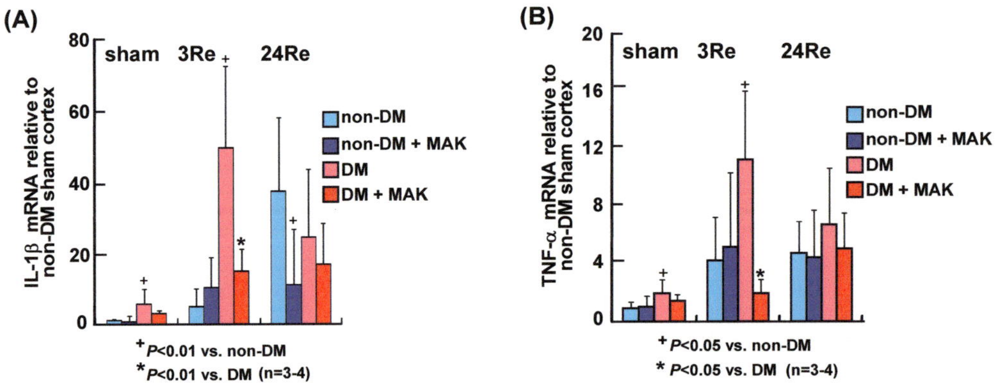

Fig. 6. Effects of MAK on expression of pro-inflammatory cytokines mRNA in the penumbral cortex after MCAO/Re in non-DM and DM rat brains.
The expression levels of IL-1β (A) and TNF-α mRNA (B) in the non-DM and DM rat penumbral cortex after MCAO/Re were determined by real-time PCR analysis.

expression of TNF-α mRNA as compared with the control non-diabetic rats. MCAO/Re increased the expression of TNF-α mRNA, which was remarkably potentiated in the diabetic group. Immunohistochemistry for these cytokines confirmed an up-regulation in biosynthesis of IL-1β and TNF-α by MCAO/Re and diabetes (Figs. 7 and 8). The expression of these pro-inflammatory cytokines was markedly accelerated in the ischemic diabetic rat cortex, whereas pretreatment of MAK significantly suppressed the augmented expression of both these cytokines.

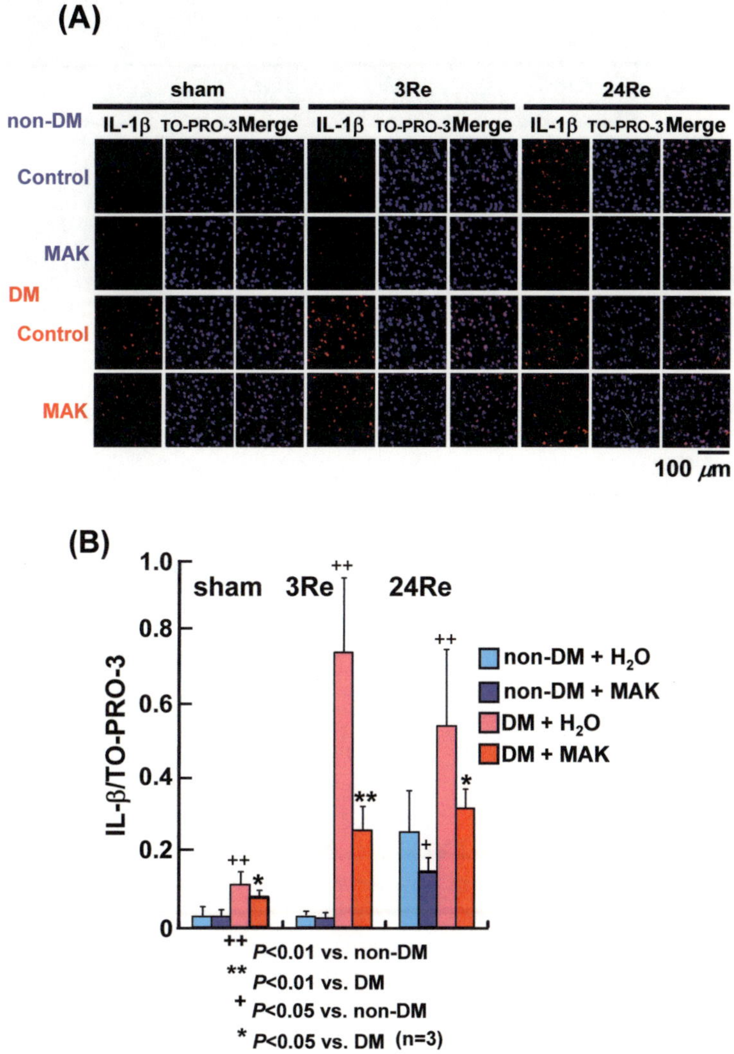

Fig. 7. Effects of MAK on expression of IL-1β in the penumbral cortex after MCAO/Re in non-DM and DM rat brains.
Representative photographs of IL-1β immunostaining (red fluorescence) and nuclei by TO-PRO-3 (blue fluorescence) in the cortex coronal sections of non-DM and DM rats. (A). Quantitative analysis of IL-1β fluorescence intensity in the cortex (B).

(A)

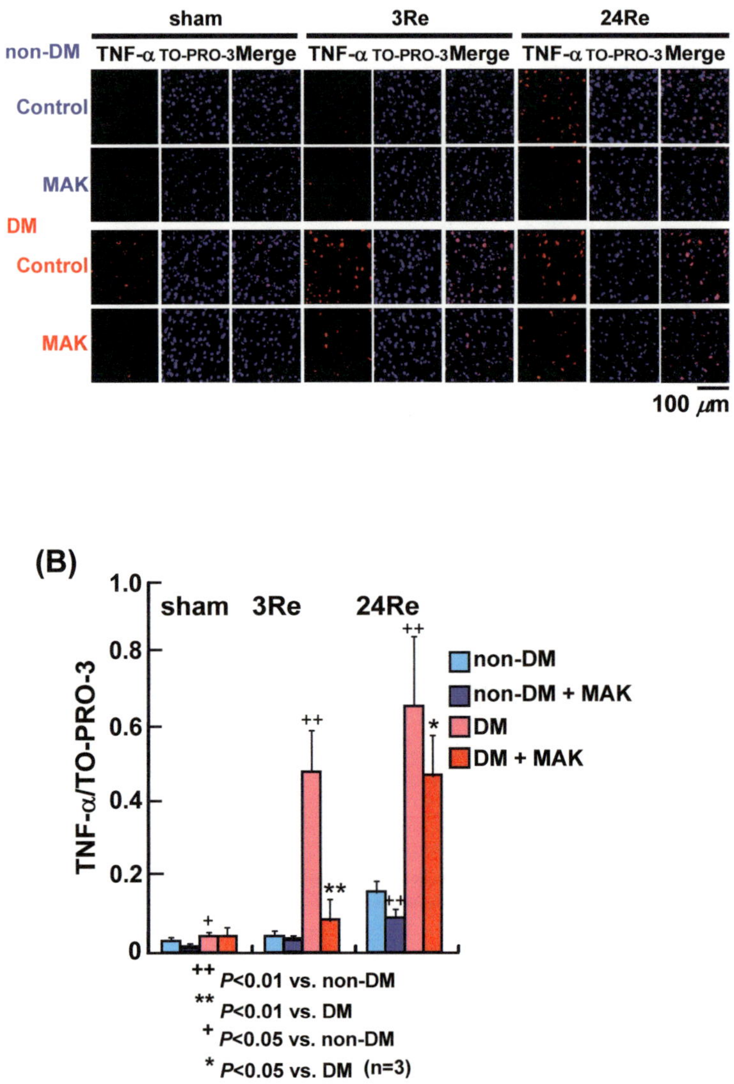

Fig. 8. Effects of MAK on expression of TNF-α in the penumbral cortex after MCAO/Re in non-DM and DM rat brains.
Representative photographs of TNF-α immunostaining (red fluorescence) and nuclei by TO-PRO-3 (blue fluorescence) in the cortex coronal sections of non-DM and DM rats. (A). Quantitative analysis of TNF-α fluorescence intensity in the cortex (B).

3.6 Activation of NF-κB in the cortex

The expression of pro-inflammatory cytokines and inflammatory mediators such as COX-2, iNOS and ICAM-1 in the cells is controlled by the transcription factor NF-κB. Thus, the activation level of NF-κB in the cortex tissue was estimated by western blotting (Fig. 9). Translocation of NF-κB from cytosol to nucleus was not detected in the cortex tissue of sham-operated non-diabetic rats. In the control non-diabetic rats submitted to MCAO/Re, there was a significant increase in NF-κB translocation. In contrast, the translocation of NF-κB was observed even in the sham-operated diabetic rat cortex and was significantly enhanced by MCAO and subsequent reperfusion. Pretreatment of MAK markedly inhibited the activation of NF-κB both in the non-diabetic and diabetic groups.

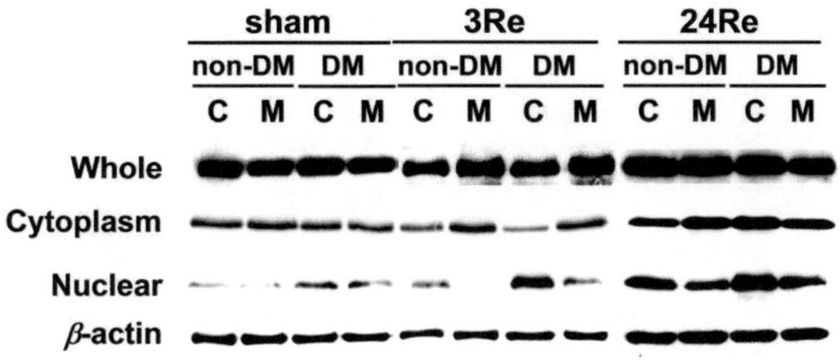

Fig. 9. Effects of MAK on NF-κB expression after MCAO/Re in non-DM and DM rat brains. Representative western blot of NF-κB in cytoplasm and nucleus extracts from the non-DM and DM rat cortex (C: control, M: MAK).

3.7 Expression of inflammatory mediators in the cortex

Figure 10 shows the effects of MAK on MCAO/Re-induced gene expression of COX-2, iNOS and ICAM-1 in the non-diabetic and diabetic rat cortex. After MCAO/Re, no distinct increase in the expression level of COX-2, iNOS and ICAM-1 mRNA was observed in the control non-diabetic group, whereas the gene expression of these inflammatory mediators was strongly enhanced in the control diabetic group. Immunohistochemistry revealed that the control diabetic rats had an increased basal expression level of COX-2 and iNOS as compared with the control non-diabetic rats (Figs. 11 and 12). The expression of ICAM-1 in endothelial cells, which indicates increased extravasation of neutrophils and macrophages/microglia into brain parenchyma, was determined using double immunostaining for ICAM-1 and endothelial cell antibody (RECA-1) (Fig. 13). The cortex of sham-operated diabetic rats had a significant up-regulated level of ICAM-1 in endothelial cells as compared with the sham-operated non-diabetic rats, which had no ICAM-1-like immunoreactive cells. MCAO/Re increased the expression of ICAM-1 both in the non-diabetic and diabetic groups, which was remarkably enhanced in the diabetic rats during 24 hrs of reperfusion. Pretreatment of MAK significantly reduced the expression of ICAM-1 both in the non-diabetic and diabetic rat cortex. Similarly, the MPO activity in the cortex was progressively increased during reperfusion, which was enhanced by diabetes and was significantly suppressed by pretreatment of MAK (Fig. 14).

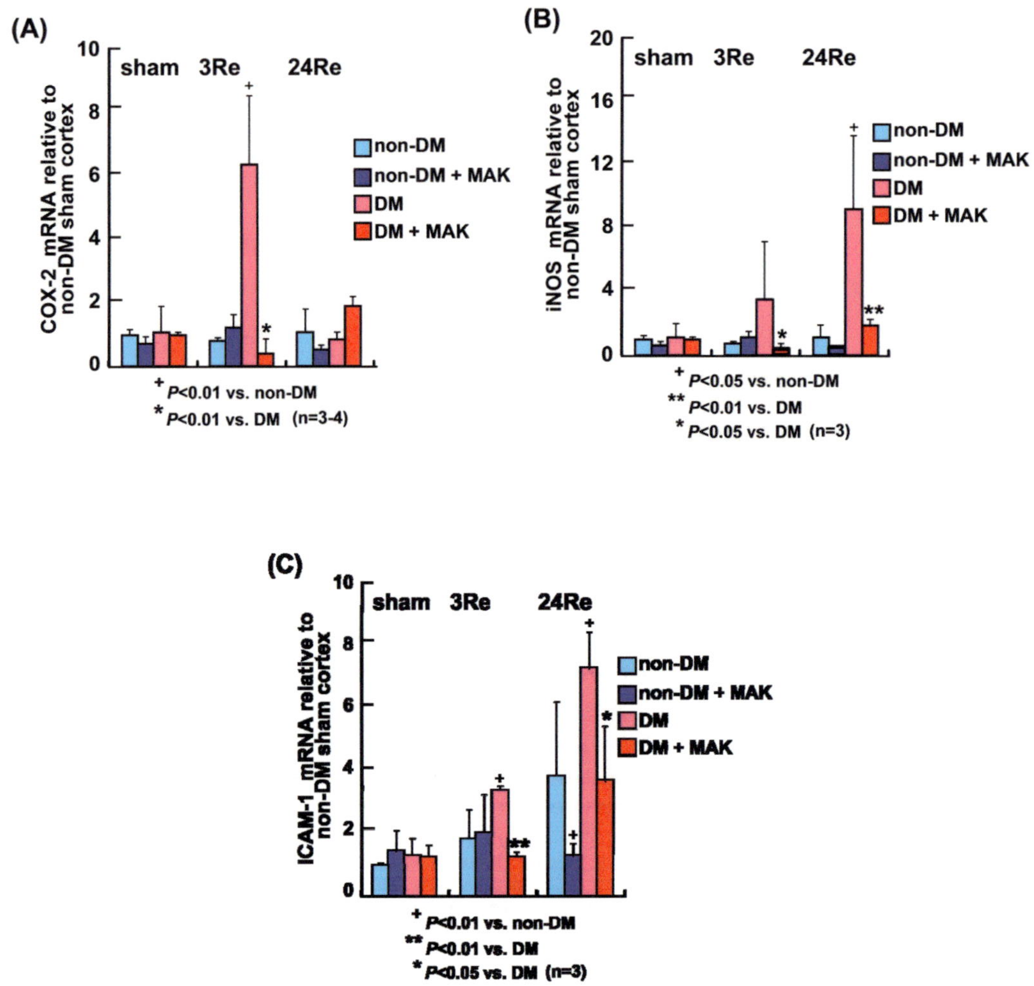

Fig. 10. Effects of MAK on expression of mRNA of inflammatory mediators in the penumbral cortex after MCAO/Re in non-DM and DM rat brains.
Expression levels of COX-2 (A), iNOS (B) and ICAM-1 mRNA (C) were determined by real-time PCR analysis in the non-DM and DM rat penumbral cortex after MCAO/Re.

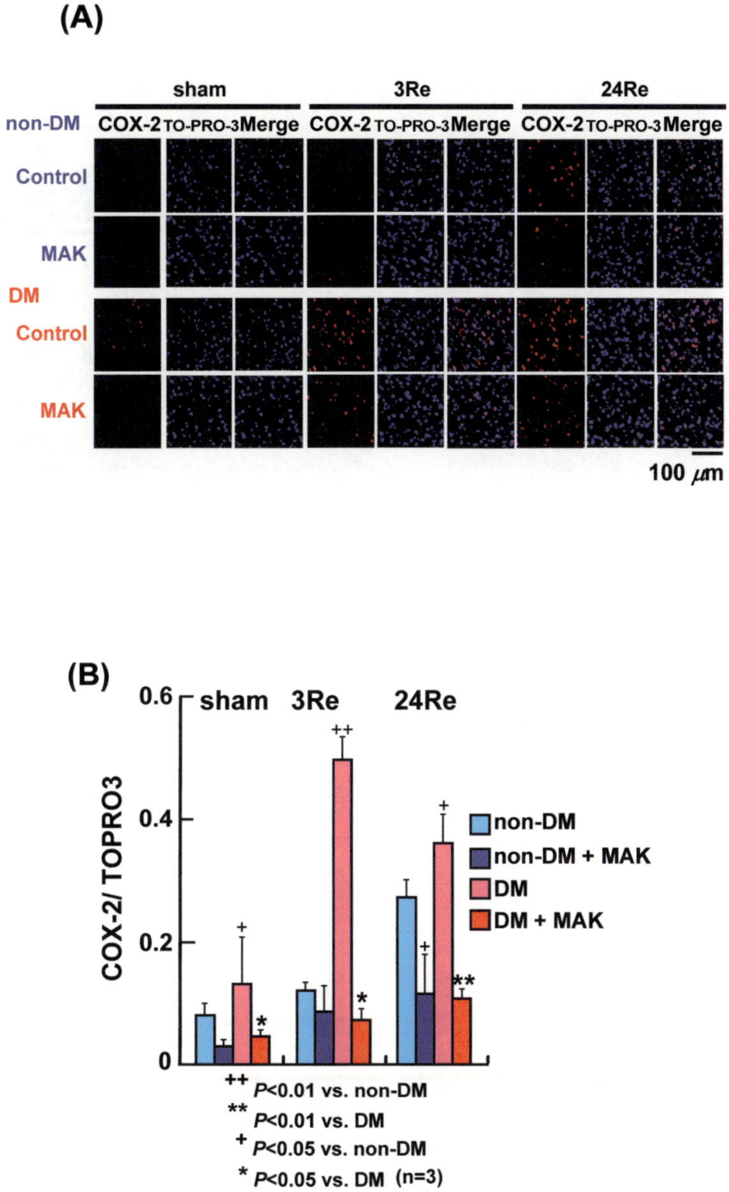

Fig. 11. Effects of MAK on expression of COX-2 in the penumbral cortex after MCAO/Re in non-DM and DM rat brains.
Representative photographs of COX-2 immunostaining (red fluorescence) and nuclei by TO-PRO-3 (blue fluorescence) in the cortex coronal sections of non-DM and DM rats. (A). Quantitative analysis of COX-2 fluorescence intensity in the cortex (B).

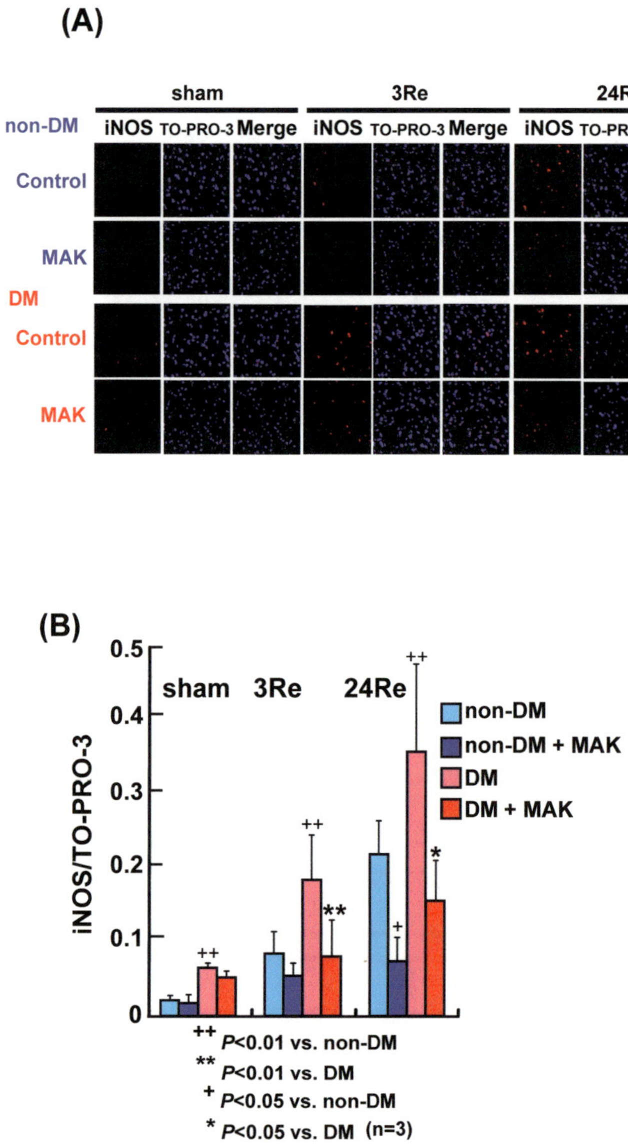

Fig. 12. Effects of MAK on expression of iNOS in the penumbral cortex after MCAO/Re in non-DM and DM rat brains.
Representative photographs of iNOS immunostaining (red fluorescence) and nuclei by TO-PRO-3 (blue fluorescence) in the cortex coronal sections of non-DM and DM rats. (A). Quantitative analysis of iNOS fluorescence intensity in the cortex (B).

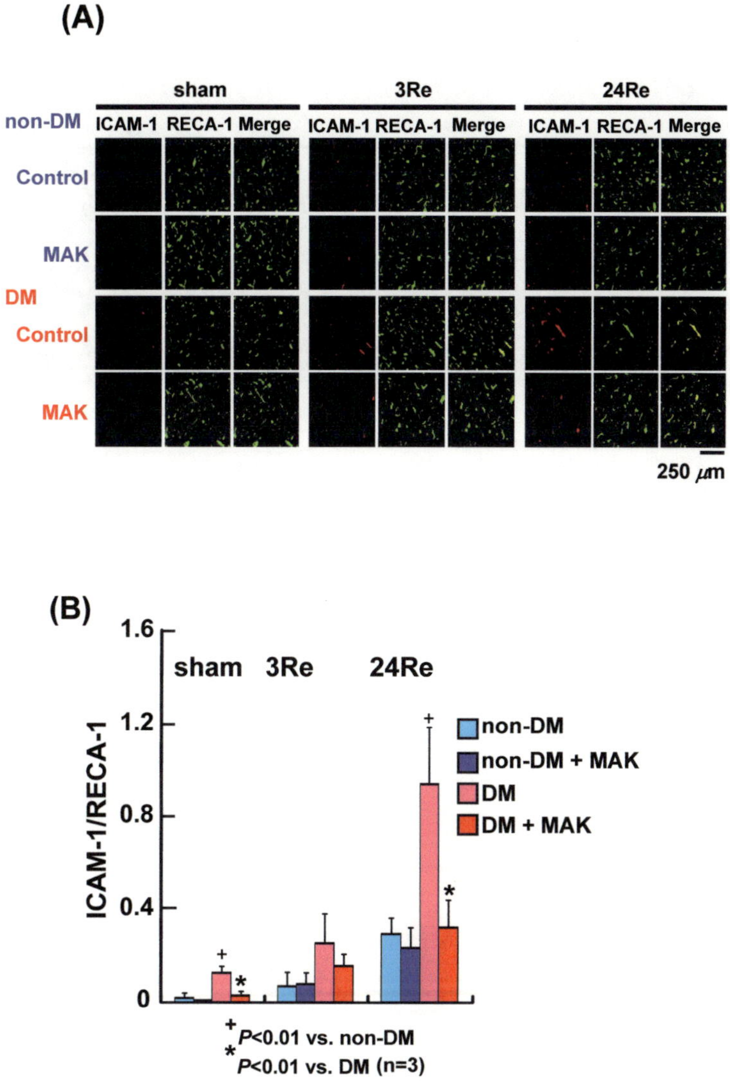

Fig. 13. Effects of MAK on expression of ICAM-1 in the penumbral cortex after MCAO/Re in non-DM and DM rat brains.
Representative photographs of ICAM-1 immunostaining (red fluorescence) and RECA-1 (green fluorescence) in the cortex coronal sections of non-DM and DM rats. (A). Quantitative analysis of ICAM-1 fluorescence intensity in the cortex (B).

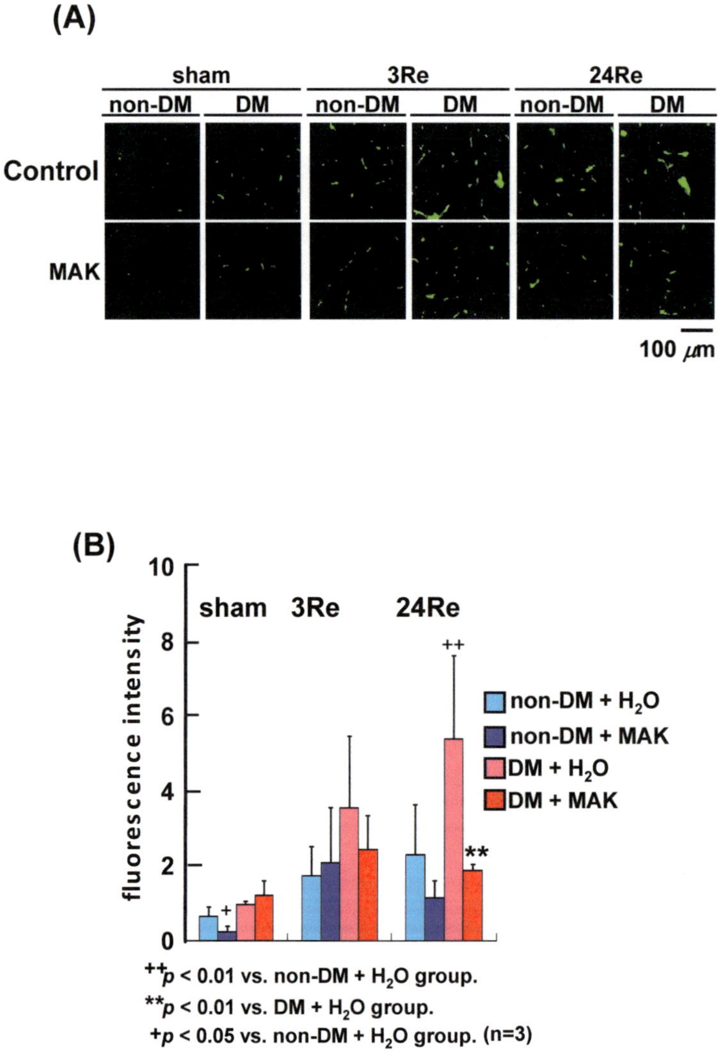

Fig. 14. Effects of MAK on MPO expression after MCAO/Re in non-DM and DM rat brains. Representative photographs of leukocytic infiltrate by MPO staining in the cortex coronal sections of non-DM and DM rats (A). Quantitative analysis of MPO fluorescence intensity in the cortex (B).

4. Discussion

The present study shows that the STZ-induced diabetic state enhanced brain infarction and neurological dysfunction caused by transient focal ischemia and subsequent reperfusion in rats. Diabetes spontaneously enhanced ROS generation and expression of pro-inflammatory cytokines and inflammatory mediators via NF-κB activation in the brain, which is accelerated after cerebral ischemia and subsequent reperfusion leading to neuronal apoptosis and inflammatory neurodegeneration. Chronic oral treatment of MAK alleviated the exacerbation of cerebral injury and neurological deficits in the diabetic state, which could be attributed to its antioxidant activity and anti-inflammatory effects.

ROS-induced oxidative stress is considered to be involved in the pathogenesis of transient cerebral ischemic injury (Fiskum et al., 2004; Saito et al., 2005; Niizuma et al., 2009). In particular, reperfusion after a long period of vessel occlusion triggers explosive generation of ROS, which causes cell death by peroxidative damage of lipids, proteins and nucleic acids (Warner et al., 2004; Anabela et al., 2006). In addition to the early necrotic cell death in the ischemic core region, ROS triggers apoptosis, a delayed death of cells, in the ischemic penumbra (Nakka et al., 2008; Niizuma et al., 2010). Furthermore, ROS induces rupture of blood brain barrier through transcriptional activation of matrix metalloproteinase and pro-inflammatory cytokines resulting in the extension of cerebral infarction and exacerbation of brain edema (Cunningham et al., 2005; Zhao et al., 2006). In this study, we observed that exacerbation of damage in the brain of diabetic rats was accelerated in a time-dependent manner during the reperfusion phase. MCAO and 3 hrs of reperfusion in the control non-diabetic rats showed little infarction in the brain and moderate neurological deficits, whereas the diabetic rats subjected to MCAO and 3 hrs of reperfusion had a large infarction that was similar in size to that in the non-diabetic rats after 24 hrs of reperfusion and severe neurological deficits. Additionally, a histochemical study revealed that generation of $O_2^{-}\cdot$ and the occurrence of apoptosis in the ischemic penumbra were markedly increased in the brain of diabetic rats. A large amount of ROS locally generated by cerebral ischemia/reperfusion induces free radical chain reactions (Saito et al., 2005), which may be enhanced by increased oxidative stress in the diabetic state. Evidence is being accumulated that oxidative stress is enhanced by hyperglycemia in the diabetic state (Kusaka et al., 2004; Rizk et al., 2005; Tsuruta et al., 2010). In the diabetic state, "glucose toxicity" caused by augmentation of intracellular glucose oxidation process and nonenzymatic glycation of protein molecules leads to over production of ROS and damage of neurons and endothelial cells (Baynes 1991). Previous studies have demonstrated that the hyperglycemic condition in cerebral ischemia without diabetes exacerbates brain injury due to enhanced production of ROS in the brain (Anabela et al., 2006; Tsuruta et al., 2010). Augmented oxidative stress involving increased ROS generation, augmented lipid peroxidation and reduction of antioxidants has been indicated in the brain, kidney, pancreas and liver of STZ-induced diabetic rats (Muralikrishna Adibhatla et al., 2006). Actually, the occurrence of apoptosis in the ischemic penumbral region has been shown to be enhanced by diabetes and correlate with serum glucose (Li et al., 1999). Antioxidant enzymes such as catalase (CAT), superoxide dismutase (SOD) and glutathione peroxidase (GPx), which scavenge ROS, are considered to contribute to the neuronal protection against ischemia/reperfusion (Warner et al.,

2004). Indeed, overexpression of SOD in transgenic mice has been shown to have a reduced infarction volume and edema after transient ischemia and reperfusion (Tsubokawa et al., 2007). Impairment of these antioxidant enzymes caused by nonenzymatic glycation is responsible for the increase of lipid peroxidation in the brain of diabetic animals. In a previous study, we also observed that the level of lipid peroxidation marker TBARS (thiobarbituric acid reactive substances) was elevated and activity of SOD, CAT and GPx was decreased in STZ-induced diabetic rat brain, which were reversed by chronic treatment of ascorbic acid (Iwata et al., 2010). Thus, the enhanced oxidative stress in diabetes is considered to cause functional impairment of antioxidant enzymes and the resulting diminution in antioxidative defense leads to further enhancement of radical reactions and other dysfunctions in the brain.

Inflammatory mechanisms that are activated after cerebral ischemia play an important role in the pathogenesis of brain injury (Caso et al., 2007; Ridder et al., 2009). The transcription factor NF-κB assumes a key role in many biological processes including cellular stress responses and regulates apoptosis and inflammation (Ridder et al., 2009). Activation of NF-κB is crucial for the inflammatory responses leading to gene expression of pro-inflammatory cytokines and mediators in immunocytes (Hu et al., 2005; Ridder et al., 2009). In this study, we demonstrated that the diabetic rats had an increased basal level of the gene expression of pro-inflammatory cytokines IL-1β and TNF-α, and inflammatory mediators COX-2 and iNOS as compared to that of non-diabetic rats. MCAO/Re increased the gene expression of these cytokines and enzymes, which was remarkably accelerated and augmented by diabetes. The result from immunoblot analysis of NF-κB in the diabetic rat cortex confirmed that the increased production of these cytokines and enzymes was mediated by the enhanced activation of NF-κB. Furthermore, we observed that the post-ischemic induction of MPO and ICAM-1, which are hallmarks of neutrophil and macrophage/microglia activation and extravasation, was significantly increased in the diabetic rat brain indicating exaggeration of inflammatory responses in ischemic injury. Our present data are in agreement with other studies describing the exacerbated inflammation in diabetic model animals (Li et al., 2004; Tsuruta et al. 2010; Tureyen et al., 2011). For example, a model of type-2 diabetes *db/db* mouse that has a point mutation of the leptin receptor showed increased brain damage and higher expression levels of IL-1β, IL-6, ICAM-1, MPO and other inflammatory markers as compared with the *db/+* control after MCAO/Re (Tureyen et al., 2011). A recent study using an electrochemical $O_2^{-}\cdot$ sensor has shown that experimental transient hyperglycemia induced by intravenous infusion of glucose increased local $O_2^{-}\cdot$ generation and exacerbated brain injury after ischemia and subsequent reperfusion in the rats (Tsuruta et al., 2010). Interestingly, high-mobility group box-1 and ICAM-1 in brain and plasma, which are induced in early inflammation and enhance inflammatory responses, were correlated with total $O_2^{-}\cdot$ generation during ischemia and reperfusion. Nevertheless, the hyperglycemia-induced overproduction of ROS may be mainly attributed to exacerbated inflammatory responses and cerebral damage after ischemia and reperfusion in diabetes.

MAK, a nutritional supplement, is a water-soluble extract from a solid culture medium composed of bagasse and defatted-rice bran overgrown with *G. lucidum* mycelia. MAK is used as a health supplement and revitalizer, and a number of studies have demonstrated its anti-tumor (Kubo et al., 2005) and immunomodulating activities (Nakagawa et al., 1999) in animals. However, the mechanistic basis and active ingredients responsible for its pharmacological effects have not been well defined. Previously, we showed that MAK inhibits the generation of $O_2^{-}\cdot$ and lipid peroxidation in a concentration dependent manner *in vitro* (Okazaki et al., 2008). Furthermore, oral administration of MAK to STZ-induced diabetic animals significantly reduced the blood glucose level and lipid peroxidation, and suppressed impairment of SOD, CAT and GPx in the brain (Iwata et al., 2008), liver and kidney (Okazaki et al., 2008). Collectively, MAK can act as an antioxidant *in vivo* and shows anti-diabetic effects by relieving diabetic-induced oxidative stress. We observed that the oral pretreatment of MAK with diabetic rats decreased the cerebral $O_2^{-}\cdot$ generation, apoptosis and subsequent inflammatory responses induced by MCAO/Re, which could be as a result of improved antioxidant status in the diabetic state. MAK had a slight effect on the elevated blood glucose level in the diabetic rats, confirming that the cerebroprotective effect of MAK could be due to its antioxidant activity. Recently, polysaccharides (Lin et al., 2010) and triterpenes (Dudhgaonkar et al., 2009), which are two major active constituents of *G. lucidum*, have been reported to suppress lipopolysaccharide-induced expression of inflammatory mediators via down-regulation of MAP kinase signaling cascade and NF-κB activity both *in vitro* and *in vivo*, whereas the mechanism of their anti-inflammatory effects remains unclear. As MAK is assumed to contain similar polysaccharides and triterpenes, it might inhibit inflammatory responses directly via its immunomodulatory effects. There are a number of factors that may explain the severe symptom of brain ischemia in the diabetes. For example, the ischemic cerebral injury in diabetic state may be aggravated by acidosis, activation of aldose reductase and NAD(P)H oxidase, enhanced production of advanced glycation end-products, protein kinase C activation induced by excessive Ca^{2+} influx, etc. The effects of MAK on these factors and identification of its active ingredients need to be further investigated.

5. Conclusion

In this study, we demonstrated that the STZ-induced diabetic state markedly aggravated MCAO/reperfusion-induced neurological deficits, infarction and apoptosis in the rat brain. Furthermore, we elucidated that the levels of $O_2^{-}\cdot$ generation and pro-inflammatory cytokines (IL-1β and TNF-α) and inflammatory mediators (COX-2 and iNOS) expression via NF-κB activation were up-regulated in the diabetic cortex, which were remarkably enhanced during reperfusion after ischemia. Post-ischemic activation of neutrophil and macrophage/microglia and extravasation estimated by ICAM-1 and MPO expression were also enhanced by diabetes. Chronic pretreatment of MAK protected the diabetic rats against the exacerbation in cerebral ischemic injury and inflammatory responses. These results suggest that daily intake of MAK relieves the exacerbation of cerebral ischemic injury in the diabetic state, which may be mainly attributed to the improvement of augmented oxidative stress by its anti-oxidant effects.

6. Acknowledgements

This study was supported by Grants-in-Aid for Scientific Research from the Japan Society for the Promotion of Science (No. 19590700, 22590663 and 23790750).

7. References

Akihisa T., Nakamura Y., Tagata M., Tokuda H., Yasukawa K., Uchiyama E., Suzuki T. & Kimura Y. (2007). Anti-inflammatory and anti-tumor-promoting effects of triterpene acids and sterols from the fungus *Ganoderma lucidum*. *Chemistry & Biodiversity*, Vol.4, No. 2, 224-231.

Anabela P. R. & Carlos M. P. (2006). Diabetes and mitochondrial function: Role of hyperglycemia and oxidative stress. *Toxicology and Applied Pharmacology*, Vol.212, No.2, 167–178.

Aragno M., Mastrocola R., Medana C., Restivo F., Catalano M.G., Pons N., Danni O. & Boccuzzi G. (2005). Up-regulation of advanced glycated products receptors in the brain of diabetic rats is prevented by antioxidant treatment. *Endocrinology*, Vol.146, No.12, 5561–5567.

Baynes J.W. (1991). Role of oxidative stress in development of complications in diabetes. *Diabetes*, Vol.40, No.4, 405-412.

Biller, J. & Love, B.B. (1993). Diabetes and stroke. *The Medical Clinics of North America*, Vol.77, No.1, 95-110.

Breckwoldt M.O., Chen J.W., Stangenberg L., Aikawa E., Rodriguez E., Qiu S., Moskowitz M.A. & Weissleder R. (2008). Tracking the inflammatory response in stroke in vivo by sensing the enzyme myeloperoxidase. *Proceedings of the National Academy of Sciences of the United States of America*, Vol.105, No.47, 18584-18589.

Brown G. C. & Neher J. J. (2010). Inflammatory neurodegeneration and mechanisms of microglial killing of neurons. *Molecular Neurobiology*, Vol.41, No.2-3, 242-247.

Caso J.R., Moro M.A., Lorenzo P., Lizasoain I. & Leza J.C. (2007). Involvement of IL-1beta in acute stress-induced worsening of cerebral ischaemia in rats. *European Neuropsychopharmacology*. Vol.17, No.9, 600-607.

Chrissobolis S., Miller A.A., Drummond G.R., Kemp-Harper B.K. & Sobey C.G. (2011). Oxidative stress and endothelial dysfunction in cerebrovascular disease. *Frontiers in Bioscience*, Vol.1, No.16, 1733-1745.

Cunningham L.A., Wetzel M. & Rosenberg G.A. (2005). Multiple roles for MMPs and TIMPs in cerebral ischemia. *Glia*, Vol.50, No.4, 329-339.

Cuzzocrea S., Riley D.P., Caputi A.P. & Salvemini D. (2001). Antioxidant therapy: a new pharmacological approach in shock, inflammation, and ischemia/reperfusion injury. *Pharmacological Reviews*, Vol.53, No.1, 135-159.

Doyle K.P., Simon R.P. & Stenzel-Poore M.P. (2008). Mechanisms of ischemic brain damage. *Neuropharmacology*, Vol.55, No.3, 310-318.

Dudhgaonkar S., Thyagarajan A. & Sliva D. (2009). Suppression of the inflammatory response by triterpenes isolated from the mushroom *Ganoderma lucidum*. *International Immunopharmacology*, Vol.9, No.11, 1272-1280.

Faraco G., Fossati S., Bianchi M.E., Patrone M., Pedrazzi M., Sparatore B., Moroni F. & Chiarugi A. (2007). High mobility group box 1 protein is released by neural cells upon different stresses and worsens ischemic neurodegeneration in vitro and in vivo. *Journal of Neurochemistry*, Vol.103, No.2, 590-603.

Fiskum G., Rosenthal R.E., Vereczki V., Martin E., Hoffman G.E., Chinopoulos C. & Kowaltowski A. (2004). Protection against ischemic brain injury by inhibition of mitochondrial oxidative stress. *Journal of Bioenergetics and Biomembranes*, Vol. 36, No. 4, 347-352.

Giacco F. & Brownlee M. (2010). Oxidative stress and diabetic complications. *Circulation Research*, Vol.107, No.9, 1058-1070.

Hu X., Nesic-Taylor O., Qiu J., Rea H.C., Fabian R., Rassin D.K. & Perez-Polo J.R. (2005). Activation of nuclear factor-kappaB signaling pathway by interleukin-1 after hypoxia/ischemia in neonatal rat hippocampus and cortex. *Journal of Neurochemistry*, Vol.93, No.1, 26-37.

Iwata, N., Okazaki, M., Kasahara, C., Kamiuchi, S., Suzuki, F., Iizuka, H. & Hibino, Y. (2008). Protective effects of a water-soluble extract from culture medium of *Ganoderma lucidum* mycelia against neuronal damage after cerebral ischemia/reperfusion in diabetic rats. *Journal of Japanese Society of Nutrition and Food Science*, Vol.61, No.3, 119-127.

Iwata, N., Okazaki, M., Kamiuchi, S. & Hibino, Y. (2010). Protective effects of oral administrated ascorbic acid against oxidative stress and neuronal damage after cerebral ischemia/reperfusion in diabetic rats. *Journal of Health Science*, Vol.56, No.1, 20-30.

Kabir Y., Kimura S. & Tamura T. (1988). Dietary effect of *Ganoderma lucidum* mushroom on blood pressure and lipid levels in spontaneously hypertensive rats (SHR). *Journal of Nutritional Science and Vitaminology (Tokyo)*, Vol.34, No.4, 433-438.

Kubo N., Myojin Y., Shimamoto F., Kashimoto N., Kyo E., Kamiya K. & Watanabe H. (2005). Protective effects of a water-soluble extract from cultured medium *Ganoderma lucidum* (Rei-shi) mycelia and Agaricus blazei murill against X-irradiation in B6C3F1 mice: increased small intestinal crypt survival and prolongation of average time to animal death. *International Journal of Molecular Medicine*, Vol.15, No.3 401-406.

Kusaka I., Kusaka G., Zhou C., Ishikawa M., Nanda A., Granger D.N., Zhang J.H. & Tang J. (2004). Role of AT1 receptors and NAD(P)H oxidase in diabetes-aggravated ischemic brain injury. *American Journal of Physiology. Heart and Circulatory Physiology*. Vol.286, No.6, 2442-2451.

Lai C.Y., Hung J.T., Lin H.H., Yu A.L., Chen S.H., Tsai Y.C., Shao L.E., Yang W.B. & Yu J. (2010). Immunomodulatory and adjuvant activities of a polysaccharide extract of *Ganoderma lucidum* in vivo and in vitro. *Vaccine*, Vol.28, No.31, 4945-4954.

Lin C.Y., Chen Y.H., Lin C.Y., Hsu H.Y., Wang S.H., Liang C.J., Kuan I.I., Wu P.J., Pai P.Y., Wu C.C. & Chen Y.L. (2010). *Ganoderma lucidum* polysaccharides attenuate endotoxin-induced intercellular cell adhesion molecule-1 expression in cultured smooth muscle cells and in the neointima in mice. *Journal of Agricultural and Food Chemistry*, Vol.58, No.17, 9563-9571.

Liu, K., Mori, S., Takahashi, H.K., Tomono, Y., Wake, H., Kanke, T., Sato, Y., Hiraga, N., Adachi, N., Yoshino, T. & Nishibori, M. (2007). Anti-high mobility group box 1 monoclonal antibody ameliorates brain infarction induced by transient ischemia in rats. *The FASEB Journal*, Vol.21, No.14, 3904-3916.

Li, P.A., Liu, G.J., He, Q.P., Floyd, R.A. & Siesjö, B.K. (1999). Production of hydroxyl free radical by brain tissues in hyperglycemic rats subjected to transient forebrain ischemia. *Free Radical Biology & Medicine*, Vol.27, No.9-10, 1033-1040.

Li, Z.G., Britton, M., Sima, A.A. & Dunbar, J.C. (2004). Diabetes enhances apoptosis induced by cerebral ischemia. *Life Sciences*, Vol.76, No.3, 249-262.

Lu H., Kyo E., Uesaka T., Katoh O. & Watanabe H. (2003). A water-soluble extract from cultured medium of *Ganoderma lucidum* (Rei-shi) mycelia suppresses azoxymethane-induction of colon cancers in male F344 rats. *Oncology Reports*, Vol.10, No.2, 375-379.

Meldrum D.R., Shenkar R., Sheridan B.C., Cain B.S., Abraham E. & Harken A.H. (1997). Hemorrhage activates myocardial NFkappaB and increases TNF-alpha in the heart. *Journal of Molecular and Cellular Cardiology*, Vol.29, No.10, 2849–2855.

Muralikrishna Adibhatla R. & Hatcher J. F. (2006). Phospholipase A2, reactive oxygen species, and lipid peroxidation in cerebral ischemia. *Free Radical Biology & Medicine*. Vol.40, No.3, 376-387.

Muranyi M., Ding C., He Q., Lin Y. & Li P. A. (2006). Streptozotocin-induced diabetes causes astrocyte death after ischemia and reperfusion injury. *Diabetes*. Vol.55, No.2, 349-355.

Nakagawa I., Hibino Y., Ohashi Y. & Suga N. (1999). Augmentation of cytolytic activity of mouse splenic cells by a heteroglycan-protein fraction from culture medium of *Ganoderma lucidum* (Rei-shi) mycelia. *Biotherapy*, Vol.13, No.5, 513-515.

Nakka V.P., Gusain A., Mehta S.L. & Raghubir R. (2008). Molecular mechanisms of apoptosis in cerebral ischemia: multiple neuroprotective opportunities. *Molecular Neurobiology*, Vol.37, No.1, 7-38.

Niizuma K., Endo H. & Chan P.H. (2009). Oxidative stress and mitochondrial dysfunction as determinants of ischemic neuronal death and survival. *Journal of Neurochemistry*, Vol.109, No.1, 133-138.

Niizuma K., Yoshioka H., Chen H., Kim G.S., Jung J.E., Katsu M., Okami N. & Chan P.H. (2010). Mitochondrial and apoptotic neuronal death signaling pathways in cerebral ischemia. *Biochimica et Biophysica Acta*, Vol.1802, No.1, 92-99.

Okazaki M., Iwata N., Horiuchi S., Kamiuchi S., Suzuki F., Iizuka H. & Hibino Y. (2008). Protective effects of a water-soluble extract from culture medium of *Ganoderma lucidum* mycelia against neuronal damage after hypoxia-ischemia in mice. *Japanese Journal of Complementary and Alternative Medicine*, Vol.5, No.2, 153-162.

Okazaki M., Tanaka A., Hatta Y., Kawahara Y., Kamiuchi S., Iwata N., Asano S., Suzuki F., Iizuka H. & Hibino Y. (2008). Antioxidant properties of a water-soluble extract from culture medium of *Ganoderma lucidum* (Rei-shi) mycelia and antidiabetic effects in streptozotocin-treated mice. *Japanese Journal of Complementary and Alternative Medicine*, Vol.5, No.3, 209-218.

Ridder D.A. & Schwaninger M. (2009). NF-kappaB signaling in cerebral ischemia. *Neuroscience*, Vol.158, No.3, 995-1006.

Rizk, N.N., Rafols, J. & Dunbar, J.C. (2005). Cerebral ischemia induced apoptosis and necrosis in normal and diabetic rats. *Brain Research*, Vol.1053, No.1-2, 1-9.

Saeed S.A., Shad K.F., Saleem T., Javed F. & Khan M.U. (2007). Some new prospects in the understanding of the molecular basis of the pathogenesis of stroke. *Experimental Brain Research*, Vol.182, No.1, 1-10.

Saito A., Maier C.M., Narasimhan P., Nishi T., Song Y.S., Yu F., Liu J., Lee Y.S., Nito C., Kamada H., Dodd R.L., Hsieh L.B., Hassid B., Kim E.E., González M. & Chan P.H. (2005). Oxidative stress and neuronal death/survival signaling in cerebral ischemia. *Molecular Neurobiology*, Vol.31, No.1-3, 105-116.

Shi Y., Sun J., He H., Guo H. & Zhang S. (2008). Hepatoprotective effects of *Ganoderma lucidum* peptides against D-galactosamine-induced liver injury in mice. *Journal of Ethnopharmacology*, Vol.117, No.3, 415-419.

Stephens, J.W., Khanolkar, M.P. & Bain, S.C. (2009). The biological relevance and measurement of plasma markers of oxidative stress in diabetes and cardiovascular disease. *Atherosclerosis*, Vol.202, No.2, 321-329.

Sugawara T., Fujimura M., Noshita N., Kim G.W., Saito A., Hayashi T., Narasimhan P., Maier C.M. & Chan P.H. (2007). Neuronal death/survival signaling pathways in cerebral ischemia. *The Journal of the American Society for Experimental NeuroTherapeutics*, Vol.1, No.1, 17-25.

Tsubokawa T., Jadhav V., Solaroglu I., Shiokawa Y., Konishi Y. & Zhang J.H. (2007). Lecithinized superoxide dismutase improves outcomes and attenuates focal cerebral ischemic injury via antiapoptotic mechanisms in rats. *Stroke*, Vol.38, No.3, 1057-1062.

Tsuruta R., Fujita M., Ono T., Koda Y., Koga Y., Yamamoto T., Nanba M., Shitara M., Kasaoka S., Maruyama I., Yuasa M. & Maekawa T. (2010). Hyperglycemia enhances excessive superoxide anion radical generation, oxidative stress, early inflammation, and endothelial injury in forebrain ischemia/reperfusion rats. *Brain Research*, Vol.1309, 155-163.

Tureyen K., Bowen K., Liang J., Dempsey R.J. & Vemuganti R. (2011). Exacerbated brain damage, edema and inflammation in type-2 diabetic mice subjected to focal ischemia. *Journal of Neurochemistry*, Vol.116, No.4, 499-507.

Vinik, A. & Flemmer, M.J. (2002). Diabetes and macrovascular disease. *Journal of Diabetes and its Complications*, Vol.16, No.3, 235-245.

Wang G.J., Deng H.Y., Maier C.M., Sun G.H. & Yenari M.A. (2002). Mild hypothermia reduces ICAM-1 expression, neutrophil infiltration and microglia/monocyte accumulation following experimental stroke. *Neuroscience*, Vol.114, No.4, 1081-1090.

Wang X. & Michaelis E.K. (2010). Selective neuronal vulnerability to oxidative stress in the brain. *Frontiers in Aging Neuroscience*, Vol.2, No.12, 1-13.

Warner D.S., Sheng H. & Batinić-Haberle I. (2004). Oxidants, antioxidants and the ischemic brain. *The Journal of Experimental Biology*, Vol.207, No.18, 3221-3231.

Wei, J. & Quast, M.J. (1998). Effect of nitric oxide synthase inhibitor on a hyperglycemic rat model of reversible focal ischemia: detection of excitatory amino acids release and hydroxyl radical formation. *Brain Research*, Vol.791, No.1-2, 146-156.

Wild S., Roglic G., Green A., Sicree R. & King H. (2004). Global prevalence of diabetes: estimates for the year 2000 and projections for 2030. *Diabetes Care*, Vol.27, No.5, 1047-1053.

Zhang H.N. & Lin Z.B. (2004). Hypoglycemic effect of *Ganoderma lucidum* polysaccharides. *Acta Pharmacologica Sinica*, Vol.25, No.2, 191-195.

Zhao B.Q., Wang S., Kim H.Y., Storrie H., Rosen B.R., Mooney D.J., Wang X. & Lo E.H. (2006). Role of matrix metalloproteinases in delayed cortical responses after stroke. *Nature Medicine*, Vol.12, No.4, 441-445.

Zhu M., Chang Q., Wong L.K., Chong F.S. & Li R.C. (1999). Triterpene antioxidants from *Ganoderma lucidum*. *Phytotherapy Research*, Vol.13, No.6, 529-531.

12

Mechanisms of Ischemic Induced Neuronal Death and Ischemic Tolerance

Jan Lehotsky, Martina Pavlikova, Stanislav Straka, Maria Kovalska, Peter Kaplan and Zuzana Tatarkova
Comenius University, Jessenius Faculty of Medicine, Department of Medical Biochemistry, Martin, Slovak Republic

1. Introduction

Stroke is the second leading cause of death and the primary cause of disability in humans. The phenomenon of ischemic tolerance perfectly describes the quote: "What does not kill you makes you stronger." Ischemic pre- or post- conditioning is actually the strongest known procedure to prevent or reverse delayed neuronal death. It works specifically in sensitive vulnerable neuronal populations, which are represented by pyramidal neurons in the hippocampal CA1 region. However, tolerance is effective in other brain cell populations as well. Although, its nomenclature is **"ischemic" tolerance (IT)** ", the tolerant phenotype can also be induced by other stimuli that lead to delayed neuronal death (intoxication). Recent data have proven further that this phenomenon is not only limited to application of sublethal stimuli before the lethal stress **(preconditioning)** but also that reversed arrangement of events, sublethal stress after lethal insult **(postconditioning),** are equally effective. Another very important term is **"cross conditioning,"** or the capability of one stressor to induce tolerance against another. Delayed neuronal death is the slow development of post-ischemic neuro-degeneration. This delay allows a therapeutic window of opportunity lasting 2–3 days to reverse the cellular death process. It seems therefore that the mechanisms of ischemic tolerance-delayed post-conditioning could be of use not only after ischemia but also in some other processes leading up to apoptosis.

This paper summarizes results of experimental studies which have shown that acute *in vivo* forebrain ischemia as well as ischemic/reperfusion injury (IRI) both alter, the expression, function and kinetic parameters of Ca^{2+} transporters as well as the physical membrane environment. Furthermore, that IRI leads to the inhibition of mitochondrial respiratory complexes I and IV. Also, that conversely, ischemic preconditioning (IPC) acts at the level of both initiation and execution of IRI-induced mitochondrial apoptosis and activates inhibition of p53 translocation to mitochondria.

Evidence is presented to show that endoplasmic reticulum (ER) is the site of complex processes such as calcium storage, synthesis and folding of proteins as well as cell response to stress. ER function is impaired in IRI which in turn induces depletion of stored calcium, the conserved stress responses linked with delayed neuronal death. In addition, IRI initiates time dependent differences in endoplasmic reticular (ER) gene expression of the key unfolded protein response (UPR), or proteins at both the mRNA and protein levels. Moreover, gene expression of the UPR proteins is affected by pre-ischemic (IPC) treatment caused by the increased expression of Ca^{2+} binding protein, GRP 78 and transcriptional factor ATF6 in reperfusion times. Thus, IPC exerts a role in the attenuation of ER stress response, which might, in turn, be involved in the neuroprotective phenomenon of ischemic tolerance. Hippocampal cells respond to the IRI by the specific expression pattern of the secretory pathways Ca^{2+} pump (SPCA1) and this pattern is affected by preischemic challenge. IPC also incompletely suppresses lipid and protein oxidation of hippocampal membranes and leads to partial recovery of the ischemic-induced depression of SPCA activity. The data suggests a correlation of SPCA function with the role of secretory pathways (Golgi apparatus) in response to preischemic challenge.

2. Ischemic stroke

Ischemic stroke arises in humans as a consequence of a cardiac arrest, the stoppage of blood flow to the brain due to embolic or thrombic occlusion of arteries. Global or focal ischemia is very severe pathogenic event with multiple, parallel, and sequential pathogenesis. Global forebrain ischemia leads to selective cell death of vulnerable pyramidal neurons in the hippocampal CA1 region. It also leads to death of cerebral cortex neurons (layers 3, 5, and 6) and the dorsolateral striatum. When blood flow decreases during focal ischemia, the area surrounding the necrotic core of ischemia, also known as "penumbra" is perfused by collateral vessels. It also undergoes fatal apoptosis of neurons (Endres et al., 2008).
Despite decades of intense research, no effective neuroprotective drugs are available to treat acute stroke or cardiac arrest. For this reason, recent attention has shifted to defining the brain's own evolutionarily conserved endogenous neuroprotective mechanisms, which occurs in **ischemic tolerance (IT) or after ischemic preconditioning (IPC).** IT induced by several paradigms represents an important phenomenon of the central nervous system (CNS) including adaptation to sublethal short-term ischemia. This results in increased tolerance of CNS to lethal ischemia (Kirino, 2002; Dirnagl et al., 2003; Gidday, 2006). The molecular mechanisms underlying IT are not yet fully understood because of its extreme complexity, involving many signaling pathways and alterations in gene expression. Additionally, a metabolic depression has also been suggested to play an important role in IT (Yenari et al., 2008).

2.1 Ischemic tolerance as a possible neuroprotective strategy

A transient, ischemia-resistant phenotype known as **"ischemic tolerance (IT)"** can be established in brain in a rapid or delayed fashion by a preceding non-injurious "preconditioning" stimulus. Thus, **ischemic preconditioning (IPC)** as one of the inducers, represents a phenomenon which eventually leads to an increase in the **tolerance** of CNS to the lethal ischemia (Dirnagl et al., 2009; Obrenovitch, 2008). Initial pre-clinical studies of this phenomenon relied primarily on brief periods of ischemia or hypoxia as the IPC stimuli, but it was later realized that many other stressors, including pharmacological agents, are also effective. Although considerably more experimentation is needed to thoroughly validate the efficacy of any already identified preconditioning agent to protect ischemic brain, the fact that some of these agents are already clinically used implies that the growing enthusiasm for translational success in the field of pharmacologic pre-conditioning may be well justified.

The mechanisms underlying ischemic tolerance are rather complex and not yet fully understood. Two windows have been identified in all multiple paradigms for IPC. One that represents very rapid and short-lasting post-translational changes and a second, which develops slowly (over days) after initial insult as a robust and long lasting transcriptional changes which culminate in prolonged neuroprotection (Dirnagl et al., 2009; Obrenovitch, 2008; Yenari et al., 2008). Differences in intensity, duration, and frequency of specific inducer/stressor determine the spectrum of responses to noxious stimuli. In other words, when the stimulus is too weak to induce any response, when it is sufficient to serve as a tolerance trigger, or when it is too strong and harmful, resulting in apoptotic or necrotic damage.

It is symptomatic that there are no clear boundaries between acquisition of tolerance and cellular apoptosis/necrosis (Dirnagl et al., 2009). Rodent and cell culture models serve as a basis for the study of the tolerance phenomenon. Mother nature presents the perfect model to help understand this better. In nature, we ubiquitously find adaptation to extreme environmental conditions, for example, the hypoxic or anoxic tolerance. Hibernation is another example of inherent adaptation to extreme low-blood perfusion in animals. As such, ischemic tolerance can be conceived as an evolutionary conserved form of cerebral plasticity (Dirnagl et al., 2009,). It is not surprising therefore that different animal species have evolved different molecular strategies to cope with anoxia and severe metabolic stress. This leads to the trigger of the neuroprotective tolerance state.

A number of common mechanisms with different relevance features can be recognized (Lehotsky et al., 2009b):

- depression of metabolic rate,
- modulation of glycolytic enzymes,
- reduction of ion channel fluxes,
- suppression of neural activity,
- expression of chaperones and heat shock proteins (Hsp),
- activation of antioxidant defense systems,
- adaptation of blood rheology and others.

At first pass, the patient population that suffers from cerebral ischemic injury due to unpredictable focal stroke, cardiac arrest, or subarachnoid hemorrhage represents, by definition, one that is unlikely to derive benefit from preconditioning research. However, the novel endogenous survival pathways identified in preclinical IT studies may ultimately become **targets for drugs** that protect the brain even when acutely administered after the precipitating event. Importantly, a significant number of other patients—those in which we can anticipate a period of cerebral ischemia following transient ischemic attack, aneurysm clipping, subarachnoid hemorrhage, carotid endarterectomy or stenting, asymptomatic carotid stenosis, coronary bypass, and cardiac valve replacement—represent defined at-risk populations ideally suited for translational **therapeutic preconditioning.** The candidate drugs that might underpin clinical trials for this latter group of patients actually comprise a relatively long and therefore promising list, particularly if the current foundation of preclinical studies is expanded with intention.

The concept of IPC in the heart was introduced in the late 80s by Murry et al. (1986) and later on in the brain by Schurr et al. (1986) and Kitagawa et al. (1991). Most stressors, including preischemia/hypoxia, induce both rapid and delayed tolerance phenotypes (Gidday, 2006). Mechanisms that are prominent during the first phases of acute ischemic insults such as excitoxicity are presumed to be induced during rapid IT. In particular, elevation of adenosine and activation of adenosine receptor with the modulation of ATP sensitive K^+ channel are paralleled by the activation of protein kinase C and other kinases in rapid tolerance. A critical role for nitric oxide signaling pathways in IPC and tolerance was also suggested (Nandagopal et al., 2001). As was recently shown by Meller et al. (2008), the selective ubiquitin-proteasome degradation of a cell death-associated protein, Bcl-2-interacting mediator of cell death (Bim) with the reduced activation of programmed cell death-associated caspases (caspase 3) could play an important role in rapid tolerance to ischemia. As mentioned earlier, IT can be induced by various stimuli that are not necessarily ischemic or hypoxic.

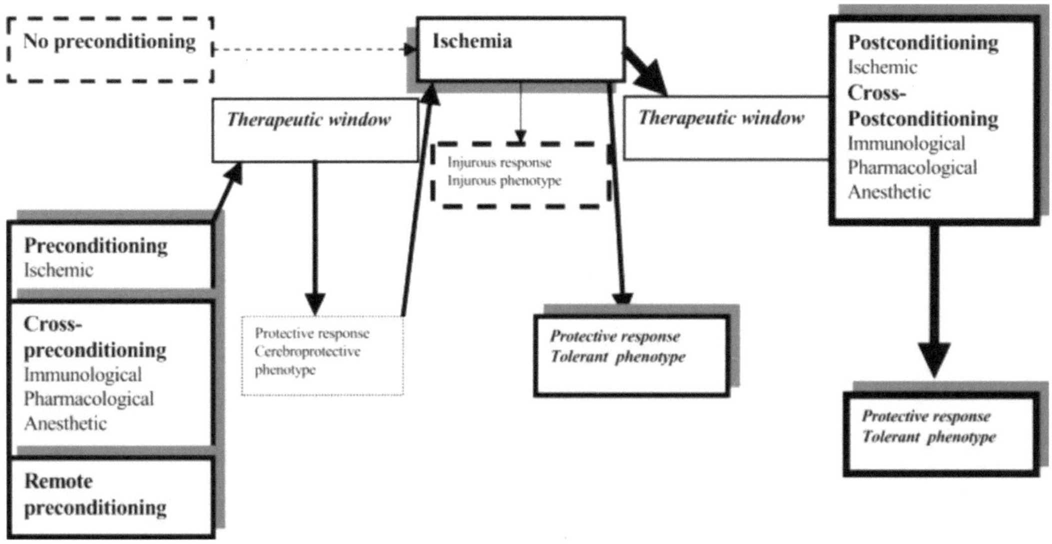

Fig. 1. Ischemic insult without any maneuvers leads to ischemic/reperfusion injured phenotype. Cerebroprotection can be induced by different types of preconditioning or postconditioning maneuvers/stimuli (ischemic, immunological, pharmacological and anesthetic). Temporary defined responses during therapeutical window may induce protective response with which subsequent ischemia serve as basis of the ischemic-tolerant phenotype. Adapted from Lehotsky et al. (2009b).

Thus, the phenomenon of cross-tolerance implies that noxious stress can initiate cellular tolerance to subsequent stress that is different in nature from the first one. Therefore, one stressor can promote cross-tolerance to another; however, the efficacy of this tolerance may be more modest, and it appears to vary with the nature and intensity of the first challenge. Additionally, the window of evolved IT may also be shifted. However, the nature of the stimulus may determine the specific protective or in worse meaning the reduced damage epiphenotype.

3. Prophylactic treatment with statins: Effect on ischemic damage

Neuronal ischemic/reperfusion damage in the brain occurs rapidly. However, significant structural changes are observed over a course of hours or days in the form of delayed neuronal death. Interruption of blood flow initiates high-energy metabolism failure, ATP depletion, ion imbalance, as well as other biochemical changes, such as an increase of free radicals, mitochondrial dysfunction, lactic acidosis, and inhibition of proteosynthesis as a consequence of endoplasmic reticular (ER) stress (DeGracia et al., 2002).

The endoplasmic reticulum of eukaryotic cell reacts to ischemic injury by **the unfolded protein response (UPR),** which can be highly variable, depending on dosage and duration of ischemic treatment (Imaizumi et al., 2001), and intensity of UPR signals (Yoshida et al., 2003). However, when ER stress is too severe and prolonged, apoptosis is induced. Various enzymes and transcription factors including the double-stranded RNA-activated protein kinase (PKR)-like ER kinase (PERK) (Harding et al., 1999), the transcription factors ATF4 and ATF6 (activating transcription factor 6) and the inositol-requiring enzyme IRE1 (Shen et al., 2001) are involved in the UPR. In the physiological state, PERK, ATF6, and IRE1 activity is suppressed by binding of the ER chaperone: glucose regulated protein 78 (GRP78). Morimoto et al. (2007) reported that induction of GRP78 prevents neuronal damage induced by ER stress, and the increase in GRP78 (BiP) expression may correlate with the degree of neuroprotection.

Statins, inhibitors of sterol synthesis, have been shown to reduce cerebrovascular events by their pleiotropic effects independent of the cholesterol lowering mechanism. Nagotani et al. (2005) found that simvastatin was the most effective statin against spontaneous stroke in human and animals. Strong liposolubility of statins may result in high permeability through the blood–brain barrier to the parenchyma, thereby protecting the neurons against ROS-induced lipid peroxidation and DNA oxidation. The neuroprotective properties of **simvastatin** in experimental stroke have been evaluated by using several rodent-simulated models of cerebral ischemia (Shabanzadeh et al., 2005; Hayashi et al., 2005). As shown by previous studies, the changes of the UPR gene expression induced by transient ischemia occur mostly during the first 24 h (Paschen 2003b) or the first few days after the insult (Qi et al., 2004). In line with this, Urban et al. (2009) have decided to measure changes in mRNA and protein levels of GRP78, ATF6, and XBP1 after 15 min of global ischemia and 1, 3, and 24 h reperfusion (UPR reaction). In addition, they have focused their attention on the effect of simvastatin pretreatment on the stress reaction of endoplasmic reticulum induced by ischemic/reperfusion insult.

Adult male Wistar rats were used as animal model for the experiment. Global forebrain ischemia was induced by the standard four-vessel occlusion model (Lehotský et al., 2004; Sivonova et al., 2008; Uríkova et al., 2006). For maximal proof of changes in mRNA levels, authors used real-time PCR. Cortexes from sham control, ischemic and simvastatin-treated animals were homogenized, and resolved by sodium dodecyl sulfate-polyacrylamide gel electrophoresis (SDS-PAGE) and level of levels of ER stress gene proteins was analyzed by Western blotting after ischemic/ reperfusion damage (I/R) in naive rats and rats pretreated with simvastatin (20 mg/kg for 14 days). In the non-treated I/R animals, the mRNA level was significantly maximal in ischemic period (43 ± 3.2% in comparison to control), followed by rapid significant decrease from the first hour of reperfusion to a minimum value reached at the third hour (57 ± 7.8% lower than control). The mRNA level at 24 h of reperfusion reached control values. The level of XBP1 protein in non-treated animals showed only slight, not significant, differences compared to controls, mainly at later reperfusion periods (3 and 24 h).

The influence of simvastatin on mRNA level was significant only in the first and the third hours of reperfusion compared to control I/R animals (about 32.8 ± 4.1% lower and two times higher in I3R, respectively). The changes in mRNA levels were not projected onto protein levels, which, in contrast to control I/R animals, was found to be significantly lower (about 37.4 ± 2.2% in ischemic phase and about 36.3 ± 5.7% lower in first hour of reperfusion). In this paper, Urban et al (2009) were interested in finding whether global ischemia induced by four vessel occlusion followed by reperfusion at different time points would initiate the unfolded protein response of ER in cortical neurons. In addition, they have proved that prophylactic simvastatin therapy affects expression of gene coding for the main proteins involved in UPR.

Clinical trials demonstrated that 3-hydroxy-3- methylglutaryl coenzyme A reductase inhibitors or statins exert beneficial effects when used as stroke prophylactic agents (Byington et al., 2001; Vaughan et al., 2001). These studies showed that statins reduce the incidence of both first and secondary events by 25– 30% and prevention is believed to be achieved mainly through their activity on blood vessel wall function. However, in addition to exerting anti-atherosclerotic and anti-thrombotic effects, statins also possess antiinflammatory and neuroprotective actions, which have been identified as cholesterol-independent or pleiotropic effects (Vaughan and Delanty, 1999; Takemoto and Liao, 2001). The findings indicated that administration of simvastatin or other statins reduced the size of brain damage (Sironi et al., 2003; Amin-Hanjan et al., 2001). The beneficial effect of simvastatin is achieved only when the drug is administered before the ischemic insult; therefore, acting as a prophylactic agent (Balduini et al., 2003). In the model of focal ischemia induced by middle carotid artery occlusion (MCAO), the size of the damaged tissue increased by 47% after 24 h and by 83% after 48 h as compared to the infarct size detected at 2 h. This time-dependent enhancement of the damage was abolished in animals pre-treated with simvastatin, as the volume of infarct was never larger than the volume reported 2 h after MCAO. (Cimino et al., 2005).

In general, I/R injury initiates suppression of global proteosynthesis (de la Vega et al., 2001; Paschen, 2003a). Ischemia is one of the strongest stimuli of gene induction in the brain. Different gene systems related to reperfusion processes of brain injury, repair, and recovery are up-regulated (Gidday, 2006). Focal ischemia shorter than 3,5 minutes and seven days of reperfusion usually causes degeneration of 75% of the neurons in the hippocampal CA1 region (Ohtsuki et al., 1996). On the other hand 6–10-minutes long global ischemia and three days of reperfusion caused death of almost all pyramidal neurons in the same hippocampal area (Coimbra and Wieloch, 1994). Urban et al., (2009) showed a significant increase of XBP1 mRNA level in ischemic phase in comparison to control (about 43% more). These findings are similar to those observed by Paschen (2003a), which showed a marked increase in processed XBP1 mRNA levels using semi-quantitative RT-PCR after focal ischemia. These changes were most pronounced in the cerebral cortex, where high levels were found throughout the entire observation period. Urban et al (2009) obtained similar results; however, the differences were smaller probably due to the different ischemic model. The rapid increase of mRNA level of XBP1 along with other genes in ischemic phase of non-treated animals was probably due to forthcoming dissociation of protein GRP78, which reached a maximum at ischemic phase and first hour of reperfusion, from bounds with sensors of UPR which quickly (ATF6) or slowly (XBP1) started transcription of effector's genes.

In simvastatin-treated animals, rapid increase of mRNA in ischemic phase was mainly a consequence of transcription factor ATF6. It has been proposed that the strong inhibition of translation induced after transient cerebral ischemia prevents the expression of key effector UPR proteins such as the XBP1, GRP78, or ATF4, thereby hindering recovery from ischemia-induced ER dysfunction (Kumar et al., 2001; Paschen, 2003a) and possibly leading to a pro apoptotic phenotype (De-Gracia and Montie, 2004). Similarly, in experiments of Urban et al. (2009), authors did not detected any significant changes in the protein level of XBP1 neither in ischemic period nor in the first 24 h of reperfusion. The results from measurements of XBP1 mRNA in simvastatin-treated animals did not show any significant changes in comparison to naive ischemic animals, i.e., the maximal differences were detected in the first and third hour of reperfusion (about 32.8 ± 4.1% lower in I1R and two times higher in I3R, respectively). A bit surprisingly, the protein level of XBP1 was generally decreased in pre-treated animals (mainly in ischemic and I1R phase than non treated group), and did not reach control levels. Recently, a novel action of statins was proven in neurons, involving cell growth and signaling as well as down-regulation of proinflammatory gene expression attenuating neurogenic inflammation (Johnson-Anuna et al., 2005; Bucelli et al., 2008).

The results of real-time PCR measurement showed an increased mRNA level of GRP78 in ischemic time and at later phases of reperfusion in non-treated animals. Probable reason is that GRP78 is a member of the 70-kDa heat shock protein family that acts as a molecular chaperone in the folding and assembly of newly synthesized proteins within the ER. Yu et al. (1999) reported that suppression of GRP78 expression enhanced apoptosis and disruption of cellular calcium homeostasis in hippocampal neurons exposed to excitotoxic and oxidative insults. This indicates that a raised level of GRP78 makes cells more resistant to the stressful conditions (Aoki et al., 2001).

In experiments of Urban et al. (2009), authors did not find any significant changes in protein levels of GRP78 neither in simvastatin-treated nor in non-treated group of animals. They have just found maximum at third hour of reperfusion in statin group and small decrease at 24 h of reperfusion in both groups. Those results are similar to the findings of Burda et al. (2003), who failed to find any differences in GRP78 protein levels at any of the reperfusion times considered (max 4 h), either in rats with or without acquired ischemic tolerance. However, in a model of ischemic preconditioning in rats (Hayashi et al., 2003; Garcıa et al., 2004) an increase in GRP78 expression was detected after 2 days of preconditioning. Authors proposed that development of tolerance includes changes in PERK/GRP78 association, which were responsible for the decrease in eIF2a phosphorylation induced by preconditioning. Other studies using distinct ischemic models also failed to detect increased levels of GRP78 protein (Paschen 2003a).

The results of Urban et al, (2009) also showed an increased mRNA expression of ATF6, however, only in ischemic time. Consequently levels of mRNA for GRP78 were increased only slightly compared to controls. The minimum level of mRNA for ATF6 was observed at third hour of reperfusion followed by increase till 24 h of reperfusion. This minimum was probably due to pro-survival mechanism through inhibition of proapoptotic protein GADD153, which usually acts as a transcription factor of UPR genes. GADD153 protein decreased during reperfusion, until the minimum was reached at the third hour of reperfusion (Kumar et al., 2003). Urban et al. (2009) also showed significant higher levels of ATF6 mRNA in statin-treated animals in comparison to non-statin animals at ischemic period and at third hour of reperfusion (about 35.2 ± 6.6% and 42 ± 2.6% higher level), which was also translated into the higher protein level, whose values had significant maximum at third hour of reperfusion (about 60% higher level than in non-treated animals).

The experimental results altogether indicate that global ischemia/reperfusion initiates time-dependent differences in endoplasmic reticular gene expression at both the mRNA and protein levels and these authors also found the generally enhanced level of mRNA in simvastatin pre-treated animals. The maximal differences between naive ischemic and pre-treated ischemic animals authors detected in protein levels of proteins ATF6 and XBP1. The level of ATF6 was 60% higher in simvastatin pre-treated animals, which might suggest that ATF6 is one of the main proteins targeted to enhance neuroprotective effect at the ER gene level during first two hours of reperfusion.

In conclusion, these data indicate that statins, in addition to their cholesterol-lowering effect may exert a neuroprotective role in the attenuation of ER stress response after acute ischemic/reperfusion insult.

4. Impact of IRI and IPC on mitochondrial calcium transport, p53 translocation and neuronal apoptosis

Mitochondria are important regulators of neuronal cell life and death through their role in metabolic energy production and involvement in apoptosis (Yuan and Yanker, 2000). Remarkably, mitochondrial dysfunction is considered to be one of the key events linking ischemic/recirculation insult with neuronal cell death (Berridge et al., 2003). In addition, mitochondria play a dual role in intracellular calcium. They are involved in the normal control of neuronal Ca^{2+} homeostasis (Berridge et al., 2003), such as Ca^{2+} signaling, Ca^{2+} -dependent exocytosis and stimulation of oxidative metabolism and ATP production (Rizzuto, 2001; Gunter et al., 2004).

Conversely, mitochondrial Ca^{2+} overload and dysfunction, due to excitotoxic activation of glutamate receptors, is a crucial early event which follows ischemic or traumatic brain injury (Nicholls et al., 2007). Evidence for mitochondrial Ca^{2+} accumulation after excitotoxic stimulation comes from experimental studies which support the idea that mitochondrial depolarization during glutamate exposure is neuroprotective (Pivovarova et al., 2004), while its reduction correlates with excitotoxicity (Ward et al., 2007). In addition, activation of apoptosis has been documented after brain ischemia in several studies (Cao et al., 2003; Endo et al., 2006), and that this phenomenon might be closely linked to mitochondrial dysfunction. In fact, mitochondrial dysfunction provoked activation of apoptotic machinery by direct triggering of cytochrome c release (Clayton et al., 2005), or induction of Bax-dependent neuronal apoptosis through mitochondrial oxidative damage (Endo et al., 2006).

Mitochondria are involved in the control of neuronal Ca^{2+} homeostasis and neuronal Ca^{2+} signaling. In a series of recent papers (Racay et al., 2007, 2009a,b,c), authors have studied the effect of global cerebral ischemia/reperfusion injury (IRI) and ischemic tolerance developed by prior ischemic non-injurious stimulus - preconditioning- ischemic preconditioning (IPC) on mitochondrial **Ca^{2+}homeostasis** and mitochondrial way of **apoptosis**. As documented by Racay et al. (2007, 2009a), global ischemia led to progressive decrease of complex I activity after IRI to 65.7% of control at 24 h after reperfusion. In preconditioned animals, the activity of complex I was also significantly inhibited after ischemia (to 65.4% of control) and ischemia/reperfusion for 1, 3, and 24 h (62-78% of control). Although the values in preconditioned animals were significantly smaller compared to naive ischemia, IPC did not protect complex I from ischemia induced inhibition. On the other hand, activity of the terminal enzyme complex of respiratory chain, complex IV were slightly protected by IPC and the net effect of IPC was the shift of its minimal activity from 1 h to 3 h after reperfusion (Racay et al., 2009c).

Mitochondrial dysfunction and oxidative stress were often implicated in pathophysiology of neurodegenerative diseases, including cerebral ischemia (Lin and Beal, 2006). Inhibition of complex I itself or in combination with elevated Ca^{2+} led to enhanced ROS production in different *in vitro* and *in vivo* systems (Yadava and Nicholls, 2007). Importantly, an enhanced production of ROS and consequent induction of p53-dependent apoptosis due to damage to neuronal DNA has also been documented after inhibition of complex I. A recent study showed that spare respiratory capacity rather then oxidative stress is involved in excitotoxic cell death (Yadava and Nicholls, 2007).

As shown by experimental and clinical studies, IRI –induced mitochondrial pathway of apoptosis is an important event leading to neuronal cell death after blood flow arrest. Impact of IRI and ischemic preconditioning on the level of apoptotic and anti-apoptotic proteins was assessed in both cortical and hippocampal mitochondria by Western blot analysis of p53, bax, and bcl-x (Racay et al., 2007, 2009b). Remarkably, IRI led to increase of p53 level in hippocampal mitochondria, with significant differences after 3 h (217.1 ± 42.2% of control), 24 h (286.8 ± 65% of control), and 72 h (232.9 ± 37.3% of control) of reperfusion. Interestingly, translocation of p53 to mitochondria was observed in hippocampus but not in cerebral cortex. However, levels of both the apoptotic proteins bax and the anti-apoptotic bcl-xl were unchanged in both hippocampal and cortical mitochondria. Ischemia-induced translocation of p53 to mitochondria was completely abolished by IPC since no significant changes in mitochondrial p53 level were observed after preconditioned ischemia. Similar to naive ischemia, the levels of both bax and bcl-xl were not affected by IPC. In addition, IPC had significant protective effect on ischemia-induced DNA fragmentation, as well as on number of positive Fluoro-Jade C staining cells. Thus, it indicates that IPC abolished almost completely both initiation and execution of mitochondrial apoptosis induced by global brain ischemia in vulnerable CA1 layer of rat hippocampus (Racay et al., 2007, 2009b).

The studies showed that ischemia induced inhibition of mitochondrial complexes I and IV, however inhibition is not accompanied by a decrease of mitochondrial Ca^{2+} uptake rate apparently due to the excess capacity of the complex I and complex IV. On the other hand, depressed activities of complex I and IV are conditions favourable of initiation of cell degenerative pathways, e.g. opening of mitochondrial permeability transition pore, ROS generation and apoptosis initiation, and might represent important mechanism of ischemic damage to neurons.

Accordingly, ischemic preconditioning acts at the level of both initiation and execution of ischemia-induced mitochondrial apoptosis affording protection from ischemia associated changes in integrity of mitochondrial membranes. IPC also activates inhibition of p53 translocation to mitochondria. Inhibition of the mitochondrial p53 pathway thus might provide a potentially important mechanism of neuronal survival in the face of ischemic brain damage (Otani, 2008).

5. Stress reaction of neuronal endoplasmic reticulum after IRI and IPC

Ischemic tolerance can be developed by prior ischemic non-injurious stimulus or preconditioning. The molecular mechanisms underlying ischemic tolerance are not yet fully understood yet. Therefore a series of papers (Urban et al., 2009; Lehotsky et al., 2009; Pavlikova et al.,2009) have focused attention at the mRNA and protein levels of **the ER stress** genes after **ischemic/reperfusion damage (IRI)** in naive and preconditioned groups of rats.

In the UPR response, an activated IRE1 specifically cuts out the coding region of X-box protein 1 (XBP1) mRNA (Calfon et al., 2002) which after translation functions as a transcription factor specific for ER stress genes including GRP78 and GRP94. In these experiments, the hippocampal mRNA for XBP1 showed elevated levels in the naive IRI group of animals during the ischemic phase (about 43%) as well as persistent non-significant changes in all other analyzed periods (Urban et al., 2009; Lehotsky et al., 2009).

Preischemic treatment (IPC) induces the level of hippocampal mRNA in ischemic phase only slight but not significant differences compared to controls, followed by significant decreases at 24 hours of reperfusion (by about 12.8 ± 1.4% compared to controls). When analyzed the translational product, the hippocampal **XBP1 protein** level in naive IRI animal group showed significant differences in ischemic phase (39.2 ± 1.6% compared to controls) and the levels were significantly elevated at later reperfusion periods (3 and 24 h) (82 ± 2.4% and 24.1± 1.6% respectively compared to controls). The influence of preischemia (IPC) on protein levels was significant mainly in later ischemic times. The protein level reached a maximum at 3 h of reperfusion (about 230% of controls) and stayed elevated in the later reperfusion (40.3 ± 4.9% compared to controls) (Urban et al., 2009; Lehotsky et al., 2009).

Endoplasmic reticular chaperone, the Ca^{2+} binding, **glucose regulated protein 78 (GRP78)** was shown to prevent neuronal damage (Morimoto et al., 2007). Under ER dysfunction and GRP78 dissociation it subsequently induced expression of ER stress genes. At the level of mRNA for GRP78 in hippocampus from naive IRI group of animals, the authors observed that maximal differences appeared in later reperfusion phases. Preischemic pretreatment (IPC) led to elevated mRNA hippocampal levels in the reperfusion period by about 11.7 ± 3.6 during the first hour and by about 8.7± 1.8% the next 24 hours of reperfusion in comparison to mRNA levels in corresponding ischemic/reperfusion times. Remarkably, the level of GRP78 protein in naive IRI showed rapid increases in ischemic time (by about 217% of controls) and remained elevated throughout 3 to 24 hours of reperfusion (about 213% and 43%, respectively, compared to controls). Increased mRNA values in preconditioned animals also corresponded with the significant increase of the levels of GRP78 protein. The changes are documented in the ischemic phase and also in all reperfusion times (by about 250% of controls and about 50% of corresponding ischemic/reperfusion times) (Urban et al., 2009; Lehotsky et al., 2009).

ATF6 works as a key transcription factor in the resolution of the mammalian UPR (Yoshida et al. 2001). As shown in this experiment, the mRNA level for ATF6 in naive IRI animals showed gradual significant increases up to 24 hours of reperfusion (9.2 ± 4 % higher than control) and preconditioning (IPC) did not significantly alter mRNA levels in all analyzed periods. Similarl to mRNA levels, the hippocampal ATF6 protein level in naive IRI animals followed the same patterns. IPC on the other hand, induced remarkable changes in the protein levels at ischemic phase achieving significant increased levels (about 170%) in comparison to controls and stayed elevated in earlier reperfusion times (about 37 and 62 % higher than in controls) and later reperfusion time (about 15% of controls).

In general, IRI initiates suppression of global proteosynthesis, which is practically recovered in the reperfusion period with the exception of the most vulnerable neurons, such as pyramidal cells of CA1 hippocampal region (de la Vega et al., 2001). Ischemia is one of the strongest stimuli of gene induction in the brain. Different gene systems related to reperfusion processes of brain injury, repair and recovery are modulated (Gidday, 2006). In fact, IRI induces transient inhibition of translation, which prevents the expression of UPR proteins and hinders recovery from ischemia-induced ER dysfunction (Kumar et al., 2001; Paschen et al., 2003a) which possibly leads to a pro-apoptotic phenotype (DeGracia and Montie, 2004). Similarly, Thuerauf et al. (2006) found that myocardial ischemia activates UPR with the increased expression of XBP1 protein and XBP1-inducible protein. They contribute to protection of the myocardium during hypoxia. Also the results of Paschen et al. (2003a) using semi-quantitative RT-PCR showed a marked increase in XBP1 mRNA levels after focal ischemia in the cerebral cortex.

Preischemia induced elevation of mRNA and protein GRP78 levels in reperfusion periods. GRP78 is a member of the 70kDa heat shock protein family that acts as a molecular chaperone in the folding and assembly of newly synthesized proteins within the ER. As shown by Yu et al. (1999) the suppression of GRP78 expression enhances apoptosis and disruption of cellular calcium homeostasis in hippocampal neurons that are exposed to excitotoxic and oxidative insults. This indicates that a raised level of GRP78 makes cells more resistant to the stressful conditions (Aoki et al. 2001). Similar results were obtained by Morimoto et al. (2007) in the focal ischemia model. Also Hayashi et al. (2003) and Garcia et al. (2004), who demonstrated an increase in GRP78 expression after 2 days of preconditioning proposed that the development of tolerance includes changes in PERK/GRP78 association, which were responsible for the decrease in eIF2a phosphorylation induced by preconditioning. On the other hand, Burda et al. (2003), failed to find any differences in the level of GRP78 protein in rats with or without acquired ischemic tolerance. This was probably due to exposure to very short reperfusion times. ATF6 is an ER-membrane-bound transcription factor activated by ER stress, which is specialized in the regulation of ER quality control proteins (Adachi et al., 2008). Haze et al. (1999) found that the overexpression of full-length ATF6 activates transcription of the GRP78 gene. Explanation of generally higher levels of protein p90ATF6 in preischemic group is probably connected to an increased promotor activity of GADD153 to UPR genes (Oyadomari et al., 2004).

The data from these experiments (Urban et al. 2009; Lehotsky et al. 2009) suggest that IRI initiates time dependent differences in **endoplasmic reticular gene expression** at both the mRNA and protein levels and that endoplasmic gene expression is affected by preischemic treatment. These data and recent experiments of Bickler et al. (2009) also suggest that preconditioning paradigm (preischemia) may exert a role in the attenuation of ER stress response and that InsP3 receptor mediated Ca^{2+} signaling is an important mediator in the neuroprotective phenomenon of acquired ischemic tolerance. Changes in gene expression of the key proteins provide an insight into ER stress pathways. It also might suggest possible targets of future therapeutic interventions to enhance recovery after stroke (Yenari et al., 2008; Pignataro et al., 2009).

6. Effect of ischemic preconditioning on secretory pathways Ca^{2+}-ATPase gene expression

The Golgi apparatus, as a part of **secretory pathways (SP)** in neural cells, represents a dynamic Ca^{2+} store. Ca^{2+} ions play an active role in processes such as secretion of neurotransmitters and secretory proteins for the growth/ reorganization of neuronal circuits, synaptic transmission, neural plasticity, and remodeling of dendrites (Michelangeli et al., 2005). In addition, SP are involved in the stress sensing, neuronal aging, and transduction of apoptotic signals (Maag et al., 2003; Sepulveda et al., 2008). On the other hand, a high luminal Ca^{2+} concentration, and Mn^{2+}, is required in the Golgi apparatus for the optimal activity of many enzymes and for post-translational processing and trafficking of the newly formed proteins. For both cytosolic and Golgi Ca^{2+} and Mn^{2+}homeostasis, **the secretory pathway Ca^{2+}-ATPases (SPCAs)** play an important role.

The SPCAs represent a subfamily of P-type ATPases related to the sarco(endo)plasmic reticulum Ca^{2+}-ATPase (SERCA) and the plasma-membrane Ca^{2+}-ATPase (PMCA) (Van Baelen et al., 2004; Murin et al., 2006). Two isoforms sharing 64% of sequence identity, namely SPCA1 and SPCA2, are expressed in mammalian cells (Wootton et al., 2004; Xiang et al., 2005). While SPCA2 expression seems to be more restricted to specific cell types, the SPCA1 is considered as a house-keeping isoform with pronounced expression in neural cells (Wootton et al., 2004; Murin et al., 2006; Sepulveda et al., 2008). The higher expression levels of SPCA1 in the brain coincide with a relatively high ratio of SPCA activity (thapsigargin insensitive) to the total activity of Ca^{2+}-dependent ATPases. Therefore, implying a significant role of SPCA-facilitated transport of Ca^{2+} for calcium storage within the brain (Wootton et al., 2004).

As shown by previous studies, the SPCA plays a pivotal role in normal neural development, neural migration, and morphogenesis (Sepulveda et al., 2007, 2008). In addition, as shown in SPCA1 knockout mice, SPCA1 deficiency caused alteration in neural tube development and Golgi stress. These animals presented structural changes in the Golgi such as dilatation and the reduction in the number of stacked leaflets (Okunade et al., 2007). In apoptosis, a morphological change in the Golgi complex, for example its fragmentation, represents an early causative step rather than a secondary event, and it is very commonly associated with several neurodegenerative diseases, such as amyotrophic lateral sclerosis, corticobasal degeneration, Alzheimer's and Creutzfeldt-Jacob diseases, and spinocerebelar ataxia type 2 (Gonatas et al., 2006).

6.1 Effect of oxidative damage on SPCA1

Collective studies confirm that reactive oxygen species contribute to neuronal cell injuries secondary to ischemia and reperfusion (Lehotsky et al., 2004; Burda et al., 2005; Danielisova et al., 2005; Shi and Liu, 2007). Oxidative burst lasting several minutes upon the onset of reperfusion is followed by dysregulation of antioxidant mechanism and moderate but persistently elevated production of oxygen radicals which might initiate cell death signaling pathways after cerebral ischemia and parallels with selective postischemic vulnerability of the brain (Valko et al., 2007; Shi and Liu, 2007).

One of the main aims of the study of Pavlikova et al. (2009) was to determine whether IRI and IPC would affect the physical and functional properties of hippocampal membrane vesicles including Golgi SP. Neuronal microsomes are vulnerable to physical and functional oxidative damage (Lehotsky et al. 1999, 2002a; Urikova et al. 2006). The nature of the effect of free radicals on SPCA1 protein is not yet known. Authors show here for the first time that SPCA activity is also selectively damaged by free radicals in vitro, the property which is similar to other P-type ATPase such as SERCA and PMCA (Lehotsky et al. 2002b). In the study, authors showed that transient ischemia for 15 min induces considerable LPO and protein oxidation in hippocampal membranes. Protein oxidation pursues disturbances in oxidant/antioxidant balance and depression of enzymatic activities of main antioxidant enzymes detected at later stages after the ischemic insult (Lehotsky et al., 2002a; Urıkova et al., 2006). Thus, oxidative alterations detected after IRI may at least partially explain functional post-ischemic disturbances of neuronal ion transport mechanisms (Lipton, 1999; Lehotsky et al., 2002a; Obrenovitch, 2008) and inhibition of global proteosynthesis (Burda et al., 2003), which both are implicated in neuronal cell damage and/or recovery from ischemic insult.

IPC caused significant reductions of LPO products and it reduced protein oxidative changes induced by ischemia in the hippocampal membranes in both the ischemic time and in reperfusion period. One of the possible explanations comes from the studies describing upregulation of defense mechanisms (antioxidant enzymes) against oxidative stress due to the preconditioning challenge (Danielisova et al., 2005; Gidday, 2006; Obrenovitch, 2008). In addition, forebrain ischemia causes small but significant drops in **the SPCA-associated Ca^{2+}-ATPase activity** (by about 9%). The activity increases in early reperfusion times. However, it did not reach the control level and reached the highest depression after 24 h reperfusion to 88% of control. In the experiments, the IPC had a partial protective effect on the SPCA-associated Ca^{2+}-ATPase activity. Ischemic insult after IPC pretreatment initiate only non-significant inhibition of Ca^{2+}-ATPase activity compared to preconditioned control. After 1 and 3 h of reperfusion, the activity exceeded the control levels and reached it again after 24 h of reperfusion. However, the changes were not statistically significant at any reperfusion time. As shown in earlier studies, preconditioning upregulates defense mechanisms against oxidative stress (Danielisova et al., 2005; Gidday, 2006; Obrenovitch, 2008), which might partially restore the depression of enzyme activity. Additionally, as shown in the study by Western blot analysis, IPC induced an elevation of SPCA protein level in comparison to corresponding naive ischemic control.

In summary, the experiments conclusively showed that cerebral IRI-induced depression of SPCA activity and lipid and protein oxidation in rat hippocampal membranes. IRI also activates induction of SPCA1 gene expression in later reperfusion periods. IPC partially suppresses oxidative changes in hippocampal membranes and also partially restores the ischemic-induced depression of SPCA activity.

In addition, IPC initiates earlier cellular response to the injury by the significant elevation of mRNA expression (to 142% comparing to 1 h of corresponding reperfusion) and to 154 and 111% comparing to 3 and 24 h of corresponding reperfusion, respectively. Similar patterns were observed on the translational level by Western blot analysis. Results of Pavlikova et al. (2009) indicate the specific SPCA1 expression pattern in injured ischemic hippocampus and might serve to understand the molecular mechanisms involved in the structural integrity and function of the Golgi complex after ischemic challenge. They also suggest for the correlation of SPCA function with the role of SP in response to preischemic challenge.

Collective studies confirm, that reactive oxygen species (ROS) contribute to neuronal cell injuries secondary to ischemia and reperfusion (Lehotsky et al., 2004; Burda et al., 2005; Danielisova et al., 2005; Shi and Liu, 2007) and might initiate cell death signaling pathways after cerebral ischemia and parallels with selective post-ischemic vulnerability of the brain (Valko et al., 2007; Shi and Liu, 2007; Otani, 2008; Dirnagl et al., 2009). As shown by measurement of steady state fluorescence of ANS in hippocampal mitochondria (Racay et al., 2007, 2009a), naive IRI induced significant increase in ANS flurescence (it binds to hydrophobic part of membrane lipids and proteins) of the forebrain in both ischemic and reperfusion periods. These results support data from previous experiments (Lehotsky et al., 2004; Babusikova et al., 2008), which showed that IRI induced structural changes on hippocampal membrane lipids and both, the lipoperoxidation dependent and the direct oxidative modifications of membrane proteins. Remarkably, preconditioning (IPC) induces significant decrease of ANS fluorescence, which indicates protective effect of IPC on mitochondrial membranes.

SP are involved in the stress sensing, neuronal aging and transduction of apoptotic signals (Maag et al., 2003; Sepulveda et al., 2008). In order to evaluate whether the severe metabolic stress induced by IRI and/or IPC affects transcription of SPCA1 gene, the mRNA and protein levels of SPCA1 was analyzed (Lehotsky, 1999, 2002a, 2004). As shown by Pavlikova et al. (2009), RT-PCR clearly detected, that hippocampal cells respond to the IRI by induction of mRNA level in reperfusion period with maximum at 3 h reperfusion (to 171% of control). Preconditioning (IPC) initiates earlier tissue response to the injury by the significant elevation of mRNA expression already at 1 h of reperfusion and the level of mRNA expression reached 142% comparing to 1 h ischemia, and to 164% comparing to control.

Neuronal microsomes are vulnerable to physical and functional oxidative damage (Lehotsky et al., 1999, 2002a, 2004; Urikova et al., 2006). The authors showed (Pavlikova et al. (2009) that SPCA activity, similar to other P-type ATPases, is also subject to ischemic damage most likely due to free radicals action (Lehotsky et al., 2002b). In addition, oxidative alterations detected in mitochondria and microsomes after IRI in our experiments, may at least partially explain functional postischemic disturbances of neuronal ion transport mechanisms (Lipton 1999; Lehotsky et al., 2002a; Obrenovitch, 2008) and inhibition of global proteosynthesis (Burda et al., 2003), which are both implicated in neuronal cell damage and/or recovery from ischemic insult, IPC-induced reduction of lipoperoxidation products and protein oxidative changes (Racay et al., 2009; Pavlikova et al., 2009). These may all be probably due to upregulation of defence mechanisms (antioxidant enzymes) against oxidative stress in the preconditioning challenge (Danielisova et al., 2005; Gidday, 2006; Obrenovitch, 2008).

One of the most pronounced morphological features following IRI is the mitochondrial and Golgi swelling and activation, which could be suppressed by neuroprotective treatment (Hicks and Machaner, 2005; Strosznajder et al., 2005; Gonatas et al., 2006). The secretory pathways are apparently involved in sensing stress and transducing signals during the execution phase of apoptosis (Maag et al., 2003; Hicks and Machamer, 2005). Data from Pavlikova (2009) showed a partial recovery of Ca^{2+}-ATPase activity and earlier hippocampal response to later ischemia by the induction of mRNA and protein expression.

Cross-talk between the function of intracellular organelles following ischemic insult and reperfusion (Fig.2) and response of the tissue to the preischemic challenge (Fig 3) is depicted bellow .

6.2 Effect of hyperhomocysteinemia on SPCA expression

Homocysteine (Hcy) is a sulfur-containing amino acid, which is derived from methionine metabolism. Hyperhomocysteinemia, condition in which Hcy concentration exceeds 16 μmol/l, is the result of perturbed Hcy metabolism and dietary deficiencies in folic acid, vitamin B6, and/or vitamin B12 (Obeid et al., 2007).

Hyperhomocysteinemia has been implicated as an independent risk factor for arteriosclerosis and coronary heart disease (Refsum et al., 1998; Thambyrajah et al., 2000). Severe forms of hyperhomocysteinemia results in convulsions and dementia (Watkins et al., 1989; van den Berg et al., 1995) corresponding multiple participation of homocysteine (Hcy) in diverse pathologies that affect the CNS. Likewise, homocysteine has also been associated with several CNS disorders, such as stroke (Obeid et al., 2007), epilepsy (Sachdev, 2004; Herrmann et al., 2007), neurodegenerative (Clarke et al., 1998; Mattson et al., 2002) and neuropsychiatric diseases (Diaz-Arrastia, 2000; Bottiglieri, 2005), as well as inborn errors of metabolism (Mudd et al., 2001). In addition, even moderate hyperhomocysteinemia is a factor stimulating the development of dementia and Alzheimer's disease (Seshadri et al., 2002).

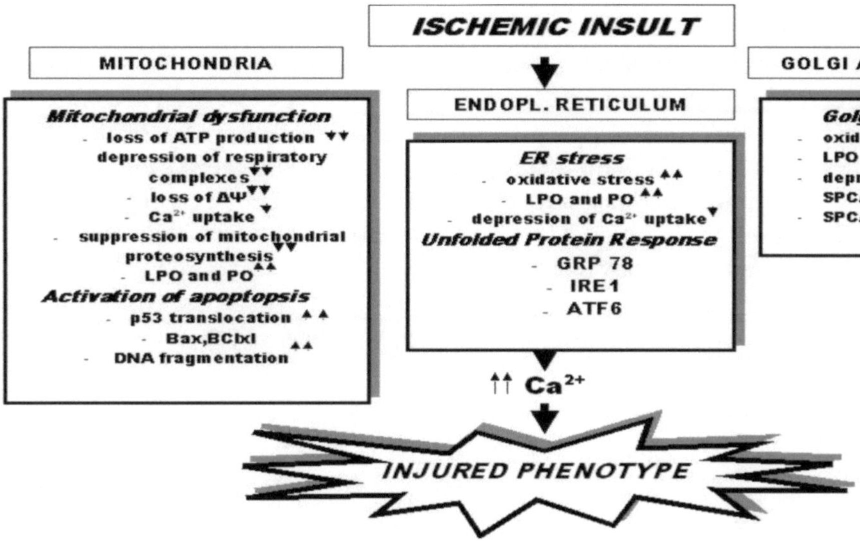

Fig. 2. Cross-talk between the fuction of intracellular organelles which follows ischemic insults and results in injured phenopyte in vulnerable neurons. Adapted from Lehotsky et al. (2009c).

Ischemic brain stroke in humans represents very complex cerebrovascular disease. A number of conventional risk factors for ischemic stroke are known, such as a previous occurrence of stroke, previous transient ischemic attack (TIA), arterial disease, atrial fibrillation, poor diet and/or obesity and physical inactivity (Prasad, 1999). It has been reported that hyperhomocysteinemia may also be associated with the incidence of ischemic brain stroke (Refsum et al., 1998), mainly due to pleiotropic activity of homocysteine and acceleration of atherosclerotic changes (Refsum et al., 1998; Thambyrajah et al., 2000). In fact, Hcy suppresses NO production by endothelial cells (Upchurch et al., 1997) and platelets (Mutus et al., 2001) and increases generation of reactive oxygen species (ROS) by the release of arachidonic acid from platelets (Signorello et al. 2002). It also inhibits glutathione peroxidase (Upchurch et al., 1997), and thus stimulates proliferation of endothelial cells (Jeremy et al., 1999; Domagala et al., 1998).

In addition, Hcy has been shown to inhibit methyltransferases, to suppress DNA reparation and to facilitate apoptosis when accumulated inside the cells (Duan et al., 2002; Kruman et al., 2002). Autooxidation of Hcy metabolites results in H_20_2 accumulation (Gortz et al., 2004; Boldyrev, 2005) and long term incubation of neurons with Hcy metabolites induces necrotic cell death (Zieminska et al., 2003; Boldyrev et al., 2004). Homocysteine has also been shown to be elevated in other disorders of the CNS, e.g. Alzheimer disease or Parkinson disease (Toohey, 2007).

A series of papers (Urban et al., 2009; Lehotsky et al., 2009b; Pavlikova et al.,2009) found that ischemia/reperfusion injury (IRI) initiates time dependent differences in endoplasmic reticular gene expression at both the mRNA and protein levels in rat hippocampus and that endoplasmic gene expression is affected by pre-ischemic treatment. More recently, Pavlikova et al. (2011) conducted an investigation into the differences between naive control and hyperhomocysteinemic control animals in each group independently. They showed for the first time that experimental 2 weeks hyperhomocysteinemia significantly decreased the level of SPCA1 mRNA gene expression in cerebral cortex which also led to the non-significantly decreased expression levels in hippocampal area. In cortex, ischemic challenge for 15 min. did not change significantly the level of mRNA SPCA1 expression in comparison to controls. Conversely, the gene response to pre-ischemic challenge was clearly shown within the homocysteine group by abrupt stimulation of the mRNA expression level to 249 % of hyperhomocysteinemic ischemic group and to 321% of hyperhomocysteinemic control. Notably, values far exceed those observed in the naive control. However, the effect of IPC challenge was not observed in the naive groups.

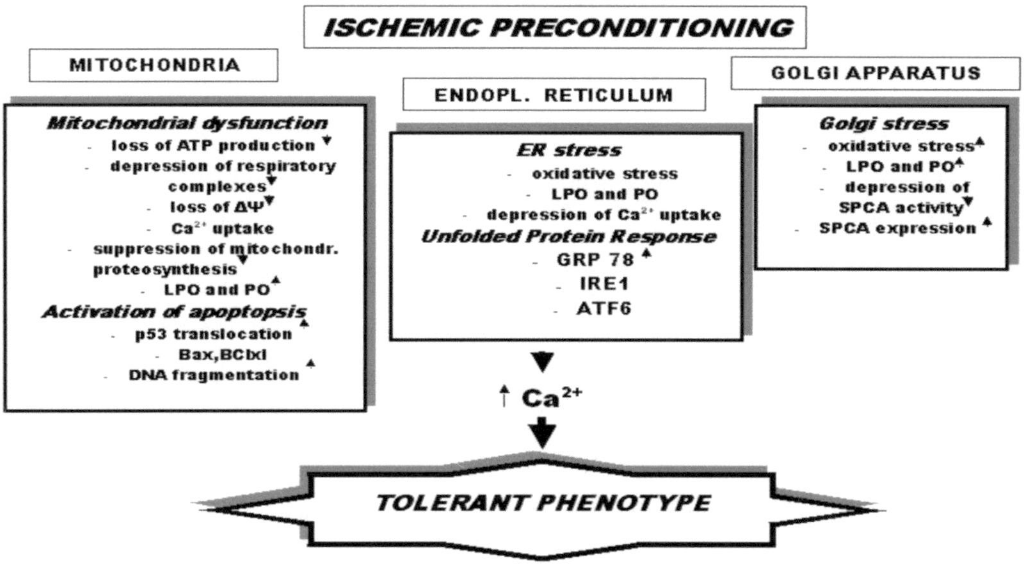

Fig. 3. Cross-talk between the fuction of intracellular organelles which follow preischemic maneuver and results in tolerant phenopyte in vulnerable neurons. Adapted from Lehotsky et al. (2009c).

The expression level decreased in the hyperhomocysteinemic control to 259% ($p<0.05$) of naive control and to 277% of control with IPC. When changes were compared between all ischemic groups, the following were observed: low level of mRNA expression in hyperhomocysteinemic ischemic group (to 201% of naive ischemia and to 185% of ischemic preconditioning. However, there were no significant differences between Hcy-control group and Hcy- ischemic group. Preischemic challenge initiated stimulation of the mRNA expression to 249% of hyperhomocysteinemic ischemic group. This response may be attributed to a part of the protective tolerant phenomenon induced by preconditioning treatment.

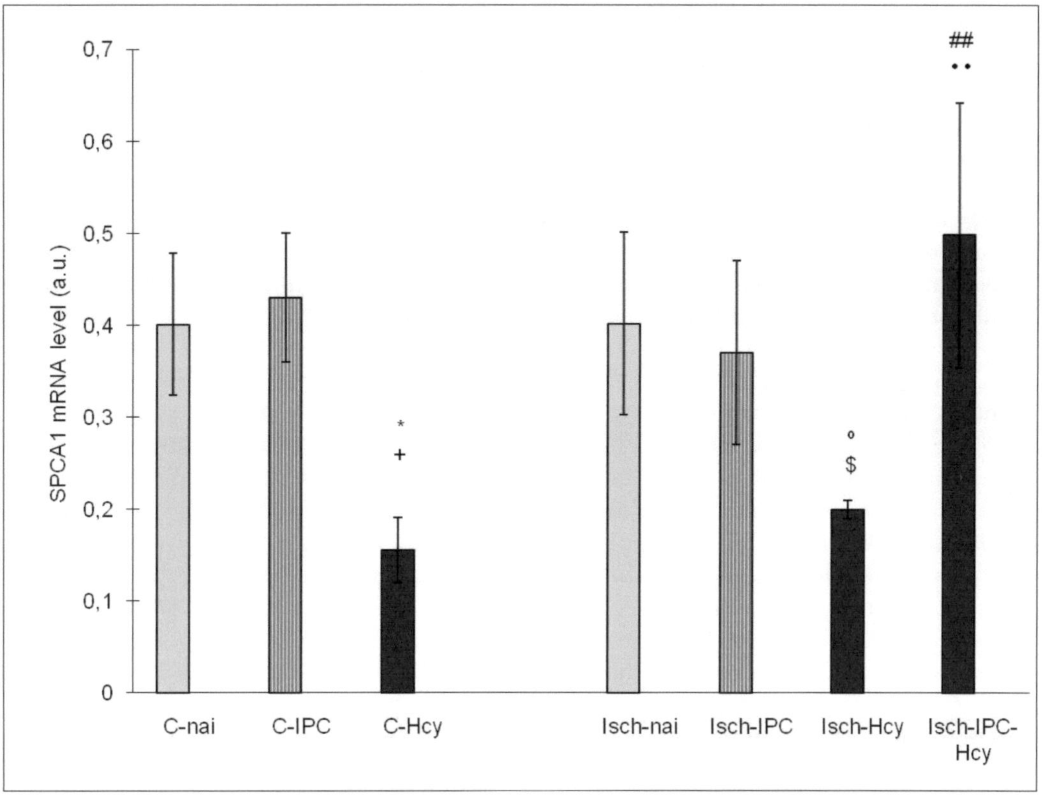

Fig. 4. Comparison of mRNA levels of SPCA1 between naive group (C-nai, Isch-nai), IPC group (C-IPC, Isch-IPC) and hyperhomocysteinemic group (C-Hcy, Isch-Hcy, Isch-IPC-Hcy) in rat cortex. Results are presented as mean ± SEM for $n = 6$. * $p < 0.05$ compared to C-nai group, + $p < 0.05$ compared to C-IPC groups, † $p < 0.05$ compared to Isch-Hcy group, ‡ $p < 0.05$ compared to C-IPC group, ## $p < 0.01$ compared to Isch-IPC-Hcy group, && $p < 0.01$ compared to Isch-IPC-Hcy group. C-nai, control naive group; Isch-nai, ischemia naive group, C-IPC, control preischemic group; Isch-IPC, preischemic group; C-Hcy, control Hcy group; Isch-Hcy, ischemia Hcy group; Isch-IPC-Hcy, preischemic Hcy group. Adapted from Pavlikova et al. (2011).

In results of mRNA SPCA1 expression in hippocampal area no statistically significant changes were found between naive control and IPC control groups. Hyperhomocysteinemia for 14 days supressed mRNA expression, however the changes were not statistically significant. Similarly, as shown in the cortex, the preischemic challenge in hippocampal region initiated stimulation of the mRNA expression by 159% of hyperhomocysteinemic control and by to 131% hyperhomocysteinemic ischemic group. The suggestion was, that this response might also be part of the protective tolerant phenomenon induced by preconditioning treatment.

The previous results showed that IRI insult alters time expression profile of SPCA1 on mRNA and protein level (Pavlikova et al. 2009), and that preischemic challenge (induction of tolerance), not only preserved majority of surviving neuron but also activates partial recovery of the secretory pathways SPCA Ca^{2+}-ATPase activity and earlier hippocampal response to later ischemia by the induction of SPCA1 mRNA and protein expression. We shown here for the first time that chemically induced experimental 2 weeks hyperhomocysteinemia significantly decreased the level of SPCA1 mRNA gene expression in cerebral cortex and also led to the non-significant decreased expression level in hippocampal area. There are no literature data on how the Hcy might affect the expression profile of the Ca^{2+}-transport proteins in neuronal cells. In fact, the general mechanism of transcriptional regulation of SPCA1 gene is not yet fully understood. The transcription factors Sp1 and YY1 were shown to be involved in the gene regulation by the cis-enhancing elements in 5′-untranslated regions (Kawada et al., 2005). Another possibility is the expression of the putative endogenous activator of SPCA or the changes in local membrane environment are suggested as a cause for the increase in SPCA activity (Sepulveda et al. 2008). In fact, hyperhomocysteinemia often results in intracellular Ca^{2+} mobilization, endoplasmic reticulum (ER) stress, with the subsequent development of apoptotic events, chronic inflammation leading to endothelial dysfunction and remodeling of the extracellular matrix. Homocysteine has also been reported to induce modulation of gene expression through alteration of the methylation status (Dionisio, 2010).

In conclusion, our results indicate that chemically induced hyperhomocysteinemia initiates supression of the SPCA1 gene expression in both brain regions cerebral cortex and hippocampus. Documented response of SPCA gene to preischemic challenge in hyperhomocysteinemic group of animals might suggest for the correlation of SPCA expression with the role of secretory pathways in the proposed phenomenon of ischemic tolerance (Dirnagl et al., 2009; Pignataro et al., 2009). This might also serve to understand the molecular mechanisms involved in the structural integrity and function of the Golgi complex after ischemic challenge.

7. Conclusion

Ischemic induced alterations of mitochondria, endoplasmic reticulum and Golgi apparatus shed more light on understanding the cross-talk between intracellular Ca^{2+} stores in cerebral ischemia/reperfusion injury. Documented neuroprotective response of intracellular organelles in the phenomenon of ischemic tolerance may also form a basis for future therapeutic interventions to enhance recovery from stroke. Finally, exploration of the protective mechanisms could lead to the recognition of newer strategies and suggestions for development of novel prophylactic/therapeutics for neuronal apoptosis-related diseases.

8. Acknowledgments

This study was supported by Grants VEGA 0049/09 from the Ministry of Education of the Slovak Republic, UK-55-15/07 from Ministry of Health of Slovak Republic, and APVV VVCE 0064-07 and by project "IDENTIFICATION OF NOVEL MARKERS IN DIAGNOSTIC PANEL OF NEUROLOGICAL DISEASES", code 26220220114, co-financed from EU sources and European Regional Development Fund. The authors are grateful to Dr N. A. Yeboah for critical reading of the manuscript.

9. References

Adachi Y, Yamamoto K, Okada T, Yoshida H, Harada A, Mori K (2008) ATF6 is a transcription factor specializing in the regulation of quality control proteins in the endoplasmic reticulum. *Cell Struct Funct,* 33: pp. 75–89. doi:10.1247/csf.07044

Amin-Hanjan S, Stagliano NE, Yamada M, Huang PL, Liao JK, Moskowitz MA (2001) Mevastatin, an HMG-CoA reductase inhibitor, reduces stroke damage and upregulates endothelial nitric oxide synthase in mice. *Stroke* pp. 32:980–986

Aoki M, Tamatani M, Taniguchi M, Yamaguchi A, Bando Y, Kasai K et al (2001) Hypothermic treatment restores glucose regulated protein 78 (GRP78) expression in ischemic brain. *Brain Res Mol Brain Res* 95(1–2): pp. 117–128. doi:10.1016/S0169-328X(01)00255-8

Babusikova E., Jesenak M., Racay P., Dobrota D., Kaplan P. (2008): Oxidative alterations in rat heart homogenate and mitochondria during ageing. *Gen. Physiol. Biophys.* 27. pp 115-120.

Balduini W, Mazzoni E, Carloni S, De Simoni MG, Perego C, Sironi L (2003) Prophylactic but not delayed administration of simvastatin protects against long-lasting cognitive and morphological consequences of neonatal hypoxicischemic brain injury, reduces interleukin-1beta and tumor necrosis factoralpha mRNA induction, and does not affect endothelial nitric oxide synthase expression. *Stroke* 34: pp. 2007–2012. doi: 10.1161/01.STR.0000080677.24419.88

Barone FC, White RF, Spera PA, Ellison J, Currie RW, Wang X, Feuerstein GZ. 1998. Ischemic preconditioning and brain tolerance:temporal histological and functional outcomes, protein synthesis requirement, and interleukin-1 receptor antagonist and early gene expression. *Stroke* 29: pp. 1937–1950; discussion pp. 1950-1951.

Berridge M. J., Bootman M. D., Roderick H. L. (2003): Calcium signalling: dynamics, homeostasis and remodelling. *Nat. Rev. Mol. Cell Biol.* 4, pp. 517–529

Bickler P. E., Fahlman C. S., Gray J., McKleroy W. (2009): Inositol 1,4,5-triphosphate receptors and NAD(P)H mediate Ca2+ signaling required for hypoxic preconditioning of hippocampal neurons. *Neuroscience* 160, pp. 51–60

Boldyrev A., Bulygina E., Makhro A. (2004): Glutamate receptors modulate oxidative stress in neuronal cells. *Neurotox. Res.* 6, pp. 581-587

Boldyrev A. (2005): Homocysteic acid causes oxidative stress in lymphocytes by potentiating toxic effect of NMDA. *Bull. Exp. Biol. Med.* 140, pp. 33-37

Bottiglieri T. (2005): Homocysteine and folate metabolism in depression. *Prog. Neuropsychopharmacol. Biol. Psychiatry* 29, pp. 1103-1112

Bucelli RC, Gonsiorek EA, Kim WY, Bruun D, Rabin RA, Higgins D et al (2008) Statins decrease expression of the proinflammatory neuropeptides calcitonin gene-related peptide and substance P in sensory neurons. *J Pharmacol Exp Ther* 324(3): pp. 1172–1180. doi:10.1124/jpet.107.132795

Burda J, Hrehorovska M, Bonilla LG, Danielisova V, Cizkova D, Burda R, Nemethova M, Fando JL, Salinas M. 2003. Role of protein synthesis in the ischemic tolerance acquisition induced by transient forebrain ischemia in the rat. *Neurochem Res* 28: pp. 1213–1219.

Burda J, Matiasova M, Gottlieb M, Danielisova V, Nemethova M, Garcia L, Salinas M, Burda R (2005) Evidence for a role of second pathophysiological stress in prevention of delayed neuronal death in the hippocampal CA1 region. *Neurochem Res* 30: pp. 1397–1405. doi:10.1007/s11064-005-8510-z

Byington RP, Davis BR, Plehn JF, White HD, Baker J, Cobbe SM (2001) Reduction of stroke events with pravastatin: the Prospective Pravastatin Pooling (PPP) Project. *Circulation* 103: pp. 387–392

Calfon M., Zeng H., Urano F., Till J. H., Hubbart S. R., Harding H.P., Clark S. G., Ron D. (2002): IRE1 couples endoplasmic reticulum load to secretory capacity by processing XBP-1 mRNA. *Nature* 415, pp. 92–96

Cao G., Clark R. S., Pei W., Yin W., Zhang F., Sun F. Y., Graham S. H., Chen J. (2003): Translocation of apoptosis-inducing factor in vulnerable neurons after transient cerebral ischemia and in neuronal cultures after oxygen-glucose deprivation. *J. Cereb. Blood Flow Metab.* 23, pp. 1137–1150

Cimino M, Balduini W, Carloni S, Gelosa P, Guerrini U, Tremoli E et al (2005) Neuroprotective effect of simvastatin in stroke: a comparison between adult and neonatal rat models of cerebral ischemia. *Neurotoxicology* 26: pp. 929–933. doi:10.1016/j.neuro.2005.03.009

Clarke R., Smith A.D., Jobst K.A., Refsum H., Sutton L., Ueland P.M. (1998): Folate, vitamin B12, and serum total homocysteine levels in confirmed Alzheimer disease. *Arch. Neurol.* 55, pp. 1449-1455

Clayton R., Clark J. B., Sharpe M. (2005): Cytochrome c release from rat brain mitochondria is proportional to the mitochondrial functional deficit: implications for apoptosis and neurodegenerative disease. *J. Neurochem.* 92, pp. 840–849

Coimbra C, Wieloch T (1994) Moderate hypothermia mitigates neuronal damage in the rat brain when initiated several hours following transient cerebral ischemia. *Acta Neuropathol* 87: pp. 325–331. doi:10.1007/BF00313599

DeGracia DJ, Kumar R, Owen CR, Krause GS, White BC (2002) Molecular pathways of protein synthesis inhibition during brain reperfusion: implications for neuronal survival or death. *J Cereb Blood Flow Metab* 22: pp. 127–141. doi:10.1097/00004647-200202000-00001

Danielisova V, Nemethova M, Gottlieb M, Burda J (2005) Changes of endogenous antioxidant enzymes during ischemic tolerance acquisition. *Neurochem Res* 30: pp. 559–565. doi:10.1007/s11064-005-2690-4

DeGracia DJ, Kumar R, Owen CR, Krause GS, White BC (2002) Molecular pathways of protein synthesis inhibition during brain reperfusion: implications for neuronal survival or death. *J Cereb Blood Flow Metab* 22: pp. 127–141. doi:10.1097/00004647-20020 2000-00001

DeGracia DJ, Montie HL (2004) Cerebral ischemia and the unfolded protein response. *J Neurochem* 91(1): pp. 1–8. doi: 10.1111/j.1471-4159.2004.02703.x

De la Vega MC, Burda J, Nemethova M, Quevedo C, Alcazar A, Martin ME et al (2001) Possible mechanisms involved in the down-regulation of translation during transient global ischaemia in the rat brain. *Biochem J* 357: pp. 819–826. doi:10.1042/0264-6021:3570819

Diaz-Arrastia R. (2000): Homocysteine and neurologic disease. *Arch. Neurol.* 57: pp. 1422-1427

Dionisio N, Jardin I., Salido G.M., Rosado J.A. (2010): Homocysteine, Intracellular Signaling and Thrombotic Disorders. *Curr.Med.Chem.* 17, pp. 3109-3119

Dirnagl U, Simon RP, Hallenbeck JM. 2003. Ischemic tolerance and endogenous neuroprotection. *Trends Neurosci* 26: pp. 248–254.

Dirnagl U, Becker K, Meisel A. Preconditioning and tolerance against cerebral ischaemia: from experimental strategies to clinical use. *Lancet Neurol.*8(4) (2009): pp. 398-412.

Domagała T.B., Undas A., Libura M., Szczeklik A. (1998): Pathogenesis of vascular disease in hyperhomocysteinaemia. *J. Cardiovasc. Risk.* 5, pp. 239-247

Duan W., Ladenheim B., Cutler R.G., Kruman I.I., Cadet J.L., Mattson M.P. (2002): Dietary folate deficiency and elevated homocysteine levels endanger dopaminergic neurons in models of Parkinson's disease. *J. Neurochem.* 80, pp. 101-110

Endo H., Kamada H., Nito C., Nishi T., Chan P. H. (2006): Mitochondrial translocation of p53 mediates release of cytochrome c and hippocampal CA1 neuronal death after transient global cerebral ischemia in rats. *J. Neurosci.* 26, pp. 7974–7983

Endres M, Engelhardt B, Koistinaho J, Lindvall O, Meairs S, Mohr JP, Planas A, Rothwell N, Schwaninger M, Schwab ME, Vivien D, Wieloch T, Dirnagl U. 2008. Improving outcome after stroke: overcoming the translational roadblock. *Cerebrovasc Dis* 25: pp. 268–278.

García L, Burda J, Hrehorovska M, Burda R, Martin E, Salinas M (2004) Ischaemic preconditioning in the rat brain: effect on the activity of several initiation factors, Akt and extracellular signal-regulated protein kinase phosphorylation, and GRP78and GADD34 expression. *J Neurochem* 88: pp. 136–147

Gidday JM. 2006. Cerebral preconditioning and ischaemic tolerance. *Nat Rev Neurosci* 7: pp. 437–448.

Gonatas N. K., Stieber A., Gonatas J. O. (2006): Fragmentation of the Golgi apparatus in neurodegenerative diseases and cell death. *J. Neurol. Sci.* pp. 246, 21–30

Gortz Ph., Hoinke A., Fleischer W., Otto F., Schwahn B., Wendel U., Siebler M. J. (2004): Implications for hyperhomocysteinemia: not homocysteine but its oxidized forms strongly inhibit neuronal network activity. *Neurol. Sci.* 218, pp. 109-114

Gunter T. E., Yule D. I., Gunter K. K., Eliseev R. A., Salter J. D.(2004): Calcium and mitochondria. *FEBS Lett.* 567, pp. 96–102

Harding H.P., Zhang Y., Ron D. (1999): Protein translation and folding are coupled by an endoplasmic reticulum-resident kinase. *Nature* 397: 271-274. doi: 10.1038/16729

Hayashi T, Saito A, Okuno S, Ferrand-Drake M, Dodd RL, Nishi T et al (2003) Oxidative damage to the endoplasmic reticulum is implicated in ischemic neuronal cell death. *J Cereb Blood Flow Metab* 23: pp. 1117–1128. doi:10.1097/ 01.WCB.0000089600.87125.AD

Hayashi T, Hamakawa K, Nagotani S, Jin G, Li F, Deguchi K et al (2005) HMG CoA reductase inhibitors reduce ischemic brain injury of Wistar rats through decreasing oxidative stress on neurons. *Brain Res* 1037(1–2): pp. 52–58. doi:10.1016/j.brainres.2004.12.051

Haze K, Yoshida H, Yanagi H, Yura T, Mori K (1999) Mammalian transcription factor ATF6 is synthesized as a transmembrane protein and activated by proteolysis in response to endoplasmic reticulum stress. *Mol Biol Cell* 10: pp. 3787–3799

Herrmann W., Lorenzl S., Obeid R. (2007): Review of the role of hyperhomocysteinemia and B-vitamin deficiency in neurological and psychiatric disorders-current evidence and preliminary recommendations. *Fortschr. Neurol. Psychiatr.* 75, pp. 515-527

Hicks S. W., Machamer C. E. (2005): Golgi structure in stress sensing and apoptosis. *Biochim. Biophys. Acta.* 1744, pp. 406–414

Imaizumi K, Katayama T, Tohyama M (2001) Presenilin and the UPR. Nat Cell Biol 3:E104. doi:10.1038/35074613 Johnson-Anuna LN, Eckert GP, Keller JH, Igbavboa U, Franke C, Fechner T et al (2005) Chronic administration of statins alters multiple gene expression patterns in mouse cerebral cortex. *J Pharmacol Exp Ther* 312(2): pp. 786–793. doi: 10.1124/jpet.104.075028

Jeremy J.Y., Rowe D., Emsley A.M., Newby A.C. (1999): Nitric oxide and the proliferation of vascular smooth muscle cells. *Cardiovasc. Res.* 43, pp. 580-594

Johnson-Anuna L.N., Eckert G.P., Keller J.H., Igbavboa U., Franke C., Fechner T., et al. (2005): Chronic administration of statins alters multiple gene expression patterns in mouse cerebral cortex. *J Pharmacol Exp Ther* 312(2): 786-793. doi: 10.1124/jpet.104.075028

Kawada H., Nishiyama C., Takagi A., Tokura T., Nakano N., Maeda K., Mayuzumi N., Ikeda S., Okumura K., Ogawa H. (2005): Transcriptional regulation of ATP2C1 gene by Sp1 and YY1 and reduced function of its promoter in Hailey-Hailey disease keratinocytes. *J. Invest. Dermatol.* 124, pp. 1206–1214

Kirino T. 2002. Ischemic tolerance. *J Cereb Blood Flow Metab* 22: pp. 1283–1296.

Kitagawa K, Matsumoto M, Kuwabara K, Tagaya M, Ohtsuki T, Hata R, Ueda H, Handa N, Kimura K, Kamada T. 1991. 'Ischemic tolerance' phenomenon detected in various brain regions. *Brain Res* 561: pp. 203–211.

Kruman I. I., Kumaravel T. S., Lohani A., Pedersen W. A., Cutler R. G., Kruman Y., Haughey N., Lee J., Evans M., Mattson M. P. (2002): Folic acid deficiency and homocysteine impair DNA repair in hippocampal neurons and sensitize them to amyloid toxicity in experimental models of Alzheimer's disease. *J. Neurosci.* 22, pp. 1752-1762

Kumar R, Azam S, Sullivan JM, Owen C, Cavener DR, Zhang P et al (2001) Brain ischemia and reperfusion activate the eukaryotic initiation factor 2a kinase, PERK. *J Neurochem* 77: pp. 1418–1421. doi:10.1046/j.1471-4159.2001.00387.x

Kumar R, Krause GS, Yoshida H, Mori K, DeGracia DJ (2003) Dysfunction of the unfolded protein response during global brain ischemia and reperfusion. *J Cereb Blood Flow Metab* 23: pp. 462- 471. doi:10.1097/00004647-200304000-00010

Lehotsky J, Kaplan P, Racay P, Matejovicova M, Drgova A, Mezesova V (1999) Membrane ion transport systems during oxidative stress in rodent brain: protective effect of stobadine and other antioxidants. *Life Sci* 65: pp. 1951–1958. doi:10.1016/ S0024-3205(99)00454-3

Lehotsky J., Kaplán P., Murín R., Raeymaekers L. (2002a): The role of plasma membrane Ca2+ pumps (PMCAs) in pathologies of mammalian cells. *Front. Biosci.* 7, pp. d53–d84

Lehotsky J., Kaplán P., Matejovicová M., Murín R., Racay P., Raeymaekers L. (2002b): Ion transport systems as targets of free radicals during ischemia reperfusion injury. *Gen. Physiol. Biophys.* 21, pp. 31–37

Lehotský J, Murín R, Strapková A, Uríková A, Tatarková Z, Kaplán P (2004) Time course of ischemia/reperfusion induced oxidative modification of neural proteins in rat forebrain. *Gen Physiol Biophys* 23(4): pp. 401–415

Lehotsky J, Pavlikova M, Urban P, Kaplan P, Cierny D, Tatarkova Z. 2008. Ischemic preconditioning affects expression of secretory pathways Ca^{2+}-ATPase (SPCA) on mRNA and protein levels after global cerebral ischemia reperfusion in rats. In: Proceedings of the 6th FENS Forum, Geneva, Poster 120.27.

Lehotsky J, Urban P, Pavlikova M, Tatarkova Z, Kaminska B, Kaplan P. (2009a). Molecular mechanisms leading to neuroprotection/ischemic tolerance: effect of preconditioning on the stress reaction of endoplasmic reticulum. *Cell Mol Neurobiol* 29: pp. 917-925

Lehotsky J, Burda J, Danielisová V, Gottlieb M, Kaplán P, et al, Ischemic tolerance: the mechanisms of neuroprotective strategy, *Anat Rec.* 292(12) (2009b): pp. 2002-12.

Lin M. T., Beal M. F. (2006): Mitochondrial dysfunction and oxidative stress in neurodegenerative diseases. *Nature* 443, pp. 787–795

Lipton P (1999) Ischemic cell death in brain neurons. *Physiol Rev* 79: pp. 1431–1568

Maag R. S., Hicks S. W., Machamer C. E. (2003): Death from within: apoptosis and the secretory pathway. *Curr. Opin. Cell Biol.* 15, pp. 456–461

Mattson M.P., Kruman I.I., Duan W. (2002): Folic acid and homocysteine in age-related disease. *Ageing Res. Rev.* 1, pp. 95-111

Mudd S.H., Levy H.L., Kraus J.P. (2001): Disorders of transsulfuration. In: Scriver C.R., Beaudet A.L., Sly W.S., Valle D. (Eds.), The metabolic & molecular bases of inherited disease. McGraw-Hill, New York: pp. 1279-1327

Meller R, Minami M, Cameron JA, Impey S, Chen D, Lan JQ, Henshall DC, Simon RP. 2005. CREB-mediated Bcl-2 protein expression after ischemic preconditioning. *J Cereb Blood Flow Metab* 25: pp. 234–246.

Meller R, Thompson SJ, Lusardi TA, Ordonez AN, Ashley MD, Jessick V, Wang W, Torrey DJ, Henshall DC, Gafken PR, Saugstad JA, Xiong ZG, Simon RP. 2008. Ubiquitin proteasome-mediated synaptic reorganization: a novel mechanism underlying rapid ischemic tolerance. *J Neurosci* 28: pp. 50–59.

Michelangeli F., Ogunbayo O. A., Wootton L. L. (2005): A plethora of interacting organellar Ca2+ stores. *Curr. Opin. Cell Biol.* 17, pp. 135–140

Mori K (2003) A time-dependent phase shift in the mammalian unfolded protein response. *Dev Cell* 4: pp. 265–271. doi:10.1016/S1534-5807(03)00022-4

Morimoto N, Oida Y, Shimazawa M, Miura M, Kudo T, Imaizumi K et al (2007) Involvement of endoplasmic reticulum stress after middle cerebral artery occlusion in mice. *Neuroscience* 147(4): pp. 957–967. doi:10.1016/j.neuro science.2007.04.017

Murin R., Verleysdonk S., Raeymaekers R., Kaplan P., Lehotsky J. (2006): Distribution of secretory pathway Ca2+ ATPase (SPCA1) in neuronal and glial cell cultures. *Cell. Mol. Neurobiol.* 26, pp. 1355–1365

Murry CE, Jennings RB, Reimer KA. 1986. Preconditioning with ischemia: a delay of lethal cell injury in ischemic myocardium. *Circulation* 74: pp. 1124–1136.

Mutus B., Rabini R.A., Staffolani R., Ricciotti R., Fumelli P., Moretti N., Martarelli D., Mazzanti L. (2001): Homocysteine-induced inhibition of nitric oxide production in platelets: a study on healthy and diabetic subjects. *Diabetologia* 44, pp. 979-982

Nagotani S, Hayashi T, Sato K, Zhang W, Deguchi K, Nagano I et al (2005) Reduction of cerebral infarction in strokeprone spontaneously hypertensive rats by statins associated with amelioration of oxidative stress. *Stroke* 36(3): pp. 670–672. doi:10.1161/01.STR.0000155732.27333.3c

Nandagopal K, Dawson TM, Dawson VL. 2001. Critical role for nitric oxide signaling in cardiac and neuronal ischemic preconditioning and tolerance. *J Pharmacol Exp Ther* 297: pp. 474–478.

Nicholls D. G., Johnson-Cadwell L., Vesce S., Jekabsons M., Yadava N. (2007): Bioenergetics of mitochondria in cultured neurons and their role in glutamate excitotoxicity. *J. Neurosci. Res.* 85, pp. 3206–3212

Obeid R., McCaddon A., Herrmann W. (2007): The role of hyperhomocysteinemia and B-vitamin deficiency in neurological and psychiatric diseases. *Clin. Chem. Lab. Med.* 45, pp. 1590-1606

Ohtsuki T, Reutzler CA, Tasaki K, Hallenbeck JM (1996) Interleukin-1 mediates induction of tolerance to global ischemia in gerbil hippocampal CA1 neurons. *J Cereb Blood Flow Metab* 16: pp. 1137–1142. doi:10.1097/00004647-199611000-00007

Okunade GW, Miller ML, Azhar M, Andringa A, Sanford LP, Doetschman T, Prasad V, Shull GE (2007) Loss of the Atp2c1 secretory pathway 22 Ca2?-ATPase (SPCA1) in mice causes Golgi stress, apoptosis, and midgestational death in homozygous embryos and squamous cell tumors in adult heterozygote. *J Biol Chem* 282: pp. 26517-26527. doi:10.1074/jbc.M703029200

Otani H. (2008): Ischemic preconditioning: from molecular mechanisms to therapeutic opportunities. *Antioxid. Redox Signal.* 10, pp. 207–247

Oyadomari S., Mori M. (2004): Roles of CHOP/GADD153 in endoplasmic reticulum stress. *Cell Death Differ.* 381, pp. 381–389

Paschen W (2003a) Endoplasmic reticulum: a primary target in various acute disorders and degenerative diseases of the brain. *Cell Calcium* 34: pp. 365–383. doi:10.1016/S0143-4160 (03)00139-8

Paschen W (2003b) Shutdown of translation: lethal or protective? Unfolded protein response versus apoptosis. *J Cereb Blood Flow Metab* 23: pp. 773–779. doi:10.1097/01.WCB. 0000075009.47474.F9

Pavlikova M, Tatarkova Z, Sivonova M, Kaplan P, Krizanova O, Lehotsky J. 2009. Alterations induced by ischemic preconditioning on secretory pathways Ca^{2+}-ATPase (SPCA) gene expression and oxidative damage after global cerebral ischemia/reperfusion in rats. *Cell Mol Neurobiol*, 29: pp. 909-916

Pavlikova M., Kovalska M., Tatarkova Z., Sivonova-Kmetova M., Kaplan P., Lehotsky J.(2011) Response of secretory pathways Ca^{2+} ATPase gene expression to hyperhomocysteinemia and ischemic preconditioning in rat forebrain. *Gen. Physiol. Biophys.*Special Issue 30; pp. 61-69

Pignataro G., Scorziello A., Di Renzo G., Annunziato L. (2009): Post-ischemic brain damage: effect of ischemic preconditioning and postconditioning and identification of potential candidates for stroke therapy. *FEBS J.* 276, pp. 46–57

Pivovarova N. B., Nguyen H. V., Winters C. A., Brantner C. A., Smith C. L., Andrews S. B. (2004): Excitotoxic calcium overload in a subpopulation of mitochondria triggers delayed death in hippocampal neurons. *J. Neurosci.* 24, pp. 5611–5622

Prasad K. (1999): Homocysteine, a risk factor for cardiovascular disease. *Int. J. Angiol.* 8, pp. 76–86

Qi X, Okuma Y, Hosoi T, Nomura Y (2004) Edaravone protects against hypoxia/ischemia-induced endoplasmic reticulum dysfunction. *J Pharmacol Exp Ther* 311: pp. 388–393. doi:10.1124/jpet. 104.069088

Racay P., Tatarkova Z., Drgova A., Kaplan P., Dobrota D. (2007): Effect of ischemic preconditioning on mitochondrial dysfunction and mitochondrial p53 translocation after transient global cerebral ischemia in rats. *Neurochem. Res.* 32, pp. 1823–1832

Racay P., Tatarkova Z., Drgova A., Kaplan P., Dobrota D. (2009a): Ischemia-reperfusion induces inhibition of mitochondrial protein synthesis and cytochrome c oxidase activity in rat hippocampus. *Physiol. Res.* 58, pp. 127–138

Racay P., Chomova M., Tatarkova Z., Kaplan P., Hatok J., Dobrota D. (2009b): Ischemia-induced mitochondrial apoptosis is significantly attenuated by ischemic preconditioning. *Cell. Mol. Neurobiol*, Exp Eye Res. 2009 Nov;89(5): pp. 782-90.doi: 10.1007/s10571-009- 9373-7, PMID: 19283470

Racay P., Tatarkova Z., Chomova M., Hatok J., Kaplan P., Dobrota D. (2009c): Mitochondrial calcium transport and mitochondrial dysfunction after global brain ischemia in rat hippocampus. *Neurochem. Res.*, Aug;34(8): pp. 1469-78. doi: 10.1007/ s11064-009-9934-7, PMID:19252983

Refsum H., Ueland P. M., Nygard O., Vollset S. E. (1998): Homocysteine and cardiovascular disease. *Annu. Rev. Med.* 49, pp. 31-62

Rizzuto R. (2001): Intracellular Ca2+ pools in neuronal signalling. *Curr. Opin. Neurobiol.* 11, pp. 306–311

Sachdev P.S. (2004): Homocysteine and neuropsychiatric disorders. *Rev. Bras. Psiquiatr.* 26, pp. 50-56

Sepúlveda M. R., Berrocal M., Marcos D., Wuytack F., Mata A. M. (2007): Functional and immunocytochemical evidence for the expression and localization of the secretory pathway Ca2+-ATPase isoform 1 (SPCA1) in cerebellum relative to other Ca2+ pumps. *J. Neurochem.* 103, pp. 1009–1018

Sepúlveda M. R., Marcos D., Berrocal M., Raeymaekers L., Mata A. M, Wuytack F. (2008): Activity and localization of the secretory pathway Ca2+-ATPase isoform 1 (SPCA1) in different areas of the mouse brain during postnatal development. *Mol. Cell. Neurosci.* 38, pp. 461–473

Seshadri S., Beiser A., Selhub J., Jacques P.F., Rosenberg I.H., D'Agostino R.B., Wilson P.W.F., Wolf P.A. (2002): Plasma homocysteine as a risk factor for dementia and Alzheimer's disease. *N. Engl. J. Med.* 346, pp. 476–483

Shabanzadeh A.P., Shuaib A., Wang C.X., (2005): Simvastatin reduced ischemic brain injury and perfusion deficits in an embolic model of stroke. *Brain Res.* 1042(1): 1-5. doi: 10.1016/j.brainres.2005.01.105

Shen X, Ellis RE, Lee K, Liu CY, Yang K, Solomon A et al (2001) Complementary signaling pathways regulate the unfolded protein response and are required for C. elegans development. *Cell* 107: pp. 893–903. doi:10.1016/S0092- 8674(01)00612-2

Shi H, Liu KJ (2007) Cerebral tissue oxygenation and oxidative brain injury during ischemia and reperfusion. *Front Biosci* 12: pp. 1318– 1328. doi:10.2741/2150

Schurr A, Reid KH, Tseng MT, West C, Rigor BM. 1986. Adaptation of adult brain tissue to anoxia and hypoxia in vitro. *Brain Res* 374: pp. 244–248.

Signorello M.G., Pascale R., Leoncini G. (2002): Effect of homocysteine on arachidonic acid release in human platelets. *Eur. J. Clin. Invest.* 32, pp. 279-284

Sironi L, Cimino M, Guerrini U, Calvio AM, Lodetti B, Asdente M (2003) Treatment with statins after induction of focal ischemia in rats reduces the extent of brain damage. *Arterioscler Thromb Vasc Biol* 23: pp. 322–327. doi: 10.1161/01.ATV.0000044458.23905.3B

Sivonova M, Kaplan P, Durackova Z, Dobrota D, Drgova A, Tatarkova Z, Pavlikova M., Halasova E., Lehotsky J. (2008) Time course of peripheral oxidative stress as consequence of global ischaemic brain injury in rats. *Cell Mol Neurobiol* 28(3): pp. 431–441. doi:10.1007/s10571-007-9246-x

Stagliano NE, Perez-Pinzon MA, Moskowitz MA, Huang PL. 1999. Focal ischemic preconditioning induces rapid tolerance to middle cerebral artery occlusion in mice. *J Cereb Blood Flow Metab* 19: pp. 757–761.

Strosznajder R, Gadamski R, Walski M (2005) Inhibition of poly(ADP-ribose) polymerase activity protects hippocampal cells against morphological and ultrastructural alteration evoked by ischemia-reperfusion injury. *Folia Neuropathol* 43: pp. 156–165

Takemoto M, Liao JK (2001) Pleiotropic effects of 3-hydroxy- 3-methylglutaryl coenzyme a reductase inhibitors. *Arterioscler Thromb Vasc Biol* 21: pp. 1712–1719. doi: 10.1161/hq1101.098486

Thambyrajah J., Townend J. N. (2000): Homocysteine and atherothrombosis – mechanisms for Injury. *Europ. Heart.* 21, pp. 967–974

Thuerauf DJ, Marcinko M, Gude N, Rubio M, Sussman MA, Glembotski CC (2006) Activation of the unfolded protein response in infarcted mouse heart and hypoxic cultured cardiac myocytes. *Circ Res* 99: pp. 275–282. doi:10.1161/01.RES.0000233317.70421.03

Toohey J.I. (2007): Mercaptopropionaldehyde from homocysteine: implications for Alzheimer's disease. *J. Alzheimer's Dis.* 12, pp. 241–3

Upchurch G.R.Jr., Welch G.N., Fabian A.J., Freedman J.E., Johnson J.L., Keaney J.F. Jr., Loscalzo, J. (1997): Homocyst(e)ine decreases bioavailable nitric oxide by a mechanism involving glutathione peroxidase. *J. Biol. Chem.* 272, pp. 17007-17012

Urban P, Pavlikova M, Sivonova M, Kaplan P, Tatarkova Z, Kaminska B, Lehotsky J. 2009. Molecular analysis of endoplasmic reticulum stress response after global forebrain ischemia/reperfusion in rats: effect of neuroprotectant simvastatin. *Cell Mol Neurobiol* 29: pp. 181–192.

Uríková A, Babusíkova E, Dobrota D, Drgová A, Kaplán P, Tatarková Z, Lehotsky J. (2006) Impact of Ginkgo Biloba Extract EGb 761 on ischemia/reperfusion-induced oxidative stress products formation in rat forebrain. *Cell Mol Neurobiol* 26: pp. 1343–1353. doi:10.1007/s10571-006-9030-3

Valko M, Leibfritz D, Moncol J, Cronin MT, Mazur M, Telser J (2007) Free radicals and antioxidants in normal physiological functions and human disease. *Int J Biochem Cell Biol* 39: pp. 44–84. doi:10.1016/j.biocel.2006.07.001

Van Baelen K., Dode L., Vanoevelen J., Callewaert G., De Smedt H., Missiaen L., Parys J. B., Raeymaekers L., Wuytack F. (2004): The Ca2+/Mn2+ pumps in the Golgi apparatus. *Biochim. Biophys. Acta* 1742, pp. 103–112

van den Berg M., van der Knaap M.S., Boers G.H., Stehouwer C.D., Rauwerda J.A., Valk J. (1995): Hyperhomocysteinaemia (with reference to its neuroradiological aspects). *Neuroradiology* 37, pp. 403-411

Vaughan CJ, Delanty N (1999) Neuroprotective properties of statins in cerebral ischemia and stroke. *Stroke* 30: pp. 1969–1973

Vaughan CJ, Delanty N, Basson CT (2001) Statin therapy and stroke prevention. *Curr Opin Cardiol* 16: pp. 219–224. doi: 10.1097/00001573-200107000-00001

Ward M. W., Huber H. J., Weisova P., Dussmann H., Nicholls D. G., Prehn J. H. (2007): Mitochondrial and plasma membrane potential of cultured cerebellar neurons during glutamate-induced necrosis, apoptosis, and tolerance. *J. Neurosci.* 27, pp. 8238–8249

Watkins D., Rosenblatt D.S. (1989): Functional methionine synthase deficiency (cblE and cblG): clinical and biochemical heterogeneity. *Am. J. Med. Genet.* 34, pp. 427-434

Wootton L. L., Argent C. C., Wheatley M., Michelangeli F. (2004): The expression, activity and localisation of the secretory pathway Ca2+-ATPase (SPCA1) in different mammalian tissues. *Biochim. Biophys. Acta* 1664, pp. 189–197

Xiang M, Mohamalawari D, Rao R (2005) A novel isoform of the secretory pathway Ca2?, Mn(2?)-ATPase, hSPCA2, has unusual properties and is expressed in the brain. *J Biol Chem* 280: pp. 11608–11614. doi:10.1074/jbc.M413116200

Yadava N., Nicholls D. G. (2007): Spare respiratory capacity rather than oxidative stress regulates glutamate excitotoxicity after partial respiratory inhibition of mitochondrial complex I with rotenone. *J. Neurosci.* 27, pp. 7310–7317

Yenari M, Kitagawa K, Lyden P, Perez-Pinzon M. 2008. Metabolic downregulation: a key to successful neuroprotection? *Stroke* 39: pp. 2910–2917.

Yoshida H., Matsui T., Yamamoto A., Okada T., Mori K. (2001): XBP1 mRNA is induced by ATF6 and spliced by IRE1 in response to ER stress to produce a highly active transcription factor. *Cell* 107, pp. 881–891

Yoshida H, Matsui T, Hosokawa N, Kaufman RJ, Nagata K, Shabanzadeh AP, Shuaib A, Wang CX (2005) Simvastatin reduced ischemic brain injury and perfusion deficits in an embolic model of stroke. *Brain Res* 1042(1): pp. 1-5. doi: 10.1016/j.brainres.2005.01.105

Yu ZW, Lou H, Fu W, Mattson MP (1999) The endoplasmic reticulum stress-responsive protein GRP78 protects neurons against excitotoxicity and apoptosis: Suppression of oxidative stress and stabilization of calcium homeostasis. *Exp Neurol* 155: pp. 302–314. doi:10.1006/exnr.1998.7002

Yuan J., Yanker B. A. (2000): Apoptosis in the nervous system. *Nature* 407, pp. 802–809

Ziemińska E, Stafiej A, Łazarewicz, J.W. (2003): Role of group I metabotropic glutamate receptors and NMDA receptors in homocysteine-evoked acute neurodegeneration of cultured cerebellar granule neurons. *Neurochem Int.* 43, pp. 481-492

13

Mitochondrial Ceramide in Stroke

Tatyana I. Gudz and Sergei A. Novgorodov
Ralph H. Johnson Veterans Affairs Medical Center and the Departments of Neuroscience and Medicine of Medical University of South Carolina, Charleston, South Carolina, USA

1. Introduction

Sphingolipids are essential structural components of cellular membranes, playing prominent roles in signal transduction that governs cell proliferation, differentiation, migration, and apoptosis. Most sphingolipids are ubiquitous, but complex sphingolipids, including sphingomyelin (SM) and glycosphingolipids (GSLs), are more abundant in the brain and are particularly abundant in myelin. Sphingolipids are defined by the presence of a long-chain sphingoid backbone, generally sphingosine. Acylation of the sphingoid base, i.e. addition of a C_{14}-C_{26} fatty acid to the amino group, yields ceramide, a building block for more complex sphingolipids. Neural cells are particularly enriched in GSLs and SM which is also a major lipid component of myelin. Sphingolipids are abundant in the plasma membranes and have unique molecular structures and conformational properties that cause them to form segregated compositional lipid domains in phospholipid bilayers (Sonnino et al., 2006). Membrane lipid domains, zones of the membrane with reduced fluidity, contain complex lipids of the cell, but are highly enriched in cholesterol and sphingolipids. Importantly, the proteins involved in signal transduction appear to segregate also in the lipid domains where they can exert their functions. Experimental evidence indicating that sphingolipids function through membrane reorganization and formation of lipid domains is summarized in a recent review by Kolesnick and Stancevic (Stancevic and Kolesnick, 2010). In addition to their role as building blocks of cellular membranes, sphingolipids have been reported to be pleotropic modulators of numerous enzymes in intracellular signaling pathways. Basic organization and specific principles of sphingolipid-mediated cell regulation have been reviewed by Hannun and Obeid (Hannun and Obeid, 2008, 2011).
After more than a decade of extensive investigations, it has become clear that ceramide is a key sphingolipid messenger regulating a diverse range of cell-stress responses, including apoptosis, cell senescence, and autophagy. Ceramide is tightly regulated in cells, and its participation in cell death signaling pathways is controlled by rapid conversion of ceramide into less deleterious sphingolipids (**Scheme 1**). Thus, ceramide can be metabolized into complex sphingolipids by glucosylceramide synthase or into SM by SM synthase, or into ceramide-1-phosphate by ceramide kinase (Hannun and Obeid, 2002; Ogretmen and Hannun, 2004), or into sphingosine-1-phosphate by ceramidase and sphingosine kinase (Hannun and Obeid, 2008). However, pathological conditions, including cerebral ischemia/reperfusion, could disturb ceramide metabolism resulting in ceramide accumulation that ultimately leads to cell death.

2. Pathways of ceramide generation

Ceramide is a family comprised of about 50 distinct molecular species characterized by various acyl chains, their desaturation, and hydroxylation. Ceramide is an N-acylsphingosine consisting of a fatty acid bound to the amino group of the sphingoid base, sphingosine. Ceramides can contain monounsaturated or saturated fatty acids of various lengths from 2 to 28 carbon atoms, and the fatty acid chain length profoundly alters ceramide's biophysical properties. Short-chain ceramides with fatty acyl chains of fewer than 12 carbons can be easily dispersed in water and serve as detergents (Sot et al., 2005b). In contrast, most ceramides found in mammalian cellular membranes contain long fatty acyl chains of 16-28 carbon atoms rendering them hydrophobic lipids lacking detergent properties. Short-chain ceramides mix much better with phospholipids, promote a positive curvature in lipid monolayers, and their capacities to increase bilayer permeability or transbilayer motion are very low or non-existent. *In situ* enzymatic generation, or external addition, of long-chain ceramides in membranes has at least three important effects: (i) the lipid monolayer has an increased tendency to adopt a negative curvature, e.g. through a transition to an inverted hexagonal structure (Graham and Kozlov, 2010), (ii) the bilayer permeability to aqueous solutes is notoriously enhanced, and (iii) a transbilayer (flip-flop) lipid motion is promoted (Goni et al., 2005).

As a result, ceramide metabolism is restricted to cellular membranes and is highly compartmentalized. Hydrophobic ceramides are generated by membrane-associated enzymes, and exert their effects either in close proximity to the generation site or require specific transport mechanisms to reach their targets in another intracellular compartment (Futerman and Riezman, 2005). Long-chain ceramides appear to be able to flip-flop across the membrane (Lopez-Montero et al., 2005); however, spontaneous inter-bilayer transfer is extremely slow (Contreras et al., 2010). Therefore, the transfer of ceramide between intracellular compartments is facilitated by vesicular transport pathways (Perry and Ridgway, 2005). Alternatively, ceramide is transported by a non-vesicular pathway involving a transfer protein, CERT, from its generation site in the endoplasmic reticulum (ER) to the Golgi where it is required for SM synthesis (Hanada et al., 2003). In addition to *de novo* biosynthesis, ceramide is generated by sphingomyelinases (SMases) from SM in two major pathways: the neutral SMase (nSMase)-dependent pathway and aSMase (aSMase)-dependent pathway or salvage (recycling) pathway (**Scheme 1**).

2.1 *De novo* ceramide biosynthesis

Remarkable progress has been made toward identifying enzymes involved in ceramide biosynthesis (Futerman and Riezman, 2005). (Dihydro) ceramide synthase (EC 2.3.1.24) is a key enzyme in *de novo* ceramide synthasis, and it utilizes fatty acid acyl CoA for N-acylation of sphinganine (dihydrosphingosine) yielding dihydroceramide that is converted to ceramide by desaturase (**Scheme 1**). In yeast, longevity assurance gene 1 (LAG1) was identified as a component of ceramide synthase. Deletion of LAG1 in haploid cells resulted in a pronounced increase (~50%) in mean and maximum life spans (D'Mello N et al., 1994).

Mammalian homologs of LAG1, which belong to the LASS (longevity assurance gene homolog) family, were cloned and characterized (Futerman and Riezman, 2005). Each of the 6 known LASS (also known as CerS) genes appears to regulate synthesis of a specific subset of ceramides, and displays a unique substrate specificity profile for chain-length and/or saturation in fatty acid acyl CoA. Over-expression of any CerS protein in mammalian cells

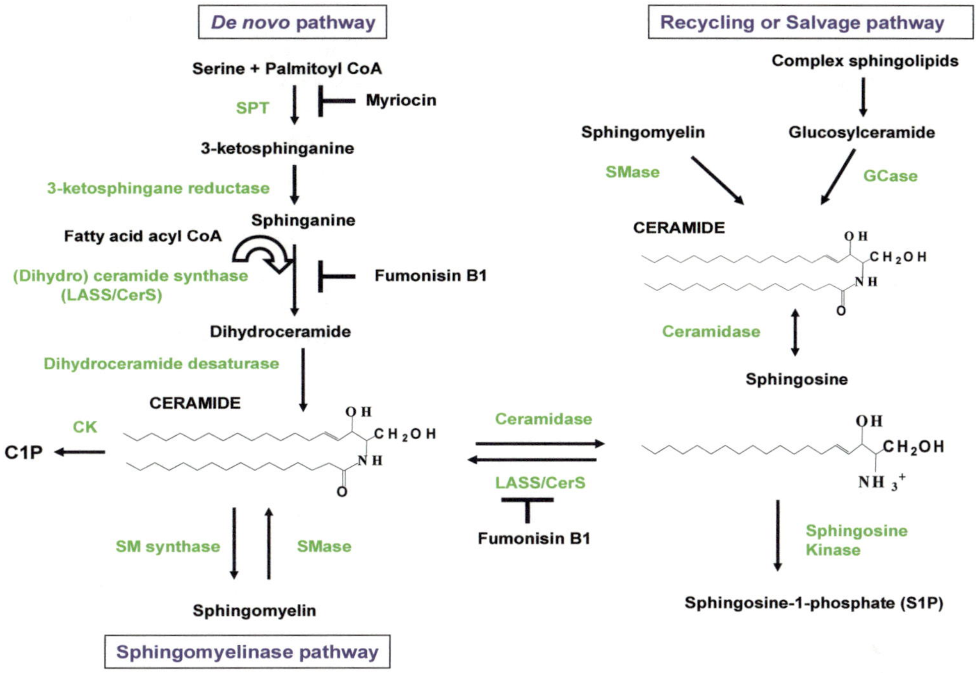

Scheme 1. Biosynthesis of ceramide and its conversion into other bioactive sphingolipids. *De novo* ceramide synthesis begins with the conversion of serine and fatty acyl CoA into 3-ketosphinganine by serine palmitoyl transferase (SPT), then 3-ketosphinganine is converted into dihydrosphingosine. Myriocin is a potent inhibitor of SPT activity. (Dihydro) ceramide synthase (LASS/CerS) acylates dihydrosphingosine to form dihydroceramide, which is then reduced to ceramide by dihydroceramide desaturase. Ceramide is also produced by SMases through SM degradation in SMase pathway. Ceramidase converts ceramide into sphingosine, which is phosphorylated by sphingosine kinase (SK) to generate sphingosine-1-phosphate. Ceramide is phosphorylated by ceramide kinase (CK) yielding ceramide-1-phosphate (C1P). In the salvage or recycling pathway, complex sphingolipids are broken down to ceramide by glucosylceramidase (GCase) and then by ceramidase to sphingosine, which is re-acylated to ceramide by LASS/CerS. Fumonisin B1 inhibits LASS/CerS activity.

resulted in increased levels of a specific subset of ceramide species. It has been demonstrated that CerS1 exhibits high specificity for $C_{18:0}$-CoA generating $C_{18:0}$-ceramide (Mizutani et al., 2005). CerS2, CerS4, and CerS3 appear to have broader specificity (Laviad et al., 2008; Mizutani et al., 2006). CerS2 or CerS4 mainly synthesizes $C_{20:0}$-, $C_{22:0}$-, $C_{24:1}$-, $C_{24:0}$-, $C_{26:1}$ and $C_{26:0}$ ceramide, but is unable to synthesize $C_{16:0}$- or $C_{18:0}$-ceramide (Laviad et al., 2008; Mizutani et al., 2005). CerS3 generates $C_{18:0}$-, $C_{20:0}$-, $C_{22:0}$- and $C_{24:0}$-ceramide (Mizutani et al., 2006). It has been shown that CerS5 generates $C_{14:0}$-, $C_{16:0}$-, $C_{18:0}$-, and $C_{18:1}$-ceramide (Lahiri and Futerman, 2005; Mizutani et al., 2005); and CerS6 produces $C_{14:0}$-, $C_{16:0}$-, and $C_{18:0}$-ceramide (Mizutani et al., 2005).

The availability of certain fatty acyl-CoA species and the characteristic distribution pattern of CerS family members in tissues seem to regulate the tissue-specificity of the ceramide species. Northern blot and real-time RT-PCR analysis revealed broad expression of CerS5, CerS4, and CerS6 genes in mammalian tissues, but CerS1 expression was limited to the brain and skeletal muscle (Laviad et al., 2008; Mizutani et al., 2006). Interestingly, CerS2 mRNA was more abundant than other CerS family members and had the broadest tissue distribution (Laviad et al., 2008). Except for a weak display in skin, CerS3 mRNA expression is limited almost solely to testis, implying that CerS3 plays an important role in this gland (Mizutani et al., 2006).

CerS are integral membrane proteins, but the exact number of transmembrane domains and their topology has not been resolved experimentally. All of the CerS genes have a highly conserved stretch of 52 amino acids known as the Lag1p motif which is essential for enzyme activity (Spassieva et al., 2006). Some of the CerS proteins are post-translationally modified, and, for instance, CerS6 is expressed as a native and an N-glycosylated form. The N-glycosylation site is conserved in CerS6, CerS2, and CerS5, but this post-translational modification is not required for ceramide synthase activity (Mizutani et al., 2005). Intriguingly, CerS1 phosphorylation appears to regulate the protein turnover (Sridevi et al., 2009). All CerS except CerS1 contain a homeobox domain, suggesting involvement in developmental regulation (Venkataraman and Futerman, 2002). *De novo* synthesis of ceramide is required for cell survival *in vivo*, and is widespread among cell types and tissues. Regulation of ceramide synthesis is only beginning to be understood. Regulation at the transcriptional level has been observed with a number of agents, including endotoxin and cytokines, UVB irradiation, and retinoic acid (Merrill, 2002).

De novo ceramide biosynthesis occurs in the endoplasmic reticulum (ER) where all the participating enzymes have been found (Hirschberg et al., 1993; Mandon et al., 1992; Michel and van Echten-Deckert, 1997). Ceramide is synthesized at the cytosolic side of the ER (Mandon et al., 1992; Merrill, 2002), serving as a precursor for the biosynthesis of glycosphingolipids and SM in the Golgi (Futerman et al., 1990; Kolter et al., 2002).

2.2 Sphingomyelin hydrolysis

SM hydrolysis by one of several SMases is another source of cellular ceramide. Three groups of SMases, acid, neutral, and alkaline, are distinguished by their primary structure, catalytic pH optimum, and localization.

2.2.1 Acid SMase

A well-characterized enzyme, acid SMase (aSMase) contributes to the catabolism of SM and ceramide formation in lysosomes (Tani et al., 2005; Tani et al., 2007). aSMase could relocate from intracellular compartments to the plasma membrane where it plays an important role in SM hydrolysis and ceramide generation within lipid rafts (Bollinger et al., 2005). aSMase is a soluble enzyme with no transmembrane domains, and the mechanism of aSMase association with the membrane, at which its substrate, SM, resides, remains unclear. aSMase is also secreted through the Golgi secretory pathway, and it is constitutively present in plasma (Spence et al., 1989) where it is involved in hydrolysis of lipoprotein-bound SM, the second most abundant lipid in human plasma. Intriguingly, aSMase hydrolyzes SM bound to oxidized LDL more effectively than SM bound to intact LDL (Schissel et al., 1998). The accelerated hydrolysis of SM could enhance LDL aggregation leading to macrophage foam cell formation, suggesting a role for secretory aSMase in the pathogenesis of arteriosclerosis (Tabas, 1999).

2.2.2 Neutral SMase

Three mammalian closely related isoforms of neutral SMase (nSMase) have been recently cloned, including nSMase1, nSMase2 and mitochondria-associated nSMase (MA-nSMase)

(Clarke et al., 2011). nSMase1 is localized to the ER and nucleus (Tomiuk et al., 2000). nSMase2 had a dynamic intracellular localization (Clarke et al., 2006), having been found in the Golgi of sub-confluent cells, at the plasma membrane at the regions of cell-cell contact (Marchesini et al., 2004) and in recycling compartments (Milhas et al., 2010). Furthermore, it appears that oxidative stress could induce nSMase2 trafficking to the plasma membrane, whereas antioxidant (glutathione) directed its translocation to the perinuclear region (Levy et al., 2006). MA-nSMase is found within the mitochondria and associated membranes (Wu et al., 2010). The physiological role of neutral SMase isoforms may be dictated by their immediate environment in the specific intracellular compartment. **Alkaline SMase** lacks homology to neutral or aSMase and its mRNA is abundant in the intestine where the enzyme plays a major role in digestion of dietary SM (Nilsson and Duan, 2006).

2.3 Recycling or salvage pathway

Ceramide is also produced during the recycling of sphingosine in the process termed the "salvage pathway" (Kitatani et al., 2008). In this process, complex sphingolipids are broken down to ceramide and then to sphingosine, which is then used by ceramide synthase to yield ceramide. SM is converted to ceramide by aSMase. Ceramide accumulation via the salvage pathway requires ceramide synthase which is important in *de novo* synthesis of ceramide. Complex sphingolipids undergo constitutive degradation in the late endosomes and the lysosomes yielding ceramide which does not leave the lysosomes (Chatelut et al., 1998) unless converted into sphingosine by acid ceramidase. Free sphingosine could be released from the lysosomes and re-acylated by ceramide synthase to form ceramide.

3. Ceramide generation in mitochondria

Mitochondria arise as important intracellular compartment for ceramide metabolism, and they have been shown to contain a variety of sphingolipids, including SM and ceramide (Ardail et al., 2001; Tserng and Griffin, 2003). Mounting evidence suggests a local action of ceramide on mitochondria in intact cells. Thus, selective hydrolysis of a mitochondrial pool of SM by overexpressed sphingomyelinase (bSMase) targeted to mitochondria resulted in apoptosis. In contrast, generation of ceramide in the plasma membrane, ER, or Golgi apparatus by bSMase targeted to these compartments had no effect on cell viability (Birbes et al., 2001). Recently, mitochondrial ceramide engagement in apoptosis has been shown using loss-of-function mutants of ceramide synthase in the germ cell line of C. *elegans* (Deng et al., 2008). In this study, an ionizing radiation-induced apoptosis of germ cells was obliterated upon inactivation of ceramide synthase, and restored upon microinjection of long-chain ceramide. Radiation-induced increase in ceramide localized to mitochondria was required for activation of CED-3 caspase and apoptosis. These studies underscore the physiological significance of the mitochondrial ceramide and SM pools (Andreyev et al., 2010; Ardail et al., 2001; Dai et al., 2004; Monette et al., 2010; Tserng and Griffin, 2003; Yabu et al., 2009).

Although several enzyme activities involved in ceramide metabolism have been demonstrated in mitochondria, the nature of enzymes generating ceramide in this organelle is still a matter of debate (Laviad et al., 2008). Mitochondria evolve as a specialized compartment of sphingolipid metabolism with their own subset of ceramide synthesizing and degrading enzymes. Three possibilities may account for ceramide generation in mitochondria.

First, experimental evidence suggests the presence of ceramide synthase activity in mitochondria. Thus, ceramide synthase activity was first detected (Morell and Radin, 1970; Ullman and Radin, 1972) and partially purified from a bovine brain mitochondria-enriched fraction (Shimeno et al., 1995) which was not characterized in terms of marker enzyme activities. Mitochondrial enzymes had almost 2-fold higher specific ceramide synthase activity than the ceramide synthase from the ER. The mitochondrial enzyme had a pH optimum around 7.5 and maximal catalytic efficiency with $C_{16:0}$- or $C_{18:0}$-acyl CoA. The addition of liposomes to the mitochondrial enzyme increased ceramide synthase activity (approx. 7.8-fold) (Shimeno et al., 1995). Purification of ceramide synthase from bovine liver mitochondria yielded two major protein bands, 62 and 72 kDa on a SDS-gel (Shimeno et al., 1998). This enzyme had an apparent Km of 146 μM and Vmax of 11.1 nmol/min/mg protein with $C_{18:0}$-acyl CoA, and corresponding values of Vmax 144 μM and 8.5 nmol/min/mg protein towards sphinganine.

Detailed analysis of ceramide synthase activity in highly purified mitochondria by Bionda *et al.* essentially confirmed previous findings (Bionda et al., 2004). Ceramide synthase activity was demonstrated in rat liver mitochondria and in the sub-compartment of the ER closely associated with mitochondria. Further sub-mitochondrial investigation of ceramide synthase activity revealed that both outer and inner mitochondrial membranes can synthesize ceramide (Bionda et al., 2004). Recent reports describing several ceramide synthase isoforms, including CerS1, CerS2, CerS4 and CerS6, in purified mouse brain mitochondria (Novgorodov et al., 2011a; Yu et al., 2007) support the notion that several ceramide synthesizing enzymes could be localized in mitochondria (Futerman, 2006). No such association was found in HeLa cells (Mesicek et al., 2010), suggesting that this might be a cell type/tissue specific event. The intra-mitochondrial localization of CerS was examined in purified brain mitochondria by immunoprecipitation (Novgorodov et al., 2011a). These studies reveal a selective CerS6 association with adenine nucleotide translocase, the inner membrane component of the mitochondrial permeability transition pore (MPTP). In contrast, CerS2 associated with the outer membrane resident protein Tom20, a receptor of the protein import complex. The data suggest CerS6/ceramide could regulate MPTP activity and mitochondrial Ca^{2+} homeostasis whereas CerS2/ceramide could modulate the mitochondrial protein import machinery.

Secondly, recent studies identified two novel SMases, which hydrolyze SM to ceramide, and phosphocholine in mitochondria from zebrafish (Yabu et al., 2009) and mouse tissues (Wu et al., 2010). Notably, in yeast, the mammalian nSMase ortholog Isc1p associates with mitochondria in the post-diauxic phase of yeast growth and regulates mitochondrial sphingolipid metabolism (Kitagaki et al., 2007; Vaena de Avalos et al., 2004).

Thirdly, the additional source of ceramide in mitochondria is a reverse reaction of a neutral ceramidase (nCDase), e.g., formation of ceramide as a result of condensation of palmitate and sphingosine (El Bawab et al., 2001). On the basis of molecular cloning and confocal microscopy data, this activity was ascribed to mitochondria (El Bawab et al., 2000), and it was demonstrated in purified mitochondria (Bionda et al., 2004). Recent studies describe the molecular mechanism of ceramide generation from palmitate and sphingosine in purified liver mitochondria that requires concerted action of two enzymes nCDase and thioesterase (which hydrolyzes palmitoyl-CoA to CoA and fatty acid)(Novgorodov et al., 2011b). Thus, mitochondria from nCDase-deficient mice have significantly decreased formation of ceramide from sphingosine and palmitoyl-CoA (or palmitate) compared to mitochondria from wild type mice, indicating that nCDase participates in ceramide formation in liver mitochondria, and that ceramide formation may occur from sphingosine and palmitoyl-CoA from coupled activities of a mitochondrial thioesterase and nCDase catalyzing the reverse reaction (**Scheme 2**). Another possibility is that ceramide could be also transported from the ER to mitochondria through the contact sites between them (Stiban et al., 2008).

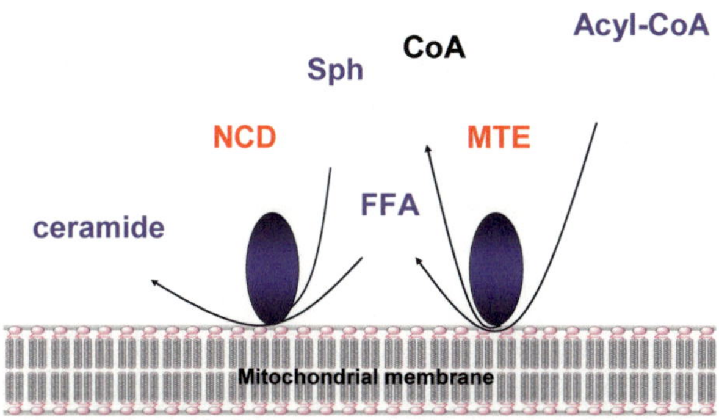

Scheme 2. Ceramide formation from Acyl-CoA and sphingosine (Sph) mediated by coupled activities of mitochondrial thioesterase (MTE) and nCDase (NCD).

4. Ceramide accumulation in Ischemia/Reperfusion (IR)

Ceramide accumulation has been demonstrated in various *in vivo* models of IR and it has been implicated as an important mediator of apoptosis in the injured tissue, but mechanisms of ceramide generation are not well-defined and the downstream targets of ceramide remain unresolved. The IR-induced accumulation of ceramide appears to be a general phenomenon for heart, kidney, liver and brain. The identification and characterization of key proteins of ceramide synthesis are expected to expand our understanding of molecular mechanisms behind ceramide's involvement in IR-induced tissue damage.

Research progress has been hampered by a lack of appropriate techniques that would allow simultaneous analysis of multiple sphingolipid species. Thus, the most common method for quantification of ceramide, the diglyceride (DG) kinase assay (Bielawska et al., 2001) has significant disadvantages including a limited separation of ceramide from dihydroceramide and the inability to determine the individual molecular species of ceramide. Recent advances in the development of new mass spectroscopy-based methods for quantitative analysis of sphingolipid molecular species may allow further dissection of ceramide specific pathways (Pettus et al., 2004; Sullards, 2000).

Increasing evidence suggests that the fatty acid chain of ceramide is an important determinant of the biological effect mediated by the individual ceramide species. Most of the experimental evidence indicating the important roles of ceramides containing distinct fatty acids is summarized in an excellent review by Futerman and his colleagues (Pewzner-Jung et al., 2006), and new studies further support the notion of distinct roles of ceramide species in cell metabolism(Hannun and Obeid, 2011). It has been demonstrated that generation of $C_{18:0}$-ceramide, and not $C_{16:0}$-ceramide repressed human telomerase reverse transcriptase promoter in lung carcinoma cells (Wooten-Blanks et al., 2007). Activation of aSMase in the salvage pathway brought about a selective accumulation of $C_{16:0}$-ceramide (Chudakova et al., 2008; Kitatani et al., 2006) due to the involvement of ceramide synthase CerS5 localized in mitochondria-associated membranes (Kitatani et al., 2006). In another study, the effects of chronic hypoxia on selected ceramide species were examined in cardiac tissue in a neonatal mouse model (Noureddine et al., 2008). The study revealed the differential involvement of the right ventricle with regard to levels of $C_{16:0}$-ceramide and its precursor, dihydro-$C_{16:0}$-ceramide. The decrease in $C_{16:0}$-ceramide observed in both hypoxic and control right ventricles over time occurred along with a significant increase in dihydro-$C_{16:0}$-ceramide in hypoxic but not control tissues suggesting a role for dihydro-$C_{16:0}$-ceramide in the adaptive tissue response to hypoxia. Although ceramide species could have different effects on biophysical properties of the membrane lipid bilayer (Sot et al., 2005a), it remains unclear how ceramides containing different fatty acids exert their effects upon cell physiology.

4.1 Cardiac ischemia

In several studies, elevated ceramide has been reported in myocardium after ischemia and IR. In the rat heart left coronary artery occlusion model, ischemia with subsequent reperfusion, but not ischemia alone, induced apoptosis in myocardial cells indicated by DNA laddering and measurement of soluble chromatin degradation products (Bielawska et al., 1997). The content of ceramide in ischemic myocardium was elevated to 155% baseline levels after 30 min ischemia, and was further increased to 250% after 3 h reperfusion. In the rabbit heart left coronary artery occlusion model, ceramide content was increased during the first minute of ischemia, peaking at 5 min with mean ceramide ~127% of baseline. However, this peak was transient because ceramide content returned to near-baseline values as soon as 10 min into the sustained ischemia (Argaud et al., 2004). In another study with the rat heart left coronary artery occlusion model, ceramide content in reperfused myocardium was found to increase up to 50%. This increase was not associated with enhanced neutral or aSMase activity, but rather with reduced activity of ceramidase, a ceramide-metabolizing enzyme (**Scheme 1**) (Zhang et al., 2001). In a global rat heart ischemia model, ceramide content was elevated about 2-fold after 30 min ischemia/30 min reperfusion which was attributed to SM hydrolysis. Thus, there was about 50% less SM in reperfused myocardium after IR (Cordis et al., 1998). This finding was confirmed in recent studies by the same group who reported an increased accumulation of ceramide in ischemic myocardium after 30 min ischemia/2 h reperfusion (Cui et al., 2004; Der et al., 2006). An inhibitor of aSMase activity desipramine prevented ceramide accumulation and provided cardioprotection. Intriguingly, a significant amount of ceramide accumulated in the caveolin-1-rich membrane microdomains after IR was abolished by pre-treatment with desipramine (Der et al., 2006). The ceramide–caveolin-1 interaction is believed to occur within lipid raft microdomains in membranes leading to rafts stabilization (Xu et al., 2001) and alteration of receptor tyrosine kinase signal transduction (Zundel et al., 2000).

In a very interesting study, analysis of cardiac tissues from mice subjected to IR revealed significant elevation of ceramide and inhibition of sphingosine kinase 1 activity (**Scheme 1**) that could ultimately result in decreased sphingosine-1-phosphate (Pchejetski et al., 2007). Furthermore, sphingosine kinase 1 inhibition, ceramide accumulation, cardiomyocyte apoptosis, and infarct size were significantly decreased in mitochondrial monoamine oxidase (MAO-A)-deficient mice after IR. MAO-A appears to play an important role in reactive oxygen species (ROS)-dependent cardiomyocytes apoptosis and postischemic cardiac damage (Bianchi et al., 2005). The data imply that the upregulation of ceramide/sphingosine-1-phosphate ratio is a critical event in MAO-A-dependent cardiac cell apoptosis in IR.

Recently, increases of specific ceramide species in the rat heart were investigated after 30 min global ischemia/30 min reperfusion. IR increased accumulation of only 7 out of 14 ceramide species identified in the heart (Beresewicz et al., 2002). Of note, the relative magnitude of IR-induced myocardial accumulation of ceramide species was not proportional to their basal tissue concentrations. For instance, although $C_{16:0}$-ceramide and $C_{18:0}$-ceramide are the most abundant in rat heart (40% and 23% of total, respectively), IR increased their content by 48–54%. However, $C_{18:2}$-ceramide, which contributes only 3.2% of total myocardial ceramides, was increased by 281%. These findings suggest the role of specific ceramide species signaling in the mechanism of post-ischemic myocardial injury.

In vitro, hypoxia/reoxygenation activated nSMase and ceramide accumulation in cardiomyocytes implicating the production of free radicals (Hernandez et al., 2000). nSMase activation could be abrogated by inhibition of a factor associated with nSMase activation (FAN) which is an adaptor protein connecting neutral SMase to the TNF receptor signaling pathway (O'Brien et al., 2003).

4.2 Liver ischemia

Ceramide was elevated in injured liver tissue after cold ischemia and warm reperfusion during liver transplantation (Bradham et al., 1997). A critical role of aSMase and ceramide accumulation was demonstrated in another study of hepatic IR injury (Llacuna et al., 2006). Hepatic ceramide transiently increased after the reperfusion phase due to activation of aSMase followed by acid ceramidase stimulation. Knocking down aSMase by *in vivo* administration of siRNA decreased ceramide generation during IR, and attenuated hepatocellular necrosis, cytochrome c release, and caspase-3 activation. The study draws attention to an important role of ceramide in IR-induced liver damage and suggests that modulation of aSMase could be of therapeutic relevance in liver transplantation.

4.3 Kidney ischemia

In the whole kidney IR model, ceramide content was increased about 1.8-fold in the injured tissue during the reperfusion phase (Zager et al., 1997) which was not accompanied by SM hydrolysis. In fact, there was no SM content change in post-IR tissue. Analysis of SMase activity revealed that ischemia induced declines (50%) in both acid and neutral SMase activity, and these persisted throughout the 24-h reperfusion period (Zager et al., 1998). $C_{16:0}$-, $C_{22:0}$-, and $C_{24:0}$-ceramides comprised 20%, 10%, and 70% of the total ceramide content in kidney tissue, respectively (Kalhorn and Zager, 1999). IR dramatically increased $C_{16:0}$-ceramide (4-fold), and all other ceramides increased modestly. Interestingly, IR induced a striking shift towards unsaturated (vs. saturated) fatty acyl within $C_{22:0}$- and $C_{24:0}$- (but not $C_{16:0}$-) ceramide pools. The data imply that IR-induced inhibition of sphingomyelin hydrolysis results in accumulation of ceramide, the substrate in sphingomyelin synthetic pathway.

4.4 Cerebral ischemia

Ischemic stroke occurs when cerebral or precerebral arteries are occluded or significantly stenosed by emboli or by local atherosclerotic disease. Within minutes of interrupted blood flow, mitochondrial energy production is shut down due to lack of oxygen resulting in membrane depolarization and excessive release of neurotransmitters, specifically, glutamate. Extracellular glutamate accumulation over-stimulates glutamate receptors, promoting cytosolic Ca^{2+} overload, the generation of ROS, and mitochondrial dysfunction leading to cell death.

A few studies reported ceramide accumulation during cerebral ischemia and IR (Kubota et al., 1989; Nakane et al., 2000), and it appears that the mechanism of ceramide accumulation depends on the severity of the insult to the brain. Thus, severe and lethal cerebral IR resulted in ceramide accumulation via activation of aSMase and SM hydrolysis (Kubota et al., 1989; Kubota et al., 1996; Nakane et al., 2000) or inhibition of ceramide utilization by glucosylceramide synthase (Takahashi et al., 2004). Consistent with these data, the extent of brain tissue damage was decreased in mice lacking aSMase (Yu et al., 2000). In a recent study, severe cerebral IR induced SM hydrolysis and increased ceramide and sphingosine in the ischemic brain (Chudakova et al., 2008). Similarly, chronic cerebral ischemia caused ceramide accumulation due to activation of SM degradation accompanied by reduced ceramide utilization via glucosylceramide synthase (Ohtani et al., 2004). The data highlight IR-induced deregulation of complex sphingolipids metabolism.

In mild IR, ceramide accumulation resulted from *de novo* ceramide biosynthesis rather from hydrolysis of SM (Yu et al., 2007). There is apparent tissue specificity in the expression of individual ceramide species that might reflect the tissue specificity of the ceramide synthases. In brain, $C_{18:0}$-, $C_{18:1}$- and $C_{24:1}$-ceramide are the major species expressed (39.5%, 34%, and 12.5% of total ceramide, respectively) whereas $C_{16:0}$- ceramide contributes only 4% of total ceramide. All ceramide species were elevated in the ischemic brain about 1.5–2-fold. The enhanced accumulation of sphingolipids seems to occur during the reperfusion phase; there were no changes in sphingolipid content after ischemia without reperfusion. This finding is in line with data which show that both ischemia and the restoration of blood flow to ischemic tissue (reperfusion) causes cellular damage by different molecular mechanisms (Chan, 2004; Gustafsson and Gottlieb, 2008).

Investigation of intracellular sites of ceramide accumulation after mild IR revealed the elevation of ceramide species both in purified mitochondria and in the ER (Yu et al., 2007). In mitochondria, only $C_{18:0}$-, $C_{18:1}$- and $C_{16:0}$-ceramides were increased, but all ceramide species increased in the ER suggesting activation of different ceramide synthases in these intracellular compartments. Indeed, several ceramide synthases were identified in mitochondria and the ER, including CerS1, CerS2, and CerS6, but CerS5 was localized only in the ER in the brain. Activity measurements indicated activation of CerS6 in ischemic mitochondria apparently via post-translational mechanisms; IR did not affect the CerS6 protein expression (Yu et al., 2007).

It appears that CerS6 is developmentally regulated and primarily generates $C_{16:0}$-ceramide in brain mitochondria (Novgorodov et al., 2011a). An investigation into the role of CerS6 in mitochondria revealed that ceramide synthase down-regulation during brain development is associated with dramatically decreased mitochondrial Ca^{2+}-loading capacity (CLC) which could be rescued by addition of ceramide. Ceramide-mediated blockade of MPTP opening seems to be the underlying mechanism of the increased CLC in brain mitochondria isolated from young animals. In fact, mitochondria maintain low cytosolic Ca^{2+} levels by sequestering Ca^{2+} inside the mitochondrial matrix complexed with phosphate. Energized mitochondria take up Ca^{2+} via the mitochondrial calcium uniporter which has been recently described as a highly selective, inwardly rectifying channel (Kirichok et al., 2004). Excessive accumulation of Ca^{2+} in the mitochondrial matrix could trigger opening of MPTP at a high conductance state, which would be accompanied by dissipation of the transmembrane potential and mitochondrial swelling. In brain mitochondria, Ca^{2+} may also activate a limited permeability state of MPTP opening (Novgorodov and Gudz, 1996) that only depolarizes mitochondria without causing swelling (Brustovetsky and Dubinsky, 2000b). This depolarization dramatically reduces the driving force for Ca^{2+} influx via mitochondrial Ca^{2+} uniporter , thus limiting the mitochondrial ability to sequester Ca^{2+}(Brustovetsky and Dubinsky, 2000a). The lower CerS6 expression and $C_{16:0}$-ceramide content were associated with reduced mitochondrial CLC in adult brain mitochondria, whereas exogenous $C_{16:0}$-ceramide restored CLC to that of young brain mitochondria. This is in line with the finding that long-chain ceramides, including $C_{16:0}$-ceramide, are potent inhibitors of MPTP activity (Novgorodov et al., 2008). This suggests that CerS6-generated ceramide could prevent MPTP opening, leading to increased Ca^{2+} accumulation in the mitochondrial matrix.

The role of CerS6 in cell survival was examined in primary oligodendrocyte (OL) precursor cells, which undergo apoptotic cell death during early postnatal brain development or following cerebral IR. Exposure of OLs to glutamate resulted in apoptosis that was prevented by inhibitors of *de novo* ceramide biosynthesis, myriocin and fumonisin B1. Knockdown of CerS6 with siRNA reduced glutamate-triggered OL apoptosis, whereas knockdown of CerS5 had no effect. Importantly, blocking mitochondrial Ca^{2+} uptake or decreasing Ca^{2+}-dependent protease calpain activity with specific inhibitors prevented OL apoptosis. Finally, knocking down CerS6 decreased calpain activation. The data suggest a novel role for CerS6 in the regulation of both mitochondrial Ca^{2+} homeostasis and calpain, which could be important in cell death after cerebral IR (**Scheme 3**). These studies illuminate a novel determinant in cerebral IR, mitochondrial ceramide synthase CerS6 which could be an important future target for neuroprotection.

In vitro, de novo synthesized ceramide increased after brief exposure of cultured brain cells to hypoxia, oxygen/glucose deprivation, or TNF (Ginis et al., 1999; Liu et al., 2000). In neuronal precursor cells, hypoxia/reoxygenation triggered a robust elevation in $C_{14:0}$- and $C_{16:0}$-ceramides, and a small increase in $C_{18:0}$-, $C_{18:1}$- and $C_{20:0}$-ceramides, and no increase in $C_{24:0}$- and $C_{24:1}$-ceramides (Jin et al., 2008). The elevations in ceramides were primarily due to the actions of aSMase and ceramide synthase CerS5, demonstrating the involvement of the salvage pathway. Interestingly, C_2-ceramide infusion protected the brain against IR injury (Chen et al., 2001; Furuya et al., 2001). However, this effect could be also attributed to the intracellular/extracellular conversion of ceramide into sphingosine-1-phosphate, which is known to protect cells from apoptosis (Hait et al., 2006; Taha et al., 2006; Tani et al., 2007).

5. Ceramide and mitochondrial injury in stroke

Although IR-induced mitochondrial injury has been extensively studied and mitochondrial functions affected by IR are characterized (Sims and Anderson, 2002), crucial information is needed regarding the cause of mitochondrial dysfunction. Our studies suggest that exogenously added ceramide could provoke mitochondrial dysfunctions similar to that occurring in cerebral IR (Yu et al., 2007). Of note, some data on mitochondrial effects of ceramide have been obtained using synthetic short-chain analogs, which may not fully mimic the properties of naturally occurring long-chain ceramides.

5.1 Respiratory chain

The restriction on mitochondrial respiratory chain function has been shown in various rodent models of stroke (Sims and Anderson, 2002). An impairment of Complex III has been

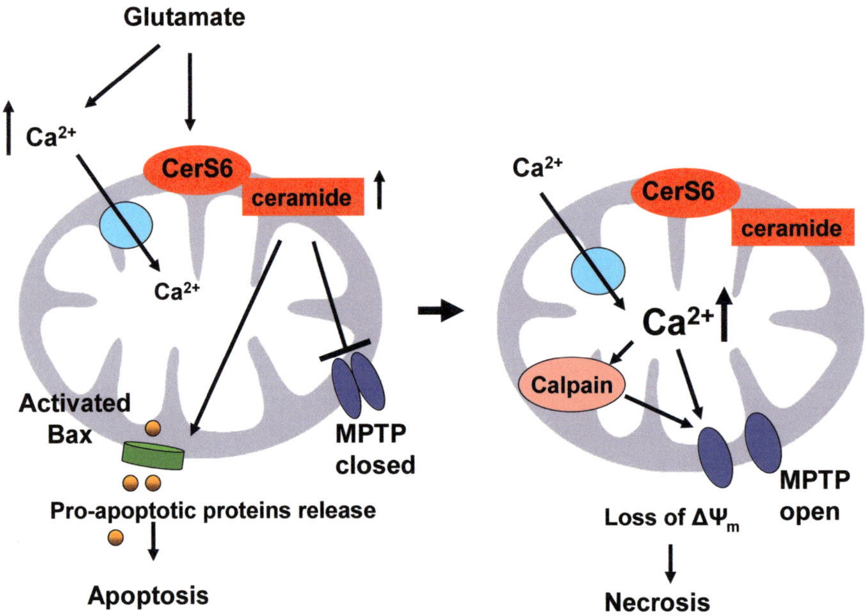

Scheme 3. Hypothetical role of CerS6/ceramide in mitochondria after cerebral IR. IR triggers glutamate-induced cytosolic Ca^{2+} influx into the mitochondria and an activation of mitochondrial CerS6 that elevates ceramide. Ceramide blocks the MPTP opening at a low conductance state, leading to increased Ca^{2+} in the mitochondrial matrix. This MPTP inactivation would allow mitochondria to support adequate ATP production for formation of the apoptosome, and might be responsible for the initial raise in ATP production (and hence $\Delta\psi$) during apoptosis (Atlante et al., 2005), an observation that corresponds well with the reported transient mitochondrial hyper-polarization in the apoptosis induced by IL-3 withdrawal (Vander Heiden et al., 1997). Rising mitochondrial Ca^{2+} activates calpain 10, which could cleave protein components of the MPTP (Arrington et al., 2006) resulting in the MPTP opening at a high conductance state, swelling, and rupture of the outer mitochondrial membrane leading to necrotic cell death.

implicated (**Scheme 4**), but the mechanisms remain unresolved, and a Complex I defect has not been ruled out. We and others have reported that short-chain ceramide could directly suppress respiratory chain Complex III activity (Di Paola et al., 2000; Gudz et al., 1997). Also, ceramide seems to participate in displacement of cytochrome c from its binding site on Complex III (Yuan et al., 2003) corresponds to an apparent mitochondrial Complex III defect in IR.

5.2 Reactive Oxygen Species (ROS)

Free radical formation occurs during cerebral IR. In fact, mitochondria are the major site of production of ROS, and are the likely source for the generation of peroxynitrite, formed from nitric oxide and superoxide during IR (Chan, 2001). Studies in isolated mitochondria indicated that Complex I and III are potential sites of superoxide formation (Votyakova and Reynolds, 2001). Complex III deficiency observed in cerebral IR strongly implicates Complex III as the major and relevant site of ROS generation; however, Complex I remains to be ruled out. Short-chain ceramide could increase the generation of ROS in isolated mitochondria (Garcia-Ruiz et al., 1997).

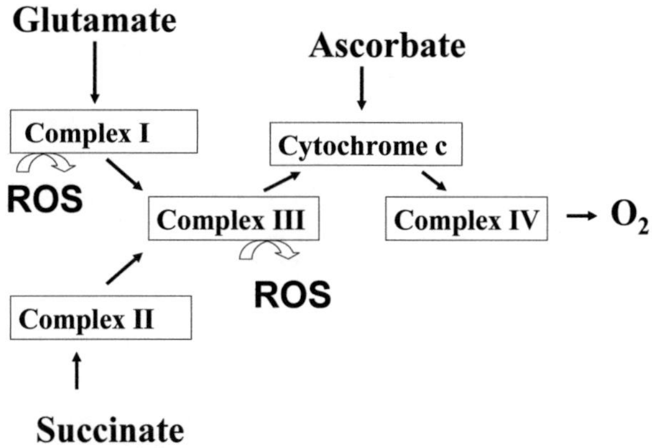

Scheme 4. Mitochondrial respiratory chain complexes. Mitochondrial respiratory chain consists of four multi-protein complexes Complex I-IV. The respiratory chain function is determined using substrates such as glutamate, succinate or ascorbate, which are oxidized via different complexes of respiratory chain. An inhibition of the electron transport through the Complex I or III could result in generation of ROS.

5.3 Mitochondrial Permeability Transition Pore (MPTP)

Excessive accumulation of Ca^{2+} in mitochondrial matrix could trigger opening of the MPTP at a high conductance state that is accompanied with dissipation of transmembrane potential and swelling of mitochondria. In brain mitochondria, Ca^{2+} may also activate a limited permeability state of MPTP opening that only depolarizes mitochondria without swelling (Novgorodov and Gudz, 1996). This depolarization dramatically reduces the driving force for Ca^{2+} influx via the uniporter channel in the inner membrane, thus limiting the mitochondrial ability to sequester Ca^{2+}.

MPTP opening at a high conductance state appears to be a crucial event leading to cell death by necrosis (Fiskum, 2000; Galluzzi et al., 2009; Kroemer et al., 1998). Severe insult causes widespread opening of the MPTP in mitochondria. Cell death proceeds through necrosis when the MPTP remains open, causing the inhibition of ATP production. If the initial insult is not too severe and MPTP does not open, cellular ATP can be maintained to support the energy demand of apoptosis. This provides an explanation for the coexistence of apoptotic and necrotic cell death in IR-injured tissue. It has been emphasized that MPTP regulates necrotic, but not apoptotic cell death in cardiac and cerebral IR (Nakagawa et al., 2005; Schinzel et al., 2005). Mice deficient in cyclophilin D (CyD), the main regulatory component of MPTP, developed up to 37% smaller brain infarcts after IR. CyD-deficient cells died normally in response to various apoptotic stimuli, but were resistant to necrotic cell death induced by ROS and Ca^{2+} overload. MPTP opening at a high conductance state has been proposed to occur in cerebral IR, but the evidence is largely indirect (Sims and Anderson, 2002; Stavrovskaya and Kristal, 2005). The opening of the MPTP at a high conductance state has been implicated as another mechanism of cytochrome c release from mitochondria due to short-chain ceramide (Arora et al., 1997; Novgorodov et al., 2005; Pastorino et al., 1999a; Szalai et al., 1999).

5.4 Release of pro-apoptotic proteins from mitochondria

Apoptosis is mediated by two major pathways: the extrinsic and the intrinsic (or mitochondrial) pathway. The release of mitochondrial cytochrome c and/or Smac, which antagonizes apoptotic protein inhibitor, into the cytosol initiates the activation of caspase-9 leading to the proteolytic activation of executioner caspase-3 and -7. Cytochrome c release from mitochondria is well documented in different models of ischemia (Galluzzi et al., 2009). Recent studies have showed caspase-independent apoptosis involving the release of mitochondrial proteins, apoptosis-inducing factor (AIF), and endonuclease G (EndoG) and their translocation to the nucleus in brain IR (Galluzzi et al., 2009; Joza et al., 2009). Emerging evidence indicates an important role of Bax in cytochrome c and Smac (but not AIF and EndoG) release from brain mitochondria (Brustovetsky et al., 2003). Importantly, mitochondrial calpain has been implicated in AIF release from mitochondria (Kar et al.). The release of mitochondrial proteins implies that the outer and /or the inner mitochondrial membrane is compromised in IR, but the precise mechanisms of the protein release remain unclear. Short-chain ceramide accelerated the release of cytochrome c and AIF from heart mitochondria (Di Paola et al., 2004), and natural C_{16}-ceramide has been shown to form large channels in the outer mitochondrial membrane permeable to cytochrome c (Siskind and Colombini, 2000).

6. Ceramide and mitochondria in cell death

Irrespective of the type of IR, IR-related physiological events have a common final consequence: alteration of mitochondrial function and release of mitochondrial proteins, leading to cell death. Cells with hallmarks of necrosis or apoptosis have been detected in animal models of IR (Li et al., 1995). The mitochondrial changes appear to be one essential step in tissue damage in IR, and treatments that ameliorate tissue infarction were associated with better recovery of mitochondrial function (Nakai et al., 1997). Multiple studies show intimate connections between ceramide signaling and functioning of mitochondria (Mimeault, 2002; Morales et al., 2007), which play central role in integration of cellular signals to determine the outcome among apoptosis, necrosis, or proliferation (Brenner and Kroemer, 2000; Ferri and Kroemer, 2001; Kroemer et al., 2007).

Several lines of evidence have implicated changes in mitochondrial function as an intermediate step in transduction of ceramide signals that culminate in apoptotic or necrotic cell death (Morales et al., 2007; Taha et al., 2006). First, ceramide-induced apoptosis is accompanied by release of pro-apoptotic proteins from mitochondria (Birbes et al., 2001; Hearps et al., 2002; Zhang et al., 2008), increased generation of mitochondrial ROS (Won and Singh, 2006), and discharge of mitochondrial transmembrane potential, $\Delta\psi$ (Gendron et al., 2001; Hearps et al., 2002; Lin et al., 2004; Zamzami et al., 1995). Second, interventions that specifically prevent mitochondrial dysfunction suppress ceramide-induced apoptosis: inhibitors of the MPTP bongkrekic acid (Gendron et al., 2001; Stoica et al., 2003) and cyclosporin A (Pacher and Hajnoczky, 2001; Pastorino et al., 1996; Stoica et al., 2003); and over-expression of Bcl-2 (Geley et al., 1997; Gendron et al., 2001; Scaffidi et al., 1999; Zamzami et al., 1995; Zhang et al., 1996). Third, TNF-α-, ischemia/reperfusion-, etoposide-, or UV-induced apoptosis is associated with simultaneous increase in mitochondrial ceramide (Birbes et al., 2005; Dai et al., 2004; Garcia-Ruiz et al., 1997; Yu et al., 2007).

Depending on cell type and stimuli, ceramide can alter mitochondrial function indirectly or directly (**Scheme 5**). Indirectly, ceramide modifies activity of pro-apoptotic and anti-apoptotic members of the Bcl-2 family of proteins that, in turn, alter the outer mitochondrial membrane permeability for cytochrome c and other pro-apoptotic molecules. Protein targets for ceramide in the cytoplasm include protein phosphatases PP1A and PP2A, protein kinases PKC ζ, raf-1, and kinase-suppressor Ras (Snook et al., 2006). In the lysosomal compartment, ceramide activates aspartate protease cathepsin D (Bidere et al., 2003; Heinrich et al., 2004; Heinrich et al., 1999; Pettus et al., 2002). Among these targets, cathepsin D, PP2A, and PP1A could propagate a pro-apoptotic ceramide signal to the level of the mitochondria (Pettus et al., 2002). Interaction of ceramide with cathepsin D results in cleavage of Bid to active tBid with subsequent activation of caspase-9 and caspase-3 (Heinrich et al., 2004). Activation by ceramides of serine/threonine protein phosphatase PP2A is involved in regulation of the apoptotic/anti-apoptotic activity of Bcl-2 family proteins by changing their phosphorylation status. Ceramide-activated PP2A increases the pro-apoptotic potential of Bcl-2 family proteins by dephosphorylation of Bax (activation) (Xin and Deng, 2006), or Bcl-2 (inactivation) (Ruvolo et al., 1999). An additional substrate for PP2A is serine/threonine kinase Akt/PKB (Pettus et al., 2002). Ceramide-dependent activation of PP2A leads to inactivation of Akt (Garcia et al., 2003; Millward et al., 1999; Pettus et al., 2002) that, in turn, results in dephosphorylation and activation of pro-apoptotic Bad, an Akt substrate (Datta et al., 1997). At the same time PP2A can directly dephosphorylate Bad, thus increasing its pro-apoptotic activity (Chiang et al., 2003). PP1A also can exert its effect on mitochondria by Bad dephosphorylation (Garcia et al., 2003). Interestingly, ceramide by itself can trigger transition of Bax into the active conformation, insertion in to the outer mitochondrial membrane with the subsequent release of cytochrome c and Smac in a cell-free system (Kashkar et al., 2005). Potentiation of Bax binding by ceramides to the outer mitochondrial membrane was shown by Birbes and colleagues (Birbes et al., 2005) and in energized mitochondria ceramide-induced Bax-dependent MPTP opening (Pastorino et al., 1999b). Critical involvement of ceramide in triggering Bax translocation to the mitochondria was demonstrated during hypoxia/reoxygenation in neuronal cells (Jin et al., 2008). Attenuation of Bax translocation by knockdown of ceramide synthase CerS5 or aSMase suggests contribution of the activated salvage pathway in ceramide upregulation; however, the mechanisms by which ceramide exerts its effect remain unknown.

Less-defined, indirect mechanisms include interaction of ceramide with protein kinases PKC δ, p38 and JNK. Short-chain ceramides induce translocation of PKC δ from the cytoplasm to the mitochondria in LNCaP cells (Sumitomo et al., 2002). The translocation of PKC δ was accompanied by cytochrome c release. Mitochondrial translocation of PKC δ and activation of kinase activity was also evident when endogenous ceramides were raised by activation of de novo and neutral SMase-dependent pathways of ceramide production. Endogenous ceramide-induced PKC δ translocation similarly promoted release of cytochrome c and caspase-9 activation. A report by Huwiler et al. (Huwiler et al., 1998) indicates that ceramide can directly target PKC δ. Thus, increased ceramide during I/R can potentially contribute to mitochondrial translocation/activation of PKC δ, which enhances cytochrome c release in heart I/R (Murriel et al., 2004). Although potential mitochondrial PKC δ targets for which phosphorylation results in cytochrome c release remain illusive, PKC δ-dependant accumulation and dephosphorylation of Bad may contribute to the initiation of apoptotic program (Murriel et al., 2004).

The member of the mitogen-activated protein kinase (MAPK) superfamily p38 MAPK was implicated in ceramide-induced apoptosis in cardiomyocytes (Kong et al., 2005). Short-chain

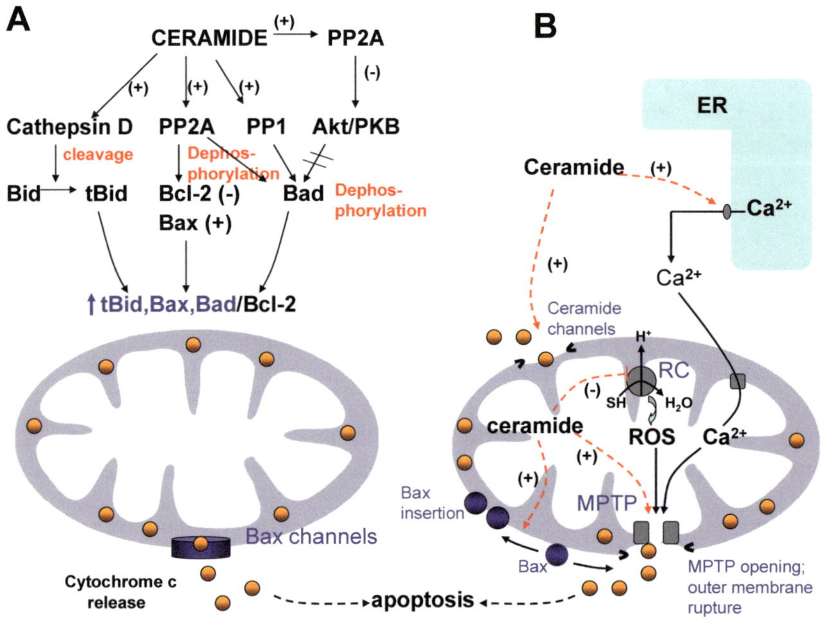

Scheme 5. Ceramide modulates mitochondrial functions through direct and indirect mechanisms. **A**. Indirect modulation of mitochondrial functions by ceramide occurs through the change in the ratio of pro-apoptotic/anti-apoptotic proteins of Bcl-2 family at the outer mitochondrial membrane. **B**. Direct modulation of mitochondrial functions by ceramide include a) formation of ceramide channels permeable for cytochrome c in the outer mitochondrial membrane; b) potentiation of mitochondrial permeability transition pore opening (MPTP) in the inner membrane in the presence of Ca^{2+} or Bax (ceramide-induced Ca^{2+} release from the endoplasmic reticulum (ER) can contribute to the processes; c) potentiation of Bax insertion (activation) in to the outer membrane, d) inhibition of the respiratory chain (RC) with a subsequent increase in ROS formation.

ceramide treatment induced phosphorylation/activation of p38 MAPK which was accompanied by release of cytochrome c from the mitochondria and by the discharge of mitochondrial membrane potential. P38 MAPK inhibitor, SB 202190, abrogated the effect of ceramide both on p38 MAPK phosphorylation and on mitochondrial dysfunction. An interesting aspect of the study was the phosphorylation of the mitochondria-associated p38 MAPK pool under the influence of ceramide. This observation might indicate local signaling in mitochondria-mediated cell death. Although mitochondria-related targets for ceramide-activated p38 MAPK are not well defined, a recent report by Capano and Crompton (Capano and Crompton, 2006) demonstrates that activation of p38 MAPK during simulated ischemia in cardiomyocytes is a key regulatory point of Bax translocation from the cytosol to the mitochondria. The evidence of p38 MAPK-dependent phosphorylation of Bim_{EL} in apoptotic cell response has been provided (Cai et al., 2006) . Another member of the MAPK superfamily, JNK, was shown to be readily activated by both endogenous ceramide generation in liver I/R (Llacuna et al., 2006) and by addition of exogenous ceramide (Kurinna et al., 2004). Activated JNK translocates to the mitochondria and initiates cytochrome c release and cell death by yet unidentified mechanisms (Eminel et al., 2004;

Kurinna et al., 2004); however, direct interaction of JNK with the mitochondrial pool of Bcl-xL was suggested (Kharbanda et al., 2000). Alternatively, activated JNK can induce mitochondrial dysfunction by phosphorylation of a pro-apoptotic member of the Bcl-2 family protein, Bim (Kurinna et al., 2004; Lei and Davis, 2003; Llacuna et al., 2006). Translocation of activated Bim to mitochondria initiates Bax-dependent cytochrome c release and apoptosis (Lei and Davis, 2003). Several other members of Bcl-2 family proteins have been proposed to mediate pro-apoptotic JNK signaling(Weston and Davis, 2007). Overall, the increased ratio of pro-apoptotic/anti-apoptotic proteins bound to mitochondria is generally considered to trigger permeabilization of the outer mitochondrial membrane for cytochrome c and other mitochondrial inter-membrane resident proteins, initiators of apoptosis (Armstrong, 2006; Kroemer et al., 2007). The increases in cell ceramide species contents are expected to contribute to the induction of apoptosis by this mechanism. Among non-protein indirect pathways, those associated with Ca^{2+} signaling attract special attention because of the well-known ability of these organelles both to respond to Ca^{2+} and to shape and propagate the Ca^{2+} signal within the cell (Giorgi et al., 2008; Szabadkai and Duchen, 2008). In this pathway, the Ca^{2+} pool of the ER is a target for ceramide (Pinton et al., 2001; Scorrano et al., 2003). Ca^{2+} released by ceramide from the ER is readily accumulated in mitochondria that, in turn, results in MPTP opening, and cytochrome c release.

Evidence is also accruing to implicate a direct action of ceramide on mitochondria. In this context, modulation by ceramide of mitochondrial functions at the level of isolated organelles has provided further evidence in support of this mechanism. It has been reported that ceramides directly suppress respiratory chain activity at the level of respiratory chain Complex III and/or Complex I (Di Paola et al., 2000; Garcia-Ruiz et al., 1997; Gudz et al., 1997; Yu et al., 2007). Suppression of the respiratory chain by ceramides results in increased production of ROS (Andrieu-Abadie et al., 2001; Di Paola et al., 2000; Garcia-Ruiz et al., 1997; Quillet-Mary et al., 1997), well-known inducers of an apoptotic cell response (Andrieu-Abadie et al., 2001; Ott et al., 2007). Increased ROS production by endothelial cells after hypoxia/reoxygenation was linked to the ceramide-induced suppression of the mitochondrial respiratory chain (Therade-Matharan et al., 2005).

Moreover, current research is focused on the ability of ceramides to release cytochrome c or other pro-apoptotic proteins from the mitochondrial inter-membrane space. Within the model of Colombini and co-workers, pro-apoptotic protein release is due to formation of large pores in the outer mitochondrial membrane by ceramide itself, whereas the inner membrane is viewed as being ceramide-insensitive. This model is supported by extensive experimental material using isolated mitochondria (Di Paola et al., 2004; Ghafourifar et al., 1999; Siskind et al., 2002, 2006) and artificial membranes (liposomes and black lipid membranes) (Montes et al., 2002; Siskind et al., 2002). Importantly, it was recently shown that anti-apoptotic Bcl-2 can disassemble ceramide channels in the outer mitochondrial membrane and black lipid membranes (Siskind et al., 2008), thus providing the mechanistic explanation for the original observation of Ghafourifar *et al.* (Ghafourifar et al., 1999) that Bcl-2 suppresses ceramide-induced cytochrome c release from isolated mitochondria. However, the formation of ceramide channels seems to be highly dependent on the conditions employed, and has been questioned in a number of publications (Kristal and Brown, 1999; Novgorodov et al., 2005; Szalai et al., 1999; Yuan H, 2003). Besides, a few reports suggest that the permeabilization of the inner mitochondrial membrane via the opening of the MPTP could be a primary event in initiation of cytochrome c release in the presence of ceramides (Pastorino et al., 1999b; Szalai et al., 1999). The switch between selective permeabilization of the outer membrane vs. permeabilization of the inner membrane in the presence of ceramide appears to depend on the composition of incubation medium and the nature of ceramide employed (Di Paola et al., 2004).

Additional direct effects of ceramide on mitochondria include modulation of the ionic permeability of the lipid component of the inner membrane (Di Paola et al., 2000) and displacement of cytochrome c from the inner membrane as a result of the direct interaction with the proteins in the respiratory chain Complex III (Ghafourifar et al., 1999; Yuan H, 2003). Emerging evidence suggests involvement of ceramides in reorganization of the mitochondrial network. Both exogenous and endogenously generated ceramides induce mitochondrial fission (Parra et al., 2008; Zeidan et al., 2008), which may contribute to apoptotic cell death (Suen et al., 2008). What particular effectors of mitochondrial fission (DRP1, Fis1, or Bax) or fusion (OPA-1, Mitofusins) machineries are the targets of ceramide in this process remains to be determined. However, in cardiomyocytes exposed to exogenous C_2-ceramide, an increased expression of mitochondrial resident Fis1 and enhanced recruitment of cytosolic DRP1 to mitochondrial fission foci may contribute to disintegration of the mitochondrial network (Parra et al., 2008).

It should be appreciated that the ceramide/mitochondria interaction in the control of apoptosis should be considered in conjunction with the effects of its pro-apoptotic metabolites such as ganglioside GD3 and sphingosine. GD3 shares with ceramide the same properties with respect to its effects on isolated mitochondria and mitochondria *in situ*. In cells, it disrupts mitochondrial membrane potential in a Bcl-2-sensitive manner (Rippo et al., 2000) and induces ROS production (Colell et al., 2001). At the level of isolated mitochondria, it inhibits the mitochondrial respiratory chain at the level of Complex III (Scorrano et al., 1999), increases ROS production (Garcia-Ruiz et al., 2000), opens the MPTP with the subsequent release of cytochrome c (Inoki et al., 2000; Kristal and Brown, 1999; Scorrano et al., 1999), and potentiates interaction of Bax with mitochondria (Pastorino et al., 1999b). Interestingly, while the effect of CD3 on ROS production is relatively nonspecific (lactosylceramide, GM1, GD1a and glucosylceramide produce a similar response (Garcia-Ruiz et al., 1997)), the effect of GD3 in the induction of apoptosis and MPTP opening shows considerable specificity. GM3, GM1 GD1, GD1a, GT1 has no or a slight inhibitory effect (Kristal and Brown, 1999; Pastorino et al., 1999b; Scorrano et al., 1999). In some instances, the effect of ceramide on mitochondria in cells can be explained by its conversion to GD3 (De Maria et al., 1997; Rippo et al., 2000).

Another pro-apoptotic ceramide derivative, sphingosine, releases cytochrome c from mitochondria that could be inhibited by over-expression of anti-apoptotic Bcl-xL (Cuvillier et al., 2000). In contrast to ceramides and GD3, sphingosine suppresses the MPTP in isolated mitochondria, and thus MPTP-dependent cytochrome c release (Broekemeier and Pfeiffer, 1995; Scorrano et al., 2001). It also inhibits ceramide channel formation in the outer mitochondrial membrane (Elrick et al., 2006). This indicates that indirect pathways of cytochrome c release, for example, by recruitment of Bax to mitochondria (Phillips et al., 2007), are predominant in the action of sphingosine on mitochondria. At the same time, similar to ceramide, sphingosine suppresses respiratory chain activity (Hassoun et al., 2006) and increases ROS production by mitochondria, although at higher concentrations (Garcia-Ruiz et al., 1997). Interaction of ceramide, sphingosine, and ganglioside pathways in the control of mitochondrial functions in the time-course of apoptosis remains to be established.

Thus, the proposed mechanisms by which ceramides may affect mitochondria vary, and the combination of direct and indirect mechanisms involved in propagation of ceramide signals to mitochondria depends on cell type and the nature of the stimuli employed.

7. Conclusion

A cardinal feature of brain tissue injury in stroke is mitochondrial dysfunction and the release of mitochondrial proteins leading to cell death. It has become increasingly clear that ceramide, a membrane sphingolipid and a key mediator of cell-stress responses, could play a critical role in cerebral IR - induced mitochondrial injury. Mitochondria are being appreciated as vital intracellular compartments for ceramide metabolism in cerebral IR. Emerging data suggest that the subcellular location of ceramide generation plays a fundamental role in dictating its downstream targets and cell responses to stress stimuli. Continued research efforts are required to better understand the pathophysiological mechanisms of cerebral IR injury, to identify and test new protective agents. Further studies of the molecular basis of the role of ceramide in the ischemic brain are warranted. Because many assumptions regarding ceramide functions in IR-induced tissue injury were based on *in vitro* studies employing artificial ceramides, we must critically evaluate the mitochondrial dysfunctions in IR-injured brain and define a possible role of long-chain ceramides as causes of the mitochondrial impairment. This will allow the discovery of novel and groundbreaking therapeutic approaches to mitigate diseases that may result from elevations in ceramide and its metabolites.

8. Acknowledgements

We thank Dr. Jennifer G. Schnellmann for help with preparation of the manuscript. This work is supported by the NIH/NCCR COBRE in Lipidomics and Pathobiology P20 RR 17677 (TIG), VA Merit Awards from BLRD and RRD Service (TIG), and SAN was supported by NIH grant AG16583.

9. References

Andreyev, A.Y., Fahy, E., Guan, Z., Kelly, S., Li, X., McDonald, J.G., Milne, S., Myers, D., Park, H., Ryan, A., *et al.* (2010). Subcellular organelle lipidomics in TLR-4-activated macrophages. J Lipid Res *51*, 2785-2797.

Andrieu-Abadie, N., Gouaze, V., Salvayre, R., and Levade, T. (2001). Ceramide in apoptosis signaling: relationship with oxidative stress. Free Radic Biol Med *31*, 717-728.

Ardail, D., Popa, I., Alcantara, K., Pons, A., Zanetta, J.P., Louisot, P., Thomas, L., and Portoukalian, J. (2001). Occurrence of ceramides and neutral glycolipids with unusual long-chain base composition in purified rat liver mitochondria. FEBS letters *488*, 160-164.

Argaud, L., Prigent, A.F., Chalabreysse, L., Loufouat, J., Lagarde, M., and Ovize, M. (2004). Ceramide in the antiapoptotic effect of ischemic preconditioning. American journal of physiology *286*, H246-251.

Armstrong, J.S. (2006). Mitochondrial membrane permeabilization: the sine qua non for cell death. Bioessays *28*, 253-260.

Arora, A.S., Jones, B.J., Patel, T.C., Bronk, S.F., and Gores, G.J. (1997). Ceramide induces hepatocyte cell death through disruption of mitochondrial function in the rat. Hepatology *25*, 958-963.

Arrington, D.D., Van Vleet, T.R., and Schnellmann, R.G. (2006). Calpain 10: a mitochondrial calpain and its role in calcium-induced mitochondrial dysfunction. American journal of physiology *291*, C1159-1171.

Atlante, A., Giannattasio, S., Bobba, A., Gagliardi, S., Petragallo, V., Calissano, P., Marra, E., and Passarella, S. (2005). An increase in the ATP levels occurs in cerebellar granule cells en route to apoptosis in which ATP derives from both oxidative phosphorylation and anaerobic glycolysis. Biochimica et biophysica acta *1708*, 50-62.

Beresewicz, A., Dobrzyn, A., and Gorski, J. (2002). Accumulation of specific ceramides in ischemic/reperfused rat heart; effect of ischemic preconditioning. J Physiol Pharmacol *53*, 371-382.

Bianchi, P., Kunduzova, O., Masini, E., Cambon, C., Bani, D., Raimondi, L., Seguelas, M.H., Nistri, S., Colucci, W., Leducq, N., *et al.* (2005). Oxidative stress by monoamine oxidase mediates receptor-independent cardiomyocyte apoptosis by serotonin and postischemic myocardial injury. Circulation *112*, 3297-3305.

Bidere, N., Lorenzo, H.K., Carmona, S., Laforge, M., Harper, F., Dumont, C., and Senik, A. (2003). Cathepsin D triggers Bax activation, resulting in selective apoptosis-inducing factor (AIF) relocation in T lymphocytes entering the early commitment phase to apoptosis. The Journal of biological chemistry *278*, 31401-31411.

Bielawska, A., Perry, D.K., and Hannun, Y.A. (2001). Determination of ceramides and diglycerides by the diglyceride kinase assay. Analytical biochemistry *298*, 141-150.

Bielawska, A.E., Shapiro, J.P., Jiang, L., Melkonyan, H.S., Piot, C., Wolfe, C.L., Tomei, L.D., Hannun, Y.A., and Umansky, S.R. (1997). Ceramide is involved in triggering of cardiomyocyte apoptosis induced by ischemia and reperfusion. The American journal of pathology *151*, 1257-1263.

Bionda, C., Portoukalian, J., Schmitt, D., Rodriguez-Lafrasse, C., and Ardail, D. (2004). Subcellular compartmentalization of ceramide metabolism: MAM (mitochondria-associated membrane) and/or mitochondria? The Biochemical journal *382*, 527-533.

Birbes, H., El Bawab, S., Hannun, Y.A., and Obeid, L.M. (2001). Selective hydrolysis of a mitochondrial pool of sphingomyelin induces apoptosis. Faseb J *15*, 2669-2679.

Birbes, H., Luberto, C., Hsu, Y.T., El Bawab, S., Hannun, Y.A., and Obeid, L.M. (2005). A mitochondrial pool of sphingomyelin is involved in TNFalpha-induced Bax translocation to mitochondria. The Biochemical journal *386*, 445-451.

Bollinger, C.R., Teichgraber, V., and Gulbins, E. (2005). Ceramide-enriched membrane domains. Biochimica et biophysica acta *1746*, 284-294.

Bradham, C.A., Stachlewitz, R.F., Gao, W., Qian, T., Jayadev, S., Jenkins, G., Hannun, Y., Lemasters, J.J., Thurman, R.G., and Brenner, D.A. (1997). Reperfusion after liver transplantation in rats differentially activates the mitogen-activated protein kinases. Hepatology (Baltimore, Md *25*, 1128-1135.

Brenner, C., and Kroemer, G. (2000). Apoptosis. Mitochondria--the death signal integrators. Science *289*, 1150-1151.

Broekemeier, K.M., and Pfeiffer, D.R. (1995). Inhibition of the mitochondrial permeability transition by cyclosporin A during long time frame experiments: relationship between pore opening and the activity of mitochondrial phospholipases. Biochemistry *34*, 16440-16449.

Brustovetsky, N., and Dubinsky, J.M. (2000a). Dual responses of CNS mitochondria to elevated calcium. J Neurosci *20*, 103-113.

Brustovetsky, N., and Dubinsky, J.M. (2000b). Limitations of cyclosporin A inhibition of the permeability transition in CNS mitochondria. J Neurosci *20*, 8229-8237.

Brustovetsky, N., Dubinsky, J.M., Antonsson, B., and Jemmerson, R. (2003). Two pathways for tBID-induced cytochrome c release from rat brain mitochondria: BAK- versus BAX-dependence. Journal of neurochemistry *84*, 196-207.

Cai, B., Chang, S.H., Becker, E.B., Bonni, A., and Xia, Z. (2006). p38 MAP kinase mediates apoptosis through phosphorylation of BimEL at Ser-65. The Journal of biological chemistry *281*, 25215-25222.

Capano, M., and Crompton, M. (2006). Bax translocates to mitochondria of heart cells during simulated ischaemia: involvement of AMP-activated and p38 mitogen-activated protein kinases. The Biochemical journal *395*, 57-64.

Chan, P.H. (2001). Reactive oxygen radicals in signaling and damage in the ischemic brain. J Cereb Blood Flow Metab *21*, 2-14.

Chan, P.H. (2004). Future targets and cascades for neuroprotective strategies. Stroke *35*, 2748-2750.

Chatelut, M., Leruth, M., Harzer, K., Dagan, A., Marchesini, S., Gatt, S., Salvayre, R., Courtoy, P., and Levade, T. (1998). Natural ceramide is unable to escape the lysosome, in contrast to a fluorescent analogue. FEBS letters *426*, 102-106.

Chen, Y., Ginis, I., and Hallenbeck, J.M. (2001). The protective effect of ceramide in immature rat brain hypoxia-ischemia involves up-regulation of bcl-2 and reduction of TUNEL-positive cells. J Cereb Blood Flow Metab *21*, 34-40.

Chiang, C.W., Kanies, C., Kim, K.W., Fang, W.B., Parkhurst, C., Xie, M., Henry, T., and Yang, E. (2003). Protein phosphatase 2A dephosphorylation of phosphoserine 112 plays the gatekeeper role for BAD-mediated apoptosis. Molecular and cellular biology *23*, 6350-6362.

Chudakova, D.A., Zeidan, Y.H., Wheeler, B.W., Yu, J., Novgorodov, S.A., Kindy, M.S., Hannun, Y.A., and Gudz, T.I. (2008). Integrin-associated Lyn kinase promotes cell survival by suppressing acid sphingomyelinase activity. The Journal of biological chemistry.

Clarke, C.J., Snook, C.F., Tani, M., Matmati, N., Marchesini, N., and Hannun, Y.A. (2006). The extended family of neutral sphingomyelinases. Biochemistry *45*, 11247-11256.

Clarke, C.J., Wu, B.X., and Hannun, Y.A. (2011). The neutral sphingomyelinase family: identifying biochemical connections. Advances in enzyme regulation *51*, 51-58.

Colell, A., Garcia-Ruiz, C., Roman, J., Ballesta, A., and Fernandez-Checa, J.C. (2001). Ganglioside GD3 enhances apoptosis by suppressing the nuclear factor-kappa B-dependent survival pathway. Faseb J *15*, 1068-1070.

Contreras, F.X., Sanchez-Magraner, L., Alonso, A., and Goni, F.M. (2010). Transbilayer (flip-flop) lipid motion and lipid scrambling in membranes. FEBS letters *584*, 1779-1786.

Cordis, G.A., Yoshida, T., and Das, D.K. (1998). HPTLC analysis of sphingomylein, ceramide and sphingosine in ischemic/reperfused rat heart. Journal of pharmaceutical and biomedical analysis *16*, 1189-1193.

Cui, J., Engelman, R.M., Maulik, N., and Das, D.K. (2004). Role of ceramide in ischemic preconditioning. Journal of the American College of Surgeons *198*, 770-777.

Cuvillier, O., Edsall, L., and Spiegel, S. (2000). Involvement of sphingosine in mitochondria-dependent Fas-induced apoptosis of type II Jurkat T cells. The Journal of biological chemistry *275*, 15691-15700.

D'Mello N, P., Childress, A.M., Franklin, D.S., Kale, S.P., Pinswasdi, C., and Jazwinski, S.M. (1994). Cloning and characterization of LAG1, a longevity-assurance gene in yeast. The Journal of biological chemistry *269*, 15451-15459.

Dai, Q., Liu, J., Chen, J., Durrant, D., McIntyre, T.M., and Lee, R.M. (2004). Mitochondrial ceramide increases in UV-irradiated HeLa cells and is mainly derived from hydrolysis of sphingomyelin. Oncogene *23*, 3650-3658.

Datta, S.R., Dudek, H., Tao, X., Masters, S., Fu, H., Gotoh, Y., and Greenberg, M.E. (1997). Akt phosphorylation of BAD couples survival signals to the cell-intrinsic death machinery. Cell *91*, 231-241.

De Maria, R., Lenti, L., Malisan, F., d'Agostino, F., Tomassini, B., Zeuner, A., Rippo, M.R., and Testi, R. (1997). Requirement for GD3 ganglioside in CD95- and ceramide-induced apoptosis. Science *277*, 1652-1655.

Deng, X., Yin, X., Allan, R., Lu, D.D., Maurer, C.W., Haimovitz-Friedman, A., Fuks, Z., Shaham, S., and Kolesnick, R. (2008). Ceramide biogenesis is required for radiation-induced apoptosis in the germ line of C. elegans. Science *322*, 110-115.

Der, P., Cui, J., and Das, D.K. (2006). Role of lipid rafts in ceramide and nitric oxide signaling in the ischemic and preconditioned hearts. Journal of molecular and cellular cardiology *40*, 313-320.

Di Paola, M., Cocco, T., and Lorusso, M. (2000). Ceramide interaction with the respiratory chain of heart mitochondria. Biochemistry *39*, 6660-6668.

Di Paola, M., Zaccagnino, P., Montedoro, G., Cocco, T., and Lorusso, M. (2004). Ceramide induces release of pro-apoptotic proteins from mitochondria by either a Ca2+ -dependent or a Ca2+ -independent mechanism. J Bioenerg Biomembr *36*, 165-170.

El Bawab, S., Birbes, H., Roddy, P., Szulc, Z.M., Bielawska, A., and Hannun, Y.A. (2001). Biochemical characterization of the reverse activity of rat brain ceramidase. A CoA-independent and fumonisin B1-insensitive ceramide synthase. The Journal of biological chemistry *276*, 16758-16766.

El Bawab, S., Roddy, P., Qian, T., Bielawska, A., Lemasters, J.J., and Hannun, Y.A. (2000). Molecular cloning and characterization of a human mitochondrial ceramidase. The Journal of biological chemistry *275*, 21508-21513.

Elrick, M.J., Fluss, S., and Colombini, M. (2006). Sphingosine, a product of ceramide hydrolysis, influences the formation of ceramide channels. Biophysical journal *91*, 1749-1756.

Eminel, S., Klettner, A., Roemer, L., Herdegen, T., and Waetzig, V. (2004). JNK2 translocates to the mitochondria and mediates cytochrome c release in PC12 cells in response to 6-hydroxydopamine. The Journal of biological chemistry *279*, 55385-55392.

Ferri, K.F., and Kroemer, G. (2001). Organelle-specific initiation of cell death pathways. Nat Cell Biol *3*, E255-263.

Fiskum, G. (2000). Mitochondrial participation in ischemic and traumatic neural cell death. J Neurotrauma *17*, 843-855.

Furuya, K., Ginis, I., Takeda, H., Chen, Y., and Hallenbeck, J.M. (2001). Cell permeable exogenous ceramide reduces infarct size in spontaneously hypertensive rats supporting in vitro studies that have implicated ceramide in induction of tolerance to ischemia. J Cereb Blood Flow Metab *21*, 226-232.

Futerman, A.H. (2006). Intracellular trafficking of sphingolipids: relationship to biosynthesis. Biochimica et biophysica acta *1758*, 1885-1892.

Futerman, A.H., and Riezman, H. (2005). The ins and outs of sphingolipid synthesis. Trends Cell Biol *15*, 312-318.

Futerman, A.H., Stieger, B., Hubbard, A.L., and Pagano, R.E. (1990). Sphingomyelin synthesis in rat liver occurs predominantly at the cis and medial cisternae of the Golgi apparatus. The Journal of biological chemistry *265*, 8650-8657.

Galluzzi, L., Blomgren, K., and Kroemer, G. (2009). Mitochondrial membrane permeabilization in neuronal injury. Nat Rev Neurosci *10*, 481-494.

Garcia-Ruiz, C., Colell, A., Mari, M., Morales, A., and Fernandez-Checa, J.C. (1997). Direct effect of ceramide on the mitochondrial electron transport chain leads to generation of reactive oxygen species. Role of mitochondrial glutathione. The Journal of biological chemistry *272*, 11369-11377.

Garcia-Ruiz, C., Colell, A., Paris, R., and Fernandez-Checa, J.C. (2000). Direct interaction of GD3 ganglioside with mitochondria generates reactive oxygen species followed by mitochondrial permeability transition, cytochrome c release, and caspase activation. Faseb J *14*, 847-858.

Garcia, A., Cayla, X., Guergnon, J., Dessauge, F., Hospital, V., Rebollo, M.P., Fleischer, A., and Rebollo, A. (2003). Serine/threonine protein phosphatases PP1 and PP2A are key players in apoptosis. Biochimie *85*, 721-726.

Geley, S., Hartmann, B.L., and Kofler, R. (1997). Ceramides induce a form of apoptosis in human acute lymphoblastic leukemia cells that is inhibited by Bcl-2, but not by CrmA. FEBS letters *400*, 15-18.

Gendron, M.C., Schrantz, N., Metivier, D., Kroemer, G., Maciorowska, Z., Sureau, F., Koester, S., and Petit, P.X. (2001). Oxidation of pyridine nucleotides during Fas- and ceramide-induced apoptosis in Jurkat cells: correlation with changes in mitochondria, glutathione depletion, intracellular acidification and caspase 3 activation. The Biochemical journal *353*, 357-367.

Ghafourifar, P., Klein, S.D., Schucht, O., Schenk, U., Pruschy, M., Rocha, S., and Richter, C. (1999). Ceramide induces cytochrome c release from isolated mitochondria. Importance of mitochondrial redox state. The Journal of biological chemistry *274*, 6080-6084.

Ginis, I., Schweizer, U., Brenner, M., Liu, J., Azzam, N., Spatz, M., and Hallenbeck, J.M. (1999). TNF-alpha pretreatment prevents subsequent activation of cultured brain cells with TNF-alpha and hypoxia via ceramide. Am J Physiol *276*, C1171-1183.

Giorgi, C., Romagnoli, A., Pinton, P., and Rizzuto, R. (2008). Ca2+ signaling, mitochondria and cell death. Current molecular medicine *8*, 119-130.

Goni, F.M., Contreras, F.X., Montes, L.R., Sot, J., and Alonso, A. (2005). Biophysics (and sociology) of ceramides. Biochemical Society symposium, 177-188.

Graham, T.R., and Kozlov, M.M. (2010). Interplay of proteins and lipids in generating membrane curvature. Current opinion in cell biology *22*, 430-436.

Gudz, T.I., Tserng, K.Y., and Hoppel, C.L. (1997). Direct inhibition of mitochondrial respiratory chain complex III by cell-permeable ceramide. The Journal of biological chemistry *272*, 24154-24158.

Gustafsson, A.B., and Gottlieb, R.A. (2008). Eat your heart out: Role of autophagy in myocardial ischemia/reperfusion. Autophagy *4*, 416-421.

Hait, N.C., Oskeritzian, C.A., Paugh, S.W., Milstien, S., and Spiegel, S. (2006). Sphingosine kinases, sphingosine 1-phosphate, apoptosis and diseases. Biochimica et biophysica acta *1758*, 2016-2026.

Hanada, K., Kumagai, K., Yasuda, S., Miura, Y., Kawano, M., Fukasawa, M., and Nishijima, M. (2003). Molecular machinery for non-vesicular trafficking of ceramide. Nature *426*, 803-809.

Hannun, Y.A., and Obeid, L.M. (2002). The Ceramide-centric universe of lipid-mediated cell regulation: stress encounters of the lipid kind. The Journal of biological chemistry *277*, 25847-25850.

Hannun, Y.A., and Obeid, L.M. (2008). Principles of bioactive lipid signalling: lessons from sphingolipids. Nature reviews *9*, 139-150.

Hannun, Y.A., and Obeid, L.M. (2011). Many Ceramides. The Journal of biological chemistry.

Hassoun, S.M., Lancel, S., Petillot, P., Decoster, B., Favory, R., Marchetti, P., and Neviere, R. (2006). Sphingosine impairs mitochondrial function by opening permeability transition pore. Mitochondrion *6*, 149-154.

Hearps, A.C., Burrows, J., Connor, C.E., Woods, G.M., Lowenthal, R.M., and Ragg, S.J. (2002). Mitochondrial cytochrome c release precedes transmembrane depolarisation and caspase-3 activation during ceramide-induced apoptosis of Jurkat T cells. Apoptosis *7*, 387-394.

Heinrich, M., Neumeyer, J., Jakob, M., Hallas, C., Tchikov, V., Winoto-Morbach, S., Wickel, M., Schneider-Brachert, W., Trauzold, A., Hethke, A., *et al.* (2004). Cathepsin D links TNF-induced acid sphingomyelinase to Bid-mediated caspase-9 and -3 activation. Cell Death Differ *11*, 550-563.

Heinrich, M., Wickel, M., Schneider-Brachert, W., Sandberg, C., Gahr, J., Schwandner, R., Weber, T., Saftig, P., Peters, C., Brunner, J., *et al.* (1999). Cathepsin D targeted by acid sphingomyelinase-derived ceramide. Embo J *18*, 5252-5263.

Hernandez, O.M., Discher, D.J., Bishopric, N.H., and Webster, K.A. (2000). Rapid activation of neutral sphingomyelinase by hypoxia-reoxygenation of cardiac myocytes. Circulation research *86*, 198-204.

Hirschberg, K., Rodger, J., and Futerman, A.H. (1993). The long-chain sphingoid base of sphingolipids is acylated at the cytosolic surface of the endoplasmic reticulum in rat liver. The Biochemical journal *290 (Pt 3)*, 751-757.

Huwiler, A., Fabbro, D., and Pfeilschifter, J. (1998). Selective ceramide binding to protein kinase C-alpha and -delta isoenzymes in renal mesangial cells. Biochemistry *37*, 14556-14562.

Inoki, Y., Miura, T., Kajimoto, T., Kawase, M., Kawase, Y., Yoshida, Y., Tsuji, S., Kinouchi, T., Endo, H., Kagawa, Y., *et al.* (2000). Ganglioside GD3 and its mimetics induce cytochrome c release from mitochondria. Biochemical and biophysical research communications *276*, 1210-1216.

Jin, J., Hou, Q., Mullen, T.D., Zeidan, Y.H., Bielawski, J., Kraveka, J.M., Bielawska, A., Obeid, L.M., Hannun, Y.A., and Hsu, Y.T. (2008). Ceramide generated by sphingomyelin hydrolysis and the salvage pathway is involved in hypoxia/reoxygenation-induced Bax redistribution to mitochondria in NT-2 cells. The Journal of biological chemistry.

Joza, N., Pospisilik, J.A., Hangen, E., Hanada, T., Modjtahedi, N., Penninger, J.M., and Kroemer, G. (2009). AIF: not just an apoptosis-inducing factor. Annals of the New York Academy of Sciences *1171*, 2-11.

Kalhorn, T., and Zager, R.A. (1999). Renal cortical ceramide patterns during ischemic and toxic injury: assessments by HPLC-mass spectrometry. The American journal of physiology *277*, F723-733.

Kar, P., Samanta, K., Shaikh, S., Chowdhury, A., Chakraborti, T., and Chakraborti, S. Mitochondrial calpain system: an overview. Archives of biochemistry and biophysics *495*, 1-7.

Kashkar, H., Wiegmann, K., Yazdanpanah, B., Haubert, D., and Kronke, M. (2005). Acid sphingomyelinase is indispensable for UV light-induced Bax conformational change at the mitochondrial membrane. The Journal of biological chemistry *280*, 20804-20813.

Kharbanda, S., Saxena, S., Yoshida, K., Pandey, P., Kaneki, M., Wang, Q., Cheng, K., Chen, Y.N., Campbell, A., Sudha, T., *et al.* (2000). Translocation of SAPK/JNK to mitochondria and interaction with Bcl-x(L) in response to DNA damage. The Journal of biological chemistry *275*, 322-327.

Kirichok, Y., Krapivinsky, G., and Clapham, D.E. (2004). The mitochondrial calcium uniporter is a highly selective ion channel. Nature *427*, 360-364.

Kitagaki, H., Cowart, L.A., Matmati, N., Vaena de Avalos, S., Novgorodov, S.A., Zeidan, Y.H., Bielawski, J., Obeid, L.M., and Hannun, Y.A. (2007). Isc1 regulates sphingolipid metabolism in yeast mitochondria. Biochim Biophys Acta *1768*, 2849-2861.

Kitatani, K., Idkowiak-Baldys, J., Bielawski, J., Taha, T.A., Jenkins, R.W., Senkal, C.E., Ogretmen, B., Obeid, L.M., and Hannun, Y.A. (2006). Protein kinase C-induced activation of a ceramide/protein phosphatase 1 pathway leading to dephosphorylation of p38 MAPK. The Journal of biological chemistry *281*, 36793-36802.

Kitatani, K., Idkowiak-Baldys, J., and Hannun, Y.A. (2008). The sphingolipid salvage pathway in ceramide metabolism and signaling. Cellular signalling *20*, 1010-1018.

Kolter, T., Proia, R.L., and Sandhoff, K. (2002). Combinatorial ganglioside biosynthesis. The Journal of biological chemistry *277*, 25859-25862.

Kong, J.Y., Klassen, S.S., and Rabkin, S.W. (2005). Ceramide activates a mitochondrial p38 mitogen-activated protein kinase: a potential mechanism for loss of mitochondrial transmembrane potential and apoptosis. Molecular and cellular biochemistry *278*, 39-51.

Kristal, B.S., and Brown, A.M. (1999). Apoptogenic ganglioside GD3 directly induces the mitochondrial permeability transition. The Journal of biological chemistry *274*, 23169-23175.

Kroemer, G., Dallaporta, B., and Resche-Rigon, M. (1998). The mitochondrial death/life regulator in apoptosis and necrosis. Annu Rev Physiol *60*, 619-642.

Kroemer, G., Galluzzi, L., and Brenner, C. (2007). Mitochondrial membrane permeabilization in cell death. Physiol Rev *87*, 99-163.

Kubota, M., Kitahara, S., Shimasaki, H., and Ueta, N. (1989). Accumulation of ceramide in ischemic human brain of an acute case of cerebral occlusion. The Japanese journal of experimental medicine *59*, 59-64.

Kubota, M., Narita, K., Nakagomi, T., Tamura, A., Shimasaki, H., Ueta, N., and Yoshida, S. (1996). Sphingomyelin changes in rat cerebral cortex during focal ischemia. Neurol Res *18*, 337-341.

Kurinna, S.M., Tsao, C.C., Nica, A.F., Jiffar, T., and Ruvolo, P.P. (2004). Ceramide promotes apoptosis in lung cancer-derived A549 cells by a mechanism involving c-Jun NH2-terminal kinase. Cancer research *64*, 7852-7856.

Lahiri, S., and Futerman, A.H. (2005). LASS5 is a bona fide dihydroceramide synthase that selectively utilizes palmitoyl-CoA as acyl donor. The Journal of biological chemistry *280*, 33735-33738.

Laviad, E.L., Albee, L., Pankova-Kholmyansky, I., Epstein, S., Park, H., Merrill, A.H., Jr., and Futerman, A.H. (2008). Characterization of ceramide synthase 2: tissue distribution, substrate specificity, and inhibition by sphingosine 1-phosphate. J Biol Chem *283*, 5677-5684.

Lei, K., and Davis, R.J. (2003). JNK phosphorylation of Bim-related members of the Bcl2 family induces Bax-dependent apoptosis. Proceedings of the National Academy of Sciences of the United States of America *100*, 2432-2437.

Levy, M., Castillo, S.S., and Goldkorn, T. (2006). nSMase2 activation and trafficking are modulated by oxidative stress to induce apoptosis. Biochemical and biophysical research communications *344*, 900-905.

Li, Y., Chopp, M., Jiang, N., and Zaloga, C. (1995). In situ detection of DNA fragmentation after focal cerebral ischemia in mice. Brain Res Mol Brain Res *28*, 164-168.

Lin, C.F., Chen, C.L., Chang, W.T., Jan, M.S., Hsu, L.J., Wu, R.H., Tang, M.J., Chang, W.C., and Lin, Y.S. (2004). Sequential caspase-2 and caspase-8 activation upstream of mitochondria during ceramideand etoposide-induced apoptosis. The Journal of biological chemistry *279*, 40755-40761.

Liu, J., Ginis, I., Spatz, M., and Hallenbeck, J.M. (2000). Hypoxic preconditioning protects cultured neurons against hypoxic stress via TNF-alpha and ceramide. American journal of physiology *278*, C144-153.

Llacuna, L., Mari, M., Garcia-Ruiz, C., Fernandez-Checa, J.C., and Morales, A. (2006). Critical role of acidic sphingomyelinase in murine hepatic ischemia-reperfusion injury. Hepatology (Baltimore, Md *44*, 561-572.

Lopez-Montero, I., Rodriguez, N., Cribier, S., Pohl, A., Velez, M., and Devaux, P.F. (2005). Rapid transbilayer movement of ceramides in phospholipid vesicles and in human erythrocytes. The Journal of biological chemistry *280*, 25811-25819.

Mandon, E.C., Ehses, I., Rother, J., van Echten, G., and Sandhoff, K. (1992). Subcellular localization and membrane topology of serine palmitoyltransferase, 3-dehydrosphinganine reductase, and sphinganine N-acyltransferase in mouse liver. The Journal of biological chemistry *267*, 11144-11148.

Marchesini, N., Osta, W., Bielawski, J., Luberto, C., Obeid, L.M., and Hannun, Y.A. (2004). Role for mammalian neutral sphingomyelinase 2 in confluence-induced growth arrest of MCF7 cells. The Journal of biological chemistry *279*, 25101-25111.

Merrill, A.H., Jr. (2002). De novo sphingolipid biosynthesis: a necessary, but dangerous, pathway. J Biol Chem *277*, 25843-25846.

Mesicek, J., Lee, H., Feldman, T., Jiang, X., Skobeleva, A., Berdyshev, E.V., Haimovitz-Friedman, A., Fuks, Z., and Kolesnick, R. (2010). Ceramide synthases 2, 5, and 6 confer distinct roles in radiation-induced apoptosis in HeLa cells. Cell Signal *22*, 1300-1307.

Michel, C., and van Echten-Deckert, G. (1997). Conversion of dihydroceramide to ceramide occurs at the cytosolic face of the endoplasmic reticulum. FEBS letters *416*, 153-155.

Milhas, D., Clarke, C.J., and Hannun, Y.A. (2010). Sphingomyelin metabolism at the plasma membrane: implications for bioactive sphingolipids. FEBS letters *584*, 1887-1894.

Millward, T.A., Zolnierowicz, S., and Hemmings, B.A. (1999). Regulation of protein kinase cascades by protein phosphatase 2A. Trends Biochem Sci *24*, 186-191.

Mimeault, M. (2002). New advances on structural and biological functions of ceramide in apoptotic/necrotic cell death and cancer. FEBS letters *530*, 9-16.

Mizutani, Y., Kihara, A., and Igarashi, Y. (2005). Mammalian Lass6 and its related family members regulate synthesis of specific ceramides. The Biochemical journal *390*, 263-271.

Mizutani, Y., Kihara, A., and Igarashi, Y. (2006). LASS3 (longevity assurance homologue 3) is a mainly testis-specific (dihydro)ceramide synthase with relatively broad substrate specificity. Biochem J *398*, 531-538.

Monette, J.S., Gomez, L.A., Moreau, R.F., Bemer, B.A., Taylor, A.W., and Hagen, T.M. (2010). Characteristics of the rat cardiac sphingolipid pool in two mitochondrial subpopulations. Biochem Biophys Res Commun *398*, 272-277.

Montes, L.R., Ruiz-Arguello, M.B., Goni, F.M., and Alonso, A. (2002). Membrane restructuring via ceramide results in enhanced solute efflux. The Journal of biological chemistry *277*, 11788-11794.

Morales, A., Lee, H., Goni, F.M., Kolesnick, R., and Fernandez-Checa, J.C. (2007). Sphingolipids and cell death. Apoptosis *12*, 923-939.

Morell, P., and Radin, N.S. (1970). Specificity in ceramide biosynthesis from long chain bases and various fatty acyl coenzyme A's by brain microsomes. The Journal of biological chemistry *245*, 342-350.

Murriel, C.L., Churchill, E., Inagaki, K., Szweda, L.I., and Mochly-Rosen, D. (2004). Protein kinase Cdelta activation induces apoptosis in response to cardiac ischemia and reperfusion damage: a mechanism involving BAD and the mitochondria. The Journal of biological chemistry *279*, 47985-47991.

Nakagawa, T., Shimizu, S., Watanabe, T., Yamaguchi, O., Otsu, K., Yamagata, H., Inohara, H., Kubo, T., and Tsujimoto, Y. (2005). Cyclophilin D-dependent mitochondrial permeability transition regulates some necrotic but not apoptotic cell death. Nature *434*, 652-658.

Nakai, A., Kuroda, S., Kristian, T., and Siesjo, B.K. (1997). The immunosuppressant drug FK506 ameliorates secondary mitochondrial dysfunction following transient focal cerebral ischemia in the rat. Neurobiol Dis *4*, 288-300.

Nakane, M., Kubota, M., Nakagomi, T., Tamura, A., Hisaki, H., Shimasaki, H., and Ueta, N. (2000). Lethal forebrain ischemia stimulates sphingomyelin hydrolysis and ceramide generation in the gerbil hippocampus. Neurosci Lett *296*, 89-92.

Nilsson, A., and Duan, R.D. (2006). Absorption and lipoprotein transport of sphingomyelin. Journal of lipid research *47*, 154-171.

Noureddine, L., Azzam, R., Nemer, G., Bielawski, J., Nasser, M., Bitar, F., and Dbaibo, G.S. (2008). Modulation of total ceramide and constituent ceramide species in the acutely and chronically hypoxic mouse heart at different ages. Prostaglandins & other lipid mediators *86*, 49-55.

Novgorodov, S.A., Chudakova, D.A., Wheeler, B.W., Bielawski, J., Kindy, M.S., Obeid, L.M., and Gudz, T.I. (2011a). Developmentally regulated ceramide synthase 6 increases mitochondrial Ca2+ loading capacity and promotes apoptosis. The Journal of biological chemistry *286*, 4644-4658.

Novgorodov, S.A., and Gudz, T.I. (1996). Permeability transition pore of the inner mitochondrial membrane can operate in two open states with different selectivities. Journal of bioenergetics and biomembranes *28*, 139-146.

Novgorodov, S.A., Gudz, T.I., and Obeid, L.M. (2008). Long-chain ceramide is a potent inhibitor of the mitochondrial permeability transition pore. The Journal of biological chemistry *283*, 24707-24717.

Novgorodov, S.A., Szulc, Z.M., Luberto, C., Jones, J.A., Bielawski, J., Bielawska, A., Hannun, Y.A., and Obeid, L.M. (2005). Positively charged ceramide is a potent inducer of mitochondrial permeabilization. The Journal of biological chemistry *280*, 16096-16105.

Novgorodov, S.A., Wu, B.X., Gudz, T.I., Bielawski, J., Ovchinnikova, T.V., Hannun, Y.A., and Obeid, L.M. (2011b). Novel Pathway of Ceramide Production in Mitochondria: THIOESTERASE AND NEUTRAL CERAMIDASE PRODUCE CERAMIDE FROM SPHINGOSINE AND ACYL-CoA. The Journal of biological chemistry *286*, 25352-25362.

O'Brien, N.W., Gellings, N.M., Guo, M., Barlow, S.B., Glembotski, C.C., and Sabbadini, R.A. (2003). Factor associated with neutral sphingomyelinase activation and its role in cardiac cell death. Circulation research *92*, 589-591.

Ogretmen, B., and Hannun, Y.A. (2004). Biologically active sphingolipids in cancer pathogenesis and treatment. Nat Rev Cancer *4*, 604-616.

Ohtani, R., Tomimoto, H., Kondo, T., Wakita, H., Akiguchi, I., Shibasaki, H., and Okazaki, T. (2004). Upregulation of ceramide and its regulating mechanism in a rat model of chronic cerebral ischemia. Brain Res *1023*, 31-40.

Ott, M., Gogvadze, V., Orrenius, S., and Zhivotovsky, B. (2007). Mitochondria, oxidative stress and cell death. Apoptosis *12*, 913-922.

Pacher, P., and Hajnoczky, G. (2001). Propagation of the apoptotic signal by mitochondrial waves. Embo J *20*, 4107-4121.

Parra, V., Eisner, V., Chiong, M., Criollo, A., Moraga, F., Garcia, A., Hartel, S., Jaimovich, E., Zorzano, A., Hidalgo, C., *et al.* (2008). Changes in mitochondrial dynamics during ceramide-induced cardiomyocyte early apoptosis. Cardiovascular research *77*, 387-397.

Pastorino, J.G., Simbula, G., Yamamoto, K., Glascott, P.A., Jr., Rothman, R.J., and Farber, J.L. (1996). The cytotoxicity of tumor necrosis factor depends on induction of the mitochondrial permeability transition. The Journal of biological chemistry *271*, 29792-29798.

Pastorino, J.G., Tafani, M., Rothman, R.J., Marcinkeviciute, A., Hoek, J.B., and Farber, J.L. (1999a). Functional consequences of the sustained or transient activation by Bax of the mitochondrial permeability transition pore. The Journal of biological chemistry *274*, 31734-31739.

Pastorino, J.G., Tafani, M., Rothman, R.J., Marcinkeviciute, A., Hoek, J.B., Farber, J.L., and Marcineviciute, A. (1999b). Functional consequences of the sustained or transient activation by Bax of the mitochondrial permeability transition pore. The Journal of biological chemistry *274*, 31734-31739.

Pchejetski, D., Kunduzova, O., Dayon, A., Calise, D., Seguelas, M.H., Leducq, N., Seif, I., Parini, A., and Cuvillier, O. (2007). Oxidative stress-dependent sphingosine kinase-1 inhibition mediates monoamine oxidase A-associated cardiac cell apoptosis. Circulation research *100*, 41-49.

Perry, R.J., and Ridgway, N.D. (2005). Molecular mechanisms and regulation of ceramide transport. Biochimica et biophysica acta *1734*, 220-234.

Pettus, B.J., Chalfant, C.E., and Hannun, Y.A. (2002). Ceramide in apoptosis: an overview and current perspectives. Biochimica et biophysica acta *1585*, 114-125.

Pettus, B.J., Kroesen, B.J., Szulc, Z.M., Bielawska, A., Bielawski, J., Hannun, Y.A., and Busman, M. (2004). Quantitative measurement of different ceramide species from crude cellular extracts by normal-phase high-performance liquid chromatography coupled to atmospheric pressure ionization mass spectrometry. Rapid Commun Mass Spectrom *18*, 577-583.

Pewzner-Jung, Y., Ben-Dor, S., and Futerman, A.H. (2006). When do Lasses (longevity assurance genes) become CerS (ceramide synthases)?: Insights into the regulation of ceramide synthesis. The Journal of biological chemistry *281*, 25001-25005.

Phillips, D.C., Martin, S., Doyle, B.T., and Houghton, J.A. (2007). Sphingosine-induced apoptosis in rhabdomyosarcoma cell lines is dependent on pre-mitochondrial Bax activation and post-mitochondrial caspases. Cancer research *67*, 756-764.

Pinton, P., Ferrari, D., Rapizzi, E., Di Virgilio, F., Pozzan, T., and Rizzuto, R. (2001). The Ca2+ concentration of the endoplasmic reticulum is a key determinant of ceramide-induced apoptosis: significance for the molecular mechanism of Bcl-2 action. Embo J *20*, 2690-2701.

Quillet-Mary, A., Jaffrezou, J.P., Mansat, V., Bordier, C., Naval, J., and Laurent, G. (1997). Implication of mitochondrial hydrogen peroxide generation in ceramide-induced apoptosis. The Journal of biological chemistry *272*, 21388-21395.

Rippo, M.R., Malisan, F., Ravagnan, L., Tomassini, B., Condo, I., Costantini, P., Susin, S.A., Rufini, A., Todaro, M., Kroemer, G., *et al.* (2000). GD3 ganglioside directly targets mitochondria in a bcl-2-controlled fashion. Faseb J *14*, 2047-2054.

Ruvolo, P.P., Deng, X., Ito, T., Carr, B.K., and May, W.S. (1999). Ceramide induces Bcl2 dephosphorylation via a mechanism involving mitochondrial PP2A. The Journal of biological chemistry *274*, 20296-20300.

Scaffidi, C., Schmitz, I., Zha, J., Korsmeyer, S.J., Krammer, P.H., and Peter, M.E. (1999). Differential modulation of apoptosis sensitivity in CD95 type I and type II cells. The Journal of biological chemistry *274*, 22532-22538.

Schinzel, A.C., Takeuchi, O., Huang, Z., Fisher, J.K., Zhou, Z., Rubens, J., Hetz, C., Danial, N.N., Moskowitz, M.A., and Korsmeyer, S.J. (2005). Cyclophilin D is a component of mitochondrial permeability transition and mediates neuronal cell death after focal cerebral ischemia. Proceedings of the National Academy of Sciences of the United States of America *102*, 12005-12010.

Schissel, S.L., Jiang, X., Tweedie-Hardman, J., Jeong, T., Camejo, E.H., Najib, J., Rapp, J.H., Williams, K.J., and Tabas, I. (1998). Secretory sphingomyelinase, a product of the acid sphingomyelinase gene, can hydrolyze atherogenic lipoproteins at neutral pH. Implications for atherosclerotic lesion development. The Journal of biological chemistry *273*, 2738-2746.

Scorrano, L., Oakes, S.A., Opferman, J.T., Cheng, E.H., Sorcinelli, M.D., Pozzan, T., and Korsmeyer, S.J. (2003). BAX and BAK regulation of endoplasmic reticulum Ca2+: a control point for apoptosis. Science *300*, 135-139.

Scorrano, L., Penzo, D., Petronilli, V., Pagano, F., and Bernardi, P. (2001). Arachidonic acid causes cell death through the mitochondrial permeability transition. Implications for tumor necrosis factor-alpha aopototic signaling. The Journal of biological chemistry *276*, 12035-12040.

Scorrano, L., Petronilli, V., Di Lisa, F., and Bernardi, P. (1999). Commitment to apoptosis by GD3 ganglioside depends on opening of the mitochondrial permeability transition pore. The Journal of biological chemistry *274*, 22581-22585.

Shimeno, H., Soeda, S., Sakamoto, M., Kouchi, T., Kowakame, T., and Kihara, T. (1998). Partial purification and characterization of sphingosine N-acyltransferase (ceramide synthase) from bovine liver mitochondrion-rich fraction. Lipids *33*, 601-605.

Shimeno, H., Soeda, S., Yasukouchi, M., Okamura, N., and Nagamatsu, A. (1995). Fatty acyl-Co A: sphingosine acyltransferase in bovine brain mitochondria: its solubilization and reconstitution onto the membrane lipid liposomes. Biol Pharm Bull *18*, 1335-1339.

Sims, N.R., and Anderson, M.F. (2002). Mitochondrial contributions to tissue damage in stroke. Neurochem Int *40*, 511-526.

Siskind, L.J., and Colombini, M. (2000). The lipids C2- and C16-ceramide form large stable channels. Implications for apoptosis. The Journal of biological chemistry *275*, 38640-38644.

Siskind, L.J., Feinstein, L., Yu, T., Davis, J.S., Jones, D., Choi, J., Zuckerman, J.E., Tan, W., Hill, R.B., Hardwick, J.M., *et al.* (2008). Anti-apoptotic Bcl-2 Family Proteins Disassemble Ceramide Channels. J Biol Chem *283*, 6622-6630.

Siskind, L.J., Kolesnick, R.N., and Colombini, M. (2002). Ceramide channels increase the permeability of the mitochondrial outer membrane to small proteins. The Journal of biological chemistry *277*, 26796-26803.

Siskind, L.J., Kolesnick, R.N., and Colombini, M. (2006). Ceramide forms channels in mitochondrial outer membranes at physiologically relevant concentrations. Mitochondrion *6*, 118-125.

Snook, C.F., Jones, J.A., and Hannun, Y.A. (2006). Sphingolipid-binding proteins. Biochimica et biophysica acta *1761*, 927-946.

Sonnino, S., Prinetti, A., Mauri, L., Chigorno, V., and Tettamanti, G. (2006). Dynamic and structural properties of sphingolipids as driving forces for the formation of membrane domains. Chemical reviews *106*, 2111-2125.

Sot, J., Aranda, F.J., Collado, M.I., Goni, F.M., and Alonso, A. (2005a). Different effects of long- and short-chain ceramides on the gel-fluid and lamellar-hexagonal transitions of phospholipids: a calorimetric, NMR, and x-ray diffraction study. Biophysical journal *88*, 3368-3380.

Sot, J., Goni, F.M., and Alonso, A. (2005b). Molecular associations and surface-active properties of short- and long-N-acyl chain ceramides. Biochimica et biophysica acta *1711*, 12-19.

Spassieva, S., Seo, J.G., Jiang, J.C., Bielawski, J., Alvarez-Vasquez, F., Jazwinski, S.M., Hannun, Y.A., and Obeid, L.M. (2006). Necessary role for the Lag1p motif in (dihydro)ceramide synthase activity. J Biol Chem.

Spence, M.W., Byers, D.M., Palmer, F.B., and Cook, H.W. (1989). A new Zn2+-stimulated sphingomyelinase in fetal bovine serum. The Journal of biological chemistry *264*, 5358-5363.

Sridevi, P., Alexander, H., Laviad, E.L., Pewzner-Jung, Y., Hannink, M., Futerman, A.H., and Alexander, S. (2009). Ceramide synthase 1 is regulated by proteasomal mediated turnover. Biochimica et biophysica acta.

Stancevic, B., and Kolesnick, R. (2010). Ceramide-rich platforms in transmembrane signaling. FEBS letters *584*, 1728-1740.

Stavrovskaya, I.G., and Kristal, B.S. (2005). The powerhouse takes control of the cell: is the mitochondrial permeability transition a viable therapeutic target against neuronal dysfunction and death? Free Radic Biol Med *38*, 687-697.

Stiban, J., Caputo, L., and Colombini, M. (2008). Ceramide synthesis in the endoplasmic reticulum can permeabilize mitochondria to proapoptotic proteins. Journal of lipid research *49*, 625-634.

Stoica, B.A., Movsesyan, V.A., Lea, P.M.t., and Faden, A.I. (2003). Ceramide-induced neuronal apoptosis is associated with dephosphorylation of Akt, BAD, FKHR,

GSK-3beta, and induction of the mitochondrial-dependent intrinsic caspase pathway. Mol Cell Neurosci *22*, 365-382.

Suen, D.F., Norris, K.L., and Youle, R.J. (2008). Mitochondrial dynamics and apoptosis. Genes & development *22*, 1577-1590.

Sullards, M.C. (2000). Analysis of sphingomyelin, glucosylceramide, ceramide, sphingosine, and sphingosine 1-phosphate by tandem mass spectrometry. Methods in enzymology *312*, 32-45.

Sumitomo, M., Ohba, M., Asakuma, J., Asano, T., Kuroki, T., and Hayakawa, M. (2002). Protein kinase Cdelta amplifies ceramide formation via mitochondrial signaling in prostate cancer cells. J Clin Invest *109*, 827-836.

Szabadkai, G., and Duchen, M.R. (2008). Mitochondria: the hub of cellular Ca2+ signaling. Physiology (Bethesda, Md *23*, 84-94.

Szalai, G., Krishnamurthy, R., and Hajnoczky, G. (1999). Apoptosis driven by IP(3)-linked mitochondrial calcium signals. Embo J *18*, 6349-6361.

Tabas, I. (1999). Secretory sphingomyelinase. Chemistry and physics of lipids *102*, 123-130.

Taha, T.A., Mullen, T.D., and Obeid, L.M. (2006). A house divided: Ceramide, sphingosine, and sphingosine-1-phosphate in programmed cell death. Biochimica et biophysica acta *1758*, 2027-2036.

Takahashi, K., Ginis, I., Nishioka, R., Klimanis, D., Barone, F.C., White, R.F., Chen, Y., and Hallenbeck, J.M. (2004). Glucosylceramide synthase activity and ceramide levels are modulated during cerebral ischemia after ischemic preconditioning. J Cereb Blood Flow Metab *24*, 623-627.

Tani, M., Igarashi, Y., and Ito, M. (2005). Involvement of neutral ceramidase in ceramide metabolism at the plasma membrane and in extracellular milieu. J Biol Chem *280*, 36592-36600.

Tani, M., Ito, M., and Igarashi, Y. (2007). Ceramide/sphingosine/sphingosine 1-phosphate metabolism on the cell surface and in the extracellular space. Cellular signalling *19*, 229-237.

Therade-Matharan, S., Laemmel, E., Carpentier, S., Obata, Y., Levade, T., Duranteau, J., and Vicaut, E. (2005). Reactive oxygen species production by mitochondria in endothelial cells exposed to reoxygenation after hypoxia and glucose depletion is mediated by ceramide. Am J Physiol Regul Integr Comp Physiol *289*, R1756-1762.

Tomiuk, S., Zumbansen, M., and Stoffel, W. (2000). Characterization and subcellular localization of murine and human magnesium-dependent neutral sphingomyelinase. The Journal of biological chemistry *275*, 5710-5717.

Tserng, K.Y., and Griffin, R. (2003). Quantitation and molecular species determination of diacylglycerols, phosphatidylcholines, ceramides, and sphingomyelins with gas chromatography. Anal Biochem *323*, 84-93.

Ullman, M.D., and Radin, N.S. (1972). Enzymatic formation of hydroxy ceramides and comparison with enzymes forming nonhydroxy ceramides. Arch Biochem Biophys *152*, 767-777.

Vaena de Avalos, S., Okamoto, Y., and Hannun, Y.A. (2004). Activation and localization of inositol phosphosphingolipid phospholipase C, Isc1p, to the mitochondria during growth of Saccharomyces cerevisiae. J Biol Chem *279*, 11537-11545.

Vander Heiden, M.G., Chandel, N.S., Williamson, E.K., Schumacker, P.T., and Thompson, C.B. (1997). Bcl-xL regulates the membrane potential and volume homeostasis of mitochondria. Cell *91*, 627-637.

Venkataraman, K., and Futerman, A.H. (2002). Do longevity assurance genes containing Hox domains regulate cell development via ceramide synthesis? FEBS letters *528*, 3-4.

Votyakova, T.V., and Reynolds, I.J. (2001). DeltaPsi(m)-Dependent and -independent production of reactive oxygen species by rat brain mitochondria. Journal of neurochemistry *79*, 266-277.

Weston, C.R., and Davis, R.J. (2007). The JNK signal transduction pathway. Current opinion in cell biology *19*, 142-149.

Won, J.S., and Singh, I. (2006). Sphingolipid signaling and redox regulation. Free radical biology & medicine *40*, 1875-1888.

Wooten-Blanks, L.G., Song, P., Senkal, C.E., and Ogretmen, B. (2007). Mechanisms of ceramide-mediated repression of the human telomerase reverse transcriptase promoter via deacetylation of Sp3 by histone deacetylase 1. Faseb J *21*, 3386-3397.

Wu, B.X., Rajagopalan, V., Roddy, P.L., Clarke, C.J., and Hannun, Y.A. (2010). Identification and characterization of murine mitochondria-associated neutral sphingomyelinase (MA-nSMase), the mammalian sphingomyelin phosphodiesterase 5. The Journal of biological chemistry *285*, 17993-18002.

Xin, M., and Deng, X. (2006). Protein phosphatase 2A enhances the proapoptotic function of Bax through dephosphorylation. The Journal of biological chemistry *281*, 18859-18867.

Xu, X., Bittman, R., Duportail, G., Heissler, D., Vilcheze, C., and London, E. (2001). Effect of the structure of natural sterols and sphingolipids on the formation of ordered sphingolipid/sterol domains (rafts). Comparison of cholesterol to plant, fungal, and disease-associated sterols and comparison of sphingomyelin, cerebrosides, and ceramide. The Journal of biological chemistry *276*, 33540-33546.

Yabu, T., Shimuzu, A., and Yamashita, M. (2009). A novel mitochondrial sphingomyelinase in zebrafish cells. J Biol Chem *284*, 20349-20363.

Yu, J., Novgorodov, S.A., Chudakova, D., Zhu, H., Bielawska, A., Bielawski, J., Obeid, L.M., Kindy, M.S., and Gudz, T.I. (2007). JNK3 signaling pathway activates ceramide synthase leading to mitochondrial dysfunction. J Biol Chem *282*, 25940-25949.

Yu, Z.F., Nikolova-Karakashian, M., Zhou, D., Cheng, G., Schuchman, E.H., and Mattson, M.P. (2000). Pivotal role for acidic sphingomyelinase in cerebral ischemia-induced ceramide and cytokine production, and neuronal apoptosis. J Mol Neurosci *15*, 85-97.

Yuan, H., Williams, S.D., Adachi, S., Oltersdorf, T., and Gottlieb, R.A. (2003). Cytochrome c dissociation and release from mitochondria by truncated Bid and ceramide. Mitochondrion *2*, 237-244.

Yuan H, W.S., Adachi S, Oltersdorf T, Gottlieb RA (2003). Cytochrome c dissociation and release from mitochondria by trancated Bid and ceramide. Mitochondrion *2*, 237-244.

Zager, R.A., Conrad, S., Lochhead, K., Sweeney, E.A., Igarashi, Y., and Burkhart, K.M. (1998). Altered sphingomyelinase and ceramide expression in the setting of ischemic and nephrotoxic acute renal failure. Kidney international *53*, 573-582.

Zager, R.A., Iwata, M., Conrad, D.S., Burkhart, K.M., and Igarashi, Y. (1997). Altered ceramide and sphingosine expression during the induction phase of ischemic acute renal failure. Kidney international *52*, 60-70.

Zamzami, N., Marchetti, P., Castedo, M., Decaudin, D., Macho, A., Hirsch, T., Susin, S.A., Petit, P.X., Mignotte, B., and Kroemer, G. (1995). Sequential reduction of mitochondrial transmembrane potential and generation of reactive oxygen species in early programmed cell death. J Exp Med *182*, 367-377.

Zeidan, Y.H., Wu, B.X., Jenkins, R.W., Obeid, L.M., and Hannun, Y.A. (2008). A novel role for protein kinase Cdelta-mediated phosphorylation of acid sphingomyelinase in UV light-induced mitochondrial injury. Faseb J *22*, 183-193.

Zhang, D.X., Fryer, R.M., Hsu, A.K., Zou, A.P., Gross, G.J., Campbell, W.B., and Li, P.L. (2001). Production and metabolism of ceramide in normal and ischemic-reperfused myocardium of rats. Basic research in cardiology *96*, 267-274.

Zhang, J., Alter, N., Reed, J.C., Borner, C., Obeid, L.M., and Hannun, Y.A. (1996). Bcl-2 interrupts the ceramide-mediated pathway of cell death. Proceedings of the National Academy of Sciences of the United States of America *93*, 5325-5328.

Zhang, X., Li, B., Zhang, Y., and Liu, J. (2008). Ceramide induces release of mitochondrial proapoptotic proteins in caspase-dependent and -independent manner in HT-29 cells. Science in China *51*, 66-71.

Zundel, W., Swiersz, L.M., and Giaccia, A. (2000). Caveolin 1-mediated regulation of receptor tyrosine kinase-associated phosphatidylinositol 3-kinase activity by ceramide. Molecular and cellular biology *20*, 1507-1514.

Part 3

Novel Approaches to Neuroprotection

14

Neuroprotection in Animal Models of Global Cerebral Ischemia

Miguel Cervantes[1], Ignacio González-Burgos[2], Graciela Letechipía-Vallejo[1], María Esther Olvera-Cortés[3] and Gabriela Moralí[4]

[1]*Laboratorio de Neurociencias. Facultad de Ciencias Médicas y Biológicas "Dr. Ignacio Chávez", Universidad Michoacana de San Nicolás de Hidalgo, Morelia, Michoacán*

[2]*Laboratorio de Psicobiología, División de Neurociencias, Centro de Investigación, Biomédica de Occidente Instituto Mexicano del Seguro Social, Guadalajara, Jalisco*

[3]*Laboratorio de Neurofisiología Experimental, Centro de Investigación Biomédica de Michoacán, Instituto Mexicano del Seguro Social, Morelia, Michoacán*

[4]*Unidad de Investigación Médica en Farmacología, UMAE Hospital de Especialidades, CMN S XXI, Instituto Mexicano del Seguro Social, México, D.F.*

Mexico

1. Introduction

The present chapter deals with some of the main lines of experimental research on global cerebral ischemia, through which a substantial knowledge has been generated, that has contributed in an important measure both to the understanding of the mechanisms of cerebral damage induced by ischemia, and of the subsequent post-ischemic neuroregenerative and cerebral plastic processes taking place in the remaining or newly differentiated neurons. Thus, data obtained from experimental designs in animal models of global cerebral ischemia, on key molecular and cellular events triggered by this condition, have provided a substantial background from which neuroprotection can be rationally approached, in order to develop strategies aimed to antagonize, to interrupt, or to slow the sequence of injurious biochemical and molecular events that would result in irreversible ischemic injury; as well as to promote brain repair and plasticity processes which can favor functional preservation or recovery after global cerebral ischemia.

Transient global cerebral ischemia, which can mainly occur during cardiac arrest and cardiopulmonary resuscitation, but also during asphyxiation, hypotensive shock, or extracorporeal circulation, is a pathophysiological condition that is associated with great morbidity and requires intensive medical treatment (Madl & Holzer, 2004). In certain clinical situations (surgical repair of the thoracic aorta, complex congenital heart lesions, and also during implantable cardiac defibrillator testing in patients with drug-resistant ventricular fibrillation) the possible occurrence of transient global cerebral ischemia, and some neuroprotective procedures, can be anticipated (Hogue et al., 2008); however, this is not the case of cardiac arrest.

Cardiopulmonary arrest remains as one among the most frequent causes of death and disability around the world. Despite quick emergency responses and better techniques of defibrillation, the chances of survival following cardiac arrest are still poor, between 20-50% of patients in whom cardiopulmonary resuscitation is attempted. A complex pathophysiological condition is elicited by cardiac arrest, since it results in whole-body ischemia which compromises systemic circulatory homeostasis and cerebral, pulmonary, renal, and cardiac functions. In the course of cardiac arrest, global cerebral blood flow is severely impaired with the consequent risk of ischemic damage of brain cells, which magnitude seems to be associated with the cumulative time staying in cardiac arrest. Thus, most deaths (60%) during the post-resuscitation period have been attributed to extensive brain injury and neuronal damage that develops as a consequence of alteration of cell processes triggered by cerebral ischemia and reperfusion, during and after cardiac arrest. In addition, it is known that transient interruption or reduction of blood flow in the whole brain, are main causes of permanent brain damage and functional disruptions in human beings, and near around a half of surviving patients show permanent impairment of cognitive functions, such as learning and memory, attention, and executive functioning, and only a small proportion (less than 10%) of those survivors are able to reassume their former usual life styles (Geocardin et al., 2008; Grubb et al., 2000; Krause et al, 1986; Schneider et al., 2009). Thus, development of effective cytoprotective therapies that may be common to the organs more sensitive to cardiac arrest, such as heart or brain, could result in improvement of survival and better outcome following this whole ischemic episode (Karanjia & Geocardin, 2011).

Experimental protocols aimed to gain relevant information regarding those pathophysiological phenomena leading to cerebral damage elicited by ischemia have included, since long time, the use of animal models of cerebral ischemia, in order to support better diagnostic, prophylactic and clinical-therapeutic procedures for ischemic cerebrovascular diseases in human beings (Ginsberg & Busto, 1989; Gupta & Briyal, 2004; Hartman et al., 2005, Hossmann, 2008; Traystman, 2003). Thus, biochemical, electrophysiological, histological, and behavioral parameters of ischemic brain damage have been included in experimental designs to evaluate the efficacy and safety of pharmacological and non pharmacological neuroprotective procedures against brain injury resulting from the significant reduction of blood supply to the whole brain, in several animal models of global cerebral ischemia.

Even though a great number of pharmacological agents have proven to exert effective neuroprotective actions against cellular events leading to ischemic brain injury in experimental models of global cerebral ischemia, unfortunately they have not had enough clinical relevance to date. On the other hand, after evaluation of its effectiveness as a neuroprotective strategy in animal models of global cerebral ischemia, hypothermia has been tested in clinical trials in patients having suffered cardiac arrest, the most frequent cause of global cerebral ischemia in human beings (Castren et al., 2009; Geocardin et al., 2008; Greer, 2006; Inamasu et al., 2010; Knapp et al., 2011; Seder & Jarrah, 2008,). It seems that new and better strategies to translate preclinical data supporting the potential clinical usefulness of neuroprotective drugs to clinical trials, must be developed.

2. Animal models of global cerebral ischemia

Animal models of global cerebral ischemia allow studying, at different levels of biological organization of the central nervous system, the development and temporal course of those processes that may result in irreversible ischemic neuronal damage, as well as in the subsequent cell repair and plasticity underlying either permanent cerebral functional impairment or recovery as a result of intrinsic brain mechanisms or neuroprotective procedures. Thus, animal-related factors (species, strain, age, sex, co-morbidities), animal-model-related factors (choice of ischemic model, anesthetic procedures, duration of ischemia, reperfusion, survival, possibility of monitoring of physiological parameters), selective vulnerability of specific neuron types in several brain structures, outcome assessment (histopathological, biochemical, functional, parameters of brain injury in specific cerebral structures), short- or long-term experimental design, pharmacological characteristics of the presumptive neuroprotective agent itself, timing and dose-response of neuroprotective drug administration with reference to starting and ending of the ischemic episode, may account for the relevance of results from these investigations.

Models of cerebral ischemia have been also developed in *in vitro* models, in particular brain tissue slices and neuronal cultures, allowing to study in detail the cellular phenomena leading either to neuronal damage or to neural recovery and plasticity after ischemia (Benítez-King, 2006; Goldberg & Choi, 1993; Kasai et al., 2003; Whittingham et al., 1984).

Several conditions have to be fulfilled by animal models of global cerebral ischemia in order to become appropriate counterparts of these pathophysiological conditions in human beings, as well as to yield reliable and valid results in supporting clinical therapeutic approaches. Thus, it could be expected that in animal models of global cerebral ischemia the ischemic episode can be induced in a constant and reproducible manner: low variation for the extent, temporal course, and magnitude of the resulting ischemic brain injury under specific experimental conditions, including duration of the ischemic episode; easy control of possible deviations of important physiological variables, feasible neurological, neuropathological, and functional evaluations; lack of influence of anesthetic drugs and surgical procedures on the mechanisms of brain injury, brain recovery and/or neuroprotection; short-, intermediate- and long-term follow up of the outcome; and economical, easily available experimental animals of those species better accepted by public animal welfare concerns to be used in experimental protocols of cerebral ischemia and neuroprotection.

2.1 Main animal models of global cerebral ischemia

Models of global cerebral ischemia have been performed in both large (monkeys, sheep, dogs, pigs, cats, rabbits) and small animals (gerbils, rats, mice). Among these, both advantages and disadvantages can be recognized according to several practical aspects: main objectives of the model; monitoring procedures to be used; nature, number and timing of simultaneous parameters to be recorded in order to evaluate the ischemic brain injury and recovery; degree of similarity of structural and functional characteristics of brains of experimental animals to those of the human brain; and updated ethical outlines for the use of experimental animals in research protocols.

Since the whole brain is exposed to transient ischemia and reperfusion as a result of cardiac arrest and the subsequent cardiorespiratory resuscitation to allow survival in human beings, animal models of global cerebral ischemia have been designed attempting to totally or partially mimic the consequences of this clinical condition on the brain (Ginsberg & Busto, 1989; Gupta & Briyal, 2004; Mc Bean & Kelly, 1998; Traystman, 2003), which are the main cause of neuronal injury to selective vulnerable brain regions, and neurological or cognitive impairment, in human beings.

Cardiac arrest (induced by injection of KCl, electric shock, thoracic compression, asphyxia, and mechanical obstruction of the ascending aorta) followed by cardiopulmonary resuscitation (by artificial ventilation, closed chest massage and electrical defibrillation), both in large experimental animals (formerly a common model, but nowadays rarely used) and also in rodents, has been a technique to produce global cerebral ischemia in an attempt to closely resemble the clinical situation of cardiac arrest, including complete ischemia and reperfusion in renal, splachnic and other peripheral organs. This technique seemed to be an excellent model of global cerebral ischemia, but it is expensive when large experimental animals are used, and intensive care (cardiopulmonary support under unconsciousness, control of blood pressure, pH, body fluids, and temperature) must be provided to the animals, especially during the first 24-48 h after the cardiac arrest. Complete acute global cerebral ischemia during cardiac arrest (8-20 min) and a variable period of incomplete cerebral ischemia during reperfusion, even after a successful cardiopulmonary resuscitation, as well as damage in those brain structures most vulnerable to ischemia, can be expected from this model (Berkowitz, et al., 1991; Bleyaert et al., 1978; Dave et al., 2004; Hossmann, 2008; Katz et al., 1995; Kofler et al., 2004; Radovsky et al., 1995; Safar et al., 1976; Todd et al., 1982). In particular, models of global cerebral ischemia in mice are currently of interest because of the availability of transgenic and knock-out strains for identification of cellular pathways of ischemic damage, and for neuroprotection studies.

Several other animal models of global cerebral ischemia have been designed in cats, monkeys, gerbils, mice, and rats, in order to circumscribe to the brain those harmful effects of the reduced blood flow that follows a cardiac arrest, avoiding affecting other vital organs in a whole body ischemia condition, as can be expected from animal models of cardiac arrest (Ginsberg & Busto, 1989).

Decapitation in small animals has been used as a model of global cerebral ischemia, only allowing the study of the immediate alterations of some biochemical and metabolic parameters elicited by ischemia in the brain contained into the head (Abe et al., 1983; Ikeda et al., 1986; Lowry et al., 1964; Yoshida et al., 1985).

A neck tourniquet or a neck cuff, whether they include or not arterial hypotension, have also been used to produce global cerebral ischemia in rats, cats, dogs, or monkeys. However, these techniques lead to variable ischemic outcomes since the produced ischemia may not be complete because of a remaining cerebral blood flow through the vertebral arteries, as well as complications due to vagal compression and venous congestion (Chopp et al., 1987, 1988; Grenell 1946; Nemoto et al., 1977; Sheller et al., 1992; Siemkowits & Gjedde, 1980; Siemkowitz & Hansen, 1978).

Reduction of cerebral blood flow near to zero has been accomplished in cats and monkeys, by occlusion of the innominate and left subclavian arteries near the aortic arch, and pharmacologically induced hypotension (below 80 mm Hg), without involvement of other organs in the ischemic phenomena. However, these experimental animals require intensive care procedures to their survival, and studies of long-term recovery are difficult to achieve (Bodsch et al., 1986; Clavier et al., 1994; Hossmann, 1971; Hossmann & Grose Ophoff, 1986; Zimmerman & Hossmann, 1975).

Gerbils usually lack of a common posterior communicating artery connecting the carotid and vertebro-basilar arterial system. Thus, the bilateral common carotid artery occlusion results in a reduction of global cerebral blood flow near to zero and injury of the most vulnerable brain structures (hippocampal CA1 pyramidal neurons after 5 min of ischemia) in most animals (Kirino, 1982). This model of forebrain global cerebral ischemia may fail in some animals in which a complete Willis circle persists, and the high susceptibility of gerbils to seizures may influence the ischemic outcome.

The four-vessel occlusion (4-VO) and the two-vessel occlusion with hypotension (2-VO) models in rats became, nowadays, the most widely used animal models that simulate the reduction of blood flow, as it would occur by effect of cardiac arrest, on the forebrain. The 4-VO model (Ginsberg & Busto, 1989; Pulsinelli & Brierley 1979; Pulsinelli & Buchan 1988; Pulsinelli & Duffy 1983; Pulsinelli et al., 1982) provides a method of reversible forebrain ischemia in awake, freely moving rats (but also in anesthetized rats). In a first step of the model procedures, vertebral arteries are permanently occluded and 24 or 48 hours later, the ischemia is produced through transient (10 - 20 min) occlusion of the common carotid arteries under light inhaled anesthesia so that the ischemic episode occurs while the animal is unanesthetized. Loss of the righting reflex, and unconsciousness persisting for at least 20 min after the onset of reperfusion have to occur for each animal to be included in the study. In this way, a reduction in cerebral blood flow to less than 5% of control values, which is followed by hyperemia during 5 to 15 min after reperfusion, and subsequent hypoperfusion lasting for 24 hr result in main ischemic neuronal damage in hippocampus, neocortex and striatum, along hours to days after ischemia, its magnitude relating to the duration of the ischemia. The effects of this insult are, however, quite variable between rat strains, as well as between those individuals surviving (survival rate, 50-75%) after having fulfilled the criteria required to be included in the experimental groups. Similar consequences in selectively vulnerable neurons in specific brain structures result from the 2-VO model of forebrain ischemia, in which bilateral common carotid artery occlusion and systemic hypotension (blood withdrawal and subsequent return with or without pharmacological procedures, leading to arterial blood pressure below 50 mm Hg) are combined to provoke reversible forebrain ischemia (Eklof & Siesjo 1972a, 1972b; Smith et al., 1984a, 1984b).

Mouse models of global cerebral ischemia have been developed through bilateral common carotid occlusion and controlled pulmonary ventilation (Traystman, 2003).

It is known that animal models of global cerebral ischemia require adequate control of certain variables, such as careful control of animal's temperature and blood glucose concentration, in order to achieve consistent pathophysiological effects and brain injury (Colbourne & Corbett, 1994; Lipton, 1999; Siemkowicz, 1981; Siemkowicz.& Gjedde 1980). Hyperthermia and hyperglycemia increase brain injury, while hypothermia results in neuroprotection by itself.

3. Cellular mechanisms of neuronal injury, neuronal repair and plasticity

Models of global cerebral ischemia in experimental animals, as well as *in vitro* models, in particular brain tissue slices and neuronal cultures, have allowed to study in detail the cellular phenomena leading either to neuronal damage, or to neural repair and plasticity after ischemia. From these studies it has been known that mechanisms of cellular damage, repair and plasticity may be the same, in general, both if reduction of blood flow to the brain tissue results from occlusion of one of the main cerebral arteries as would occur in focal ischemia, and if it is the result of reduction of blood flow to the whole brain as it would occur after a cardiorrespiratory arrest.

3.1 Cellular mechanisms of neuronal injury

Interruption of blood flow and hence, of glucose and oxygen supply to the brain, results in an immediate severe energy failure in terms of ATP depletion that leads to alterations of the cell membrane ionic gradients and a severe breakdown in cellular homeostasis. Several mechanisms of neuronal damage are triggered and evolve both in cascade and as parallel pathways (Gwag et al, 2002; Lakhan et al, 2009; Lipton, 1999; Mehta et al, 2007; Schneider et al, 2009; Sugawara et al, 2004; Warner et al., 2004). In particular, a massive accumulation of intracellular calcium and sodium occurs because of failure of their energy-dependent efflux processes, and anoxic depolarization. This further leads to accumulation of lactate and hydrogen ions, and as a consequence, to decreased pH.

As a result of anoxic depolarization, excitatory aminoacids such as glutamate and aspartate are released, activating ligand-gated calcium and sodium channels with a further influx of these ions into the cells. Calcium is also released from intracellular pools, and its excessive, unregulated intracellular overload causes direct Ca^{2+}-dependent activation of lipases, proteases, and endonucleases leading to breakdown of structural and functional proteins, and damage to cytoskeleton and macromolecules including nucleic acids. A result of these phenomena is, among others, cell membrane lipoperoxidation.

Excessive intracellular calcium activate abnormal cell processes promoting functional derangements of mitochondria and an increased production of free radicals, exceeding the neuronal antioxidant reserves, and imposing risks to the structural and functional integrity of neuronal cells. The brain is highly susceptible to oxidative damage as a consequence of its high lipid and metal content, as well as other biochemical characteristics (Margaill et al., 2005; Reiter et al., 2005; Warner el al., 2004). Reperfusion and reoxygenation of the ischemic tissue, which must be reestablished within minutes in an effort to prevent severe neurological damage and favor survival of individuals, also may provide chemical substrates for further increasing cellular alterations, neuronal death and neurological deficits (Margaill et al., 2005).

Free radicals also contribute to the breakdown of the blood-brain barrier and brain edema. Reactive oxygen and nitrogen species including superoxide, hydroxyl free radical, and peroxylnitrite anion are also important mediators of inflammatory tissue damage, of activation and secretion of inflammatory cytokines such as tumor necrosis factor α, interleukin-1, and interleukin-6, and of expression of cyclo-oxigenase (COX)-2, and inducible nitric oxide synthase generating nitric oxide that also contributes to neuronal damage. These changes favor inflammatory reactions soon after cerebral ischemia/reperfusion (Barone & Feuerstein, 1999; Lakhan et al, 2009; Lipton, 1999; Mehta et al, 2007).

Calcium overload may additionally lead to mitochondrial damage and trigger an apoptotic cascade. The pro-apoptotic cascade involves nuclear factor κB- and p53-dependent pathways, changes in the Bcl-2 to Bax ratio, opening of the mitochondrial transition pore, release of cytochrome *c*, and activation of caspases (Chan, 2001; Chinopoulos & Adam-Vizi, 2006). In addition, caspase-independent pathways may also contribute to neuronal apoptosis.

Several gene families such as immediate early genes, heat-shock proteins, and inflammation-and apoptosis-related genes, are known to be differentially expressed during cerebral ischemia, and some neuropathologic processes triggered by ischemia seem to be mediated in part by alterations of molecular transcriptional and translational activities (Mehta et al, 2007).

Activation of DNA fragmentation enzymes and energy-consuming DNA repair enzymes, finally lead to DNA breakdown, interruption of protein synthesis, and cell death (Iadecola & Alexander, 2001; Leker & Shohami, 2002).

In addition to the above mentioned cellular processes of ischemic damage, brain ischemia/reperfusion may also trigger cellular mechanisms for neuronal repair, and functional recovery through neuronal plasticity involving remaining neurons in vulnerable damaged or undamaged brain structures (Barone & Feuerstein, 1999; Bendel et al., 2005; Crepel et al., 2003; Hurtado et al., 2006; Jourdain et al., 2002; Ruan et al., 2006). The different ischemia/reperfusion induced cellular mechanisms leading either to brain injury and neuronal death, or to neuronal repair, as well as plasticity and brain functional recovery, may occur in a sequential or simultaneous manner. Their latencies and temporal course, from minutes to weeks, are important references in attempting to establish their differential relevance in those critical periods for neuronal damage and death, as well as the "window of opportunity" for specific neuroprotective procedures (Barone & Feuerstein, 1999; Lipton, 1999; Leker & Shohami, 2002; Pulsinelli et al., 1997).

3.2 Differential neuronal vulnerability in animal models of global cerebral ischemia

Brain injury is expected to occur when cerebral blood flow is reduced to less than 10-20% of the normal value; the greater the reduction and/or longer lasting, the worst damage. Under these conditions, damage to specific brain structures due to immediate or delayed death of highly vulnerable neuronal groups, including the pyramidal neurons of the CA1 subfield of the hippocampus, and to a lesser degree those in layers 3 and 5 of the cerebral cortex, the Purkinje cells of the cerebellum, and spiny neurons in the striatum, take place after global cerebral ischemia (Ginsberg & Busto, 1989; Pulsinelli, 1985). Experimental models of global cerebral ischemia have allowed to know some neuronal characteristics that seem to account for selective vulnerability to ischemia, including a high density of excitatory glutamatergic synapses; low antioxidant enzyme reserves; high content of transition metals; increased expression of pro-apoptotic Bax protein; thus leading to differential susceptibility of some cell processes (Ca^{2+} homeostasis, oxidative-antioxidative balance, functional mitochondrial stability) to become out of physiological control under ischemia (Arai et al., 2001; Araki et al., 1989; Chen et al., 1996; Lipton 1999; Schmidt-Kastner et al., 2001; Sugawara et al., 1999). Brain injury after global ischemia/reperfusion is finally evidenced by neuronal death, affecting the neuronal population, circuit connectivity and functioning in specific brain structures involved in the neural integration of cognitive brain functions and behavior.

3.3 Cellular mechanisms of neuronal plasticity and repair

Cellular mechanisms of neuronal repair and plasticity have been observed to occur in vulnerable brain structures in which damage or death of neurons resulted from a sequence of pathophysiological phenomena triggered by global cerebral ischemia and the subsequent reperfusion. Thus, structural and functional characteristics of those neuronal components of circuits in the hippocampus and prefrontal cortex, which are identified, among others, as highly vulnerable to ischemia, and their correlation with the integration of specific cerebral functions (mainly cognitive functions) after global cerebral ischemia, have been analyzed. In this sense, short- and long-term structural alterations have been shown to occur in the remaining pyramidal neurons of the hippocampus after ischemia; thus, axonal degeneration as well as reduction of dendritic length and arborizations, of number and shape of dendritic spines, and of number of synapses, are usually related to impairment of cognitive functions and recognized as degenerative changes. By contrast, cytoarchitectural adjustments such as axonal and dendritic sprouting, increase of number of dendritic spines and synapses, changes in the relative proportion of spine types, are interpreted as compensatory plastic responses of surviving neurons. They contribute to neuronal circuit remodeling and functional recovery, and have been correlated with preservation of cognitive functions after the ischemic insult, even in absence of neuroprotective procedures (Briones et al., 2006; Jourdain et al., 2002; Mudrick & Baimbridge, 1989; Neigh et al., 2004; Onodera et al., 1990; Ruan et al., 2006; Skibo & Nikonenko, 2010; Sorra & Harris, 2000). In addition, neurogenesis and integration of newly differentiated neurons into neuronal circuits in the Ammon's horn may contribute to recovery of hippocampal-dependent cognitive functions (Bendel et al., 2005; Bernabeu & Sharp, 2000).

Similarly, reductions of dendritic length, arborization, and dendritic spine density have also been described, among various cytoarchitectural adjustments, in sensorymotor cortex pyramidal neurons following global cerebral ischemia (Akulinin et al., 1997, 1998, 2004). These cytoarchitectural alterations could be influenced by the extent of neuronal remaining connections; thus, either reduction or increase of afferent connections may result in changes in dendritic arborizations and spine density (Fiala et al., 2002; Johansson & Belinchenko, 2002). It has been emphasized the functional relevance of neuronal connections from the hippocampus to the prefrontal cortex for synaptogenesis and neuronal plasticity accounting for learning and memory (González-Burgos, 2009; Laroche et al., 2000). Thus, a permanent deafferentation of pyramidal neurons at cortical layer V after the extensive reduction of pyramidal neuron population of the CA1 subfield of the Ammon's horn as expected to occur after global ischemia (Letechipía-Vallejo et al., 2007), may lead to changes in neuronal activity, which may in turn affect the cytoarchitectural characteristics of pyramidal prefrontal cortex neurons (García-Chávez et al., 2008; Wellman & Sengelaub, 1991).

These dendritic restructuring (Neigh el al., 2004; Ruan el al., 2006) and reactive synaptogenesis (Briones et al., 2005; Crepel et al., 2003; Jourdain et al., 2002, Kovalenko et al., 2006) among other phenomena including the activation of a variety of potential growth-promoting processes (Arvidsson et al., 2001; Gobbo & O´Mara, 2004; Schmidt-Kastner et al., 2001), that occur in neurons surviving to the ischemic insult in vulnerable brain structures, seem to be a part of mechanisms of adaptive changes, probably accounting for neuronal conditions favoring synaptic plasticity and functional recovery. In fact, a long-term progressive continuous plastic reorganization of the dendritic tree and dendritic spines, initially altered by acute global cerebral ischemia, has been shown to occur in pyramidal neurons at layers 3 and 5 of the sensorymotor cortex of the rat (Akulinin et al., 1997, 1998, 2004).

Thus, preservation or recovery of hippocampal- and pre-frontal cortex- dependent functions after global cerebral ischemia, may involve long-term cytoarchitectural modifications in those remaining hippocampal CA1 and prefronto-cortical (layers 3 and 5) pyramidal neurons, since their morpho-functional organization is critical for normal learning and memory performance (Block, 1999; McDonald & White, 1993; McNamara & Skelton, 1993; Olsen et al., 1994; Olvera-Cortés et al., 2002; Silva et al., 1998), on the basis of the major role played by the CA1 region for the output of information flowing through the hippocampus, via the tri-synaptic circuit (Herreras et al., 1987). It is well known that the prefrontal cortex is directly involved in the organization of sequenced motor actions during working-memory performance (Fuster, 1999; I. Lee & Kesner, 2003), and that hippocampal projections supply of spatial information to the prefrontal cortex allowing suitability of motor responses in the spatial context (Jung et al., 1998). These phenomena may be altered not only by gross lesions of the prefrontal cortex, but fine alterations of its neuronal circuits may also result in impairment of the spatial working memory (Fritts et al., 1998; Lambe et al., 2000; I. Lee & Kesner, 2003; Olvera-Cortés et al., 2001; Taylor et al., 2003). Experimental data have shown that variations in cognitive behavioral performance are related to plastic changes in dendritic spines (Pérez-Vega et al., 2000). In addition, excitatory information flows mostly through dendritic spines-mediated synaptic contacts (Gray, 1959), which are highly sensitive to electrical stimulation and yet to mnemonic activity-related electrical phenomena (Harris, 1999; Hartman et al., 2005; Onodera et al., 1990).

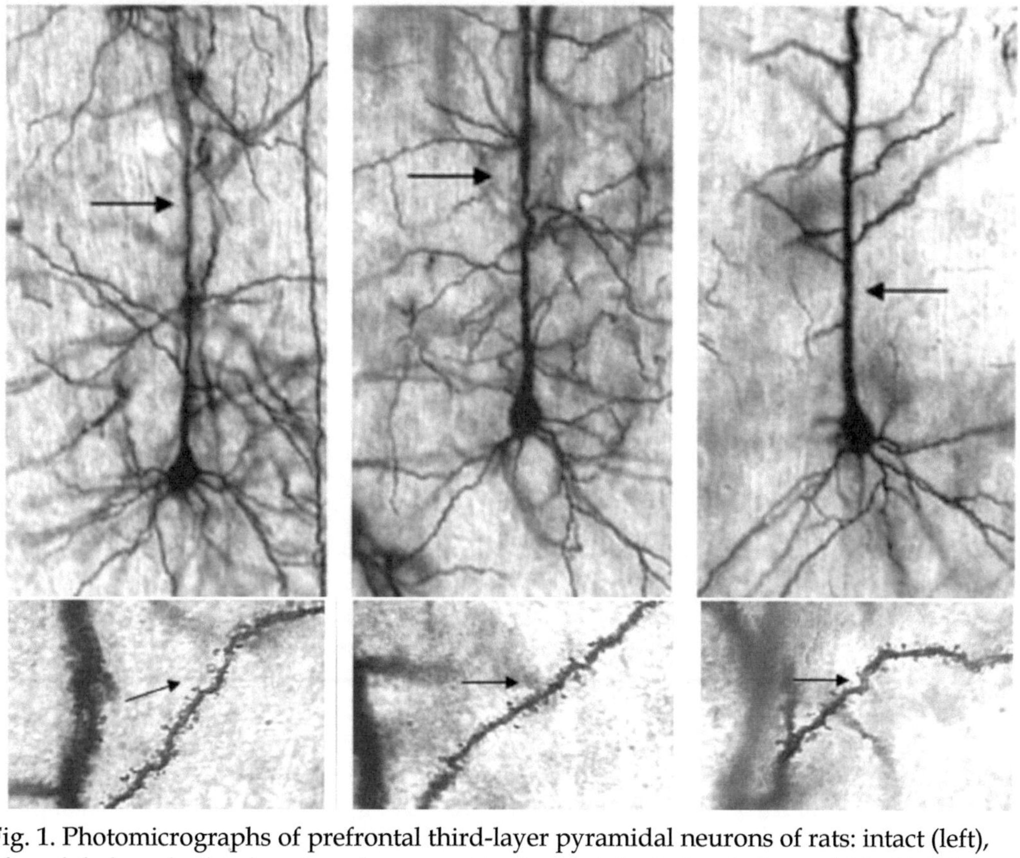

Fig. 1. Photomicrographs of prefrontal third-layer pyramidal neurons of rats: intact (left), after global cerebral ischemia and neuroprotective melatonin (centre) or vehicle (right) treatment. Note the reduction in dendritic arborization protruding from the apical dendrite, and dendritic spine reduction (arrows) in the ischemic and non treated cell in comparison with neurons from intact, and ischemia melatonin treated rats.
(Modified from: García-Chávez et al., 2008).

Since long-term preservation of the neuronal substrate in cerebral vulnerable structures underlying functional recovery after cerebral ischemia has been considered to be a major end point of neuroprotective strategies (STAIR, 1999) it can be expected that experimental designs for neuroprotection studies may lead to reliable interpretations of the efficiency of neuroprotective agents, in view of the proven capability of intrinsic cerebral mechanisms to promote , by themselves, neuronal repair and plasticity after ischemia.
Some neuronal proteins that are involved in structural and functional aspects of synaptic connectivity and neuronal circuits remodeling have been evaluated as parameters of ischemic damage and neuroprotection. In this sense, synaptophysin has been shown to be reduced in the frontal motor and temporal cortex of human beings that have been survived for 1 week to 1 year after a cardiac arrest (Akulinin et al., 1998). Besides, a reduction of synaptophysin 2, Munc-18-interacting proteins, 1-3 days after global cerebral ischemia in mice has been related to delayed neuronal death (Nishimura et al., 2000). On the other hand it has been proposed that progesterone-induced increase (3-35 days after ischemia) in the expression of synaptophysin and growth-associated protein 43, and the effects of venlafaxine preventing the decrease of synaptophysin, in the rat hippocampus are evidences of the neuroprotective effects of these drugs (Fang et al., 2010; Zhao et al., 2011).

4. Approaches to neuroprotection in animal models of global cerebral ischemia

The experimental approach to neuroprotection aimed to influence, through pharmacological and non pharmacological procedures, those early and late neural phenomena accounting either for brain damage or for neuronal repair, plasticity and functional recovery after global cerebral ischemia and reperfusion, has resulted in a considerable amount of reliable information along the last 40 years.
Different strategies of neuroprotection attempting to prevent, reduce, or stop the progress of the ischemic brain damage have been assayed in animal models of global cerebral ischemia, under the premise of an opposition relationship between the mechanism(s) of action of the presumptive neuroprotective drugs or non pharmacological procedures, and the pathophysiological mechanisms of brain damage, which has been maintained as targets of neuroprotective strategies.
Neuroprotection studies in animal models of global cerebral ischemia have maintained the main objective of support proposals of pharmacological and non-pharmacological neuroprotective procedures to be incorporated as a matter for clinical trials aimed to a better management of human beings exposed to global cerebral ischemia, frequently as a consequence of a cardiorespiratory arrest. Translation of knowledge about neuroprotection obtained from models in experimental animals, to clinical practice has not been successful. This situation has been also observed in the case of focal cerebral ischemia, leading to consensus meetings (Fisher et al., 2009; STAIR, 1999) attempting to establish the better conditions for preclinical studies of neuroprotection as to give reliable results to be applied in clinical conditions. If opinion of these consensuses may be recognized as applicable to preclinical studies of global cerebral ischemia, it is apparent that some factors must be taken in account for designing and carrying of the respective experimental protocols. Thus, studies in animal models of global cerebral ischemia should give information on effective neuroprotective doses in the case of drugs being tested; hence, dose-response relationships should be investigated. Routes of drug administration and pharmacokinetic characteristics

should also be taken in account as to be compatible with their potential use in human beings.

The time window of opportunity for the effective neuroprotective treatment is an important factor to be considered in preclinical models that may predict the timing of neuroprotective procedures in clinical situations with reference to the onset of global cerebral ischemia and subsequent reperfusion. The initial hypothesis that opportunity window for neuroprotective procedures would be limited to a short period after the ischemic episode has been changed in view of experimental evidence. Thus, different drugs or neuroprotective procedures having predominant mechanisms of action against specific cellular processes of ischemia damage occurring lately within the pathophysiological cascade, may allow to neuroprotection even when administered hours or days after ischemia. Besides, the opportunity time window may be further extended when it is expected that neuroprotective procedures act through promotion of cellular processes of neuronal repair and plasticity.

In view of the multiple pathophysiological processes occurring both in sequence and simultaneously after ischemia and reperfusion, it is considered as an advantage for presumptive neuroprotective drugs to have multiple cellular or molecular mechanisms of action, as occurring with some originally endogenous compounds, namely melatonin, estradiol and progesterone (El-Abhar et al, 2002; Hurn et al, 1995; Jover-Mengual et al, 2010; Lebesgue et al, 2009; Reiter et al, 2005; Wang et al, 2008). By contrast, most synthetic drugs only have one mechanism of action accounting for neuroprotection. Attempting to counteract several mechanisms of ischemic brain injury would require the simultaneous administration of several drugs (Hicks et al, 1999; Matsumoto et al, 1993; Pazos et al, 1999; del Pilar Fernández et al, 1998; Sánchez-Casado et al, 2007; Zapater et al, 1997) (Table 1).

Recommendations arisen from these consensuses of opinion have also highlighted the importance of long-term studies to identify whether functional preservation or recovery may be attributed to effects of the neuroprotective procedures, and/or to intrinsic mechanisms of plasticity and repair triggered by ischemia *per se*. Reliable parameters of long-term structural and functional outcome may allow to evaluate the final result of the neuroprotective procedures on cerebral structures vulnerable to ischemia. Thus, evaluation of neuronal population, cytoarchitectonic characteristics, and connectivity of the neural circuits in these vulnerable structures, as well as different aspects of cognitive functions depending on them should be included as a part of experimental designs of neuroprotection.

It has been described that the neuronal population of remaining neurons in CA1 at survival times of 2-3 weeks may be less than that evaluated 3-4 months after the ischemic episode, suggesting that, without exogenous intervention, CA1 neurons may have been repopulate, became integrated to the hippocampal neuronal circuits, and contribute to functional recovery (Bendel, et al 2005; von Euler et al., 2006, Hartman et al, 2005, Nakatomi et al., 2002). Obviously, the potential repopulation complicates the interpretation of learning and memory studies after global cerebral ischemia, because short-term studies may not give an adequate end point of the cognitive alteration after global cerebral ischemia, which seems to require a long-term follow up.

Experimental designs to evaluate the potential of neuroprotective drugs or hypothermia may have not met all requirements set by these consensuses in a single study, but integration of results of the many experimental studies may give enough information as to support proposals for their clinical usefulness.

Main Mechanism of Action	Neuroprotective Agent	References
PHARMACOLOGICAL AGENTS		
Increase of energy reserve	Creatine	Lensman et al., 2006; Otellin et al., 2003.
Calcium channel blockers	Nimodipine	Cervantes et al., 1992; Choi SK et al., 2011; Haddon et al., 1988; Lazarewicz et al., 1990; Lazarewicz et al., 1993; del Pilar Fernández et al., 1998; Rami & Krieglstein, 1994; Zornow et al, 1996.
	Levemopamil	Block & Schwarz 1998.
	Dantrolene	Nakayama et al, 2002
	Flunarizine	Lee Y.S. et al., 1999.
K^+ channel activators	Linoleic acid	Blondeau et al., 2002.
Glutamate antagonists	Dizocilpine	Bernabeu, R., & Sharp, 2000; Hicks et al., 1999; Janac et al., 2008; Kwon et al., 2000; Montero et al., 2007; Stevens & Yaksh, 1990; Selakovic et al., 2010; Zhang et al., 2009.
	Dextromethorphan	Block & Schwarz, 1998.
	Lamotrigine	Conroy et al., 1999 ; Crumrine et al., 1997; Lee Y.S. et al., 1999 ; Morimoto et al., 2002 ; Shuaib et al., 1995b ; Wiard et al., 1995.
	Lubeluzole	Koinig et al., 2001; Mueller et al., 2003; Haseldonckx et al., 1997
	$MgSO_4$	Meloni et al., 2009; Miles et al., 2001; Sirin et al., 1998.
	Zinc	Matsushita et al., 1996.
	Antiepileptic agents	Stepień et al., 2005.
GABAergic agents	Clomethiazole	Clarkson et al., 2005; Chaulk et al, 2003; Cross et al, 1995; Liang et al, 1997; Shuaib et al., 1995a; Sydserff et al., 2000.
	Diacepam	Corbett et al, 2008; Dowden et al, 1999; Hall et al, 1998; Johansen FF, Diemer, 1991; Schwartz et al, 1995.
	Thiopental	Kofke et al., 1979; Pappas & Mironovich, 1981; Todd et al, 1982 .
	Propofol	Cai et al., 2011 ; Cervantes et al., 1995 ; Ergün et al, 2002.
	Progesterone, allopregnanolone	Aggarwal et al., 2008 ; Cervantes et al., 2002 ; González-Vidal et al., 1998 ; Moralí et al., 2005 ; Moralí et al., 2011a, 2011b; Ozacmak & Sayan, 2009 ; J.M. Wang et al, 2008 ; Zhao et al, 2011.

Main Mechanism of Action	Neuroprotective Agent	References
Antioxidants	Tirilazad	Li et al., 2010; del Pilar Fernández et al., 2008; Selakovic et al., 2010; Stevens & Yaksh, 1990.
	Pentoxifylline	Sirin et al., 1998; Tuong et al., 1994.
	Edaravone	Kubo et al., 2009 ; Otani et al., 2005.
	Methylene blue	Wiklund et al., 2007.
	Melatonin	Cervantes et al., 2008; Cho et al, 1997; El-Abhar et al., 2002; García-Chávez et al., 2008; González-Burgos et al., 2007; Letechipía-Vallejo et al., 2001; Letechipía-Vallejo et al., 2007; Rennie et al., 2008; Weil et al., 2009.
	Other	Bashkatova et al, 2001; Fang et al, 2010; Gaur & Kumar, 2010; Nanri et al, 1998; Pazos et al., 1999; Sinha et al., 2001; Warner et al, 2004.
	Human albumin	Belayev et al., 1999.
Antiapoptotic agents	Estradiol	Dai et al., 2007 ; He et al., 2002 ; Hurn et al., 1995 ; Jover-Mengual et al, 2010; Koh et al., 2006 ; Lebesgue et al., 2009 ; Littleton-Kearney et al, 2005 ; Lu et al., 2002 ; Wang et al., 2006 ; Wappler et al., 2010.
Other mechanisms	Delta 9-tetrahydro-cannabinol	Zani et al., 2007.
	Linoleic acid and other PUFA's	Blondeau et al., 2002; Fernandes et al., 2008; Lauritzen et al., 2000; Ma et al., 2008; Plamondon & Roberge, 2008.
Cell proliferation stimulants	Erythropoietin	Cotena et al, 2008 ; Givehchian et al., 2010; Incagnioli et al., 2009; Zhang et al, 2007.
Growth Factors	BDNF	D'Cruz et al., 2002; Kiprianova et al., 1999a, 1999b; Larsson et al., 1999; Popp et al., 2004.
NON-PHARMACOLOGICAL AGENTS		
Reduction of: cerebral metabolism and oxygen demands, reactive oxygen species, release of excitatory aminoacids, apoptosis, inflammatory reactions. Enhancement of BDNF	Hypothermia	Asai et al., 2000; Baumann et al, 2009; Chopp et al, 1988; Colbourne & Corbett, 1994; Dong et al, 2001; Noguchi et al., 2011; Silasi & Colbourne, 2011; Webster et al., 2009; Zhang H. et al., 2010; Zhang Z, et al., 2001.

Main Mechanism of Action	Neuroprotective Agent	References
ASSOCIATION OF PHARMACOLOGICAL AND NON-PHARMACOLOGICAL AGENTS		
	Hypothermia + $MgSO_4$	Meloni et al., 2009.
	Hypothermia + $MgSO_4$ + tirilazad	Sánchez Casado et al., 2007

Table 1. Main pharmacological and non-pharmacological agents showing neuroprotective effects through molecular, biochemical , histopathological, behavioral, neurologic, and cognitive parameters.

These strategies have allowed identifying the neuroprotective characteristics of many agents, including non-pharmacological procedures like hypothermia, that have been tested in animal models of global cerebral ischemia from the knowledge of an opposition relationship between their mechanism(s) of action, and the nature of the pathophysiological phenomena of ischemic damage. They may be grouped in relation to their main predominant mechanism of action against ischemic damage: calcium channel blockers, glutamate antagonists, GABAergic drugs, antioxidant agents, anti-inflammatory compounds, etc. Many of these compounds are products of chemical synthesis; but endogenous compounds (melatonin, estradiol, progesterone, allopregnanolone, etc.) playing important physiological roles in mammals, have also been shown to exert potent neuroprotective effects. Table 1 presents some examples of the various groups of neuroprotective agents.

4.1 Outcome assessment of brain injury and neuroprotection in animal models of global cerebral ischemia

Assessment of brain injury and neuroprotection in animal models of global cerebral ischemia can be effected at different levels of biological organization of the central nervous system, from molecular and cellular phenomena to brain functions requiring highly integrated, behavioral expressions. In general, parameters of cellular and molecular processes leading to ischemic brain damage or neuroprotection require obtaining brain tissue samples at a selected time point after ischemia for these phenomena to be evaluated. On the other hand, a follow-up of damage and/or recovery through repeated bioelectrical, behavioral, and cognitive measurements is possible to be done in the same animal along extended periods. Parameters that allow evaluating the presence and magnitude of ischemic brain injury at the different levels of biological organization are also reliable indexes of neuroprotective actions, as they are induced by ischemia and may be counteracted by neuroprotective procedures. A similar consideration can be done regarding cell repair and plasticity mechanisms triggered by the ischemic insult, which are expected to be favored by neuroprotective agents.

Measurements have been done of parameters of each of the various phenomena affected by ischemia which constitute the starting point of ischemic brain injury. These include timely and topographically appropriate evaluation of ionic changes, release of neurotransmitters, modification of receptor molecular structure, excitotoxicy, morphological and functional mitochondrial alterations, reactive oxygen and nitrogen species, antioxidant enzymes and lipoperoxidation, activation of pro- and antiapoptotic cascades, DNA breakdown, pro- and

anti-inflammatory processes, among others (Lakhan et al, 2009; Lipton, 1999; Mehta et al, 2007; Schneider et al, 2009).
Neurological, behavioral, electrophysiological and histopathological correlates of the outcome after global cerebral ischemia being end points of cellular processes triggered by ischemia, give information about ischemic brain injury and neuroprotection.

4.1.1 Neurological assessment

Global cerebral ischemia usually does not result in long lasting focal neurological deficits in rats. Thus neurological deficit scores resulting from sensorimotor tests assessing motor-sensory functions in rats, including placement reactions, righting and flexion reflexes, equilibrium, spontaneous motility, among others may be altered shortly after (24 h) global cerebral ischemia, but they appear recovered 7 days after ischemia. These transient neurological deficits have been interpreted as functional alteration of hippocampus and striatum; though correlation between neurological deficit scores and ischemic neuronal damage in these structures, not always were found (Block, 1999; Hartman et al., 2005; Kofler et al, 2004).

4.1.2 Mood and behavioral assessment

Elevated, four (two open and two closed) arms plus maze, and open field tests have been used, among other to evaluate anxiety after global cerebral ischemia especially in rodents. Thus scores of latency to enter to open arms, the number of open and closed arms entries and rears are taken as parameters of anxiety in the elevated plus maze, while in the open field (circular arena 80 cm in diameter, three concentric rings and lines radiating from the center) tests, the number of segments entered with all the four paws, the number of rears, and the number of *faecal boli* are indexes of anxiety (Nelson et al., 1997).

4.1.3 Cognitive functions assessment

Since the clinical consequences of cardiac arrest, as the main cause of global cerebral ischemia, have been consistently described as long-term alterations of cognitive functions, it can be expected that similar cognitive deficits may be elicited by global cerebral ischemia in experimental animals. In fact, the most vulnerable neurons to ischemia are located in brain structures involved in cognitive processes (Ginsberg & Busto, 1989; Gionet et al., 1991; Pulsinelli, 1985); thus, evaluation of cognitive functions mainly dependent on hippocampus, striatum and prefrontal cortex, and its electrophysiological and morphological correlates may be reliable parameters of brain injury and neuroprotection after global cerebral ischemia.
The magnitude and type of cognitive deficits in experimental animals submitted to global cerebral ischemia may vary considerably depending on the animal model, the survival times of testing, and the specific behavioral tests that could have been used. Among these procedures to evaluate cognitive functions, the Morris water maze, the eight-arms radial Olton maze, and the T maze, have been widely used in assessing learning and memory in both 2VO and 4VO models in rats, and its correlation with neuronal loss (Block, 1999; Hartmann et al., 2005; Olsen et al., 1994; Volpe et al., 1984), and functional and morphological characteristics of the neural substrate underlying cognitive functions in brain structures vulnerable to ischemia. Novel object recognition tests have been shown to be a reliable index of cognitive functions since rats or mice normally spend more time exploring novel objects, whereas animals with recognition memory deficits will explore novel and

familiar objects equally (Hartman et al., 2005). Cognitive functions have also been assessed in rodents through conditioned avoidance tasks (Block, 1999; Kofler et al., 2004; Langdon et al., 2008).

Several paradigms in the Morris water maze and in the eight-arms radial Olton maze, that have been used in most of neuroprotection studies in which cognitive functions are assessed, have proven to be useful for testing hippocampal, striatum and prefrontal cortex functioning as end points of brain damage or neuroprotection after global cerebral ischemia (Morris, 1984; Olton et al, 1982).

Hippocampal functioning has been evaluated in rats and mice through some behavioral paradigms that require the integrity of this brain structure and related structures in the temporal lobe (Barnes, 1979; Morris et al., 1982, 1990), in order to configure cognitive spatial representations, i.e., a cognitive spatial map (Cassels, 1998; Jarrad, 1993; McDonald and White, 1994; 1995; Moser et al, 1993). Thus parameters of spatial learning training to locate a hidden platform, (escape latency: time spent by the animal to reach the platform; swimming path length: distance swam until reaching the platform; searching strategy: pattern of the swimming path towards the platform) and probe trial to evaluate retention of spatial learning (time spent, or the distance traveled by the animal in each of the four quadrants of the maze; number of crossings over the former platform location) in the Morris water maze including extra maze spatial clues, have been used in testing the morpho-functional state of the hippocampus (Dalm et al 2000; D'Hooge & De Deyn, 2001; Eichenbaum et al, 1990; Morris, 1984; Myhrer, 2003)..

Under these training conditions and since there are no intra maze clues to guide the animal's behavior, it is assumed that, to achieve the goal, the animal has to build the cognitive map and thus, a hippocampal processing of information occurs (Gallagher and Pelleymounter, 1988, O'Keffe & Nadel 1978). For this reason, studies of neuroprotection use the spatial learning in the Morris water maze paradigm, as a reliable index of the hippocampal functioning.

However, in addition to place learning, spatial navigation in the water maze may occur through at least, two additional strategies not depending on the hippocampus but on the striatum: signal learning and egocentric learning (Brandeis et al 1989; Gallagher & Pelleymounter, 1988; O'Keefe & Nadel 1978). Signal learning is displayed when the animal reaches a visible platform, or a visible stimulus indicating (signaling) the location of the platform within the maze. Learning of the association between the stimulus and the response is established and depends on the functioning of the striatum (McDonald & White, 1994). The egocentric learning occurs when the animal develops stereotyped motor patterns to locate the invisible platform on the basis of the proprioceptive information provided by its own movement. It is also an ability that depends on the memory system to which the striatum belongs (McDonald & White, 1994; McDonald & White 1995; Oliveira et al., 1997). Results obtained when evaluating both adult and aged male rats, show that some adult rats may use either place, hippocampal dependent allocentric, or striatum-dependent, egocentric strategies; on the other hand, aged rats use egocentric, as their main swimming strategy to solve the task (Dalm et al., 2000; Olvera-Cortés et al, 2011). Thus, deficits in the performance of this task may indicate an alteration of any of these two abilities, place and egocentric learning, so that different parameters should be evaluated to assess the mechanism underlying the observed deficit (D'Hooge & De Deyn, 2001). A qualitative analysis of the swimming paths both during the training period and the probe trial may allow a better determining of the strategy used by the rat in solving the task in the water maze.

Spatial working memory can be evaluated by using the 8-arms Olton radial maze (Myhrer, 2003; Olton, 1983, 1987; Olton et al., 1982; Shibata et al., 2007). For a daily standard evaluation all eight arms are baited and the rat is allowed to collect food from each arm; the number of errors, defined as a re-entry into an arm that had already been visited, is recorded in order to evaluate withholding and updating of information about each arm visited and rewarding obtained. An alternative maze configuration in which only some of the eight arms are baited allows to evaluate reference memory besides working memory through recording of the number of reference memory errors (number of entries into unbaited arms) and working memory errors (re-entry into an already visited arm). Performance in the Olton maze requires an adequate functioning of hippocampal-prefrontocortical neuronal circuits, and is a reliable parameter of morpho-functional integrity of these brain structures after ischemia and neuroprotection (Cassel et al., 1998; Fritts et al., 1998; Izaki et al., 2008; Kolb, 1990, Kolb et al 1982; Laroche et al., 2000; Olton et al., 1982; Seamans et al., 1995; Winocur, 1982). An aquatic version of the 8-arm radial maze has also been described (Kolb et al, 1982), and used to correlate hippocampal pyramidal neurons damage and working memory performance (Nelson et al. 1997).

4.1.4 Histopathological assessment

Neuronal population of different neuron types in brain vulnerable structures has been considered as a reliable parameter of ischemia brain damage and neuroprotection. Thus, pyramidal neuron population in the Ammon´s horn of the hippocampus and in the neocortex (Bleayert et al, 1978; Colbourne & Corbett, 1994; García-Chávez et al., 2008; Hartman et al, 2005; Johansen & Diemer, 1991; Kirino, 1982; Letechipía-Vallejo et al., 2007; Moralí et al., 2011b; Pulsinelli, 1985; Schmidt-Kastner & Freund, 1991; Shuaib et al, 1995), or different neuron types in other brain vulnerable structures (Block & Schwartz, 1998; Cervantes et al., 2002), have been evaluated through the number and proportion of surviving neurons. However, most of these studies deal with histopathological assessment of the hippocampus, the highest vulnerable brain region to global cerebral ischemia. Usually four separate counts of surviving neurons in selected areas of the Ammon´s horn are obtained from each of five coronal sections of the hippocampus per rat, stained with cresyl violet for a total of 20 counts per animal, under the different experimental conditions (Hartman et al., 2005). Similar procedures are followed for neuronal counting in other brain structures vulnerable to ischemia.

Immunohistochemical staining techniques have been also used in animal models of global cerebral ischemia and neuroprotection in order to identify specific proteins or fluorescent DNA labels that may selectively mark cells undergoing an acute necrotic or apoptotic process, as well as the activation of specific cellular processes involved in neuronal damage or repair and survival. Immunohistochemical marks (c-fos/c-jun, heat shock proteins, Bcl-2/Bax immunoreactivity, among others) allow to identify neuron types and neuroanatomical regions where ischemia-induced phenomena take place. Besides, immunohistochemical markers of glial fibrillary acidic protein (GFAP) as well as microglia cell surface components lead to identification of reactive gliosis in the hippocampus, as a consequence of global cerebral ischemia and ischemic neuronal death, which elicited activation of microglial cells and interleukine 1 release that may trigger an astrocyte reaction mainly located in the *stratum lacunosum-moleculare, stratum moleculare,* and *hilus,* and persisting for weeks after ischemia (Buffo et al., 2010; Choi JS et al, 2008; Mori et al, 2008; Morioka et al., 1991, 1992; Nikonenko et al., 2009; Petito & Halaby, 1993). The efficacy of neuroprotective agents can also be determined on the basis of the success in preventing the occurrence of necrosis, apoptosis, heat shock expression, gliosis, etc., as indicated by the immunohistochemical biomarkers (Scallet, 1995). Different parameters of the glial reaction elicited by global cerebral ischemia have been used as indexes of brain damage or neuroprotection (Cervantes et al., 2002; de Yebra et al., 2006; Duan et al., 2011; Korzhevskii et al., 2005; Piao et al., 2002; Soltys et al., 2003).

Neuronal cytoarchitecture and fine structure parameters of synaptic connectivity have also been used for histopathological assessment after brain damage and neuroprotection (Briones et al., 2006; García-Chávez et al., 2008; González-Burgos et al., 2007; Johansson & Belichenko, 2002; Kovalenko et al., 2006, Moralí et al., 2011a; Nikonenko et al., 2009; Ruan et al., 2006).

4.2 Therapeutic opportunity window in animal models of global cerebral ischemia

In any case, recognition of a "therapeutic opportunity window" or "therapeutic time window" in relation to the timing of the ischemic episode, the temporal course of the mechanisms of brain damage and/or repair, and the exerting of actions of presumptive pharmacological or non pharmacological neuroprotective agents, has been a relevant aspect in the approach to neuroprotection in experimental models of global cerebral ischemia (Pulsinelli et al., 1997; Barone & Feuerstein, 1999). In these, the beginning and the extent of this therapeutic window can be expected to be different according to the actions of neuroprotective procedures against immediate or late cellular mechanisms of brain damage, or in favor of later long-lasting cerebral processes of repair and plasticity.

Thus optimal neuroprotective effectiveness may require a schedule of drug administration in which drug actions are coincident with the therapeutic opportunity window, that have to be established for different drugs according to their specific mechanisms of action and pharmacokinetic characteristics. In this sense, counteracting of immediate cell mechanisms of neuronal damage may require the administration of neuroprotective drugs before the ischemic episode, though its administration has to be continued afterwards for variable periods. By contrast, drug-promoting repair or plasticity processes admit the starting of neuroprotective treatment hours or days after ischemia.

Accordingly, designs of neuroprotective studies in experimental animals in supporting proposals of neuroprotection for patients exposed to global cerebral ischemia due to cardiorespiratory arrest, should take in account that this clinical condition usually occurs unexpectedly, and requires cardiorespiratory resuscitation maneuvers; thus neuroprotection procedures have to be installed soon, but after the ischemic episode. Experimental designs of neuroprotection studies assessing neuroprotective procedures against late neuronal damage processes or promoting neuronal repair and plasticity, favoring functional preservation and recovery, may lead supporting to a wideness of the therapeutic opportunity window, for neuroprotection in human beings.

4.2.1 Prophylactic neuroprotection

Transient global cerebral ischemia can occur during certain clinical situations which can either be anticipated, occur during intraoperative emergencies, or even induced, like extracorporeal circulation for cardiac surgery. Under these conditions, prophylactic neuroprotection as that provided by intraoperative hypothermia and pharmacological neuroprotection are possible alternatives to prevent or reduce the risk of ischemic neuronal damage (Savitz & Fisher, 2007; Weigl et al, 2005). This has stimulated designing of experimental studies on prophylactic neuroprotection to assess the effectiveness of several agents and their clinical potential. Some neuroprotective agents have proven to be more effective when applied before the ischemic insult than when given later in time, in particular those agents affecting the early cellular phenomena induced by ischemia, such as calcium channel blockers, GABAergic and anti-excitotoxic agents, as well as antioxidant drugs (Weigl et al, 2005). Pharmacological treatments (antihypertensive, antidiabetic, antithrombotic, antiatherogenic drugs) effective in modifying in the long term the risk for cardiac arrest or cardiac infarct which may result in global cerebral ischemia or in severe hypoperfusion have also been proposed as prophylactic neuroprotection procedures (Savitz & Fisher, 2007).

5. Conclusion

Though an increasing number of drugs have proven to be effective neuroprotective agents in experimental models of global cerebral ischemia, data supporting proposals for their clinical use have not been enough to influence clinical management and outcome of patients exposed to global cerebral ischemia in clinical trials. However, after its evaluation in animal models of global cerebral ischemia, special interest has been paid to carry out clinical trials with a non-pharmacological procedure, hypothermia, as a part of the intensive care of patients after a cardiorespiratory arrest. Nevertheless, the wide perspectives to gain information on neuroprotection through experimental designs including animal models of global cerebral ischemia are maintained to date, despite the tendency to preferentially conduct studies on rodents; in particular if differences between experimental animals and human beings are taken into account, and attention is paid to reproduce those components mainly accounting for brain damage after global cerebral ischemia.

6. Acknowledgement

Partially supported by Instituto Mexicano del Seguro Social, MEXICO (2006/1A/I/029; FIS/IMSS/PROT/196).

7. References

Abe, K.; Yoshida, S.; Watson, B.D.; Busto, R.; Kogure, K. & Ginsberg, M.D. (1983). Alpha-Tocopherol and Ubiquinones in Rat Brain Subjected to Decapitation Ischemia. *Brain Research*, Vol.273, No.1, (August 1983), pp. 166-169, ISSN 0006-8993

Aggarwal, R.; Medhi, B.; Pathak, A.; Dhawan, V. & Chakrabarti, A. (2008). Neuroprotective Effect of Progesterone on Acute Phase Changes Induced by Partial Global Cerebral Ischaemia in Mice. *Journal of Pharmacy and Pharmacology*, Vol.60, No.6, (May 2008), pp. 731-737, ISSN 0022-3573

Akulinin, V.A.; Belichenko, P.V. & Dahlstrom, A. (1998). Quantitative Analysis of Synaptophysin Immunoreactivity in Human Neocortex after Cardiac Arrest: Confocal Laser Scanning Microscopy Study. *Resuscitation*, Vol.39, No.3, (March 1999), pp. 207-213, ISSN 0300-9572

Akulinin, V.A.; Semchenko, V.V.; Stepanov, S.S. & Belichenko, P.V. (2004). Structural Changes in the Dendritic Spines of Pyramidal Neurons in Layer III of the Sensorimotor Cortex of the Rat Cerebral Cortex in the Late Post-Ischemic Period. *Neuroscience and Behavioral Physiology,*Vol.34, No.3, (May 2004), pp. 221-227, ISSN 0097-0549

Akulinin, V.A.; Stepanov, S.S.; Semchenko, V.V. & Belichenko, P.V. (1997). Dendritic Changes of the Pyramidal Neurons in Layer V of Sensory-motor Cortex of the Rat Brain During the Postresuscitation Period. *Resuscitation,*Vol.35, No.2, (October 1997), pp. 157-164, ISSN 0300-9572

Arai, K.; Ikegaya, Y.; Nakatani, Y.; Kudo, I.; Nishiyama, N. & Matsuki, N. (2001). Phospholipase A2 Mediates Ischemic Injury in the Hippocampus: a Regional Difference of Neuronal Vulnerability. *European Journal of Neuroscience,* Vol.13, No.12, (June 2001), pp. 2319-2323, ISSN 1460-9568

Araki, T.; Kato, H. & Kogure, K. (1989). Selective Neuronal Vulnerability Following Transient Cerebral Ischemia in the Gerbil: Distribution and Time Course. *Acta Neurologica Scandinavica,*Vol.80, No.6, (December 1989), pp. 548-553, ISSN 0001-6314

Asai, S.; Zhao, H.; Kohno, T.; Takahashi, Y.; Nagata, T. & Ishikawa, K. (2000). Quantitative Evaluation of Extracellular Glutamate Concentration in Postischemic Glutamate Re-uptake, Dependent on Brain Temperature, in the Rat Following Severe Global Brain Ischemia. *Brain Research,* Vol.864, No.1, (May 2000), pp. 60-68, ISSN 0006-8993

Arvidsson, A.; Kokaia, Z.; Airaksinen, M.S.; Saarma, M. & Lindvall, O. (2001). Stroke Induces Widespread Changes of Gene Expression for Glial Cell Line-derived Neurotrophic Factor Family Receptors in the Adult Rat Brain. *Neuroscience,*Vol.106, No.1, (September 2001), pp. 27-41, ISSN 0306-4522

Barnes, C.A. (1979). Memory Deficits Associated With Senescence: A Neurophysiological and Behavioral Study in the Rat. *Journal of Comparative & Physiological Psychology,*Vol.93, No.1, (February 1979), pp. 74-104, ISSN 0021-9940

Barone, F.C. & Feuerstein, G.Z. (1999). Inflammatory Mediators and Stroke: New Opportunities for Novel Therapeutics. *Journal of Cerebral Blood Flow & Metabolism,*Vol.19, No.8, (August 1999), pp. 819-834, ISSN 0271-678X

Bashkatova, V.G.; Koshelev, V.B.; Fadyukova, O.E.; Alexeev, A.A.; Vanin, A.F.; Rayevsky, K.S.; Ashmarin, I.P. & Armstrong, D.M. (2001). Novel Synthetic Analogue of ACTH 4-10 (Semax) but not Glycine Prevents the Enhanced Nitric Oxide Generation in Cerebral Cortex of Rats with Incomplete Global Ischemia. *Brain Research,*Vol.894, No.1, (March 2001), pp. 145-149, ISSN 0006-8993

Baumann, E.; Preston, E.; Slinn, J. & Stanimirovic, D. (2009). Post-ischemic Hypothermia Attenuates Loss of the Vascular Basement Membrane Proteins, Agrin and SPARC, and the Blood-brain Barrier Disruption After Global Cerebral Ischemia. *Brain Research,* Vol.1269, No.1, (May 2009), pp. 185-97, ISSN 0006-8993

Belayev, L.; Saul, I.; Huh, P.W.; Finotti, N.; Zhao, W.; Busto, R. & Ginsberg, M.D. (1999). Neuroprotective Effect of High-dose Albumin Therapy Against Global Ischemic Brain Injury in Rats. *Brain Research,* Vol.845, No.1, (October n 1999), pp. 107-111, ISSN 0006-8993

Bendel, O.; Bueters, T.; von Euler, M.; Ove Ogren, S.; Sandin, J. & von Euler, G. (2005). Reappearance of Hippocampal CA1 Neurons after Ischemia is Associated with

Recovery of Learning and Memory. *Journal of Cerebral Blood Flow and Metabolism*, Vol.25, No.12, (December 2005), pp. 1586-1595, ISSN 0271-678X

Benítez-King, G. (2006). Melatonin as a Cytoskeletal Modulator: Implications for Cell Physiology and Disease. *Journal of Pineal Research*,Vol.40, No.1, (November 2005), pp. 1-9, ISSN 0742-3098

Berkowitz, I.D.; Gervais, H.; Schleien, C.L.; Koehler, R.C.; Dean, J.M. & Traystman, R.J. (1991). Epinephrine Dosage Effects on Cerebral and Myocardial Blood Flow in an Infant Swine Model of Cardiopulmonary Resuscitation. *Anesthesiology*,Vol.75, No.6, (December 1991), pp. 1041-1050, ISSN 0003-3022

Bernabeu, R. & Sharp, F.R. (2000). NMDA and AMPA/Kainate Glutamate Receptors Modulate Dentate Neurogenesis and CA3 Synapsin-I in Normal and Ischemic Hippocampus. *Journal of Cerebral Blood Flow & Metabolism*,Vol.20, No.12, (December 2000), pp. 1669-1680, ISSN 0271-678X

Bleyaert, A.L.; Nemoto, E.M.; Safar, P.; Stezoski, S.M.; Mickell, J.J.; Moossy, J. & Rao, G.R. (1978). Thiopental Amelioration of Brain Damage After Global Ischemia in Monkeys. *Anesthesiology*,Vol.49, No.6, (December 1978), pp. 390-398, ISSN 0003-3022

Block, F. (1999). Global Ischemia and Behavioural Deficits. *Progress in Neurobiology*,Vol.58, No.3, (May 1999), pp. 279-295, ISSN 0301-0082

Block, F. & Schwarz, M. (1998). Global Ischemic Neuronal Damage Relates to Behavioural Deficits: A Pharmacological Approach. *Neuroscience*,Vol.82, No.3, (March 1998), pp. 791-803, ISSN 0306-4522

Blondeau, N.; Widmann, C.; Lazdunski, M. & Heurteaux, C. (2002). Polyunsaturated Fatty Acids Induce Ischemic and Epileptic Tolerance. *Neuroscience*,Vol.109, No.2, (January 2002), pp. 231-241, ISSN 0306-4522

Bodsch, W.; Barbier, A.; Oehmichen, M.; Grosse Ophoff, B. & Hossmann, K.A. (1986). Recovery of Monkey Brain After Prolonged Ischemia. II. Protein Synthesis and Morphological Alterations. *Journal of Cerebral Blood Flow & Metabolism*,Vol.6, No.1, (February 1986), pp. 22-33, ISSN 0271-678X

Bortolotto, Z.A.; Collett, V.J.; Conquet, F.; Jia, Z.; van der Putten, H. & Collingridge, G.L. (2005). The Regulation of Hippocampal LTP by the Molecular Switch, a Form of Metaplasticity, Requires mGlu5 Receptors. *Neuropharmacology*,Vol.49, Suppl 1, (July 2005), pp. 13-25, ISSN 0028-3908

Briones, T.L.; Suh, E.; Jozsa, L.; Rogozinska, M.; Woods, J. & Wadowska, M. (2005). Changes in Number of Synapses and Mitochondria in Presynaptic Terminals in the Dentate Gyrus Following Cerebral Ischemia and Rehabilitation Training. *Brain Research*,Vol.1033, No.1, (February 2005), pp. 51-57, ISSN 0006-8993

Briones, T.L.; Suh, E.; Jozsa, L. & Woods, J. (2006). Behaviorally Induced Synaptogenesis and Dendritic Growth in the Hippocampal Region Following Transient Global Cerebral Ischemia are Accompanied by Improvement in Spatial Learning. *Experimental Neurology*,Vol.198, No.2, (February 2006), pp. 530-538, ISSN 0014-4886

Buffo, A.; Rolando, C. & Ceruti, S. (2010). Astrocytes in the Damaged Brain: Molecular and Cellular Insights into their Reactive Response and Healing Potential. *Biochemical Pharmacology*, Vol.79, No.2, (January 2010), pp. 77-89, ISSN 0006-2952

Cai, J.; Hu, Y.; Li, W.; Li, L.; Li, S.; Zhang, M. & Li, Q. (2011). The Neuroprotective Effect of Propofol against Brain Ischemia is Mediated by the Glutamatergic Signaling

Pathway in Rats. *Neurochemical Research*, Vol.36, No.10, (October 2011), pp. 1724-1731, ISSN 0364-3190

Cassel, J.C.; Cassel, S.; Galani, R.; Kelche, C.; Will, B. & Jarrard, L. (1998). Fimbria-Fornix vs Selective Hippocampal Lesions in Rats: Effects on Locomotor Activity and Spatial Learning and Memory. *Neurobiology of Learning and Memory,*Vol.69, No.1, (June 1998), pp. 22-45, ISSN 1074-7427

Castren, M.; Silfvast, T.; Rubertsson, S.; Niskanen, M.; Valsson, F.; Wanscher, M. & Sunde, K. (2009). Scandinavian Clinical Practice Guidelines for Therapeutic Hypothermia and Post-resuscitation Care After Cardiac Arrest. *Acta Anaesthesiologica Scandinavica,*Vol.53, No.3, (February 2009), pp. 280-288, ISSN 1399-6576

Cervantes, M.; Chávez-Carrillo, I. & Antonio-Ocampo, A. (1992). Effects of Nimodipine on Multiunit Activity of Several Brain Structures Following Acute Global Cerebral Ischemia-anoxia in Cats. *Boletín de Estudios Médicos y Biológicos* Vol.40, No.1-4, (January-December 1992), pp. 21-30, ISSN 0067-9666

Cervantes, M.; González-Vidal, M.D.; Ruelas, R.; Escobar, A. & Moralí, G. (2002). Neuroprotective Effects of Progesterone on Damage Elicited by Acute Global Cerebral Ischemia in Neurons of the Caudate Nucleus. *Archives of Medical Research,*Vol.33, No.1, (February 2002), pp. 6-14, ISSN 0188-4409

Cervantes, M.; Moralí, G. & Letechipía-Vallejo, G. (2008). Melatonin and Ischemia-reperfusion Injury of the Brain. *Journal of Pineal Research,*Vol.45, No.1, (January 2008), pp. 1-7, ISSN 1600-079X

Cervantes, M.; Ruelas, R.; Chávez-Carrillo, I.; Contreras-Gómez, A. & Antonio-Ocampo, A. (1995). Effects of Propofol on Alterations of Multineuronal Activity of Limbic and Mesencephalic Structures and Neurological Deficit Elicited by Acute Global Cerebral Ischemia. *Archives of Medical Research,*Vol.26, No.4, (January 1995), pp. 385-395, ISSN 0188-4409

Chan, P.H. (2001), Reactive Oxygen Radicals in Signalling and Damage in the Ischemic Brain. *Journal of Cerebral Blood Flow & Metabolism* Vol. 21, No. 1, (January 2001), pp. 2-14, ISSN 0271-678X

Chaulk, D.; Wells, J.; Evans, S.; Jackson, D. & Corbett, D. (2003). Long-term Effects of Clomethiazole in a Model of Global Ischemia. *Experimental Neurology,*Vol.182, No.2, (August 2003), pp. 476-482, ISSN 0014-4886

Chen, J.; Zhu, R.L.; Nakayama, M.; Kawaguchi, K.; Jin, K.; Stetler, R.A.; Simon, R.P. & Graham, S.H. (1996). Expression of the Apoptosis-effector Gene, Bax, is Up-regulated in Vulnerable Hippocampal CA1 Neurons Following Global Ischemia. *Journal of Neurochemistry,*Vol.67, No.1, (July 1996), pp. 64-71, ISSN 0022-3042

Chinopoulos, C. & Adam-Vizi, V. (2006). Calcium, mitochondria and Oxidative Stress in Neuronal Pathology. Novel Aspects of an Enduring Theme. *FEBS Journal,* Vol. 273, No. 3, (February 2006), pp. 433-450, ISSN

Cho, S.; Joh, T.H.; Baik, H.H.; Dibinis, C. & Volpe, B.T. (1997). Melatonin Administration Protects CA1 Hippocampal Neurons After Transient Forebrain Ischemia in Rats. *Brain Research,*Vol.755, No.2, (May 1997), pp. 335-338, ISSN 0006-8993

Choi, S.K.; Lee, G.J.; Choi, S.; Kim, Y.J.; Park, H.K. & Park, B.J. (2011). Neuroprotective Effects by Nimodipine Treatment in the Experimental Global Ischemic Rat Model: Real Time Estimation of Glutamate. *Journal of Korean Neurosurgical Society* Vol.49, No.1, (April 2011), pp. 1-7, ISSN 1598-7876

Choi, J.S.; Shin, Y.J.; Cha, J.H.; Kim, H.Y.; Choi, J.Y.; Chun, M.H. & Lee, M.Y. (2008). Induction of Suppressor of Cytokine Signaling-3 in Astrocytes of the Rat Hippocampus Following Transient Forebrain Ischemia. *Neuroscience Letters,* Vol.441, No.3, (August 2008), pp. 323-327, ISSN 0304-3940

Chopp, M.; Frinak, S.; Walton, D.R.; Smith, M.B. & Welch, K.M. (1987). Intracellular Acidosis During and After Cerebral Ischemia: in Vivo Nuclear Magnetic Resonance Study of Hyperglycemia in Cats. *Stroke,*Vol.18, No.5, (September 1987), pp. 919-923, ISSN 0039-2499

Chopp, M.; Welch, K.M.; Tidwell, C.D.; Knight, R. & Helpern, J.A. (1988). Effect of Mild Hyperthermia on Recovery of Metabolic Function After Global Cerebral Ischemia in Cats. *Stroke,*Vol.19, No.12, (December 1988), pp. 1521-1525, ISSN 0039-2499

Clarkson, A.N.; Liu, H.; Rahman, R.; Jackson, D.M.; Appleton, I. & Kerr, D.S. (2005). Clomethiazole: Mechanisms Underlying Lasting Neuroprotection Following Hypoxia-ischemia. *FASEB Journal,*Vol.19, No.8, (April 2005), pp. 1036-1038, ISSN 1530-6860

Clavier, N.; Kirsch, J. R.; Hurn, P.D. & Traystman, R.J. (1994). Effect of Postischemic Hypoperfusion on Vasodilatory Mechanisms in Cats. *American Journal of Physiology,*Vol.267, No.5 Pt 2, (November 1994), pp. H2012-2018, ISSN 0002-9513

Colbourne, F. & Corbett, D. (1994). Delayed and Prolonged Post-ischemic Hypothermia is Neuroprotective in the Gerbil. *Brain Research,*Vol.654, No.2, (August 1994), pp. 265-272, ISNN 0006-8993

Conroy, B.P.; Black, D.; Lin, C.Y.; Jenkins, L.W.; Crumrine, R.C.; DeWitt, D.S. & Johnston, W.E. (1999). Lamotrigine Attenuates Cortical Glutamate Release during Global Cerebral Ischemia in Pigs on Cardiopulmonary Bypass. *Anesthesiology,*Vol.90, No.3, (March 1999), pp. 844-854, ISSN 0003-3022

Corbett, D.; Larsen, J. & Langdon, K.D. (2008) Diazepam Delays the Death of Hippocampal CA1 Neurons Following Global Ischemia. *Experimental Neurology,* Vol.214, No.2, (December 2008), pp. 309-14, ISSN

Cotena, S.; Piazza, O. & Tufano, R. (2008). The Use of Erythtropoietin in Cerebral Diseases. *Panminerva Medica,*Vol.50, No.2, (July 2008), pp. 185-192, ISSN 0031-0808

Crepel, V.; Epsztein, J. & Ben-Ari, Y. (2003). Ischemia Induces Short- and Long-Term Remodeling of Synaptic Activity in the Hippocampus. *Journal of Cellular and Molecular Medicine,*Vol.7, No.4, (February 2004), pp. 401-407, ISSN 1582-1838

Cross, A.J.; Jones, J.A.; Snares, M.; Jostell, K.G.; Bredberg, U. & Green, A.R. (1995). The Protective Action of Chlormethiazole against Ischaemia-induced Neurodegeneration in Gerbils when Infused at Doses Having Little Sedative or Anticonvulsant Activity. *British Journal of Pharmacology* Vol.114, No.8, (April 1995), pp. 1625-1630, ISSN 0007-1188

Crumrine, R.C.; Bergstrand, K.; Cooper, A.T.; Faison, W.L. & Cooper, B.R. (1997). Lamotrigine Protects Hippocampal CA1 Neurons from Ischemic Damage after Cardiac Arrest. *Stroke,*Vol.28, No.11, (November 1997), pp. 2230-2236, ISSN 0039-2499

D'Cruz, B.J.; Fertig, K.C.; Filiano, A.J.; Hicks, S.D.; DeFranco, D.B. & Callaway, C.W. (2002). Hypothermic Reperfusion After Cardiac Arrest Augments Brain-Derived Neurotrophic Factor Activation. *Journal of Cerebral Blood Flow & Metabolism,* (July 2002), Vol.22, No.7, pp. 843-851, ISSN 0271-678X

D'Hooge, R. & De Deyn, P.P. (2001). Applications of the Morris Water Maze in the Study of Learning and Memory. *Brain Research Brain Research Reviews*,Vol.36, No.1, (August 2001), pp. 60-90, ISSN 0006-8993

Dai, X.; Chen, L. & Sokabe, M. (2007). Neurosteroid Estradiol Rescues Ischemia-induced Deficit in the Long-term Potentiation of Rat Hippocampal CA1 Neurons. *Neuropharmacology*,Vol.52, No.4, (January 2007), pp. 1124-1138, ISSN 0028-3908

Dalm, S.; Grootendorst, J.; de Kloet, E.R. & Oitzl, M.S. (2000). Quantification of Swim Patterns in the Morris Water Maze. *Behavior Research Methods, Instruments, & Computers*,Vol.32, No.1, (April 2000), pp. 134-139, ISSN 0743-3808

Dave, K.R.; Raval, A.P.; Prado, R.; Katz, L.M.; Sick, T.J.; Ginsberg, M.D.; Busto, R. & Perez-Pinzon, M.A. (2004). Mild Cardiopulmonary Arrest Promotes Synaptic Dysfunction in Rat Hippocampus. *Brain Research*,Vol.1024, No.1-2, (September 2004), pp. 89-96, ISSN 0006-8993

De Yebra, L.; Malpesa, Y.; Ursu, G.; Pugliese, M.; Lievéns, J.C.; Goff, L.K. & Mahy, N. (2006). Dissociation Between Hippocampal Neuronal Loss, Astroglial and Microglial Reactivity after Pharmacologically Induced Reverse Glutamate Transport. *Neurochemistry International*, Vol.49, No.7, (December 2006), pp. 691-697, ISSN 0197-0186

Dong, H.; Moody-Corbett, F.; Colbourne, F.; Pittman, Q. & Corbett, D. (2001). Electrophysiological Properties of CA1 Neurons Protected by Postischemic Hypothermia in Gerbils. *Stroke*, Vol.32, No.3, (March 2001), pp. 788-95, ISSN 0039-2499

Dowden, J.; Reid, C.; Dooley, P. & Corbett, D. (1999). Diazepam-Induced Neuroprotection: Dissociating the Effects of Hypothermia Following Global Ischemia. *Brain Research*, Vol.829, No.1-2, (May 1999), pp. 1-6, ISSN 0006-8993

Duan, Y.L.; Wang, S.Y.; Zeng, Q.W.; Su, D.S.; Li, W.; Wang, X.R. & Zhao, Z. (2011). Astroglial Reaction to Delta Opioid Peptide [D-Ala2, D-Leu5] Enkephalin Confers Neuroprotection Against Global Ischemia in the Adult Rat Hippocampus. *Neuroscience*, Vol.192, (September 2011), pp. 81-90, ISSN 0306-4522

Eichenbaum, H.; Stewart, C. & Morris, R. G. (1990). Hippocampal Representation in Place Learning. *Journal of Neuroscience*, Vol.10, No.11, (November 1990), pp. 3531-3542, ISSN 0270-6474

Eklof, B. & Siesjo, B.K. (1972a). The Effect of Bilateral Carotid Artery Ligation Upon Acid-base Parameters and Substrate Levels in the Rat Brain. *Acta Physiologica Scandinavica*,Vol.86, No.4, (December 1972), pp. 528-538, ISSN 0001-6772

Eklof, B. & Siesjo, B.K. (1972b). The Effect of Bilateral Carotid Artery Ligation Upon the Blood Flow and the Energy State of the Rat Brain. *Acta Physiologica Scandinavica*,Vol.86, No.2, (October 1972), pp. 155-165, ISSN 0001-6772

El-Abhar, H.S.; Shaalan, M.; Barakat, M. & El-Denshary, E.S. (2002). Effect of Melatonin and Nifedipine on some Antioxidant Enzymes and Different Energy Fuels in the Blood and Brain of Global Ischemic Rats. *Journal of Pineal Research*,Vol.33, No.2, (August 2002), pp. 87-94, ISSN 0742-3098

Ergün, R.; Akdemir, G.; Sen, S.; Taşçi, A. & Ergüngör. F. (2002). Neuroprotective Effects of Propofol Following Global Cerebral Ischemia in Rats. *Neurosurgical Review*, Vol.25, No.1-2, (March 2002), pp. 95-98, ISSN 0344-5607 von Euler, M.; Bendel, O.; Bueters, T.; Sandin, J. & von Euler, G. (2006).Profound but Transient Deficits in Learning and memory after Global Cerebral Ischemia Using a Novel Water Maze Test. *Behavioral Brain research*, Vol.166, No.2, (January 2006), pp. 204-210, ISSN 0166-4328

Fang, S.; Yan, B.; Wang, D.; Bi, X.; Zhang, Y.; He, J.; Xu, H.; Yang, Y.; Kong, J.; Wu, J. & Li, X.M. (2010). Chronic Effects of Venlafaxine on Synaptophysin and Neuronal Cell Adhesion Molecule in the Hippocampus of Cerebral Ischemic Mice. *Biochemistry and Cell Biology* Vol.88, No.4, (July 2010), pp. 655-663, ISSN 1208-6002

Fernandes, J.S.; Mori, M.A.; Ekuni, R.; Oliveira, R.M. & Milani, H. (2008). Long-term Treatment with Fish Oil Prevents Memory Impairments but not Hippocampal Damage in Rats Subjected to Transient, Global Cerebral Ischemia. *Nutrition Research* Vol.28, No.11, (December 2008), pp. 798-808, 1879-0739

Fiala, J.C.; Spacek, J. & Harris, K.M. (2002). Dendritic Spine Pathology: Cause or Consequence of Neurological Disorders? *Brain Research Reviews,*Vol.39, No.1, (June 2002), pp. 29-54, ISSN 0165-0173

Fisher, M.; Feuerstein, G.; Howells, D.W.; Hurn, P.D.; Kent, T.A.; Savitz, S.I. & Lo, E.H. (2009). Update of the Stroke Therapy Academic Industry Roundtable Preclinical Recommendations. *Stroke,*Vol.40, No.6, (February 2009), pp. 2244-2250, ISSN 0039-2499

Fritts, M.E.; Asbury, E.T.; Horton, J.E. & Isaac, W.L. (1998). Medial Prefrontal Lesion Deficits Involving or Sparing the Prelimbic Area in the Rat. *Physiology & Behavior,*Vol.64, No.3, (September 1998), pp. 373-380, ISSN 0031-9384

Fuster, J.M. (1997). *The Prefrontal Cortex. Anatomy, Physiology, and Neuropsychology of the Frontal Lobe,* Lippincott-Raven, ISBN 978-0881674668, New York, USA

Fuster, J.M. (1999). Synopsis of Function and Dysfunction of the Frontal Lobe. *Acta Psychiatrica Scandinavica,* Vol.395, Supplementum, (May 1999), pp. 51-57, ISSN 0065-159

Gallagher, M. & Pelleymounter, M.A. (1988). Spatial Learning Deficits in Old Rats: a Model for Memory Decline in the Aged. *Neurobiology of Aging,*Vol.9, No.5-6, (September 1988), pp. 549-556, ISSN 0197-4580

García-Chávez, D.; González-Burgos, I.; Letechipía-Vallejo, G.; López-Loeza, E.; Moralí, G. & Cervantes, M. (2008). Long-term Evaluation of Cytoarchitectonic Characteristics of Prefrontal Cortex Pyramidal Neurons, Following Global Cerebral Ischemia and Neuroprotective Melatonin Treatment, in Rats. *Neuroscience Letters,*Vol.448, No.1, (October 2008), pp. 148-152, ISSN 0304-3940

Gaur, V. & Kumar, A. (2010). Protective Effect of Desipramine, Venlafaxine and Trazodone against Experimental Animal Model of Transient Global Ischemia: Possible Involvement of NO-cGMP Pathway. *Brain Research,*Vol.1353, (July 2010), pp. 204-212, ISSN 0006-8993

Geocadin, R.G.; Koenig, M.A.; Jia, X.; Stevens, R.D. & Peberdy, M.A. (2008). Management of Brain Injury After Resuscitation from Cardiac Arrest. *Neurologic Clinics,*Vol.26, No.2, (June 2008), pp. 487-506, ix, ISSN 0733-8619

Ginsberg, M.D. & Busto, R. (1989). Rodent Models of Cerebral Ischemia. *Stroke,*Vol.20, No.12, (December 1989), pp. 1627-1642, ISSN 0039-2499

Gionet, T.X.; Thomas, J.D.; Warner, D.S.; Goodlett, C.R.; Wasserman, E.A. & West, J.R. (1991). Forebrain Ischemia Induces Selective Behavioral Impairments Associated with Hippocampal Injury in Rats. *Stroke,*Vol.22, No.8, (August 1991), pp. 1040-1047, ISSN 0039-2499

Givehchian, M.; Beschorner, R.; Ehmann, C.; Frauenlob, L.; Morgalla, M.; Hashemi, B.; Ziemer, G. & Scheule, A.M. (2010). Neuroprotective Effects of Erythropoietin During Deep Hypothermic Circulatory Arrest. *European Journal of Cardio-thoracic Surgery,*Vol.37, No.3, (September 2009), pp. 662-668, ISSN 1873-734X

Gobbo, O.L. & O'Mara, S.M. (2004). Impact of Enriched-environment Housing on Brain-derived Neurotrophic Factor and on Cognitive Performance After a Transient Global Ischemia. *Behavioral Brain Research,*Vol.152, No.2, (June 2004), pp. 231-241, ISSN 0166-4328

Goldberg, M.P. & Choi, D.W. (1993). Combined Oxygen and Glucose Deprivation in Cortical Cell Culture: Calcium-dependent and Calcium-independent Mechanisms of Neuronal Injury. *Journal of Neuroscience,*Vol.13, No.8, (August 1993), pp. 3510-3524, ISSN 0270-6474

González-Burgos, I. (2009). Dendritic Spines Plasticity and Learning/Memory Processes: Theory, Evidence and Prospectives, In: *Dendritic Spines. Biochemistry, Modelling and Properties.* L.R. Baylon, (Ed.), pp. 163-186. Nova Science Publishers, Inc, ISBN 978-1607414605, New York, USA

González-Burgos, I.; Letechipía-Vallejo, G.; López-Loeza, E.; Moralí, G. & Cervantes, M. (2007). Long-term Study of Dendritic Spines from Hippocampal CA1 Pyramidal Cells, After Neuroprotective Melatonin Treatment Following Global Cerebral Ischemia in Rats. *Neuroscience Letters,*Vol.423, No.2, (August 2007), pp. 162-166, ISSN 0304-3940

González-Vidal, M.D.; Cervera-Gaviria, M.; Ruelas, R.; Escobar, A.; Moralí, G. & Cervantes, M. (1998). Progesterone: Protective Effects on the Cat Hippocampal Neuronal Damage Due to Acute Global Cerebral Ischemia. *Archives of Medical Research,*Vol.29, No.2, (July 1998), pp. 117-124, ISSN 0188-4409

Gray, E.G. (1959). Electron Microscopy of Synaptic Contacts on Dendrite Spines of the Cerebral Cortex. *Nature,*Vol.183, No.4675, (June 1959), pp. 1592-1593, ISSN 0028-0836

Greer, D.M. (2006). Hypothermia for Cardiac Arrest. *Current Neurology and Neuroscience Reports,*Vol.6, No.6, (November 2006), pp. 518-524, ISSN 1528-4042

Grenell, R.G. (1946). Central Nervous System Resistance; the Effects of Temporary Arrest of Cerebral Circulation for Periods of Two to Ten Minutes. *Journal of Neuropathology & Experimental Neurology,*Vol.5, (April 1946), pp. 131-154, ISSN 0022-3069

Grubb, N.R.; Fox, K.A.; Smith, K.; Best, J.; Blane, A.; Ebmeier, K.P.; Glabus, M.F. & O'Carroll, R.E. (2000). Memory Impairment in Out-of-Hospital Cardiac Arrest Survivors is Associated with Global Reduction in Brain Volume, not Focal Hippocampal Injury. *Stroke,*Vol.31, No.7, (July 2000), pp. 1509-1514, ISSN 0039-2499

Gupta, Y.K. & Briyal, S. (2004). Animal Models of Cerebral Ischemia for Evaluation of Drugs. *Indian Journal of Physiology and Pharmacology,*Vol.48, No.4, (May 2005), pp. 379-394, ISSN 0019-5499

Gwag, B.J.; Won, S.J. & Kim, D.Y. (2002). Excitotoxicity, Oxidative Stress, and Apoptosis in Ischemic Neuronal Death, In: *New Concepts in Cerebral Ischemia. Methods and New Frontiers In Neuroscience,* R.C.S. Lin, (Ed.), 79-112, CRC Press, ISBN 0-8493-0119-X, Boca Raton, USA

Haddon, W.S.; Prough, D.S.; Kong, D. & Petrozza, P. (1988). Effects of Nimodipine on the Production of Thromboxane A2 Following Total Global Cerebral Ischemia. *Journal of Neurosurgery*,Vol.69, No.3, (September 1988), pp. 416-420, ISSN 0022-3085

Hall, E.D.; Fleck, T.J. & Oostveen, J.A. (1998). Comparative Neuroprotective Properties of the Benzodiazepine Receptor Full Agonist Diazepam and the Partial Agonist PNU-101017 in the Gerbil Forebrain Ischemia Model. *Brain Research*, Vol.798, No.1-2, (July 1998), pp. 325-329, ISSN 0006-8993

Harris, K.M. (1999). Calcium From Internal Stores Modifies Dendritic Spine Shape. *Proceedings of the National Academy of Sciences of the United States of America*,Vol.96, No.22, (October 1999), pp. 12213-12215, ISSN 0027-8424

Hartman, R.E.; Lee, J.M.; Zipfel, G.J. & Wozniak, D.F. (2005). Characterizing Learning Deficits and Hippocampal Neuron Loss Following Transient Global Cerebral Ischemia in Rats. *Brain Research*,Vol.1043, No.1-2, (May 2005), pp. 48-56, ISSN 0006-8993

Haseldonckx, M.; Van Reempts, J.; Van de Ven, M.; Wouters, L. & Borgers, M. (1997). Protection with Lubeluzole Against Delayed Ischemic Brain Damage in Rats. A Quantitative Histopathologic Study. *Stroke*,Vol.28, No.2, (February 1997), pp. 428-432, ISSN 0039-2499

He, Z.; He, Y.J.; Day, A.L. & Simpkins, J.W. (2002). Proestrus Levels of Estradiol During Transient Global Cerebral Ischemia Improves the Histological Outcome of the Hippocampal CA1 Region: Perfusion-dependent and-independent Mechanisms. *Journal of the Neurological Sciences*,Vol.193, No.2, (January 2002), pp. 79-87, ISSN 0022-510X

Herreras, O.; Solis, J.M.; Martin del Rio, R. & Lerma, J. (1987). Characteristics of CA1 Activation Through the Hippocampal Trisynaptic Pathway in the Unanaesthetized Rat. *Brain Research*,Vol.413, No.1, (June 1987), pp. 75-86, ISSN 0006-8993

Hicks, C.A.; Ward, M.A.; Swettenham, J.B. & O'Neill, M.J. (1999). Synergistic Neuroprotective Effects by Combining an NMDA or AMPA Receptor Antagonist with Nitric Oxide Synthase Inhibitors in Global Cerebral Ischaemia. *European Journal of Pharmacology*,Vol.381, No.2-3, (November 1999), pp. 113-119, ISSN 0014-2999

Hogue, C.W.; Gottesman, R.F. & Stearns, J. (2008). Mechanisms of Cerebral Injury from Cardiac Surgery. *Critical Care Clinics*,Vol.24, No.1, (February 2008), pp. 83-98, viii-ix, ISSN 0749-0704

Hossmann, K.A. (1971). Cortical Steady Potential, Impedance and Excitability Changes During and After Total Ischemia of Cat Brain. *Experimental Neurology*,Vol.32, No.2, (August 1971), pp. 163-175, ISSN 0014-4886

Hossmann, K.A. (2008). Cerebral Ischemia: Models, Methods and Outcomes. *Neuropharmacology*,Vol.55, No.3, (January 2008), pp. 257-270, ISSN 0028-3908

Hossmann, K.A. & Grosse Ophoff, B. (1986). Recovery of Monkey Brain After Prolonged Ischemia. I. Electrophysiology and Brain Electrolytes. *Journal of Cerebral Blood Flow & Metabolism*,Vol.6, No.1, (February 1986), pp. 15-21, ISSN 0271-678X

Hurn, P.D.; Littleton-Kearney, M.T.; Kirsch, J.R.; Dharmarajan, A.M. & Traystman, R.J. (1995). Postischemic Cerebral Blood Flow Recovery in the Female: Effect of 17 Beta-Estradiol. *Journal of Cerebral Blood Flow & Metabolism*,Vol.15, No.4, (July 1995), pp. 666-672, ISSN 0271-678X

Hurtado, O.; Pradillo, J.M.; Alonso-Escolano, D.; Lorenzo, P.; Sobrino, T.; Castillo, J.; Lizasoain, I. & Moro M.A. (2006). Neurorepair versus Neuroprotection in Stroke. *Cerebrovascular Diseases,* Vol. 21, (Suppl. 2), pp. 54-63, ISSN 1015-9770

Iadecola, C. & Alexander, M. (2001) Cerebral Ischemia and Inflammation. *Current Opinion in Neurology,* Vol. 14, No.1 , (February 2001), pp. 89-94, ISSN 0959-4388

Ikeda, M.; Yoshida, S.; Busto, R.; Santiso, M. & Ginsberg, M.D. (1986). Polyphosphoinositides as a Probable Source of Brain Free Fatty Acids Accumulated at the Onset of Ischemia. *Journal of Neurochemistry,*Vol.47, No.1, (July 1986), pp. 123-132, ISSN 0022-3042

Inamasu, J.; Nakatsukasa, M.; Suzuki, M. & Miyatake, S. (2010). Therapeutic Hypothermia for Out-of-Hospital Cardiac Arrest: An Update for Neurosurgeons. *World Neurosurgery,* Vol. 74, No. 1, (July 2010), pp. 120-128, ISSN 1878-8750

Incagnoli, P.; Ramond, A.; Joyeux-Faure, M.; Pepin, J.L.; Levy, P. & Ribuot, C. (2009). Erythropoietin Improved Initial Resuscitation and Increased Survival After Cardiac Arrest in Rats. *Resuscitation,*Vol.80, No.6, (May 2009), pp. 696-700, ISSN 1873-1570

Izaki, Y.; Takita, M. & Akema, T. (2008). Specific Role of the Posterior Dorsal Hippocampus-Prefrontal Cortex in Short-Term Working Memory. *European Journal of Neuroscience,*Vol.27, No.11, (June 2008), pp. 3029-3034, ISSN 1460-9568

Janac, B.; Selakovic, V. & Radenovic, L. (2008). Temporal Patterns of Motor Behavioural Improvements by MK-801 in Mongolian Gerbils Submitted to Different Duration of Global Cerebral Ischemia. *Behavioural Brain Research,*Vol.194, No.1, (July 2008), pp. 72-78, ISSN 0166-4328

Jarrard, L.E. (1993). On the Role of the Hippocampus in Learning and Memory in the Rat. *Behavioral and Neural Biology,*Vol.60, No.1, (July 1993), pp. 9-26, ISSN 0163-1047

Johansen, F.F. & Diemer, N.H. (1991). Enhancement of GABA Neurotransmission After Cerebral Ischemia in the Rat Reduces Loss of Hippocampal CA1 Pyramidal Cells. *Acta Neurologica Scandinavica,* Vol.84, No.1, (July 1991), pp. 1-6. ISSN

Johansson, B.B. & Belichenko, P.V. (2002). Neuronal Plasticity and Dendritic Spines: Effect of Environmental Enrichment on Intact and Postischemic Rat Brain. *Journal of Cerebral Blood Flow & Metabolism,*Vol.22, No.1, (January 2002), pp. 89-96, ISSN 0271-678X

Jourdain, P.; Nikonenko, I.; Alberi, S. & Muller, D. (2002). Remodeling of Hippocampal Synaptic Networks by a Brief Anoxia-hypoglycemia. *Journal of Neuroscience,*Vol.22, No.8, (April 2002), pp. 3108-3116, ISSN 1529-2401

Jover-Mengual, T.; Miyawaki, T.; Latuszek, A.; Alborch, E.; Zukin, R.S. & Etgen, A.M. (2010). Acute Estradiol Protects CA1 Neurons from Ischemia-induced Apoptotic Cell Death Via the PI3K/Akt Pathway. *Brain Research,*Vol.1321, (February 2010), pp. 1-12, ISSN 1872-6240

Jung, M.W.; Qin, Y.; McNaughton, B.L. & Barnes, C.A. (1998). Firing Characteristics of Deep Layer Neurons in Prefrontal Cortex in Rats Performing Spatial Working Memory Tasks. *Cerebral Cortex,*Vol.8, No.5, (August 1998), pp. 437-450, ISSN 1047-3211

Karanjia, N. & Geocadin, R.G. (2011). Post-cardiac Arrest Syndrome: Update on Brain Injury Management and Prognostication. *Current Treatment Options in Neurology,*Vol.13, No.2, (January 2011), pp. 191-203, ISSN 1534-3138

Kasai, H.; Matsuzaki, M.; Noguchi, J.; Yasumatsu, N. & Nakahara, H. (2003). Structure-Stability-Function Relationships of Dendritic Spines. *Trends in Neurosciences,*Vol.26, No.7, (July 2003), pp. 360-368, ISSN 0166-2236

Katz, L.; Ebmeyer, U.; Safar, P.; Radovsky, A. & Neumar, R. (1995). Outcome Model of Asphyxial Cardiac Arrest in Rats. *Journal of Cerebral Blood Flow & Metabolism*,Vol.15, No.6, (November 1995), pp. 1032-1039, ISSN 0271-678X

Kiprianova, I.; Freiman, T.M.; Desiderato, S.; Schwab, S.; Galmbacher, R.; Gillardon, F. & Spranger, M. (1999a). Brain-Derived Neurotrophic Factor Prevents Neuronal Death and Glial Activation After Global Ischemia in the Rat. *Journal of Neuroscience Research*, Vol.56, No.1, (April 1999), pp. 21-27, ISSN 0270-6474

Kiprianova, I.; Sandkühler, J.; Schwab, S.; Hoyer, S. & Spranger, M. (1999b). Brain-Derived Neurotrophic Factor Improves Long-Term Potentiation and Cognitive Functions After Transient Forebrain Ischemia in the Rat. *Experimentsal Neurology*, (October 1999), Vol.159, No.2, pp. 511-519, ISSN

Kirino, T. (1982). Delayed Neuronal Death in the Gerbil Hippocampus Following Ischemia. *Brain Research*, Vol.239, No.1, (May 1982), pp. 57-69, ISSN 0006-8993

Knapp, J.; Heinzmann, A.; Schneider, A.; Padosch, S.A.; Böttiger, B.W.; Teschendorf, P. & Popp, E. (2011). Hypothermia and Neuroprotection by Sulfide After Cardiac Arrest and Cardiopulmonary Resuscitation. *Resuscitation*, Vol.82, No.8, (August 2011) pp. 1076-1080, ISSN

Kofke, W.A.: Nemoto, E.M.; Hossmann, K.A.; Taylor, F.; Kessler, P.D. & Stezoski, S.W. (1979). Brain Blood Flow and Metabolism after Global Ischemia and Post-Insult Thiopental Therapy in Monkeys. *Stroke*, (September-October 1979), Vol.10, No.5, pp. 554-560, ISSN 0039-2499

Kofler, J.; Hattori, K.; Sawada, M.; DeVries, A.C.; Martin, L.J.; Hurn, P.D. & Traystman, R.J. (2004). Histopathological and Behavioral Characterization of a Novel Model of Cardiac Arrest and Cardiopulmonary Resuscitation in Mice. *Journal of Neuroscience Methods*,Vol.136, No.1, (May 2004), pp. 33-44, ISSN 0165-0270

Koh, P.O.; Cho, G.J. & Choi, W.S. (2006). 17beta-Estradiol Pretreatment Prevents the Global Ischemic Injury-Induced Decrease of Akt Activation and Bad Phosphorylation in Gerbils. *Journal of Veterinary Medical Science*,Vol.68, No.10, (November 2006), pp. 1019-1022, ISSN 0916-7250

Koinig, H.; Vornik, V.; Rueda, C. & Zornow, M. H. (2001). Lubeluzole Inhibits Accumulation of Extracellular Glutamate in the Hippocampus During Transient Global Cerebral Ischemia. *Brain Research*, Vol.898, No.2, (April 2001), pp. 297-302, ISSN 0006-8993

Kolb, B. (1990) In: *The Cerebral Cortex of the Rat*. B. Kolb & R.C. Tees, (Eds.), 437-458, MIT Press, ISBN: 978-026-2610-64-3, Cambridge, Massachussetts, USA

Kolb, B.; Pittman, K.; Sutherland, R.J. & Whishaw, I.Q. (1982). Dissociation of the Contributions of the Prefrontal Cortex and Dorsomedial Thalamic Nucleus to Spatially Guided Behavior in the Rat. *Behavioural Brain Research*, Vol.6, No.4, (December 1982), pp. 365-378, ISSN 0166-4328

Kolb, B.; Teskey, G.C. & Gibb, R. (2010). Factors Influencing Cerebral Plasticity in the Normal and Injured Brain. *Frontiers in Human Neuroscience*, Vol.4, (November 2010), pp. 1-12, ISSN 1662-5161

Korzhevskii, D.E.; Otellin, V.A.; Grigor'ev, I.P.; Kostkin, V.B.; Polenov, S.A.; Lentsman, M.V. & Balestrino, M. (2005). Structural Organization of Astrocytes in the Rat Hippocampus in the Post-ischemic Period. *Neuroscience & Behavioral Physiology*, Vol.35, No.4, (May 2005), pp. 389-392, ISSN 0097-0549

Kovalenko, T.; Osadchenko, I.; Nikonenko, A.; Lushnikova, I.; Voronin, K.; Nikonenko, I.; Muller, D. & Skibo, G. (2006). Ischemia-Induced Modifications in Hippocampal CA1 Stratum Radiatum Excitatory Synapses. *Hippocampus,* Vol.16, No.10, (August 2006), pp. 814-825, ISSN 1050-9631

Krause, G.S.; Kumar, K.; White, B.C.; Aust, S.D. & Wiegenstein, J.G. (1986). Ischemia, Resuscitation, and Reperfusion: Mechanisms of Tissue Injury and Prospects for Protection. *American Heart Journal,* Vol.111, No.4, (April 1986), pp. 768-780, ISSN 0002-8703

Kubo, K.; Nakao, S.; Jomura, S.; Sakamoto, S.; Miyamoto, E.; Xu, Y.; Tomimoto, H.; Inada, T. & Shingu, K. (2009). Edaravone, a Free Radical Scavenger, Mitigates Both Gray and White Matter Damages After Global Cerebral Ischemia in Rats. *Brain Research,* Vol. 1279, No. 3, (July 2009), pp. 139-46, ISSN ISSN 0006-8993

Kwon, Y.B.; Yang, I.S.; Kang, K.S.; Han, H.J.; Lee, Y.S. & Lee, J.H. (2000). Effects of Dizocilpine Pretreatment on Parvalbumin Immunoreactivity and Fos Expression after Cerebral Ischemia in the Hippocampus of the Mongolian Gerbil. *Journal of Veterinary Medical Science,*Vol.62, No.2, (March 2000), pp. 141-146, ISSN 0916-7250

Lakhan, S.E.; Kirchgessner, A. & Hofer, M. (2009). Inflammatory Mechanisms in Ischemic Stroke: Therapeutic Approaches. *Journal of Translational Medicine,*Vol.7, (November 2009), pp. 97, ISSN 1479-5876

Lambe, E.K.; Goldman-Rakic, P.S. & Aghajanian, G.K. (2000). Serotonin Induces EPSCs Preferentially in Layer V Pyramidal Neurons of the Frontal Cortex in the Rat. *Cerebral Cortex,*Vol.10, No.10, (September 2000), pp. 974-980, ISSN 1047-3211

Langdon, K.D.; Granter-Button, S. & Corbett, D. (2008). Persistent Behavioral Impairments and Neuroinflammation Following Global Ischemia in the Rat. *European Journal of Neuroscience,*Vol.28, No.11, (November 2008), pp. 2310-2318, ISSN 1460-9568

Laroche, S.; Davis, S. & Jay, T. M. (2000). Plasticity at Hippocampal to Prefrontal Cortex Synapses: Dual Roles in Working Memory and Consolidation. *Hippocampus,*Vol.10, No.4, (September 2000), pp. 438-446, ISSN 1050-9631

Larsson, E.; Nanobashvili, A.; Kokaia, Z & Lindvall, O. (1999) Evidence for Neuroprotective Effects of Endogenous Brain-Derived Neurotrophic Factor After Global Forebrain Ischemia in Rats. *Journal of Cerebral Blood Flow & Metab,* Vol.19, No.11, (November 1999), pp. 1220-1228, ISSN

Lauritzen, I.; Blondeau, N.; Heurteaux, C.; Widmann, C.; Romey, G. & Lazdunski, M. (2000). Polyunsaturated Fatty Acids are Potent Neuroprotectors. *EMBO Journal,*Vol.19, No.8, (April 2000), pp. 1784-1793, ISSN 0261-4189

Lazarewicz, J.W.; Pluta, R.; Puka, M. & Salinska, E. (1990). Diverse Mechanisms of Neuronal Protection by Nimodipine in Experimental Rabbit Brain Ischemia. *Stroke,* Vol.21, (12 Supplement), (December 1990), pp. IV108-110, ISSN 0039-2499

Lazarewicz, J.W.; Pluta, R.; Puka, M. & Salinska, E. (1993). Local Nimodipine Application Improves Early Functional Recovery in the Rabbit Hippocampus After 15-min Global Cerebral Ischemia. *Acta Neurobiologiae Experimentalis* Vol.53, No.4, (January 1993), pp. 499-510, ISSN 0065-1400

Lebesgue, D.; Chevaleyre, V.; Zukin, R.S. & Etgen, A.M. (2009). Estradiol Rescues Neurons from Global Ischemia-Induced Cell Death: Multiple Cellular Pathways of Neuroprotection. *Steroids,* Vol.74, No.7, (May 2009), pp. 555-561, ISSN 0039-128X

Lee, I. & Kesner, R. P. (2003). Time-dependent Relationship between the Dorsal Hippocampus and the Prefrontal Cortex in Spatial Memory. *Journal of Neuroscience,* Vol.23, No.4, (February 2003), pp. 1517-1523, ISSN 1529-2401

Lee, Y.S.; Yoon, B.W. & Roh, J.K. (1999). Neuroprotective Effects of Lamotrigine Enhanced by Flunarizine in Gerbil Global Ischemia. *Neuroscience Letters,* Vol.265, No.3, (May 1999), pp. 215-217, ISSN 0304-3940

Leker, R.R. & Shohami, E. (2002). Cerebral Ischemia and Trauma – Different Ethiologies yet Similar Mechanisms: Neuroprotective Opportunities. *Brain Research Brain Research Reviews,* Vol. 39, No. 1, (January 2002), pp. 55-73, ISSN 0165-0173

Lensman, M.; Korzhevskii, D.E.; Mourovets, V.O.; Kostkin, V.B.; Izvarina, N.; Perasso L.; Gandolfo C.; Otellin, V.A.; Polenov, S.A. & Balestrino, M. (2006). Intracerebroventricular Administration of Creatine Protects against Damage by Global Cerebral Ischemia in Rat. *Brain Research.* Vol. 1114, No. 1, (October 2006), pp. 187-194, ISSN 0006-8993

Letechipía-Vallejo, G.; González-Burgos, I. & Cervantes, M. (2001). Neuroprotective Effect of Melatonin on Brain Damage Induced by Acute Global Cerebral Ischemia in Cats. *Archives of Medical Research,* Vol.32, No.3, (June 2001), pp. 186-192, ISSN 0188-4409

Letechipía-Vallejo, G.; López-Loeza, E.; Espinoza-González, V.; González-Burgos, I.; Olvera-Cortés, M. E.; Moralí, G. & Cervantes, M. (2007). Long-term Morphological and Functional Evaluation of the Neuroprotective Effects of Post-ischemic Treatment with Melatonin in Rats. *Journal of Pineal Research,* Vol.42, No.2, (February 2007), pp. 138-146, ISSN 0742-3098

Li, R.C.; Guo, S.Z.; Lee, S.K. & Gozal, D. (2010). Neuroglobin Protects Neurons Against Oxidative Stress in Global Ischemia. *Journal of Cerebral Blood Flow & Metabolism,* Vol.30, No.11, (June 2010), pp. 1874-1882, ISSN 1559-7016

Liang, S.P.; Kanthan, R.; Shuaib, A., & Wishart, T. (1997). Effects of Clomethiazole on Radial-arm Maze Performance Following Global Forebrain Ischemia in Gerbils. *Brain Research,* Vol.751, No.2, (March 1997), pp. 189-195, ISSN 0006-8993

Lipton, P. (1999). Ischemic Cell Death in Brain Neurons. *Physiology Reviews,* Vol.79, No.4, (October 1999), pp. 1431-1568, ISSN 0031-9333

Littleton-Kearney, M.T.; Gaines, J.M.; Callahan, K.P.; Murphy, S.J. & Hurn, P.D. (2005). Effects of Estrogen on Platelet Reactivity after Transient Forebrain Ischemia in Rats. *Biological Research for Nursing,* Vol.7, No.2, (November 2005), pp. 135-145, ISSN 1099-8004

Lowry, O.H.; Passonneau, J.V.; Hasselberger, F.X. & Schulz, D.W. (1964). Effect of Ischemia on Known Substrates and Cofactors of the Glycolytic Pathway in Brain. *Journal of Biological Chemistry,* Vol.239, (January 1964), pp. 18-30, ISSN 0021-9258

Lu, A.; Ran, R.Q.; Clark, J.; Reilly, M.; Nee, A. & Sharp, F.R. (2002). 17-beta-Estradiol Induces Heat Shock Proteins in Brain Arteries and Potentiates Ischemic Heat Shock Protein Induction in Glia and Neurons. *Journal of Cerebral Blood Flow & Metabolism,* Vol.22, No.2, (February 2002), pp. 183-195, ISSN 0271-678X

Ma, D.; Lu, L.; Boneva, N.B.; Warashina, S.; Kaplamadzhiev, D.B.; Mori, Y.; Nakaya, M.A.; Kikuchi, M.; Tonchev, A.B.,; Okano, H. & Yamashima, T. (2008). Expression of Free Fatty Acid Receptor GPR40 in the Neurogenic Niche of Adult Monkey Hippocampus. *Hippocampus,* Vol.18, No.3, (December 2007), pp. 326-333, ISSN 1098-1063

Madl, C. & Holzer, M. (2004). Brain Function after Resuscitation from Cardiac Arrest. *Current Opinion in Critical Care,* Vol.10, No.3, (May 2004), pp. 213-217, ISSN 1070-5295

Margaill, I.; Plotkine, M. & Lerouet, D. (2005). Antioxidant Strategies in the Treatment of Stroke. *Free Radical Biology & Medicine,* Vol. 39, No.4 , (August 2005), pp. 429-443, ISSN 0891-5849

Matsumoto, M.; Scheller, M.S.; Zornow, M.H. & Strnat, M.A. (1993). Effect of S-emopamil, Nimodipine, and Mild Hypothermia on Hippocampal Glutamate Concentrations after Repeated Cerebral Ischemia in Rabbits. *Stroke,* Vol.24, No.8, (August 1993), pp. 1228-1234, ISSN 0039-2499

Matsushita, K.; Kitagawa, K.; Matsuyama, T.; Ohtsuki, T.; Taguchi, A.; Mandai, K.; Mabuchi, T.; Yagita, Y.; Yanagihara, T. & Matsumoto, M. (1996). Effect of Systemic Zinc Administration on Delayed Neuronal Death in the Gerbil Hippocampus. *Brain Research,* Vol.743, No.1-2, (December 1996), pp. 362-365, ISSN 0006-8993

McBean, D.E. & Kelly, P.A. (1998). Rodent Models of Global Cerebral Ischemia: a Comparison of Two-vessel Occlusion and Four-vessel Occlusion. *General Pharmacology,* Vol.30, No.4, (April 1998), pp. 431-434, ISSN 0306-3623

McDonald, R.J. & White, N.M. (1993). A Triple Dissociation of Memory Systems: Hippocampus, Amygdala, and Dorsal Striatum. *Behavior Neuroscience,* Vol.107, No.1, (February 1993), pp. 3-22, ISSN 0735-7044

McDonald, R.J. & White, N.M. (1994). Parallel Information Processing in the Water Maze: Evidence for Independent Memory Systems Involving Dorsal Striatum and Hippocampus. *Behavioral and Neural Biology,* Vol.61, No.3, (May 1994), pp. 260-270, ISSN 0163-1047

McDonald, R.J. & White, N.M. (1995). Hippocampal and Nonhippocampal Contributions to Place Learning in Rats. *Behavioral Neuroscience,* Vol.109, No.4, (August 1995), pp. 579-593, ISSN 0735-7044

McNamara, R.K. & Skelton, R.W. (1993). The Neuropharmacological and Neurochemical Basis of Place Learning in the Morris Water Maze. *Brain Research Brain Research Reviews,* Vol.18, No.1, (January 1993), pp. 33-49, ISSN 0165-0173

Mehta, S.L.; Manhas, N. & Raghubir, R. (2007). Molecular Targets in Cerebral Ischemia for Developing Novel Therapeutics. *Brain Research Reviews,* Vol.54, No.1, (January 2007), pp. 34-66, ISSN 0165-0173

Meloni, B.P.; Campbell, K.; Zhu, H. & Knuckey, N.W. (2009). In Search of Clinical Neuroprotection after Brain Ischemia: the Case for Mild Hypothermia (35 Degrees C) and Magnesium. *Stroke,* Vol.40, No.6, (April 2009), pp. 2236-2240, ISSN 0039-2499

Miles, A.N.; Majda, B.T.; Meloni, B.P. & Knuckey, N.W. (2001). Postischemic Intravenous Administration of Magnesium Sulfate Inhibits Hippocampal CA1 Neuronal Death after Transient Global Ischemia in Rats. *Neurosurgery,* Vol.49, No.6, (February 2002), pp. 1443-1450, ISSN 0148-396X

Montero, M.; Nielsen, M.; Ronn, L.C.; Moller, A.; Noraberg, J. & Zimmer, J. (2007). Neuroprotective Effects of the AMPA Antagonist PNQX in Oxygen-glucose Deprivation in Mouse Hippocampal Slice Cultures and Global Cerebral Ischemia in Gerbils. *Brain Research,* Vol.1177, (September 2007), pp. 124-135, ISSN 0006-8993

Moralí, G.; Letechipía-Vallejo, G.; López-Loeza, E.; Montes, P.; Hernández-Morales, L. & Cervantes, M. (2005). Post-ischemic Administration of Progesterone in Rats Exerts Neuroprotective Effects on the Hippocampus. *Neuroscience Letters,* Vol.382, No.3, (May 2005), pp. 286-290, ISSN 0304-3940

Moralí, G.; Montes, P.; González-Burgos, I.; Velázquez-Zamora, D.A. & Cervantes, M. (2011a). Cytoarchitectural Characteristics of Hippocampal CA1 Pyramidal Neurons of Rats, Four Months After Global Cerebral Ischemia and Progesterone Treatment. *Restorative Neurology and Neuroscience,* (September 2011), ISSN 0922-6028 [Epub ahead of print]

Moralí, G.; Montes, P.; Hernández-Morales, L.; Monfil, T.; Espinosa-García, C. & Cervantes, M. (2011b). Neuroprotective Effects of Progesterone and Allopregnanolone on Long-term Cognitive Outcome after Global Cerebral Ischemia. *Restorative Neurology and Neuroscience,* Vol.29, No.1, (February 2011), pp. 1-15, ISSN 0922-6028

Mori, T.; Tan, J.; Arendash, G.W.; Koyama, N.; Nojima, Y. & Town, T. (2008). Overexpression of Human S100B Exacerbates Brain Damage and Periinfarct Gliosis after Permanent Focal Ischemia. *Stroke,* Vol.39, No.7, (July 2008), pp. 2114-2121, ISSN 0039-2499

Morimoto, Y.; Kwon, J. Y.; Deyo, D. J. & Zornow, M. H. (2002). Effects of Lamotrigine on Conditioned Learning after Global Cerebral Ischemia in Rabbits. *Journal of Anesthesia,*Vol.16, No.4, (October 2003), pp. 349-353, ISSN 0913-8668

Morioka, T.; Kalehua, A.N. & Streit, W.J. (1991). The Microglial Reaction in the Rat Dorsal Hippocampus Following Transient Forebrain Ischemia. *Journal of Cerebral Blood Flow & Metabolism,* Vol.11, No.6, (November 1991), pp. 966-973, ISSN 0271-678X

Morioka, T.; Kalehua, A.N. & Streit, W.J. (1992). Progressive Expression of Immunomolecules on Microglial Cells in Rat Dorsal Hippocampus Following Transient Forebrain Ischemia. *Acta Neuropathologica (Berlin),* Vol.83, No.2, (February 1992), pp. 149-157, ISSN 0001-6322

Morris, R. (1984). Development of a Water-maze Procedure for Studying Spatial Learning in the Rat. *Journal of Neuroscience Methods,* Vol.11, No.1, (May 1984), pp. 47-60, ISSN 0165-0270

Morris, R.G.; Garrud, P.; Rawlins, J.N. & O'Keefe, J. (1982). Place Navigation Impaired in Rats with Hippocampal Lesions. *Nature,* Vol.297, No.5868, (June 1982), pp. 681-683, ISSN 0028-0836

Morris, R.G.; Schenk, F.; Tweedie, F. & Jarrard, L E. (1990). Ibotenate Lesions of Hippocampus and/or Subiculum: Dissociating Components of Allocentric Spatial Learning. *European Journal of Neuroscience,*Vol.2, No.12, (January 1990), pp. 1016-1028, ISSN 1460-9568

Moser, E.; Moser, M.B. & Andersen, P. (1993). Spatial Learning Impairment Parallels the Magnitude of Dorsal Hippocampal Lesions, but is Hardly Present Following Ventral Lesions. *Journal of Neuroscience,* Vol.13, No.9, (September 1993), pp. 3916-3925, ISSN 0270-6474

Mudrick, L.A. & Baimbridge, K.G. (1989). Long-term Structural Changes in the Rat Hippocampal Formation Following Cerebral Ischemia. *Brain Research,* Vol.493, No.1, (July 1989), pp. 179-184, ISSN 0006-8993

Mueller, R.N.; Deyo, D.J.,; Brantley, D.R.; Disterhoft, J.F. & Zornow, M.H. (2003). Lubeluzole and Conditioned Learning after Cerebral Ischemia. *Experimental Brain Research,*Vol.152, No.3, (August 2003), pp. 329-334, ISSN 0014-4819

Myhrer, T. (2003). Neurotransmitter Systems Involved in Learning and Memory in the Rat: a Meta-analysis Based on Studies of Four Behavioral Tasks. *Brain Research Brain Research Reviews,* Vol.41, No.2-3, (March 2003), pp. 268-287, ISSN 0165-0173

Nakatomi, H.; Kuriu, T.; Okabe, S.; Yamamoto, S.; Hatano, O.; Kawahara, N.; Tamura, A.; Kirino, T. & Nakafuku, M. (2002). Regeneration of Hippocampal Pyramidal Neurons after Ischemic Brain Injury by Recruitment of Endogenous Neural Progenitors. *Cell,* Vol.110, No.4, (August 2002), pp. 429-441, ISSN 0092-8674

Nakayama, R.; Yano, T.; Ushijima, K.; Abe, E. & Terasaki, H. (2002). Effects of Dantrolene on Extracellular Glutamate Concentration and Neuronal Death in the Rat Hippocampal CA1 Region Subjected to Transient Ischemia. *Anesthesiology,* Vol.96, No.3, (March 2002), pp. 705-710, ISSN 0003-3022

Nanri, K.; Montecot, C.; Springhetti, V.; Seylaz, J. & Pinard, E. (1998). The Selective Inhibitor of Neuronal Nitric Oxide Synthase, 7-nitroindazole, Reduces the Delayed Neuronal Damage Due to Forebrain Ischemia in Rats. *Stroke,* Vol.29, No.6, (June 1998), pp. 1248-1253; discussion 1253-1244, ISSN 0039-2499

Neigh, G.N.; Glasper, E.R.; Kofler, J.; Traystman, R.J.; Mervis, R.F.; Bachstetter, A. & DeVries, A.C. (2004). Cardiac Arrest with Cardiopulmonary Resuscitation Reduces Dendritic Spine Density in CA1 Pyramidal Cells and Selectively Alters Acquisition of Spatial Memory. *European Journal of Neuroscience,* Vol.20, No.7, (September 2004), pp. 1865-1872, ISSN 0953-816X

Nelson, A.; Lebessi, A.; Sowinski, P. & Hodges, H. (1997). Comparison of Effects of Global Cerebral Ischaemia on Spatial Learning in the Standard and Radial Water Maze: Relationship of Hippocampal Damage to Performance. *Behavioral Brain Research,* Vol.85, No.1, (April 1997), pp. 93-115, ISSN 0166-4328

Nemoto, E.M.; Bleyaert, A.L.; Stezoski, S.W.; Moossy, J.; Rao, G.R. & Safar, P. (1977). Global Brain Ischemia: a Reproducible Monkey Model. *Stroke,* Vol.8, No.5, (September 1977), pp. 558-564, ISSN 0039-2499

Nikonenko, A.G.; Radenovic, L.; Andjus, P.R. & Skibo, G.G. (2009). Structural Features of Ischemic Damage in the Hippocampus. *The Anatomical Record,* Vol.292, No.12, (December 2009), pp. 1914-1921, ISSN 1932-8486

Nishimura, H.; Matsuyama, T.; Obata, K.; Nakajima, Y.; Kitano, H.; Sugita, M. & Okamoto, M. (2000). Changes in Mint1, a Novel Synaptic Protein, after Transient Global Ischemia in Mouse Hippocampus. *Journal of Cerebral Blood Flow & Metabolism,* Vol.20, No.10, (November 2000), pp. 1437-1445, ISSN 0271-678X

Noguchi, K.; Matsumoto, N.; Shiozaki, T.; Tasaki, O.; Ogura, H.; Kuwagata, Y.; Sugimoto, H. & Seiyama A. (2011). Effects of Timing and Duration of Hypothermia on Survival in an Experimental Gerbil Model of Global Ischaemia. *Resuscitation,* Vol.82, No.4, (April 2011), pp. 481-486, ISSN 0300-9572

O'Keefe, J. & Nadel, L. (1978). *The Hippocampus as a Cognitive Map,* Oxford University Press, ISBN 0-19-857206-9, New York, USA

Oliveira, M.G.; Bueno, O.F.; Pomarico, A.C. & Gugliano, E.B. (1997). Strategies Used by Hippocampal- and Caudate-Putamen-Lesioned Rats in a Learning Task.

Neurobiology of Learning and Memory, Vol.68, No.1, (July 1997), pp. 32-41, ISSN 1074-7427

Olsen, G.M.; Scheel-Kruger, J.; Moller, A. & Jensen, L.H. (1994). Relation of Spatial Learning of Rats in the Morris Water Maze Task to the Number of Viable CA1 Neurons Following Four-vessel Occlusion. *Behavioral Neuroscience,*Vol.108, No.4, (August 1994), pp. 681-690, ISSN 0735-7044

Olton, D.S. (1983). Memory Functions and the Hippocampus, In: *Neurobiology of the Hippocampus,* W. Seifer, (Ed.), 335-373, Academic Press, ISBN 0126348804, New York, USA

Olton, D.S. (1987). The Radial Arm Maze as a Tool in Behavioral Pharmacology. *Physiology & Behavior,* Vol. 40, No. 6, (December 1987), pp. 793-797, ISSN 0031-9384

Olton, D.S.; Walker, J.A. & Wolf, W.A. (1982). A Disconnection Analysis of Hippocampal Function. *Brain Research,* Vol.233, No.2, (February 1982), pp. 241-253, ISSN 0006-8993

Olvera-Cortés, E.; Barajas-Pérez, M.; Morales-Villagrán, A. & González-Burgos, I. (2001). Cerebral Serotonin Depletion Induces Egocentric Learning Improvement in Developing Rats. *Neuroscience Letters,* Vol.313, No.1-2, (October 2001), pp. 29-32, ISSN 0304-3940

Olvera-Cortés, E.; Cervantes, M. & González-Burgos, I. (2002). Place-learning, but not Cue-learning Training, Modifies the Hippocampal Theta Rhythm in Rats. *Brain Research Bulletin,* Vol.58, No.3, (July 2002), pp. 261-270, ISSN 0361-9230.

Olvera-Cortés, M.E.; García-Alcántar, I.; Gutiérrez-Guzmán, B.E.; Hernández-Pérez, J.J.; López-Vázquez, M.A. & Cervantes, M. (2012). Differential Learning-Related Changes in Theta Activity During Place Learning in Young and Old Rats. Behavioural Brain Research, *Behavioural Brain Research,* Vol.226, No.2, (January 2012), pp. 555-562, ISSN 0166-4328 (In Press)

Onodera, H.; Aoki, H.; Yae, T. & Kogure, K. (1990). Post-ischemic Synaptic Plasticity in the Rat Hippocampus After Long-term Survival: Histochemical and Autoradiographic Study. *Neuroscience,* Vol.38, No.1, (January 1990), pp. 125-136, ISSN 0306-4522

Otani, H.; Togashi, H.; Jesmin, S.; Sakuma, I.; Yamaguchi, T.; Matsumoto, M.; Kakehata, H. & Yoshioka, M. (2005). Temporal Effects of Edaravone, a Free Radical Scavenger, on Transient Ischemia-induced Neuronal Dysfunction in the Rat Hippocampus. *European Journal of Pharmacology,* Vol. 512, No. 2-3, (April 2005), pp. 129-37, ISSN 0014-2999

Otellin, V.A.; Korzhevskii, D.E.; Kostkin, V.B.; Balestrino, M.; Lensman, M.V. & Polenov, S.A. (2003). The Neuroprotective Effect of Creatine in Rats with Cerebral Ischemia. *Doklady Biological Sciences,* Vol. 390, No. 3, (May-Jun 2003), pp. 197-199, ISSN 0012-4966

Ozacmak, V.H. & Sayan, H. (2009). The Effects of 17beta Estradiol, 17alpha Estradiol and Progesterone on Oxidative Stress Biomarkers in Ovariectomized Female Rat Brain Subjected to Global Cerebral Ischemia. *Physiological Research,* Vol.58, No.6, (December 2008), pp. 909-912, ISSN 0862-8408

Pappas, T.N. & Mironovich, R.O. (1981). Barbiturate-Induced Comma to Protect Against Cerebral Ischemia and Increased Intracranial Pressure. *American Journal of Hospital Pharmacy,* (April 1981), Vol.38, No.4, pp. 494-498, ISSN 0002-9289

Pazos, A.J.; Green, E.J.; Busto, R.; McCabe, P.M.; Baena, R.C.; Ginsberg, M.D.; Globus, M.Y.; Schneiderman, N. & Dietrich, W.D. (1999). Effects of Combined Postischemic Hypothermia and Delayed N-tert-butyl-alpha-pheylnitrone (PBN) Administration on Histopathological and Behavioral Deficits Associated with Transient Global Ischemia in Rats. *Brain Research,* Vol.846, No.2, (November 1999), pp. 186-195, ISSN 0006-8993

Pérez-Vega, M.I.; Feria-Velasco, A. & González-Burgos, I. (2000). Prefrontocortical Serotonin Depletion Results in Plastic Changes of Prefrontocortical Pyramidal Neurons, Underlying a Greater Efficiency of Short-term Memory. *Brain Research Bulletin,* Vol.53, No.3, (December 2000), pp. 291-300, ISSN 0361-9230

Petito, C.K. & Halaby, I.A. (1993). Relationship Between Ischemia and Ischemic Neuronal Necrosis to Astrocyte Expression of Glial Fibrillary Acidic Protein. *International Journal of Developmental Neuroscience,* Vol.11, No.2, (April 1993), pp. 239-47, ISSN 0736-5748

Piao, C.S.; Che, Y.; Han, P.L. & Lee, J.K. (2002). Delayed and Differential Induction of p38 MAPK Isoforms in Microglia and Astrocytes in the Brain after Transient Global Ischemia. *Brain Research. Molecular Brain Research,* Vol.107, No.2, (November 2002), pp. 137-144, ISSN 0169-328X

del Pilar Fernández, M., Meizoso, M.J., Lodeiro, M.J. & Belmonte, A. (1998). Effect of Desmethyl Tirilazad, Dizocilpine Maleate and Nimodipine on Brain Nitric Oxide Synthase Activity and Cyclic Guanosine Monophosphate During Cerebral Ischemia in Rats. *Pharmacology,*Vol.57, No.4, (September 1998), pp. 174-179, ISSN 0031-7012

Plamondon, H. & Roberge, M.C. (2008). Dietary PUFA Supplements Reduce Memory Deficits But not CA1 Ischemic Injury in Rats. *Physiology & Behavior,*Vol.95, No.3, (August 2008), pp. 492-500, ISSN 0031-9384

Popp, E.; Padosch, S.A.; Vogel, P.; Schäbitz, W.R.; Schwab, S. & Böttiger, B.W. (2004). Effects of Intracerebroventricular Application of Brain-Derived Neurotrophic Factor on Cerebral Recovery After Cardiac Arrest in Rats. *Critical Care Medicine,* (September 2004), Vol.32, (9 Suppl), pp. S359-65, ISSN 0090-3493

Pulsinelli, W.A. (1985). Selective Neuronal Vulnerability: Morphological and Molecular Characteristics. *Progress in Brain Research,* Vol.63, (January 1985), pp. 29-37, ISSN 0079-6123

Pulsinelli, W.A. & Brierley, J.B. (1979). A New Model of Bilateral Hemispheric Ischemia in the Unanesthetized Rat. *Stroke,* Vol.10, No.3, (May 1979), pp. 267-272, ISSN 0039-2499

Pulsinelli, W.A. & Buchan, A.M. (1988). The Four-vessel Occlusion Rat Model: Method for Complete Occlusion of Vertebral Arteries and Control of Collateral Circulation. *Stroke,* Vol.19, No.7, (July 1988), pp. 913-914, ISSN 0039-2499

Pulsinelli, W.A. & Duffy, T.E. (1983). Regional Energy Balance in Rat Brain after Transient Forebrain Ischemia. *Journal of Neurochemistry,* Vol.40, No.5, (May 1983), pp. 1500-1503, ISSN 0022-3042

Pulsinelli, W.A.; Jacewicz, M.; Levy, D.E.; Petito, C.K. & Plum, F. (1997). Ischemic Brain Injury and the Therapeutic Window. *Annals of the New York Academy of Sciences,* Vol.835, (June 1998), pp. 187-193, ISSN 0077-8923

Pulsinelli, W.A.; Levy, D.E. & Duffy, T.E. (1982). Regional Cerebral Blood Flow and Glucose Metabolism Following Transient Forebrain Ischemia. *Annals of Neurology,* Vol.11, No.5, (May 1982), pp. 499-502, ISSN 0364-5134

Radovsky, A.; Safar, P.; Sterz, F.; Leonov, Y.; Reich, H. & Kuboyama, K. (1995). Regional Prevalence and Distribution of Ischemic Neurons in Dog Brains 96 Hours After Cardiac Arrest of 0 to 20 Minutes. *Stroke,* Vol.26, No.11, (November 1995), pp. 2127-2133; discussion 2133-2124, ISSN 0039-2499

Rami, A. & Krieglstein, J. (1994). Neuronal Protective Effects of Calcium Antagonists in Cerebral Ischemia. *Life Sciences,* Vol.55, No.25-26, (January 1994), pp. 2105-2113, ISSN 0024-3205

Reiter, R.J.; Tan, D.X.; Leon, J.; Kilic, U. & Kilic, E. (2005). When Melatonin Gets on your Nerves: Its Beneficial Actions in Experimental Models of Stroke. *Experimental Biology & Medicine (Maywood),* Vol.230, No.2, (February 2005), pp. 104-117 ISSN 1535-3702

Rennie, K.; de Butte, M.; Frechette, M. & Pappas, B.A. (2008). Chronic and Acute Melatonin Effects in Gerbil Global Forebrain Ischemia: Long-term Neural and Behavioral Outcome. *Journal of Pineal Research,* Vol.44, No.2, (February 2008), pp. 149-156, ISSN 1600-079X

Roberge, M.C.; Hotte-Bernard, J.; Messier, C. & Plamondon, H. (2008). Food Restriction Attenuates Ischemia-induced Spatial Learning and Memory Deficits Despite Extensive CA1 Ischemic Injury. *Behavioral Brain Research,* Vol.187, No.1, (October 2007), pp. 123-132, ISSN 0166-4328

Robinson, T.E. & Kolb, B. (2004). Structural Plasticity Associated with Exposure to Drugs of Abuse. *Neuropharmacology,* Vol.47, Suppl 1, (October 2004), pp. 33-46, ISSN 0028-3908

Ruan, Y.W.; Zou, B.; Fan, Y.; Li, Y.; Lin, N.; Zeng, Y.S.; Gao, T.M.; Yao, Z. & Xu, Z.C. (2006). Dendritic Plasticity of CA1 Pyramidal Neurons After Transient Global Ischemia. *Neuroscience,* Vol.140, No.1, (March 2006), pp. 191-201, ISSN 0306-4522

Safar, P.; Stezoski, W. & Nemoto, E.M. (1976). Amelioration of Brain Damage after 12 Minutes' Cardiac Arrest in Dogs. *Archives of Neurology,* Vol.33, No.2, (February 1976), pp. 91-95, ISSN 0003-9942

Sánchez-Casado, M.; Sánchez-Ledesma, M.J.; Goncalves-Estella, J.M.; Abad-Hernández, M.M.; García-March, G. & Broseta-Rodrigo, J. (2007). Effect of Combination Therapy with Hypothermia, Magnesium and Tirilazad in an Experimental Model of Diffuse Cerebral Ischemia]. *Medicina Intensiva,* Vol.31, No.3, (April 2007), pp. 113-119, ISSN 0210-5691

Savitz, S.I. & Fisher, M. (2007). Prophylactic Neuroprotection. *Current Drug Targets,* Vol.8, No.7, (July 2007), pp. 846-849, ISSN 1389-4501

Scallet, A.C. (1995). Quantitative Histological Evaluation of Neuroprotective Compounds. *Annals of the New York Academy of Sciences,* Vol.765, (September 1995), pp. 47-61, ISSN 0077-8923, Book: ISBN 0-89766-946-0

Scheller, M.S.; Grafe, M.R.; Zornow, M.H. & Fleischer, J.E. (1992). Effects of Ischemia Duration on Neurological Outcome, CA1 Histopathology, and Nonmatching to Sample Learning in Monkeys. *Stroke,*Vol.23, No.10, (October 1992), pp. 1471-1476; discussion 1477-1478, ISSN 0039-2499

Schmidt-Kastner, R. & Freund, T.F. (1991). Selective Vulnerability of the Hippocampus in Brain Ischemia. *Neuroscience*, Vol.40, No.3, (March 1991), pp. 599-636, ISSN 0306-4522

Schmidt-Kastner, R.; Truettner, J.; Lin, B.; Zhao, W.; Saul, J.; Busto, R. & Ginsberg, M.D. (2001). Transient Changes in Brain-Derived Neurotrophic Factor (BDNF) mRNA Expression in Hippocampus During Moderate Ischemia Induced by Chronic Bilateral Common Carotid Artery Occlussion in the Rat. *Molecular Brain Research*, Vol. 92, No.1-2, (August 2001), pp. 157-166, ISSN 0169-328X

Schneider, A.; Bottiger, B.W. & Popp, E. (2009). Cerebral Resuscitation after Cardiocirculatory Arrest. *Anesthesia and Analgesia*, Vol.108, No.3, (February 2009), pp. 971-979, ISSN 1526-7598

Schwartz, R.D.; Yu, X.; Katzman, M.R.; Hayden-Hixson, D.M. & Perry, J.M. (1995). Diazepam, Given Postischemia, Protects Selectively Vulnerable Neurons in the Rat Hippocampus and Striatum. *Journal of Neuroscience*, Vol.15, (1 Pt 2), (January 1995), pp. 529-39, ISSN 0270-6474

Seamans, J.K.; Floresco, S.B. & Phillips, A.G. (1995). Functional Differences Between the Prelimbic and Anterior Cingulate Regions of the Rat Prefrontal Cortex. *Behavioral Neuroscience*, Vol.109, No.6, (December 1995), pp. 1063-1073, ISSN 0735-7044

Seder, D.B. & Jarrah, S. (2008). Therapeutic Hypothermia for Cardiac Arrest: a Practical Approach. *Current Neurology and Neuroscience Reports*, Vol.8, No.6, (October 2008), pp. 508-517, ISSN 1534-6293

Selakovic, V.; Janac, B. & Radenovic, L. (2010). MK-801 Effect on Regional Cerebral Oxidative Stress Rate Induced by Different Duration of Global Ischemia in Gerbils. *Molecular and Cellular Biochemistry*, Vol.342, No.1-2, (April 2010), pp. 35-50, ISSN 1573-4919

Shibata, M.; Yamasaki, N.; Miyakawa, T.; Kalaria, R.N.; Fujita, Y.; Ohtani, R.; Ihara, M.; Takahashi, R. & Tomimoto, H. (2007). Selective Impairment of Working Memory in a Mouse Model of Chronic Cerebral Hypoperfusion. *Stroke*, Vol.38, No.10, (September 2007), pp. 2826-2832, ISSN 0039-2499

Shuaib, A.; Ijaz, S. & Kanthan, R. (1995a). Clomethiazole Protects the Brain in Transient Forebrain Ischemia When Used up to 4 h After the Insult. *Neuroscience Letters*, Vol. 197, No. 2, (September 1995), pp. 109-12, ISSN 0304-3940

Shuaib, A.; Mahmood, R.H.; Wishart, T.; Kanthan, R.; Murabit, M.A.; Ijaz, S.; Miyashita, H. & Howlett, W. (1995b). Neuroprotective Effects of Lamotrigine in Global Ischemia in Gerbils. A Histological, in Vivo Microdialysis and Behavioral Study. *Brain Research*, Vol.702, No.1-2, (December 1995), pp. 199-206, ISSN 0006-8993

Siemkowicz, E. (1981). Hyperglycemia in the Reperfusion Period Hampers Recovery from Cerebral Ischemia. *Acta Neurologica Scandinavica*, Vol.64, No.3, (September 1981), pp. 207-216, ISSN 0001-6314

Siemkowicz, E. & Gjedde, A. (1980). Post-ischemic Coma in Rat: Effect of Different Pre-ischemic Blood Glucose Levels on Cerebral Metabolic Recovery after Ischemia. *Acta Neurologica Scandinavica*,Vol.110, No.3, (November 1980), pp. 225-232, ISSN 0001-6772

Siemkowicz, E. & Hansen, A.J. (1978). Clinical Restitution Following Cerebral Ischemia in Hypo-, Normo- and Hyperglycemic Rats. *Acta Neurologica Scandinavica*,Vol.58, No.1, (July 1978), pp. 1-8, ISSN 0001-6314

Silasi, G. & Colbourne, F. (2011). Therapeutic Hypothermia Influences Cell Genesis and Survival in the Rat Hippocampus Following Global Ischemia. *Journal of Cerebral Blood Flow and Metab*, Vol.31, No.8, (August 2011), pp. 1725-35, ISSN

Silva, A.J.; Giese, K.P.; Fedorov, N.B.; Frankland, P.W. & Kogan, J.H. (1998). Molecular, Cellular, and Neuroanatomical Substrates of Place Learning. *Neurobiology of Learning and Memory*, Vol.70, No.1-2, (October 1998), pp. 44-61, ISSN 1074-7427

Sinha, J.; Das, N. & Basu, M. K. (2001). Liposomal Antioxidants in Combating Ischemia-reperfusion Injury in Rat Brain. *Biomedicine and Pharmacotherapy*, Vol.55, No.5, (June 2001), pp. 264-271, ISSN 0753-3322

Sirin, B.H.; Coskun, E.; Yilik, L.; Ortac, R.; Sirin, H. & Tetik, C. (1998). Neuroprotective Effects of Preischemia Subcutaneous Magnesium Sulfate in Transient Cerebral Ischemia. *European Journal of Cardio-thoracic Surgery*,Vol.14, No.1, (September 1998), pp. 82-88, ISSN 1010-7940

Sirin, B.H.; Yilik, L.; Coskun, E.; Ortac, R. & Sirin, H. (1998). Pentoxifylline Reduces Injury of the Brain in Transient Ischaemia. *Acta Cardiologica*, Vol.53, No.2, (July 1998), pp. 89-95, ISSN 0001-5385

Skibo, G.G. & Nikonenko, A.G. (2010). Brain Plasticity after Ischemic Episode. *Vitamins & Hormones*, Vol.82, (May 2010), pp. 107-127, ISSN 0083-6729

Smith, M.L.; Auer, R.N. & Siesjo, B.K. (1984a). The Density and Distribution of Ischemic Brain Injury in the Rat Following 2-10 min of Forebrain Ischemia. *Acta Neuropathologica*,Vol.64, No.4, (January 1984), pp. 319-332, ISSN 0001-6322

Smith, M.L.; Bendek, G.; Dahlgren, N.; Rosen, I.; Wieloch, T. & Siesjo, B.K. (1984b). Models for Studying Long-term Recovery Following Forebrain Ischemia in the Rat. 2. A 2-Vessel Occlusion Model. *Acta Physiologica Scandinavica*,Vol.69, No.6, (June 1984), pp. 385-401, ISSN 0001-6314

Soltyz, Z.; Janeczko, K.; Orzylowska-Sliwinska, O.; Zaremba, M.; Januszewski, S. & Aderfeld-Nowak, B. (2003). Morphological Ttransformation of Cells Immunopositive to GFAP, TrkA or p75 in CA1 Hippocampal Area Following Transient Global Ischemia in the Rat. A Quantitative Study. *Brain Research*, Vol.987, No.2, (October 2003), pp. 186-193, ISSN 0006-8993

Sorra, K.E. & Harris, K.M. (2000). Overview on the Structure, Composition, Function, Development, and Plasticity of Hippocampal Dendritic Spines. *Hippocampus*, Vol.10, No.5, (November 2000), pp. 501-511, ISSN 1050-9631

STAIR. (1999). Recommendations for Standards Regarding Preclinical Neuroprotective and Restorative Drug Development. *Stroke*, Vol.30, No.12, (December 1999), pp. 2752-2758, ISSN 0039-2499

Stepień, K.; Tomaszewski, M. & Czuczwar, S.J. (2005). Profile of Anticonvulsant Activity and Neuroprotective Effects of Novel and Potential Antiepileptic Drugs -- An Update. *Pharmacological Reports*,Vol.57, No.6, (December 2005), pp. 719-733, ISSN 1734-1140

Stevens, M.K. & Yaksh, T.L. (1990). Systematic Studies on the Effects of the NMDA Receptor Antagonist MK-801 on Cerebral Blood Flow and Responsivity, EEG, and Blood-brain Barrier Following Complete Reversible Cerebral Ischemia. *Journal of Cerebral Blood Flow & Metabolism*, Vol.10, No.1, (January 1990), pp. 77-88, ISSN 0271-678X

Sugawara, T.; Fujimura, M.; Morita-Fujimura, Y.; Kawase, M. & Chan, P.H. (1999). Mitochondrial Release of Cytochrome c Corresponds to the Selective Vulnerability of Hippocampal CA1 Neurons in Rats After Transient Global Cerebral Ischemia. *Journal of Neuroscience*, Vol. 19, No. 22, (November 1999), pp. RC39 1-6. ISSN 1529-2401

Sugawara, T.; Fujimura, M.; Noshita, N.; Kim, G.W.; Saito, A.; Hayashi, T.; Narasimhan, P.; Maier, C.M. & Chan, P.H. (2004). Neuronal Death/Survival Signaling Pathways in Cerebral Ischemia. *NeuroRx*, Vol.1, No.1, (February 2005), pp. 17-25, ISSN 1545-5343

Sydserff, S.G.; Cross, A.J.; Murray, T.K.; Jones, J.A. & Green, A.R. (2000). Clomethiazole is Neuroprotective in Models of Global and Focal Cerebral Ischemia when Infused at Doses Producing Clinically Relevant Plasma Concentrations. *Brain Research*, Vol.862, No.1-2, (May 2000), pp. 59-62, ISSN 0006-8993

Tarelo-Acuna, L.; Olvera-Cortés, E. & González-Burgos, I. (2000). Prenatal and Postnatal Exposure to Ethanol Induces Changes in the Shape of the Dendritic Spines from Hippocampal CA1 Pyramidal Neurons of the Rat. *Neuroscience Letters*, Vol.286, No.1, (May 2000), pp. 13-16, ISSN 0304-3940

Taylor, C.L.; Latimer, M.P. & Winn, P. (2003). Impaired Delayed Spatial Win-shift Behaviour on the Eight Arm Radial Maze Following Excitotoxic Lesions of the Medial Prefrontal Cortex in the Rat. *Behavioral Brain Research*, Vol.147, No.1-2, (December 2003), pp. 107-114, ISSN 0166-4328

Todd, M.M.; Chadwick, H.S.; Shapiro, H.M.; Dunlop, B.J.; Marshall, L.F. & Dueck, R. (1982). The Neurologic Effects of Thiopental Therapy Following Experimental Cardiac Arrest in Cats. *Anesthesiology*, Vol.57, No.2, (August 1982), pp. 76-86, ISSN 0003-3022

Toung, T.J.; Kirsch, J.R.; Maruki, Y. & Traystman, R.J. (1994). Effects of Pentoxifylline on Cerebral Blood Flow, Metabolism, and Evoked Response after Total Cerebral Ischemia in Dogs. *Critical Care Medicine*, Vol.22, No.2, (February 1994), pp. 273-281, ISSN 0090-3493

Traystman, R.J. (2003). Animal Models of Focal and Global Cerebral Ischemia. *Institute for Laboratory Animal Research*, Vol.44, No.2, (March 2003), pp. 85-95, ISSN 1084-2020

Volpe, B.T.; Pulsinelli, W.A.; Tribuna, J. & Davis, H.P. (1984). Behavioral Performance of Rats Following Transient Forebrain Ischemia. *Stroke*, Vol.15, No.3, (May 1984), pp. 558-562, ISSN 0039-2499

Wang, J.M.; Liu, L.; Irwin, R.W.; Chen, S. & Diaz-Brinton, R. (2008). Regenerative Potential of Allopregnanolone. *Brain Research Reviews*, Vol.57, No.2, (March 2008), pp. 398-409, ISSN 0165-0173

Wang, R.; Zhang, Q.G.; Han, D.; Xu, J.; Lu, Q. & Zhang, G. Y. (2006). Inhibition of MLK3-MKK4/7-JNK1/2 Pathway by Akt1 in Exogenous Estrogen-induced Neuroprotection against Transient Global Cerebral Ischemia by a Non-genomic Mechanism in Male Rats. *Journal of Neurochemistry*, Vol.99, No.6, (October 2006), pp. 1543-1554, ISSN 0022-3042

Wappler, E.A.; Felszeghy, K.; Szilagyi, G.; Gal, A.; Skopal, J.; Mehra, R.D.; Nyakas, C. & Nagy, Z. (2010). Neuroprotective Effects of Estrogen Treatment on Ischemia-induced Behavioural Deficits in Ovariectomized Gerbils at Different Ages. *Behavioral Brain Research*, Vol.209, No.1, (January 2010), pp. 42-48, ISSN 1872-7549

Warner, D.S.; Sheng, H. & Batinie-Haberle, I. (2004). Oxidants, Antioxidants and the Ischemic Brain. *Journal of Experimental Biology*, Vol. 207, Pt.18, (August 2004), pp. 3221-3231, ISSN 0022-0949

Webster, C.M.; Kelly, S.; Koike, M.A.; Chock, V.Y.; Giffard, R.G. & Yenari, M.A. (2009). Inflammation and NFkappaB Activation is Decreased by Hypothermia Following Global Cerebral Ischemia. *Neurobiology of Disease*, Vol.33, No.2, (February 2009), pp. 301-312, ISSN 0969-9961

Weigl, M.; Tenze, G.; Steinlechner, B.; Skhirtladze, K.; Reining, G.; Bernardo, M.; Pedicelli, E. & Dworschak, M. (2005). A Systematic Review of Currently Available Pharmacological Neuroprotective Agents as a Sole Intervention before Anticipated or Induced Cardiac Arrest. *Resuscitation*, Vol.65, No.1, (April 2005), pp. 21-39, ISSN 0300-9572

Weil, Z.M.; Karelina, K.; Su, A.J.; Barker, J.M.; Norman, G.J.; Zhang, N.; Devries, A.C. & Nelson, R.J. (2009). Time-of-day Determines Neuronal Damage and Mortality after Cardiac Arrest. *Neurobiology of Disease*, Vol.36, No.2, (August 2009), pp. 352-360, ISSN 0969-9961

Wellman, C.L. & Sengelaub, D.R. (1991). Cortical Neuroanatomical Correlates of Behavioral Deficits Produced by Lesion of the Basal Forebrain in Rats. *Behavioral and Neural Biology*, Vol.56, No.1, (July 1991), pp. 1-24, ISSN 0163-1047

Whittingham, T.S.; Lust, W.D. & Passonneau, J.V. (1984). An in Vitro Model of Ischemia: Metabolic and Electrical Alterations in the Hippocampal Slice. *Journal of Neuroscience*, Vol.4, No.3, (March 1984), pp. 793-802, ISSN 0270-6474

Wiard, R.P.; Dickerson, M.C.; Beek, O.; Norton, R. & Cooper, B.R. (1995). Neuroprotective Properties of the Novel Antiepileptic Lamotrigine in a Gerbil Model of Global Cerebral Ischemia. *Stroke*, Vol.26, No.3, (March 1995), pp. 466-472, ISSN 0039-2499

Wiklund, L.; Basu, S.; Miclescu, A.; Wiklund, P.; Ronquist, G. & Sharma, H.S. (2007). Neuro- and Cardioprotective Effects of Blockade of Nitric Oxide Action by Administration of Methylene Blue. *Annals of the New York Academy of Sciences*, Vol.1122, (December 2007), pp. 231-244, ISSN 0077-8923

Winocur, G. (1982). Radial-arm-maze Behavior by Rats with Dorsal Hippocampal Lesions: Effect of Cuing. *Journal of Comparative and Physiological Psychology*, Vol.96, No.2, (April 1982), pp. 155-169, ISSN 0021-9940

Yoshida, S.; Busto, R.; Watson, B.D.; Santiso, M. & Ginsberg, M.D. (1985). Postischemic Cerebral Lipid Peroxidation in Vitro: Modification by Dietary Vitamin E. *Journal of Neurochemistry,*Vol.44, No.5, (May 1985), pp. 1593-1601, ISSN 0022-3042

Zani, A.; Braida, D.; Capurro, V. & Sala, M. (2007). Delta9-tetrahydrocannabinol (THC) and AM 404 Protect against Cerebral Ischaemia in Gerbils through a Mechanism Involving Cannabinoid and Opioid Receptors. *British Journal of Pharmacology* Vol.152, No.8, (October 2007), pp. 1301-1311, ISSN 0007-1188

Zapater, P.; Moreno, J. & Horga, J.F. (1997). Neuroprotection by the Novel Calcium Antagonist PCA50938, Nimodipine and Flunarizine, in Gerbil Global Brain Ischemia. *Brain Research,*Vol.772, No.1-2, (December 1997), pp. 57-62, ISSN 0006-8993

Zhang, Z.; Sobel, R.A.; Cheng, D.; Steinberg, G.K. & Yenari, M.A. (2001). Mild Hypothermia Increases Bcl-2 Protein Expression Following Global Cerebral Ischemia. *Brain Research Molecular Brain Research*, Vol.95, No.1-2, (November 2001), pp. 75-85, ISSN

Zhang, F.; Wang, S.; Cao, G.; Gao, Y. & Chen, J. (2007). Signal Transducers and Activators of Transcription 5 Contributes to Erythropoietin-mediated Neuroprotection Against

Hippocampal Neuronal Death after Transient Global Cerebral Ischemia. *Neurobiology of Disease*, Vol.25, No.1, (September 2006), pp. 45-53, ISSN 0969-9961

Zhang, Q.G.; Wang, R.M.; Han, D.; Yang, L.C.; Li, J. & Brann, D.W. (2009). Preconditioning Neuroprotection in Gobal Cerebral Ischemia Involves NMDA Receptor-mediated ERK-JNK3 Crosstalk. *Neuroscience Research*, Vol.63, No.3, (April 2009), pp. 205-212, ISSN 0168-0102

Zhang, H.; Xu, G.; Zhang, J.; Murong, S.; Mei, Y. & Tong E. (2010). Mild Hypothermia Reduces Ischemic Neuron Death via Altering the Expression of p53 and bcl-2. *Neurological Research*, Vol.32, No.4, (May 2010), pp. 384-9, ISSN 0161-6412

Zhao, Y.; Wang, J.; Liu, C.; Jiang, C.; Zhao, C. & Zhu, Z. (2011). Progesterone Influences Postischemic Synaptogenesis in the CA1 Region of the Hippocampus in Rats. *Synapse*, Vol.65, No.9, (February 2011), pp. 880-891, ISSN 1098-2396

Zimmermann, V. & Hossmann, K.A. (1975). Resuscitation of the Monkey Brain after One Hour's Complete Ischemia. II. Brain Water and Electrolytes. *Brain Research*, Vol.85, No.1, (February 1975), pp. 1-11, ISSN 0006-8993

Zornow, M.H. & Prough, D.S. (1996). Neuroprotective Properties of Calcium-channel Blockers. *New Horizons*, Vol.4, No.1, (February 1996), pp. 107-114, ISSN 1063-7389

15

Nrf2 Activation, an Innovative Therapeutic Alternative in Cerebral Ischemia

Carlos Silva-Islas, Ricardo A. Santana, Ana L. Colín-González and Perla D. Maldonado
Patología Vascular Cerebral, Instituto Nacional de Neurología y Neurocirugía Manuel Velasco Suárez
México

1. Introduction

Cerebrovascular disease is the second cause of death and the most frequent cause of non-traumatic disability in adults worldwide, according to the World Health Organization (WHO, 2005). Noteworthy, acute ischemic stroke accounts for about 85% of all cases (Diez-Tejedor et al., 2001). The most common cause of stroke is a sudden occlusion of a blood vessel, resulting in activation of a series of biochemical events eventually leading to neuronal death (Dirgnal et al., 1999). Although return of blood flow (reperfusion) in ischemic brain tissue is essential for restoring normal function, paradoxically it can result in a secondary damage, where oxidative stress mediators play a critical role (Wong & Crack, 2008).

Antioxidant therapies have been used to determine whether oxidative stress may constitute a valuable therapeutic target in cerebral ischemia. Indeed, free radical scavengers (direct antioxidants) and agents that decrease free radicals production reduce damage in experimental models of cerebral ischemia. Despite experimental evidence supports the concept that free radicals production represents a valuable therapeutic target in stroke, negative results have been obtained in a number of clinical trials when some direct antioxidant agents have been evaluated (Aguilera et al., 2007). At present, this discrepancy is unclear; however, administration of treatment outside the temporal window of efficacy and difficulties in the establishment of the onset of ischemia and reperfusion in humans (Hsu et al., 2000) are factors that likely contributing to these differences. Clearly, development of preclinical testing must consider these factors in order to improve successful transition to clinical studies.

NF-E2-Related Factor-2 (Nrf2) is a transcription factor that play a crucial role in the cellular protection against oxidative stress. Nrf2 is referred to as the "master regulator" of the antioxidant response due to the fact that it modulates the expression of several genes including phase 2 and antioxidant enzymes playing an important role in detoxification of reactive oxygen species (ROS) and electrophilic species, including heme oxygenase-1, NAD(P)H:quinone oxidoreductase, glutathione-S-transferase, gamma-glutamyl cysteine ligase, glutathione reductase, etc. Recent studies demonstrate that dysfunction of Nrf2-driven pathways impairs cellular redox state thus oxidative stress.

Since ischemia and reperfusion insults generate an oxidative stress state, and considering that up to date there is no effective treatment to reverse morphological and behavioral alterations induced by stroke, it is conceivable that administration of antioxidants may limit oxidative damage and ameliorate progression of the disease. In this context, Nrf2 inducers are promising indirect antioxidant agents that are effective to attenuate oxidative stress and tissue/cell damage in different *in vivo* and *in vitro* experimental paradigms; therefore, here we review some compounds capable of inducing cellular antioxidant responses in order to understand their usefulness in prevention and treatment of cerebral ischemia-induced damage through activation of the Nrf2/ARE pathway.

2. Mechanism related to cerebral ischemic damage

Brain tissue requires high and constant supply of oxygen and glucose provided for the vascular system to maintain its viability and normal functions. Vascular obstruction - either transitory or permanent - of cerebral blood flow (ischemia) is accompanied by an immediate drop in neurological activity ultimately leading to cell death. The brain is not affected homogeneously and so, cerebral ischemia generates differentially damaged areas. Complete loss of blood flow produces an *infarct zone* where necrotic cell death is observed. The infarct area is surrounded by a *penumbra zone*, which is located between the *infarct zone* and the non-damaged area, or normally irrigated tissue. Cells belonging to the *penumbra zone* are still irrigated by collateral arteries, which maintain them viable for a variable period of time, although not functional (Figure 1). This is the area that shall be rescued, and the potential target for intervention with neuroprotective treatments (Dirgnal et al., 1999).

The return of blood flow (reperfusion) is associated with a decrease in the infarct size and clinical outcome. Although reperfusion is determinant for cell function recovery, after prolonged periods of ischemia, it also exerts negative side-effects. If blood flow is not restored within hours, the penumbra region will become part of the infarct zone. In some patients, reperfusion may exacerbate brain injury (*e.g.*, some patients show edema or intracranial hemorrhage) (Kuroda & Siesjo, 1997). In animal models, reperfusion can induce larger infarct areas that can be associated with permanent vessel occlusion (Aronowski et al., 1997).

The reduction and return of blood flow triggers a cascade of events further leading to neuronal death (Dirgnal et al., 1999; Durukan & Tatlisumak, 2007). Such sequence includes:

1. *Energy failure.* This is the first event of the ischemic cascade. Cells need oxygen and glucose to undergo oxidative phosphorylation for energy production, consequently during ischemia ATP production is decreased (Figure 2).
2. *Depolarization of membrane.* The impairment of ATP production disrupts Na^+/K^+-ATPase and Ca^{2+}/H^+-ATPase pumps and reverses the Na^+/Ca^{2+}-transporter. Upon these conditions, cells are unable to maintain membrane potential and Ca^{2+} voltage-dependent channels are activated, leading to depolarization of cellular membrane (Figure 3).
3. *Excitotoxicity and increase in intracellular Ca^{2+} levels.* After depolarization, excitotoxic amino acids - mostly glutamate - are released to the synaptic cleft. Glutamate activates N-methyl-D-aspartic acid (NMDA), α-amino-3-hydroxy-5-methylisoxazole-4-propionic acid (AMPA), and metabotropic glutamate receptors, thereby increasing intracellular

Ca^{2+} levels. In turn, voltage gated Ca^{2+} channels together with reverse operation of the Na^+/Ca^{2+} exchanger also increase intracellular Ca^{2+} levels (Figure 3). Once in the cytoplasmic domain, Ca^{2+} activates a variety of Ca^{2+} dependent enzymes, including protein kinase C, phospholipase A2, phospholipase C, cyclooxygenase-2, Ca^{2+}-dependent nitric oxide synthase, proteases and endonucleases, hence triggering protein phosphorylation, proteolysis, and mitochondrial damage.

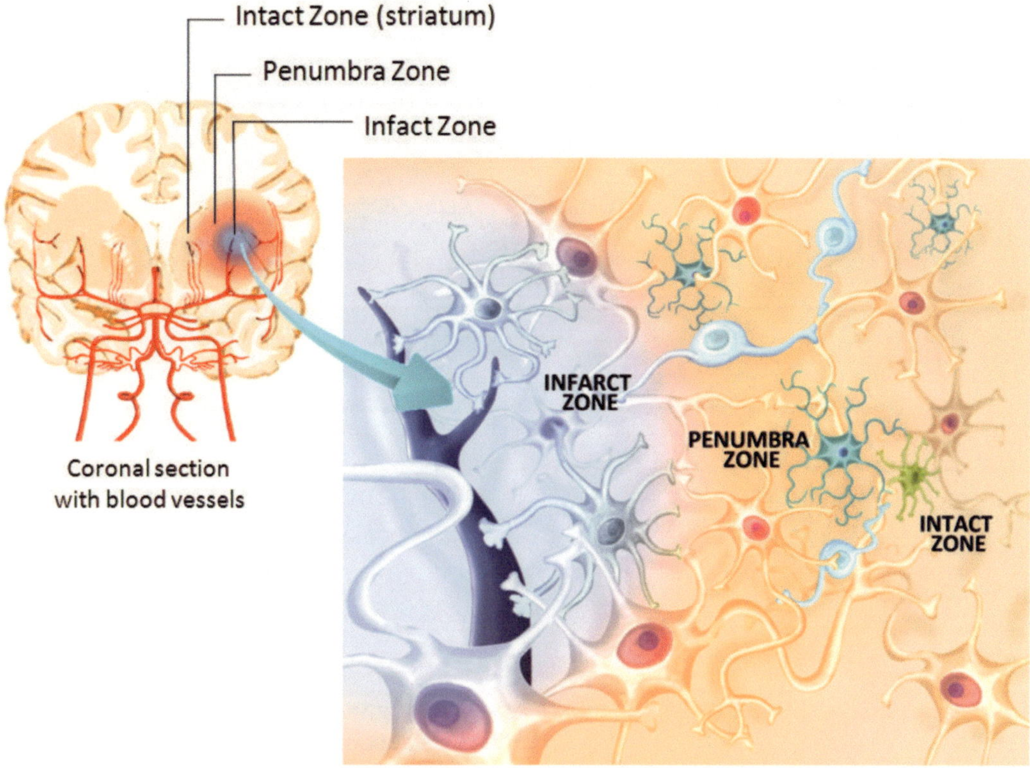

Fig. 1. Vascular obstruction of cerebral blood flow (ischemia) is accompanied by an immediate drop in neurological activity ultimately leading to cell death (*infarct zone*). Infarct core is surrounded by an area supplied with oxygen and glucose by collateral blood vessels (*penumbra zone*). Cells from the penumbra area are not functional; however, they remain viable for a variable period of time.

4. *Generation of free radicals and oxidative stress.* Reactive oxygen (ROS) and nitrogen (RNS) species generation is increased during ischemia, but particularly during reperfusion, and they eventually lead to oxidative stress. ROS and RNS cause lipid peroxidation, membrane injury, disruption of cellular processes, and DNA damage. Moreover, oxidative stress contributes to the disruption of the blood-brain barrier, hence allowing the infiltration of neutrophils and other cells (see below) (Chan, 2001).
5. *Inflammation and apoptosis.* Cerebral injury is a potent triggering of inflammatory cytokines and proteases secretion by microglia, leukocytes and resident cells of the neurovascular unit. Once the neurovascular barriers are breached, multiple neuroinflammatory cascades are activated, further leading to secondary brain injury

(Danton & Dietrich, 2003). Post-ischemic inflammation contributes to brain injury and has been linked to apoptosis. Cell death in cerebral ischemia is mainly dependent of the localization of the cells. For instance, in the core region, cell death is caused mainly by necrosis, while apoptosis predominates in the penumbra area.

ISCHEMIA

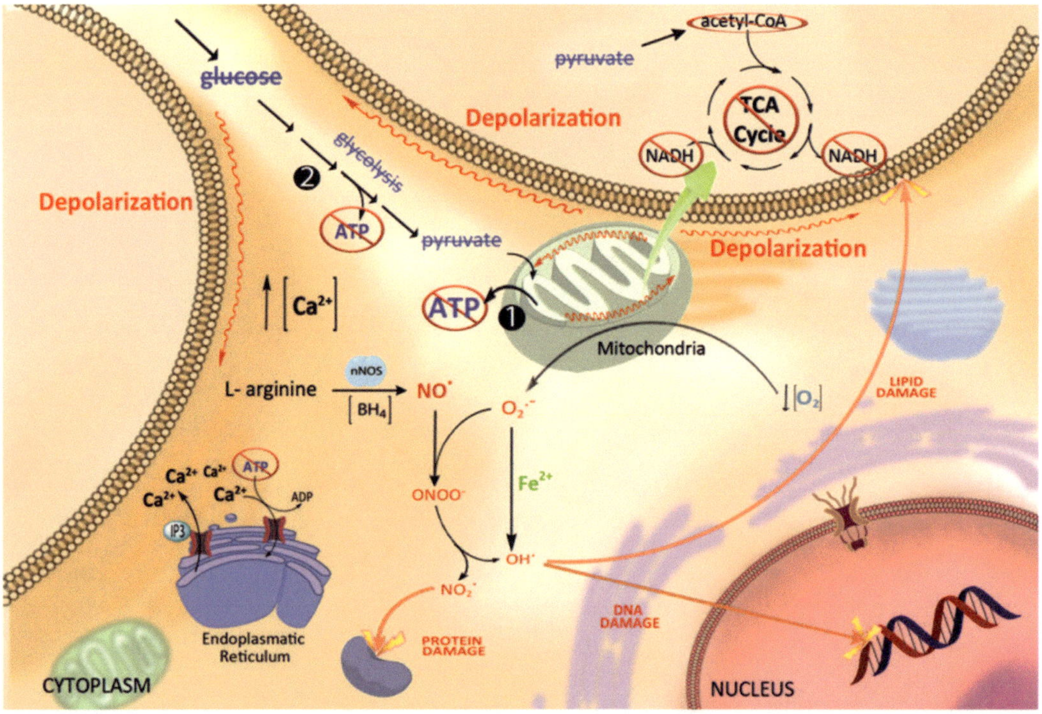

Fig. 2. The reduction of blood flow decreases oxygen and glucose levels; consequently, ATP production *(Energy failure)* (❶), glycolysis(❷) and ATP-dependent processes are blocked. Upon these conditions, oxidative damage is generated by residual oxygen in mitochondria. Pathways that are inhibited during ischemia are crossed out in the image. TCA cycle, tricarboxylic acid cycle; nNOS, neuronal nitric oxide synthase.

3. Oxidative stress is one of the most important events in ischemia/reperfusion-induced cerebral damage

In cells, the predominant ROS and RNS produced are superoxide anion ($O_2^{-\bullet}$), hydrogen peroxide (H_2O_2), hydroxyl radical ($^\bullet OH$), nitric oxide ($^\bullet NO$), peroxynitrite anion (ONOO-), and nitrogen dioxide ($^\bullet NO_2$). In normal conditions, natural defense against ROS and RNS is provided by antioxidant molecules such as glutathione (GSH), ascorbic acid, α-tocopherol, and a number of antioxidant enzymes, including superoxide dismutase (SOD), glutathione peroxidase (GPx), and catalase (CAT). SOD converts $O_2^{-\bullet}$ to H_2O_2, whereas GPx and CAT convert H2O2 to H2O. However, an imbalance in the formation and clearance of ROS and RNS can lead to oxidative stress and subsequent changes affecting the cell dynamics (Aguilera et al., 2007; Margaill et al., 2005).

ISCHEMIA

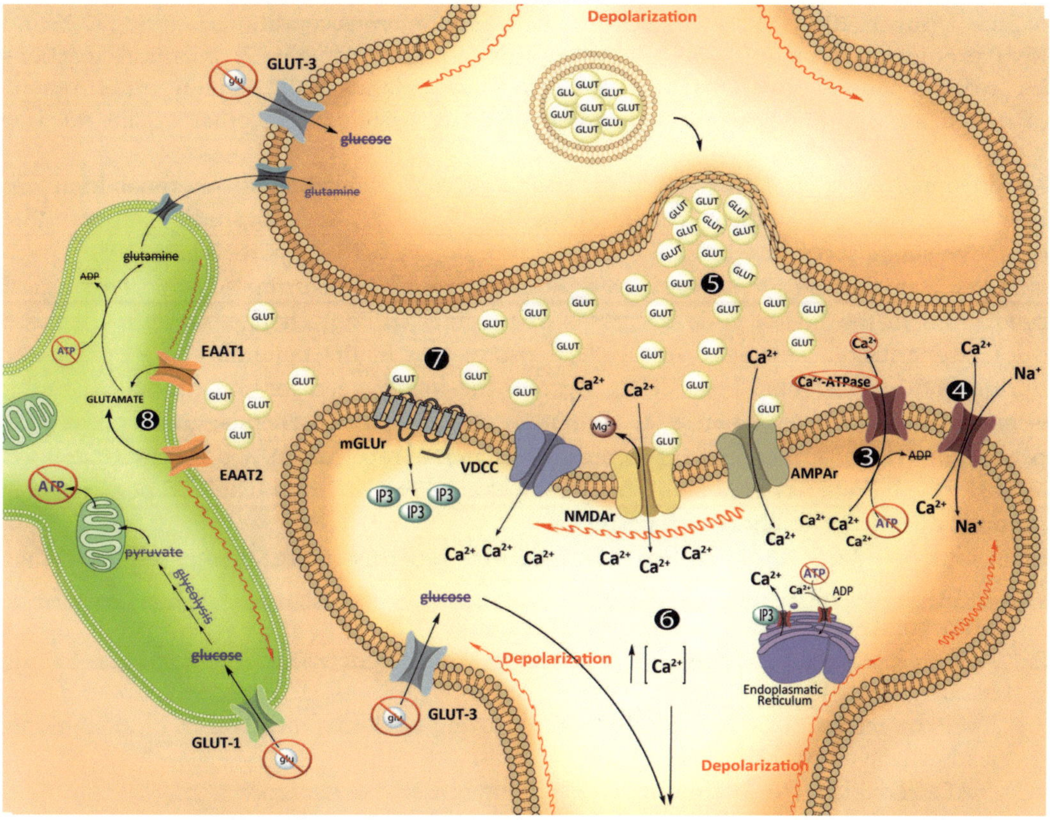

Fig. 3. Reduction of blood flow decreases ATP production, disrupts ATP-dependent pumps (❸) and reverses the Na^+/Ca^{2+} transporter (❹). Upon these conditions, cells are unable to maintain membrane potential *(Depolarization of membrane)*. After depolarization, glutamate (GLUT) is released and activates N-methyl-D-aspartic acid (NMDAr) and α-amino-3-hydroxy-5-methylisoxazole-4-propionic acid (AMPAr) receptors(❺, *Excitotoxicity)*, hence directly increasing intracellular Ca^{2+} levels (❻). On one hand, GLUT activates metabotropic glutamate receptors (mGLUr) (❼), which releases inositol 1,4,5-triphosphate (IP3), a molecule that binds to its receptor at the endoplasmatic reticulum to release more Ca^{2+} (❻, *Increase of intracellular Ca^{2+} level*). On the other hand, voltage gated Ca^{2+} channels (VDCC) and the reverse operation of the $Na+/Ca^{2+}$-exchanger increase intracellular Ca^{2+} levels. Energy disruption also affects astrocytes, causing a deficient activity of glutamate transporters (EAAT1 and EAAT2) (❽).

ROS and RNS produce cellular damage through lipid peroxidation, nucleic acid alteration and inactivation of enzymes (Figure 4); they also modify cellular signaling and gene regulation, contributing to breakdown of the blood-brain barrier and edema generation (Moro et al., 2005). Oxidative stress can ultimately induce neuronal damage, leading to neuronal death by apoptosis or necrosis (Loh et al., 2006).

The brain is particularly sensitive to oxidative stress since 20% of the total oxygen consumed by the body is used by this organ, which constitutes only 2% of the total body weight. This feature makes the brain the major generator of ROS and RNS when compared with other organs (Dringen, 2000). Moreover, in brain there are numerous conditions favoring ROS and RNS production, including: 1) a high unsaturated lipid content, 2) chemical reactions involving dopamine oxidation (Heiss, 2002; Hou & MacManus, 2002), 3) high concentrations of iron in various regions, and 4) lower antioxidant systems than other organs such as kidney or liver (Dringen, 2000).

As previously described, physiopathological mechanisms leading to neuronal injury in cerebral stroke are complex and multifactorial. However, several studies suggest that oxidative stress, secondary to ROS and RNS production, actively participates during post-ischemic brain damage (Peters et al., 1998; Rodrigo et al., 2005). During ischemia, free radical production in the infarct zone decreases or remains without change, while it increases during reperfusion. However, free radical production in the penumbral zone increases during both events (Liu et al., 2003). Despite the low oxygen tension produced during ischemia, exist an increase in ROS formation after 1.6 h of ischemia, the highest ROS production ($489 \pm 330\%$ of control) occurs after 20 min of reperfusion, and remains increased at least for 3 h (Peters et al., 1998). Christensen et al. (1994) reported that ROS production is maximal during the first hour of reperfusion.

Main sources of ROS, RNS, and free radicals during reperfusion are summarized as follows (Aguilera et al., 2007; Margaill et al., 2005):

1. Mitochondrial respiratory chain generates $O_2^{-\bullet}$.
2. Xanthine oxidase produces $O_2^{-\bullet}$ when it catalyzes oxidation of hypoxhantine to uric acid.
3. Cyclooxygenase 2 (COX-2) produces $O_2^{-\bullet}$ during oxidative metabolism of arachidonic acid, a delayed process in ischemia reperfusion.
4. NADPH oxidase (NOX) produces $O_2^{-\bullet}$ during NADPH oxidation.
5. Nitric oxide synthases (NOS) produce $^{\bullet}NO$ in normal conditions. $^{\bullet}NO$ produced can react with $O_2^{-\bullet}$ and generate the strong oxidant $ONOO^-$. Tetrahydrobiopterin (BH4) is an important regulator of NOS function because it is required to maintain enzymatic coupling. Loss or oxidation of BH4 to 7,8-dihydrobiopterin (BH2) is associated with NOS uncoupling, resulting in the production of $O_2^{-\bullet}$ rather than $^{\bullet}NO$ (Crabtree & Channon, 2011) (Figure 4).

4. Direct and indirect antioxidants

Living systems have developed multiple lines of defense against oxidative stress. Cellular protection against oxidative stress is a process more complex than cellular protection against electrophiles. In this process two types of molecules participate (Dinkova-Kostova et al., 2007):

1. *Direct antioxidants.* Compounds of low molecular weight (ascorbate, glutathione, tocopherols, lipoid acid, ubiquinones, carotenes) that can undergo redox reactions and scavenge reactive oxidation products (peroxides), as well as ROS and RNS ($^{\bullet}OH$, $ONOO^-$). Direct antioxidants are consumed or modified in the process of their antioxidant action (ROS scavenger). Thus, it is necessary to replenish or regenerate them.
2. *Indirect antioxidants.* These agents may or may not have redox activity, and exert many of their effects through upregulation of phase 2 and antioxidant enzymes. In turn, theses enzymes act catalytically, exhibit long half-lives, and display a wide variety of antioxidant activities, in addition to their capacities to detoxify electrophiles.

REPERFUSION

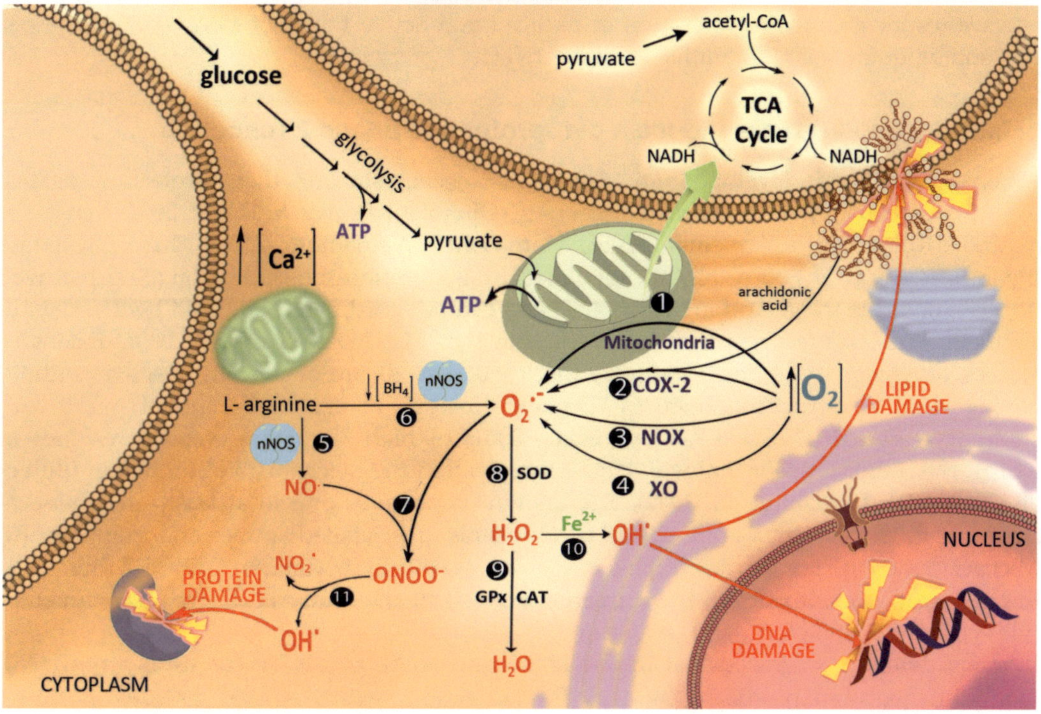

Fig. 4. Main sources of superoxide anion ($O_2^{-\bullet}$) during reperfusion are summarized as follows: mitochondrial respiratory chain ❶; cyclooxygenase-2 (COX-2) ❷; NADPH oxidase (NOX) ❸; xanthine oxidase (XO) ❹; and nitric oxide synthase (NOS), responsible for nitric oxide ($^{\bullet}NO$) formation ❺, or $O_2^{-\bullet}$ if tetrahydrobiopterin (BH4) is deficient ❻. $O_2^{-\bullet}$ can react with $^{\bullet}NO$ to generate peroxynytrite anion ($ONOO^-$) ❼, or be degraded by superoxide dismutase (SOD) to hydrogen peroxide (H_2O_2) ❽. Then, H_2O_2 can be catabolized by glutathione peroxidase (GPx) or catalase (CAT) to H_2O ❾, or react with Fe^{2+} to form hydroxyl radicals ($^{\bullet}OH$) via the Fenton reaction ❿. $ONOO^-$ can be degraded to nitrogen dioxide radical ($NO_2^{\bullet}$) and $^{\bullet}OH$ (**11**), responsible for damaging lipids, proteins and DNA.

However, the distinction between direct and indirect antioxidants is complicated by a close reciprocal relation between these two types of agents, as is showed in the following examples (Dinkova-Kostova et al., 2007):

1. Whilst glutathione is the main protective direct antioxidant present in high concentrations (mM) in tissues, its rate of synthesis is controlled by γ-glutamate cysteine ligase (GCL), a typical phase 2 enzyme that is upregulated by phase 2 inducers which are, by definition, indirect antioxidants. The complexity of this reciprocal relation is further enhanced by the mandatory participation of glutathione in activities of several antioxidant enzymes (glutathione peroxidase, glutathione-S-transferases, glutathione reductase).
2. At least one phase 2 enzyme, heme oxygenase-1 (HO-1) generates carbon monoxide and biliverdin/biliruvin, which are small direct antioxidant molecules.
3. Some direct antioxidants are inducers of the phase 2 response; e.g., the vicinal dithiol lipoic acid and reduced Michale reaction acceptors such as hydroquinones.

4. Phase 2 enzymes NADPH:quinone oxidoreductase-1 (NQO1) and glutathione reductase are responsible for regeneration of reduced and active forms of oxidized tocopherols, and ubiquinone and glutathione, respectively.

5. Indirect antioxidants induce a cytoprotective phase 2 response

Aerobic cells have developed an elaborated mechanism for their protection against oxidative stress, known as "phase 2 response" (Dinkova-Kostova & Talaly, 2008; Kensler et al., 2007; Kobayashi & Yamamoto, 2006; Motohashi & Yamamoto, 2004). Phase 2 response involves a group of genes that are regulated by a common molecular signaling pathway depending of the transcription factor Nrf2, and can be coordinately induced by a variety of synthetic and natural agents (Dinkova-Kostova et al., 2005a; Talalay, 2000). Extensive studies on chemistry of inducers have disclosed that all are chemically reactive without having common structural features (Dinkova-Kostova et al., 2004), and all react with sulfhydryl groups (Dinkova-Kostova et al., 2001) of highly reactive cysteine residues of Keap1, the cellular sensor that is integrally involved in the mechanism of induction (Itoh et al., 2003; Wakabayashi et al., 2004). The known inducers belong to at least nine chemical classes (Dinkova-Kostova et al., 2004): (i) diphenols, phenylenediamines and quinones; (ii) Michael reaction acceptors; (iii) isothiocyanates/dithiocarbamates; (iv) 1,2-dithiole-3-thiones/oxathiolene oxides; (v) hydroperoxides; (vi) trivalent arsenicals; (vii) heavy metals; (viii) vicinal dimercaptans; and (ix) carotenoids.

It is now widely recognized that the up-regulation of the phase 2 response is a powerful, highly efficient and promising strategy for protection against several diseases including ischemic stroke (Alfieri et al., 2011; Talalay, 2000). Experimental evidence shows the powerful protective effects of phase 2 response: (*i*) its up-regulation protects cells, animals, and humans against a wide variety of damaging agents including ROS, RNS, carcinogens, electrophiles, and radiation (Kensler et al., 2007; Kobayashi & Yamamoto, 2006; Motohashi & Yamamoto, 2004; Talalay et al., 2007); (*ii*) when the phase 2 response is disrupted, cells are much more susceptible to oxidative damage; and (*iii*) numerous anticarcinogens have been identified and isolated from natural sources by bioassays that monitor induction of Nrf2-dependent enzymes such as NAD(P)H:quinone oxidoreductase (NQO1) (Kang & Pezzuto, 2004; Zhang et al., 1992).

5.1 Phase 2 proteins and enzymes

In the past, enzymatic protection against oxidants focused largely on classical enzymes such as SOD, CAT, and various types of peroxidases (Halliwell & Gutteridge, 1999), now this is changing. Phase 2 proteins were originally perceived as only promoters of xenobiotic conjugation with endogenous ligands (e.g., glutathione, glucuronic acid) to generate more water-soluble and easily excretable products. This restricted view of the nature and functions of phase 2 proteins and enzymes has gradually been expanded. Nowadays, several genes are considered part of the phase 2 response. Enzymes encoded by these genes have chemically versatile antioxidant properties, share common regulatory mechanisms, and are highly inducible by a variety of agents including dietary components (Ramos-Gomez et al., 2001; Talalay, 2000).

Phase 2 proteins catalyze diverse reactions that collectively result in broad protection against the continuous damaging effects of ROS, RNS and electrophiles. They are expressed at low basal levels, but can be markedly elevated by various small molecules (indirect antioxidants).

Using an oligonucleotide microarray analysis, Lee et al. (2003a) reported that *tert*-butylhydroquinone (t-BHQ), a well know Nrf2 inducer, stimulated a group of genes responsible for conferring protection against oxidative stress or inflammation in primary cortical astrocytes. The major functional categories are detoxification enzymes, antioxidant proteins, NADPH-producing proteins, growth factors, defense/immune/inflammation-related proteins, and signaling proteins (Table 1). It has been proposed that proteins within these functional categories are vital to cell's defense system, suggesting that an orchestrated change in the modulation of Nrf2/ARE pathway would stimulate a synergistic protective effect.

Proteins and enzymes directly related with an antioxidant protective effect can be divided into 3 major groups (Lee et al., 2003a):

Group 1. Genes involved in glutathione (GSH) homeostasis. GSTs catalyze the nucleophilic addition of GSH to an electrophilic group of a broad spectrum of xenobiotic compounds. GPx and PRx metabolize H_2O_2 to H_2O and oxidized GSH (GSSG), and GR regenerates GSH. Ideally, in association with an increased utilization of GSH, there would also be an increased production of GSH. The rate-limiting step in the GSH biosynthesis is mediated by GCLM/GCLC. The coordinate regulation of these genes can evoke a synergistic effect in the maintenance of GSH levels, as well as in detoxification of reactive intermediates (Figure 5).

Group 2. Genes involved in H_2O_2 detoxification and iron homeostasis. SOD and HO-1 are very important for cellular defense against oxidative stress. SOD detoxifies $O_2^{-\bullet}$ resulting H_2O_2, and HO-1 generates a potent radical scavenger, bilirubin. However, SOD and HO-1 can induce more oxidative stress because they increase the cellular concentrations of H_2O_2 and free iron, respectively; which together can generate •OH through the Fenton reaction. For complete detoxification of superoxide, H_2O_2 should be further metabolized to H_2O by GPx, CAT, or PRx. CAT directly detoxifies H_2O_2, whereas PRx uses GSH (Figure 6) and/or thioredoxin (Trx) as an electron donor for peroxidation of H_2O_2, resulting in generation of GSSG or oxidized thioredoxin, respectively (Figure 6). GSSG and oxidized thioredoxin are converted to their reduced forms by GR and TXNRD1, respectively. In addition, proper management of free iron is also important for minimizing oxidative stress, and this can be best achieved by ferritin. Ferritin converts Fe^{2+} to Fe^{3+} (ferroxidase activity) and sequesters it, thereby avoiding the participation of Fe^{2+} in the Fenton reaction (Orino et al., 2001). Thus, up-regulation of HO-1 together with ferritin constitutes a physiological strategy to increase the antioxidant potential while $^{\bullet}OH$ formation is minimized.

Group 3. Genes involved in NADPH homeostasis. NQO1, GR, and TXNRD1 are important in detoxifying quinones and maintaining the cellular redox balance. One common feature of these proteins is the fact that they use NADPH as an electron donor. So, for efficient detoxification and maintenance of cellular redox status, it would be beneficial to up-regulate these proteins together with the appropriate reducing potential (NADPH) to support enzymatic reactions. G6PD/malic enzyme can directly generate NADPH, and transketolase/transaldolase can increase NADPH production by regenerating substrates for G6PD (Figure 7). These Nrf2-dependent genes would also contribute to cell's detoxification potential and cellular redox balance.

GENE	GENE	GENE
Detoxification ✓ NAD(P)H:quinone oxidoreductase-1 (NQO1)[a] ✓ Glutathione-S-transferase (GST) A4[a] ✓ GST Pi2[a] ✓ GST Mu1[a] ✓ GST Mu3[a] ✓ GST Omega1[a] ✓ GST microsomal-1[a] ✓ UDP glycosyltransferase 1A6[a] ✓ Epoxide hydrolase-1[a] ✓ Aldehyde dehydrogenase-2 ✓ Aldehyde dehydrogenase-9 ✓ Aldehyde oxidase-1 ✓ Cytochrome P450 1B1 ***Signaling*** ✓ Protein kinase, cAMP-dependent regulatory, type Iβ ✓ AW125016 4 1.9 0.07 NR ✓ Mitogen-activated protein kinase-10	***Antioxidant/reducing potential*** ✓ γ-glutamate cysteine ligase modifier subunit (GCLM)[a] ✓ γ-glutamate cysteine ligase catalytic subunit (GCLC)[a] ✓ Hemo oxygenase-1 (HO-1) (decycling)[a] ✓ Thioredoxin reductase-1 (TXNRD-1) ✓ Thioredoxin (Trx)[a] ✓ Ferritin light chain-1[a] ✓ Ferritin H subunit[a] ✓ Type I peroxiredoxin (PRx) ✓ 1-Cys PRx protein-2 ✓ Transferrin receptor ✓ Cu, Zn superoxide dismutase (CuZnSOD)[a] ✓ Catalase-1 (CAT) ✓ Glutathione peroxidase-4 (GPx) ✓ Glutathione reductase-1 (GR) ✓ Glucose-6-phosphate dehydrogenase (G-6PD), X-linked ✓ G-6PDH-2 ✓ Transaldolase-1 ✓ Transketolase ✓ Solute carrier family-1/4 ✓ Glycine transporter- ✓ Malic enzyme, supernatant[a]	***Transcription*** ✓ CCAAT/enhancer-binding protein-β ✓ Zinc finger protein of cerebellum-2 ✓ TG-interacting factor ✓ MafG ✓ Activating transcription factor-4 ***Growth*** ✓ Proliferin ✓ Proliferin-2 ✓ Nerve growth factor- β ✓ Platelet-derived growth factor-α ***Defense/immune/ inflammation*** ✓ Macrophage C-type lectin ✓ EST, similar to dithiolethione-inducible-1 ✓ PAF acetylhydrolase ✓ P lysozyme structural ✓ Lysozyme M ✓ Prostaglandin-endoperoxide synthase-2 ✓ Matrix metalloproteinase-12

[a]Known to contain or to potentially have an ARE sequence.
Modified of Lee et al., 2003a.

Table 1. Nrf2-dependent genes induced by *tert*-butylhydroquinone in primary cortical astrocytes

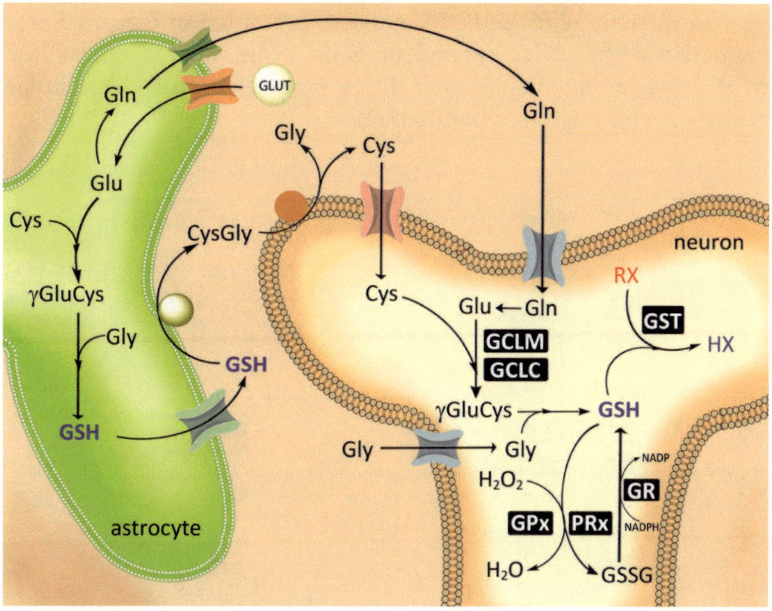

Fig. 5. Genes involved in glutathione (GSH) homeostasis are indicated in black boxes. GST, glutathione-S-transferase; GCLM, γ-glutamate cysteine ligase modifier subunit; GCLC, γ-glutamate cysteine ligase catalytic subunit; GPx, glutathione peroxidase; PRx, peroxiredoxin; GR, glutathione reductase.

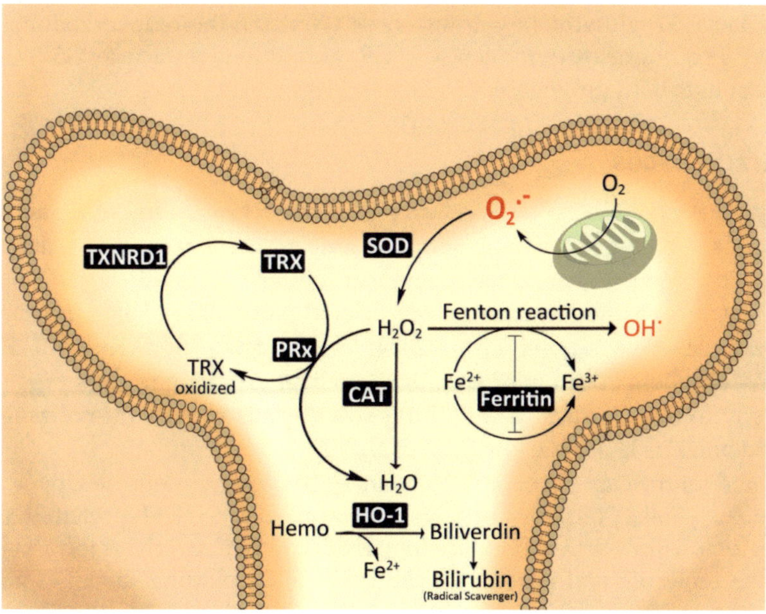

Fig. 6. Genes involved in H_2O_2 detoxification and iron homeostasis are indicated in black boxes. SOD, superoxide dismutase; CAT, catalase; PRx, peroxiredoxin; Trx, thioredoxin; HO-1, hemo oxygenase-1; TXNRD1, thioredoxin reductase-1.

Together, these coordinately regulated gene clusters presented in Figures 5, 6 and 7 strongly support the hypothesis that Nrf2-dependent gene expression is crucial for an efficient detoxification of reactive metabolites and ROS, as well as for the cellular capacity to counteract stressing events such as inflammation.

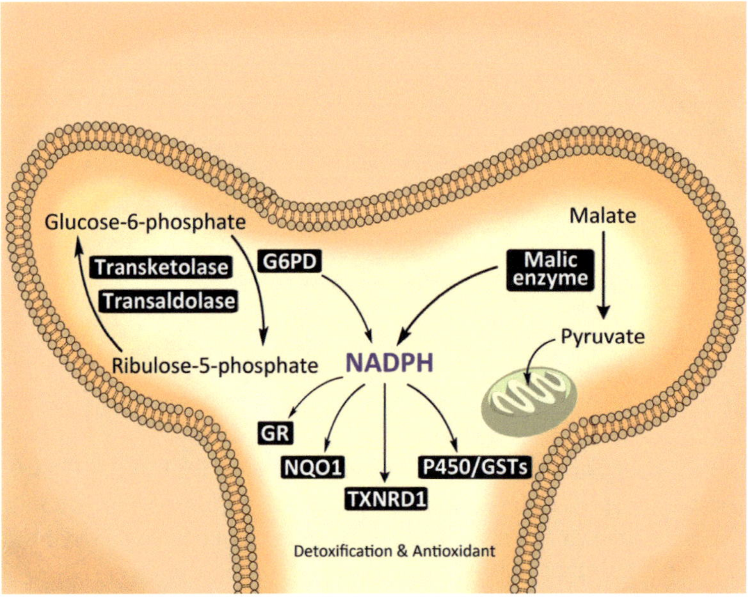

Fig. 7. Genes involved in NADPH homeostasis are indicated in black boxes. P450, cytochrome P450; GST, glutathione-S-transferase; TXNRD1, thioredoxin reductase-1; NQO1, NAD(P)H:quinone oxidoreductase-1; GR, glutathione reductase; G6PD, glucose-6-phosphate dehydrogenase.

6. Nrf2 characteristics

The transcription factor Nrf2 (Nuclear factor-E2-related factor 2) is the guardian of redox homeostasis because it regulates basal and inducible expression of array ride of antioxidant and cytoprotective genes, providing a level of protection required for normal cellular activities and against various oxidative stress-related pathologies, including ischemic stroke (Cho & Kleeberger, 2009; Nguyen et al., 2004; Van Muiswinkel & Kuiperij, 2005). Nrf2 is highly expressed in detoxification organs - such as liver and kidney - and organs exposed to the external environment - such as skin, lung and digestive tract - (Motohashi et al., 2002), whereas in the brain its levels are low (Moi et al., 1994).

Nrf2 is a member of the cap 'n' collar (CNC) family basic region-leucine zipper transcription factor (Katsuoka et al., 2005; Sykiotis & Bohmann, 2010). Nrf2 protein has six highly conserved regions, called Nrf2-ECH homology (Neh) domains. Neh1 is located in the half C-terminal of the molecule and constitutes the basic DNA binding domain and the leucine zipper for dimerization. Neh2 domain is located in the proximal N-terminus of Nrf2 and represents the region through which Nrf2 associates with the cytoplasmic protein Keap1 (kelch-like ECH-associated protein 1) (Itoh et al., 1999). Neh6 is a redox-insensitive degron, which is essential for maximal turnover of Nrf2 in stressed cells, as well as for its degradation (McMahon et al., 2004). Neh3 domain is required for transcriptional activation of the protein (Nioi et al., 2005). Neh4 and Neh5 domains are required for its binding to ARE (Figure 8, *upper panel*).

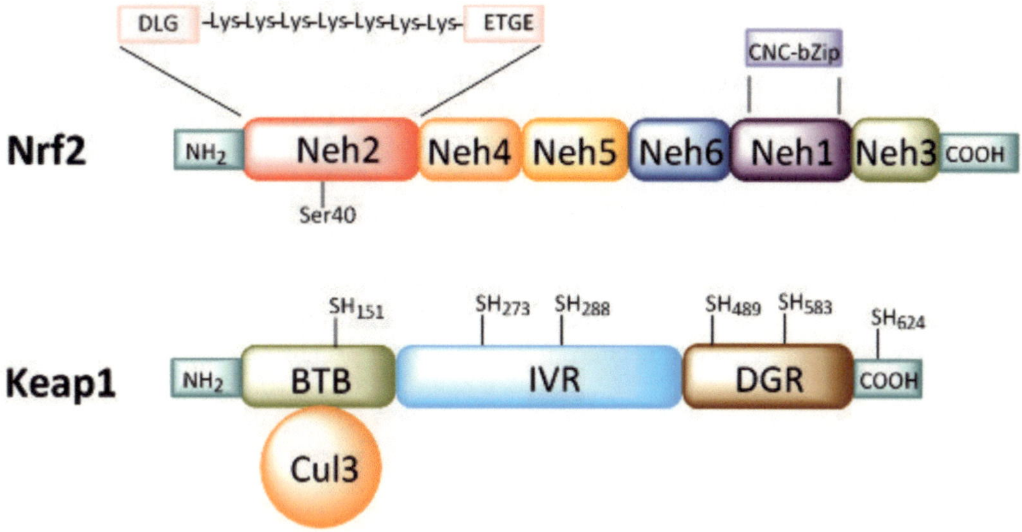

Fig. 8. Nrf2 and Keap1 domains. *Upper panel*: in Nrf2, Neh1 is the basic DNA binding domain and the leucine zipper for dimerization. Neh2 is the Keap1 (kelch-like ECH-associated protein 1) binding domain. Neh3 is required for transcriptional activation of the protein. Neh4 and Neh5 domains are required for the binding to ARE. Neh6 is essential for both Nrf2 turnover in stressed cells and for its degradation. *Lower panel*: in Keap1, BTB domain functions as a substrate adaptor protein for a Cul3-dependent ubiquitin ligase complex. IVR domain is a domain of intervention which is distinguished for its high number of cysteine residues. DGR domain is associated with actin filaments, giving stability to Keap1.

Under oxidant conditions, Nrf2 binds with high affinity to the *cis*-acting enhancer sequence called Antioxidant Response Element (ARE, 5´-GTGACnnnGC-3´), located in the 5´-flanking regions of a broad range of antioxidant and cytoprotective genes that act against oxidative/electrophilic damage (Nguyen et al., 2004; Rushmore et al., 1991). The binding of Nrf2 to ARE requires its heterodimerization with small Maf proteins (Katsuoka et al., 2005), which stimulates transcription of downstream genes, with participation of transcriptional co-activators - mainly CREB-binding protein (CBP) -, through the Neh4 and Neh5 domains (Figure 8, *upper panel*) in the transcription factor. These co-activators act synergistically to attain maximum its activity (Katoh et al., 2001).

7. Regulation of Nrf2: Keap1 (ARE elements)

Nrf2 activity is primarily regulated by suppressor protein Keap1 (Figure 8, *lower panel*), a member of the BTB (Broad complex/Tramtrack/Bric-a-brac)-Kelch protein family (Cullinan et al., 2004), that under normal conditions (unstressed) forms a complex with Nrf2 within the cytosol. This complex is associated with actin filaments through its double glycine repeat

(DGR) domain (Figure 10, *left panel*), which plays an important role in retention of Nrf2 (Kang et al., 2004).

BTB domain of Keap1 functions as an adaptor for Cul3-dependent E3 ubiquitin ligase complex that interacts with the seven lysine residues located in the Neh2 domain of Nrf2, promoting its ubiquitination (Kobayashi et al., 2004; Zhang et al., 2004) and its continuous degradation by 26S proteasome (Nguyen et al., 2003). This is supported by the relatively short half-life of Nrf2 (10-30 min) in absence of cellular stress (McMahon et al., 2003). Upon oxidative stress conditions, the interaction between Nrf2 and Keap1 is disrupted through changes in certain domains of Keap1, hence promoting the release of Nrf2 (Eggler et al., 2005).

The human Keap1 protein contains 27 cysteine residues, some of which are highly reactive to a wide variety of chemical stimuli. Furthermore, a large amount of evidence has emerged suggesting that certain cysteines of Keap1 may be targets of Nrf2 inducers such as sulforaphane, which reacts with thiol groups of Keap1 to form resistant thionoacyl adducts by hydrolysis and transacylation reactions (Hong et al., 2005) (Figure 9).

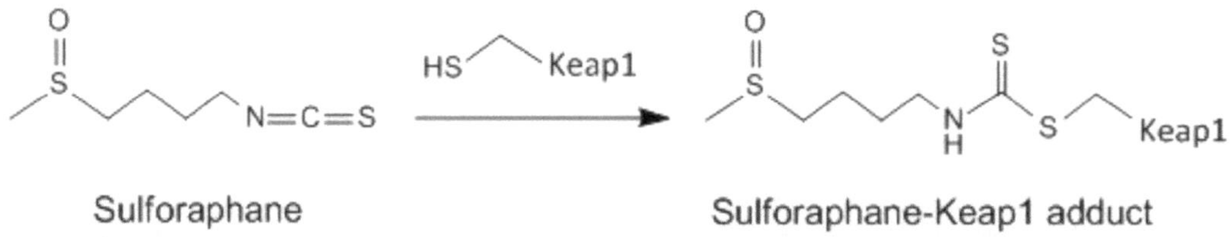

Fig. 9. Formation of adducts between sulforaphane and Keap1.

It has been reported that Cys151 in BTB domain of Keap1 is required for inhibition of Keap1-dependent Nrf2 degradation stimulated by sulforaphane and oxidative stress (Zhang & Hannink, 2003). Cys273 and Cys288, located in the IVR domain of Keap1, are essential for its repressive activity under basal conditions. It has been suggested that this effect also responds to sulforaphane (Kobayashi et al., 2006). On the other hand, it has been reported that Cys489, Cys583, and Cys624 were most reactive toward sulforaphane (Hong et al., 2005). Therefore, the responsiveness of Nrf2 to inducers, such as sulforaphane, involves redox-dependent alterations of thiol groups in several domains of Keap1, which acts like a sensor responding to oxidative and environment stress through dynamic changes in cystein reducing status (Jung & Kwak, 2010). In turn, Keap1 is considered as a zinc metalloprotein because the chemical modification of critical cysteine residues is modulated by thiol-bound zinc (approximately 1 mol per subunit), which is displaced by the reaction with inducers or other classical sulfhydryl reagents, such as sulforaphane (Dinkova-Kostova et al., 2005b).

Another important event in the activation of Nrf2 may be its phosphorylation. The protein kinase-dependent signal transduction pathways have been implicated in the release of Nrf2 from Keap1-mediated repression, mainly by protein kinase C, whose target is a single serine residue, Ser40 (Bloom & Jaiswal, 2003; Huang et al., 2002). To explain how Keap1/Nrf2 complex respond to basal or inducible stimuli, it has been proposed the "hinge and latch" model (Tong et al., 2006a), which suggests that a single Nrf2 molecule makes contacts with two domains of Keap1 homodimer (McMahon et al., 2006; Tong et al., 2006a). Neh2 domain of Nrf2 contains two sites for Keap1 binding, termed motifs DLG and ETGE. These motifs exhibit different affinity for Keap1; the affinity of ETGE is greater than DLG (Tong et al., 2006b). The term "hinge" indicates that the interaction of high affinity is not affected by inducers; in contrast, inducers abolish the low-affinity interaction mediated by the "latch", thereby disrupting the presentation of Nrf2 to the ubiquitination machinery of Keap1 (Li & Kong, 2009) (Figure 10, *right panel*). Other models that describe the interaction between Nrf2 and Keap1 have provided conflicting information when contrasted with the "hinge and latch" model (Lo & Hannink, 2006; 2008).

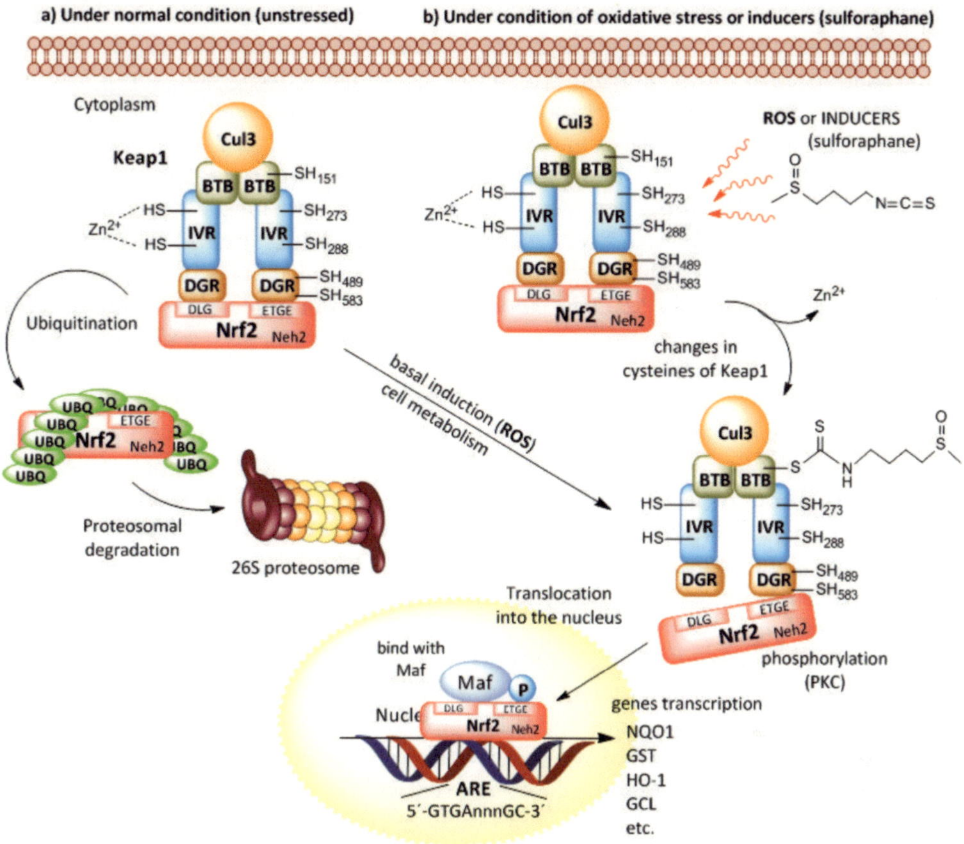

Fig. 10. Effect of sulforaphane on Nrf2/Keap1 complex. *Left panel*: Upon unstressed conditions, this complex is dissociated and Nrf2 can either suffer proteosomal degradation or respond to stimuli typical of basal cell metabolism. In the later, Nrf2 is phosphorylated and translocated to the nucleus forming heterodimers with Maf and acting on ARE. *Right panel*: Under stress oxidative conditions, or in the presence of inducers, several cysteine residues suffer changes inducing its Nrf2 dissociation and further translocation of this factor to nucleus, where it will induce phase 2 genes transcription.

Sulforaphane induces a phase 2 response as a result of gene expression modulation through Nrf2/ARE pathway. ARE-driven targets include NAD(P)H:quinone oxidereductase (NQO1), heme oxygenase-1 (HO-1) and γ-glutamylcysteine ligase (γGCL). The induction of these enzymes has been observed both in *in vivo* and *in vitro* experiments after sulforaphane treatment.

8. Nrf2 in cerebral ischemia

Nrf2 has been detected in neuronal and glial cells (Chen et al., 2011; Li et al., 2011; Shah et al., 2010; Yang et al., 2009). Previous studies using gel-shift assay found that ischemic brains selectively upregulates ARE-mediated gene expression, whereas binding activities of other stress response elements were unchanged, including metal response element, interleukin-6, and STAT (signal transducer and activator of transcription) response elements (Campage et al., 2000).

Middle cerebral artery occlusion (permanent or transient) is a classical and well-characterized model inducing cerebral ischemia in rats that involves a cytotoxic response occurring within few minutes from the onset of cerebral ischemia, and encompasses oxidative stress, pro-inflammatory responses and cell death (Ikeda et al., 2003; Longa et al., 1989; Simonyi et al., 2005). Yang et al. (2009) used permanent focal ischemia to detect the expression of Nrf2. They found that Nrf2 protein and mRNA were upregulated when is compared with normal control, showing a peak at 24 h and localizing with nuclei and cytoplasm of neurons and astrocytes. Alternatively, Nrf2 was presented in the injured regions of cortices with cerebral ischemic/reperfusion, and markedly increased in both cytoplasm and nuclei (Li et al., 2011). Meanwhile, Keap1 immunoreactivity was significantly reduced. Besides, an altered expression of thioredoxin, glutathione, and heme oxigenase was detected (Tanaka et al., 2011).

Oligemia is another model that was used to determine Nrf2 localization. It consists in a reduction in the mean arterial pressure to 30-40 mm Hg, resulting in a 50% reduction in cerebral blood flow after reperfusion. This blood flow reduction presents an increase in oxidative stress through lipid peroxidation (Heim et al., 1995; Läer et al., 1993) and an augmented •OH production during the reperfusion phase (Heim et al., 2000). In this model, Nrf2 was specifically upregulated 1 h after the surgery. Nrf2-positive neurons were found in the Purkinje cells of the cerebellar cortex and in the pyramidal neurons of the cingulate cortex (Liverman et al., 2004).

Additionally, Nrf2 knockout ($Nrf2^{-/-}$) mice have been used to understand the role of Nrf2 during ischemia-mediated oxidative brain insult.

In vitro studies showed that neurons and astrocytes from Nrf2 knockout ($Nrf2^{-/-}$) mice were more sensitive to oxidative stress, Ca^{2+} influx and mitochondrial toxicity than neurons and astrocytes from wild type animals; however, when the cells were transfected with a functional Nrf2 construct, they became less prone to oxidative stress (Kraft et al., 2004; Lee et al., 2003a; Lee and Johnson, 2004). Consistent with these results, dominant negative-Nrf2 stable cells and Nrf2-sensitized neuroblastoma cells silenced with siRNA were more amenable to apoptosis induced by nitric oxide (Dhakshinamoorthy & Porter, 2004). Also, increasing Nrf2 activity in mixed neuronal/glial cultures was highly neuroprotective in *in vitro* models that simulated components of stroke damage, such as oxidative glutamate toxicity, H_2O_2 exposure, metabolic inhibition by rotenone, and Ca^{2+} overload (Duffy et al., 1998; Kraft et al., 2004; Lee et al., 2003b; Murphy et al., 1991; Shih et al., 2003).

In vivo, using permanent middle cerebral artery occlussion by cauterization, Shih et al. (2005) did not observe significant difference in infarct size between $Nrf2^{-/-}$ and $Nrf2^{+/+}$ mice 24 h after stroke. However, 7 days after permanent focal ischemia, they observed a two-fold increase in infarct volume with $Nrf2^{-/-}$ mice, while the infarct size of Nrf2 $^{+/+}$ mice did not increase in size between 24 h and 7 days. On the other hand, Nrf2 knockout ($Nrf2^{-/-}$) mice subjected to 90 min middle cerebral artery occlusion followed by 24 h reperfusion, showed

an infarct volume and neurological deficit significantly larger than in wild type mice (Shah et al., 2007).
Taking together, these data suggest that Nrf2 is upregulated in permanent ischemia and ischemic/reperfusion, an augment that is related with a decreased expression of Keap1 and an altered expression of antioxidant proteins. Thus, this upregulation may be due to an alteration in the redox state, a mechanism through which cells active an antioxidant response to protect themselves from future oxidant damage. Moreover, it has been demonstrated that Nrf2 activation induces the expression of the Nrf2 gene itself (Lee et al., 2005), indicating that the administration of Nrf2 inducers may be an important neuroprotective antioxidant mechanism that can limit stroke damage.

9. Effect of Nrf2 inducers in cerebral ischemia

A wide range of dietary phytochemicals or supplements with medicinal properties have been reported to activate adaptive stress responses related with the induction of cytoprotective genes through Nrf2 induction (Surh et al., 2008). The mechanism of action of such phytochemicals can therefore be considered as a form of hormesis where a stressor triggers an adaptive response which increases resistance to more severe stress and disease (Calabrese et al., 2007). Unfortunately, few of these compounds have been tested in brain ischemic models; some of them are sulforaphane, curcumin and ter-butilhydroquinone, among others.

Sulforaphane

Sulforaphane is a natural dietary isothiocyanate present in cruciferous vegetables of the genus *Brassica* such as broccoli, brussel sprouts, cauliflower, cabbage, etc. Several studies have shown the neuroprotective properties of sulforaphane against ischemia/reperfusion damage. It has been found that sulforaphane (5 mg/kg) reduced the cerebral infarct volume in a carotid/middle cerebral artery occlusion common model in rodents when it was administered 15 min after injury (Zhao et al., 2006). Other groups reported that an injection of sulforaphane (5 mg/kg) 30 min before the onset of ischemia reduced the infarct size in a neonatal hypoxia-ischemia model (Ping et al., 2010). In both studies, the protective effects of sulforaphane were associated with its well-known capacity to induce the expression of HO-1 mRNA and protein through Nrf2/ARE pathway.
Other *in vivo* studies support the ability of sulforaphane as inducer of phase II enzymes in brain increasing HO-1, NQO1 and GST mRNA levels (Chen et al., 2011). It has also shown in *in vitro* studies that pretreatment and post-treatment with sulforaphane reduced hippocampal death of astrocytes and neurons induced by transient exposure to O_2 and glucose deprivation. This protective effect was associated with nuclear accumulation of Nrf2 accompanied by an increase in NQO1, HO-1 and GCL mRNA levels, and a decrease in DNA oxidation (Danilov et al., 2009; Soane et al., 2010). Altogether, these studies indicate that sulforaphane could be considered as a useful tool for pre- and post-treatment of brain injury due its well-know capacity as inducer of Nrf2.

Curcumin

Curcumin is a diferuloylmethane derived from the rhizomes of turmeric (*Curcuma longa* Linn, Zingiberaceae) widely used in Indian curry with a favorable safe profile. Its chemopreventive effects have been related with its antioxidant and anti-inflammatory properties (Surh & Chun, 2007; Thangapazham et al., 2006). However, its mechanism of action is still poorly understood.

Curcumin has a protective effect against neurodegeneration in cerebral ischemia through the preservation of the blood-brain barrier integrity, and a decrease of the ischemia-induced lipid peroxidation, mitochondrial dysfunction and anti-apoptotic effects (Sun et al., 2008).

Yang et al., (2009) observed that the systematic administration of curcumin (100 mg/kg) 15 min after middle cerebral artery permanent occlusion increased Nrf2 nuclear translocation and Nrf2 and HO-1 gene and protein levels at 24 h onset of reperfusion. Curcumin reduced neurologic deficit, brain edema and infarct volume at 24 h after stroke. These results show that curcumin maybe an effective therapeutic drug for the treatment of brain injury toward a potential mechanism of upregulation Nrf2/ARE pathway at gene and protein levels.

However, the bioavailability of curcumin is very limited due to poor absorption, rapid metabolism and quick systemic elimination. Moreover, it has a poor blood-brain barrier penetration following acute administration. To improve its bioavailability, pharmacokinetics and interaction with multiple viable targets, new curcumin derivatives are being synthesized (Lapchak, 2001).

tert-Butylhydroquinone (t-BHQ)

tert-butylhydroquinone (t-BHQ), a metabolite of the widely used food antioxidant butylated hydroxyanisole, has already been approved for human use (Food and Agriculture Organization of the United Nations/World Health Organization, 1999; National Toxicology Program, 1997). t-BHQ possesses an oxidizable 1,4 diphenolic structure that confers its potent ability to dissociate Keap1/Nrf2 complex (Van Ommen et al., 1992). T-BHQ can protect neuronal cells against the oxidative insult initiated by dopamine, H_2O_2, *tert*-butyl hydroperoxide, NMDA and glutamate (Duffy et al., 1998; Kraft et al., 2004; Li et al., 2002; Murphy et al., 1991; Shah et al., 2007).

Shih et al., (2005) determined the neuroprotective effect of tBHQ in ischemic injury in two different ischemia/reperfusion models - middle cerebral artery occlusion and endothelin-1 vasoconstriction - in rats and mice, using different routes of administration: intacerebroventricular, intraperitoneal, and dietary. Intracerebroventricular administration of t-BHQ (1 μL/h) during 3 days before rats were subjected to 1.5 h of ischemia and 24 h reperfusion showed a significant reduction of infarction in the cortex and a significant reduction in the neuronal scores. Intraperitoneal administration of t-BHQ (16.7 mg/Kg; 3 times/8h) 24 h before middle cerebral artery occlusion improved functional recovery up to 1 month after MCAO, showing a long-term benefit in ischemic damage and sensimotor deficit. $Nrf2^{+/+}$ and $Nrf2^{+/-}$ mice fed with 1% t-BHQ during one week before permanent focal ischemia did not show changes in infarct area after 7 days, while $Nrf2^{-/-}$ mice were less tolerant to the diet, losing 20% body weight and showing a continuous growth of infarct area, thus suggesting that loss of Nrf2 function promotes peri-infact zone. Finally, $Nrf2^{+/+}$ and $Nrf2^{-/-}$ mice were fed with t-BHQ after endothelin-1 administration into cortical parenchyma. $Nrf2^{+/+}$ mice showed a decrease in endothelin-1-induced infarction while $Nrf2^{-/-}$ mice showed an exacerbated injury (Shih et al., 2003; 2005).

Collectively, these data suggest that t-BHQ may have a therapeutic potential for ischemic injury by increasing brain antioxidant capacity though the up-regulation of Nrf2 expression.

10. Presumable protective effect of garlic compounds in cerebral ischemia

Numerous studies have shown that garlic and its compounds exhibit a diverse biological activity, including anti-tumorigenic, anti-atherosclerosis, detoxification, anti-inflammatory, and antioxidant (Aguilera et al., 2010; Ali et al., 2000; Fisher et al., 2007; Fukushima et al., 1997; Mathew & Biju, 2008). The effect of different garlic preparations (aged garlic extract, aqueous garlic extract, garlic oil) and isolated compounds (S-allylcysteine) in cerebral ischemia, has been associated to its ability to scavenge ROS, acting as direct antioxidants (Kim et al., 2006a).

Gupta et al. (2003) found that garlic oil administration 90 min before the ischemia/reperfusion diminished the infarct area and associated this effect to its antioxidant properties. Saleem et al. (2006) showed that aqueous garlic extract treatment increased neurobehavioral score, decreased malondialdehyde levels, increased GSH content, and prevented the depletion in GPx, GR, GST and Na^+/K^+-ATPasa activities. Moreover, CAT and SOD activities were increased by aqueous garlic extract. Aguilera et al. (2010) reported that the major protective effect exerted by aged garlic extract was observed when it was administered at the onset of reperfusion. In this work, aged garlic extract prevented the ischemia/reperfusion-induced increase in nitrotyrosine levels and the decrease in GPx, SOD and CAT activities both in cortex and striatum.

Numagami et al. (1996) demonstrated that aged garlic extract compounds that present a thioallyl group (particularly S-allylcysteine) exhibited a strong antioxidant capacity in a model of cerebral ischemia in rats. Indeed, S-allylcysteine reduced the infarct volume and brain edema, while prevented $ONOO^-$ formation and lipid peroxidation (Numagami & Ohnishi, 2001). More recently, S-allylcysteine (300 mg/kg, i.p.) produced a protective effect on cerebral ischemic injury in rats due to the inhibition of extracellular signal-regulated kinase activity (Kim et al., 2006a). The fact that S-allylcysteine can cross the blood-brain barrier turned it soon of potential interest to be tested in neurotoxic models. In fact, the prophylactic impact and rescue properties of S-allylcysteine in ischemia/reperfusion injury are being recently discussed and reinforced (Sener et al., 2007). In addition, S-allylcysteine is a stable compound (Lawson, 1998) and is easily absorbed by gastrointestinal tract after oral administration (Kodera et al., 2002). One of its advantages in regard to other garlic compounds, such as allicin and dialyl sulfide, is its limited toxicity established by its higher lethal oral dose (Amagase et al., 2001). Pharmacokinetic studies demonstrate fast absorption and distribution phases followed by a slow elimination phase for oral administration, as well as fast distribution and slow elimination phases for i.v. administration (Nagae et al., 1994; Yan & Zeng, 2005). Pharmacokinetics of S-allylcysteine in humans by oral garlic administration revealed a half-life of 10 h and clearance time of 30 h (Kodera et al., 2002), suggesting a high bioavailability. After its oral administration, S-allylcysteine is absorbed by gastrointestinal tract, and its higher concentrations are detected in plasma and kidney up to 8 h post-intake (Nagae et al., 1994; Yan & Zeng, 2005).

On the other hand, garlic oil-derived organosulfur compounds such as diallyl trisulfide, dialyl disulfide, and dialyl sulfide provide significant protection against carcinogenesis, and this protection is likely related with their antioxidant properties (Maldonado et al., 2009). Moreover, the lipophilic characteristics of these compounds allow crossing the blood-brain barrier as follows: dialyl sulfide crosses the blood-brain barrier easier than dialyl disulfide > diallyl trisulfide > S-allylcysteine (Kim et al., 2006b).

Recently, it has been reported that some garlic compounds (diallyl trisulfide, dialyl disulfide, dialyl sulfide and S-ally-L-cysteine) are able to activate Nrf2 factor in liver, kidney, intestine and lung. (Chen et al., 2004; Fisher et al., 2007; Fukao et al., 2004; Gong et al., 2004; Guyonnet et al., 1999; Kalayarasan et al., 2008; 2009; Wu et al., 2002). However, there is no information on Nrf2 induction by these garlic compounds in the brain.
Altogether, these data indicate that S-ally-L-cysteine, diallyl trisulfide, dialyl disulfide, and dialyl sulfide may be alternative treatments for cerebral ischemia through Nrf2 upregulation.

11. Conclusion

Nowadays is widely recognized that up-regulation of phase 2 response is a powerful, highly efficient and promising antioxidant strategy for protection against several diseases, including ischemic stroke. A wide range of dietary phytochemicals with medicinal properties have been reported to activate adaptive stress responses related with the induction of cytoprotective genes through Nrf2/ARE pathway. Unfortunately, few of these compounds (sulforaphane, curcumin, ter-butilhydroquinone) have been tested in cerebral ischemia experimental models. Moreover, these compounds have characteristics that limit their use as therapeutic agents in ischemic stroke. For example, sulforaphane is expensive, while curcumin poorly crosses the blood-brain barrier. Due to this, new agents should be evaluated. In this context, some garlic compounds (diallyl sulfide, diallyl disulfide, diallyl trisulfide and S-allylcysteine) could be promising agents for treatment of ischemic stroke because their physicochemical properties are promising, their absorption is high and most of them can easily cross the blood-brain barrier. Moreover, they have the ability to active Nrf2 factor and induce a phase 2 response in several models of hepatic and renal damage.

12. Acknowledgements

This study was supported by CONACYT (Grant No. 103527 to PDM).

13. Abbreviation list

ARE	Antioxidant Response Element
BH2	Dihydrobiopterin
BH4	Tetrahydrobiopterin
CAT	Catalase
G6PD	Glucose-6phosphate dehydrogenase
GCLC	Glutamate cysteine ligase catalitic subunit
GCLM	Glutamate cysteine ligase modifier subunit
GPx	Glutathione Peroxidase
GSH	Reduced Glutathione
GSSG	Oxidized Glutathione
HO-1	Heme oxygenase-1
NQO1	NADPH:quinone oxidoreductase-1
Keap1	Kelch-like ECH-associated protein 1
Nrf2	Nuclear Factor-E2-related Factor 2
RNS	Reactive Nitrogen Species

ROS	Reactive Oxygen Species
SOD	Superoxide Dismutase
tBHQ	tert-butylhydroquinone
TXNRD1	Thioredoxine Reductase-1

14. References

Aguilera, P.; Chánez-Cárdenas, M.E. & Maldonado, P.D. (2007). Recent Advances in the Use of Antioxidant Treatments in Cerebral Ischemia, In: *New Perspectives on Brain Cell Damage, Neurodegeneration and Neuroprotective Strategies*, A. Santamaría & M.E. Jiménez-Capdeville, (Ed.), 145–159, Research Signpost, ISBN 81-308-0164-7, Kerala, India.

Aguilera, P.; Chánez-Cárdenas, M.E.; Ortiz-Plata, A.; León-Aparicio, D.; Barrera, D.; Ezpinoza-Rojo, M.; Villeda-Hernández, J.; Sánchez-García, A. & Maldonado P.D. (2010). Aged Garlic Extract Delays the Appearance of Infarct Area in Cerebral Ischemia Model, an Effect Likely Conditioned by the Celular Antioxidant System. *Phytomedicine*, Vol.17, No.4-3, (March), pp. 241-247, ISSN 0944-7113 (Print)

Alfieri, A.; Srivastava, S.; Siow, R.C.; Modo, M.; Fraser, P.A. & Mann, G.E. (2011). Targeting the Nrf2-Keap1 Antioxidant Defence Pathway for Neurovascular Protection in Stroke. *Journal of Physiologie*, Vol.589, No.Pt17, (September), pp. 4125-4136, ISSN 0022-3751 (Print)

Ali, M.; Al-Qattan, K.K.; Al-Enezi, F.; Khanafer, R.M. & Mustafa, T. (2000). Effect of Allicin From Garlic Powder on Serum Lipids and Blood Pressure in Rats Fed With a High Cholesterol Diet. *Prostaglandins, leukotrienes, and essential fatty acids*, Vol.62, No.4, (April), pp. 253-259, ISSN 0952-3278 (Print)

Amagase, H.; Petesch, B.L.; Matsuura, H.; Kasuga, S. & Itakura, Y. (2001). Intake of Garlic and Its Bioactive Components. *Journal of Nutrition*, Vol.131, No.3s, (March), pp. 955S-962S, ISSN 0022-3166 (Print)

Aronowski, J.; Strong, R. & Grotta, J.C. (1997). Reperfusion Injury: Demonstration of Brain Damage Produced by Reperfusion After Transient Focal Ischemia in Rats. *Journal of Cerebral Blood Flow and Metabolism*, Vol.17, No.10, (October), pp. 1048–1056, ISSN 0271-678X (Print)

Bloom, D.A. & Jaiswal, A.K. (2003). Phosphorylation of Nrf2 at Ser40 by Protein Kinase C in Response to Antioxidants Leads to the Release of Nrf2 From INrf2, but is not Required for Nrf2 Stabilization/Accumulation in the Nucleus and Transcriptional Activation of Antioxidant Response Element-Mediated NAD(P)H:Quinone Oxidoreductase-1 Gene Expression. *The Journal of Biological Chemistry*, Vol.278, No.45, (November), pp. 44675-44682, ISSN 0021-9258 (Print)

Calabrese, E.J.; Bachmann, K.A.; Bailer, A.J.; Bolger, P.M.; Borak, J.; Cai, L.; Cedergreen, N.; Cherian, M.G.; Chiueh, C.C.; Clarkson, T.W.; Cook, R.R.; Diamond, D.M.; Doolittle, D.J.; Dorato, M.A.; Duke, S.O.; Feinendegen, L.; Gardner, D.E.; Hart, R.W.; Hastings, K.L.; Hayes, A.W.; Hoffmann, G.R.; Ives, J.A.; Jaworowski, Z.; Johnson, T.E.; Jonas, W.B.; Kaminski, N.E.; Keller, J.G.; Klaunig, J.E.; Knudsen, T.B.; Kozumbo, W.J.; Lettieri, T.; Liu, S.Z.; Maisseu, A.; Maynard, K.I.; Masoro, E.J.; McClellan, R.O.; Mehendale, H.M.; Mothersill, C.; Newlin, D.B.; Nigg, H.N.; Oehme, F.W.; Phalen, R.F.; Philbert, M.A.; Rattan, S.I.; Riviere, J.E.; Rodricks, J., Sapolsky, R.M.; Scott, B.R.; Seymour, C.; Sinclair, D.A.; Smith-Sonneborn, J.; Snow,

E.T.; Spear, L.; Stevenson, D.E.; Thomas, Y.; Tubiana, M.; Williams, G.M. & Mattson, M.P. (2007). Biological Stress Response Terminology: Integrating the Concepts of Adaptive Response and Preconditioning Stress Within a Hormetic Dose-Response Framework. *Toxicology and Applied Pharmacology*, Vol.222, No.1, (July), pp. 122-128, ISSN 0041-008X (Print)

Campagne, M.V.; Thibodeaux, H.; van Bruggen, N.; Cairns, B. & Lowe, D.G. (2000). Increased Binding Activity at an Antioxidant-Responsive Element in the Metallothionein-1 Promoter and Rapid Induction of Metallothionein-1 and -2 in Response to Cerebral Ischemia and Reperfusion. *The Journal of Neuroscience: the Official Journal of the Society for Neuroscience*, Vol.20, No.14, (July), pp. 5200-5207, ISSN 0270-6474 (Print)

Chan, P.H. (2001). Reactive oxygen radicals in signaling and damage in the ischemic brain. *Journal of Cerebral Blood Flow and Metabolism*, Vol. 21, No. 1, (January), pp. 2-14, ISSN 0271-678X (Print)

Chen, C.; Pung, D.; Leong, V.; Hebbar, V.; Shen, G.; Nair, S.; Li, W. & Kong, A.N. (2004). Induction of Detoxifying Enzymes by Garlic Organosulfur Compounds Through Transcription Factor Nrf2: Effect of Chemical Structure and Stress Signals. *Free Radical Biology & Medicine*, Vol.37, No.10, (November), pp. 1578-1590, ISSN 0891-5849 (Print)

Chen, G.; Fang, Q.; Zhang, J.; Zhou, D. & Wang, Z. (2011). Role of the Nrf2-ARE Pathway in Early Brain Injury After Experimental Subarachnoid Hemorrhage. *Journal of Neuroscience Research*, Vol.89, No.4, (April), pp. 515-523, ISSN 0360-4012 (Print)

Cho, H.Y. & Kleeberger, S.R. (2009). Nrf2 Protects Against Airway Disorders. *Toxicology and Applied Pharmacology*, Vol.244, No.1, (April), pp. 43-56, ISSN 0041-008X (Print)

Christensen, T.; Bruhn, T.; Balchen, T. & Diemer, N.H. (1994). Evidence for Formation of Hydroxyl Radicals During Reperfusion After Global Cerebral Ischaemia in Rats Using Salicylate Trapping and Microdialysis. *Neurobiology of Disease*, Vol.1, No.3, (December), pp. 131–138, ISSN 0969-9961 (Print)

Crabtree, M.J. & Channon, K.M. (2011). Synthesis and Recycling of Tetrahydrobiopterin in Endothelial Function and Vascular Disease. *Nitric Oxide*, Vol.25, No.2, (August), pp. 81-88, ISSN 1089-8603 (Print)

Cullinan, S.B.; Gordan, J.D.; Jin, J.; Harper, J.W. & Diehl, J.A. (2004). The Keap1-BTB Protein is an Adaptor That Bridges Nrf2 to a Cul3-Based E3 Ligase: Oxidative Stress Sensing by a Cul3-Keap1 Ligase. *Molecular and Cellular Biology*, Vol.24, No.19, (October), pp. 8477-8486, ISSN 0270-7306 (Print)

Danilov, C.A.; Chandrasekaran, K.; Racz, J.; Soane, L.; Zielke, C. & Fiskum, G. (2009). Sulforaphane Protects Astrocytes Against Oxidative Stress and Delayed Death Caused by Oxygen and Glucose Deprivation. *Glia*, Vol.57, No.6, (April), pp. 645-656, ISSN 0894-1491 (Print)

Danton, G.H. & Dietrich, W.D. (2003). Inflammatory Mechanism After Ischemia and Stroke. *Journal of Neuropathology and Experimental Neurology*, Vol.62, No.2, (February), pp. 127-136, ISSN 0022-3069 (Print)

Dhakshinamoorthy, S. & Porter, A.G. (2004). Nitric Oxide-Induced Transcriptional Up-Regulation of Protective Genes by Nrf2 Via the Antioxidant Response Element Counteracts Apoptosis of Neuroblastoma Cells. *The Journal of Biological Chemistry*, Vol.279, No.19, (May), pp. 20096–20107, ISSN 0021-9258 (Print)

Díez-Tejedor, E.; Del Brutto, O.; Álvarez-Sabín, J.; Muñoz, M. & Abiusi, G. (2001). Classification of the Cerebrovascular Diseases. *Revista de Neurologia*, Vol.33, No.5, (September), pp. 455-464, ISSN 0210-0010 (Print)

Dinkova-Kostova, A.T.; Massiah, M.A.; Bozak, R.E.; Hicks, R.J. & Talalay, P. (2001). Potency of Michael Reaction Acceptors as Inducers of Enzymes That Protect Against Carcinogenesis Depends on Their Reactivity With Sulfhydryl Groups. *Proceedings of the National Academy of Sciences of the United States of America*, Vol.98, No.6, (March), pp. 3404-3409, ISSN 0027-8424 (Print)

Dinkova-Kostova, A.T.; Fahey, J.W. & Talalay, P. (2004) Chemical Structures of Inducers of Nicotinamide Quinone Oxidoreductase 1 (NQO1). *Methods in Enzymology*, Vol.382, pp. 423-448, ISSN 0076-6879 (Print)

Dinkova-Kostova, A.T.; Holtzclaw, W.D. & Kensler, T.W. (2005a) The Role of Keap1 in Celular Protective Responses. *Chemical Research in Toxicology*, Vol.18, No.12, (December), pp. 1779-1791. ISSN 0893-228X (Print)

Dinkova-Kostova, A.T.; Holtzclaw, W.D. & Wakabayashi, N. (2005b). Keap1, the Sensor for Electrophiles and Oxidants That Regulates the Phase 2 Response, is a Zinc Metalloprotein. *Biochemistry*, Vol.44, No.18, (May), pp. 6889-6899, ISSN 0006-2960 (Print)

Dinkova-Kostova, A.T.; Cheah, J.; Samouilov, A.; Zweier, J.L.; Bozak, R.E.; Hicks, R.J. & Talalay, P. (2007). Phenolic Michael Reaction Acceptors: Combined Direct and Indirect Antioxidant Defenses Against Electrophiles and Oxidants. *Medicinal Chemistry*, Vol.3, No.3, (May), pp. 261-268, ISSN 1573-4064 (Print)

Dinkova-Kostova, A.T. & Talalay, P. (2008). Direct and Indirect Antioxidant Properties of Inducers of Cytoprotective Proteins. *Molecular Nutrition & Food Ressearch*, Vol.52, No.Suppl1, (June), pp. S128–S138, ISSN 1613-4125 (Print)

Dirnagl, U.; Iadecola, C. & Moskowitz, M.A. (1999). Pathobiology of Ischaemic Stroke: An Integrated View. *Trends in Neuroscience*, Vol.22, No.9, (September), pp. 391-397, ISSN 0166-2236 (Print)

Dringen, R. (2000). Metabolism and Functions of Glutathione in Brain. *Progress in Neurobiology*, Vol.62, No.6, (December), pp. 649-671, ISSN 0301-0082 (Print)

Duffy, S.; So, A. & Murphy, T.H. (1998). Activation of Endogenous Antioxidant Defenses in Neuronal Cells Prevents Free Radical-Mediated Damage. *Journal of Neurochemistry*, Vol.71, No.1, (July), pp. 69–77, ISSN 0022-3042 (Print)

Durukan, A. & Tatlisumak, T. (2007). Acute Ischemic Stroke: Overview of Major Experimental Rodent Models, Pathophysiology, and Therapy of Focal Cerebral Ischemia. *Pharmacology, Biochemistry, and Behavior*, Vol.87, No.1, (May), pp. 179-197, ISSN 0091-3057 (Print)

Eggler, A.L.; Liu, G.; Pezzuto, J.M.; van Breemen, R.B. & Mesecar, A.D. (2005). Modifying Specific Cysteines of the Electrophile-Sensing Human Keap1 Protein is Insufficient to Disrupt Binding to the Nrf2 Domain Neh2. *Proceedings of the National Academy of Sciences of the United States of America*, Vol.102, No.29, (July), pp. 10070-10075, ISSN 0027-8424 (Print)

Fisher, C.D., Augustine, L.M.; Maher, J.M.; Nelson, D.M.; Slitt, A.L.; Klaassen, C.D.; Lehman-McKeeman, L.D. & Cherrington, N.J. (2007). Induction of Drug Metabolizing Enzymes by Garlic and Allyl Sulfide Compounds Via Activation of Constitutive Androstane Receptor and Nuclear Factor E2-Related Factor 2. *Drug*

Metabolism and Disposition: The Biological Fate of Chemicals, Vol. 35, No. 6, (June), pp. 995-1000, ISSN 0090-9556 (Print)

Food and Agriculture Organization of the United Nations/World Health Organization. (1999). Evaluation of certain food additives and contaminants (forty-ninth report of the Joint FAO/WHO Expert Committee on Food Additives). World Health Organ Tech Rep Ser 884:i-viii, pp. 1–96.

Fukao, T.; Hosono, T.; Misawa, S.; Seki, T. & Ariga, T. (2004). The Effects of Allyl Sulfides on the Induction of Phase II Detoxification Enzymes and Liver Injury by Carbon Tetrachloride. *Food and Chemical Toxicology: An International Journal Publisher for the British Industrial Biological Research Association*, Vol42, No.5, (May), pp. 743-749, ISSN 0278-6915 (Print)

Fukushima, S.; Takada, N.; Hori, T. & Wanibuchi, H. (1997). Cancer Prevention by Organosulfur Compounds From Garlic and Onion. *Journal of Cellular Biochemistry. Supplement*, Vol.27, pp. 100-105, ISSN 0733-1959 (Print)

Gong, P.; Hu, B. & Cederbaum, A.I. (2004). Diallyl Sulfide Induces Heme Oxygenase-1 Through MAPK Pathway. *Archives of Biochemistry and Biophysics*, Vol.432, No.2, (December), pp. 252-260, ISSN 0003-9861 (Print)

Gupta, R.; Singh, M. & Sharma, A. (2003). Neuroprotective Effect of Antioxidants on Ischemia and Reperfusion-Induced Cerebral Injury. *Pharmacological Research: the Official Journal of the Italian Pharmacological Society*, Vol.48, No.2, (August), pp. 209-215, ISSN 1043-6618 (Print)

Guyonnet, D.; Siess, M.H.; Le Bon, A.M. & Suschetet, M. (1999). Modulation of Phase II Enzymes by Organosulfur Compounds From Allium Vegetables in Rat Tissues. *Toxicology and Applied Pharmacology*, Vol.154, No.1, (January), pp. 50-58, ISSN 0041-008X (Print)

Halliwell, B. & Gutteridge, J. (1999). *Free Radicals in Biology and Medicine*, Oxford Univ. Press, ISBN 13 9780198568698, New York

Heim, C.; Melzacka, M.; Kolasiewicz, W.; Jaros, T.; Sieklucka, M.; Wesemann, W. & Sontag, K.H. (1995). Cerebral Oligemic Hypoxia and Iron Toxicity in the Mesolimbic System of Rats. *Journal of Neural Transmission. Supplementum*, Vol.46, pp. 165-173, ISSN 0303-6995 (Print)

Heim, C.; Zhang, J.; Lan, J.; Sieklucka, M.; Kurz, T.; Riederer, P.; Gerlach, M. & Sontag K.H. (2000). Cerebral Oligaemia Episode Triggers Free Radical Formation and Late Cognitive Deficiencies. *The European Journal of Neuroscience*, Vol.12, No.4, (February), pp. 715-725, ISSN 0953-816X (Print)

Heiss, W.D. (2002). Stroke--Acute Interventions. *Journal of Neural Transmission. Supplementum*, Vol.63, pp. 37-57, ISSN 0303-6995 (Print)

Hong, F.; Freeman, M.L. & Liebler, D.C. (2005). Identification of Sensor Cysteines in Human Keap1 Modified by the Cancer Chemopreventive Agent Sulforaphane. *Chemical Research in Toxicolog*, Vol.18, No.12, (December), pp. 1917-1926, ISSN 0893-228X (Print)

Hou, ST. & MacManus, J.P. (2002). Molecular Mechanisms of Cerebral Ischemia-Induced Neuronal Death. *International Review of Cytology*, Vol.221, pp. 93-148, ISSN 0074-7696 (Print)

Huang, H.C.; Nguyen, T. & Pickett. C.B. (2002). Phosphorylation of Nrf2 at Ser-40 by Protein Kinase C Regulates Antioxidant Response Element-Mediated Transcription. *The*

Journal of Biological Chemistry, Vol.277, No.45, (November), pp. 42769-42774, ISSN 0021-9258 (Print)

Hsu, C.Y.; Ahmed, S.H. & Lees, K.R. (2000). The Therapeutic Time Window--Theoretical and Practical Considerations. *Journal of Stroke and Cerebrovascular Diseases: The Official Journal of National Stroke Association*, Vol.9, No.6 Pt2, (November), pp. 24–31, ISSN 1052-3057 (Print)

Ikeda, K.; Negishi, H. & Yamori, Y. (2003). Antioxidant Nutrients and Hypoxia/Ischemia Brain Injury in Rodents. *Toxicology*, Vol.189, No.1-2, (July), pp. 55–61, ISSN 0300-483X (Print)

Itoh, K.; Wakabayashi, N.; Katoh, Y.; Ishii, T.; Igarashi, K.; Engel, J.D. & Yamamoto, M. (1999). Keap1 Represses Nuclear Activation of Antioxidant Responsive Elements by Nrf2 Through Binding to the Amino-Terminal Neh2 Domain. *Genes & Development*, Vol.13, No.1, (January), pp. 76-86, ISSN 0890-9369 (Print)

Itoh,K.; Wakabayashi,N.; Katoh,Y.; Ishii,T.; O'Connor,T. & Yamamoto, M. (2003). Keap1 Regulates Both Cytoplasmic--Nuclear Shuttling and Degradation of Nrf2 in Response to Electrophiles. *Genes to Cells: Devoted to Molecular & Cellular Mechanisms*, Vol.8, No.4, (April), pp. 379—391, ISSN 1356-9597 (Print)

Jung, K.A. & Kwak, M.K. (2010). The Nrf2 System as a Potential Target for the Development of Indirect Antioxidants. *Molecules*, Vol.15, No.10, (Octuber), pp. 7266-7291, ISSN 1420-3049 (Electronic)

Kalayarasan, S.; Sriram, N.; Sureshkumar, A. & Sudhandiran, G. (2008). Chromium (VI)-Induced Oxidative Stress and Apoptosis is Reduced by Garlic and Its Derivative S-allylcysteine Through the Activation of Nrf2 in the Hepatocytes of Wistar Rats. *Journal of Applied Toxicology: JAT*, Vol.28, No.7, (Octuber), pp. 908-919, ISSN 0260-437X (Print)

Kalayarasan, S.; Prabhu, P.N.; Sriram, N.; Manikandan, R.; Arumugam, M.,& Sudhandiran, G. (2009). Diallyl Sulfide Enhances Antioxidants and Inhibits Inflammation Through the Activation of Nrf2 Against Gentamicin-Induced Nephrotoxicity in Wistar Rats. *European Journal of Pharmacology*, Vol.606, No.1-3, (March), pp. 162-171, ISSN 0014-2999 (Print)

Kang, M.I.; Kobayashi, A.; Wakabayashi, N.; Kim, S.G. & Yamamoto, M. (2004). Scaffolding of Keap1 to the Actin Cytoskeleton Controls the Function of Nrf2 as Key Regulator of Cytoprotective Phase 2 Genes. *Proceedings of the National Academy of Sciences of the United States of America*, Vol.101, No.7, (February), pp. 2046-2051, ISSN 0027-8424 (Print)

Kang, Y.H. & Pezzuto, J.M. (2004). Induction of Quinone Reductase as a Primary Screen for Natural Product Anticarcinogens. *Methods in Enzymology*, Vol.382, pp. 380–414, ISSN 0076-6879 (Print)

Katoh, Y.; Itoh, K.; Yoshida, E.; Miyagishi, M.; Fukamizu, A. & Yamamoto, M. (2001). Two Domains of Nrf2 Cooperatively Bind CBP, a CREB Binding Protein, and Synergistically Activate Transcription. *Genes to Cells: Devoted to Molecular & Cellular Mechanisms*, Vol.6, No.10, (October), pp. 857-868, ISSN 1356-9597 (Print)

Katsuoka, F.; Motohashi, H.; Ishii, T.; Aburatani, H.; Engel, J.D. & Yamamoto, M. (2005). Genetic Evidence That Small Maf Proteins are Essential for the Activation of Antioxidant Response Element-Dependent Genes. *Molecular and Cellular Biology*, Vol.25, No.18, (September), pp. 8044-8051, ISSN 0270-7306 (Print)

Kensler, T.W.; Wakabayashi, N. & Biswal, S. (2007). Cell Survival Responses to Environmental Stresses Via the Keap1-Nrf2-ARE Pathway. *Annual Review of Pharmacology and Toxicology*, Vol.47, pp. 89–116, ISSN 0362-1642 (Print)

Kim, J. M.; Chang, N.; Kim, W.K. & Chun, H.S. (2006a). Dietary S-allyl-L-Cysteine Reduces Mortality With Decreased Incidence of Stroke and Behavioral Changes in Stroke-Prone Spontaneously Hypertensive Rats. *Bioscience, Biotechnology, and Biochemistry*, Vol.70, No.8, (August), pp. 1969-1971, ISSN 0916-8451 (Print)

Kim, J.M., Chang, H.J.; Kim, W.K.; Chang, N. & Chun, H.S. (2006b). Structure-Activity Relationship of Neuroprotective and Reactive Oxygen Species Scavenging Activities for Allium Organosulfur Compounds. *Journal of Agricultural and Food Chemistry*, Vol.54, No.18, (September), pp. 6547-6553, ISSN 0021-8561 (Print)

Kobayashi, A.; Kang, M.I.; Okawa, H.; Ohtsuji, M.; Zenke, Y.; Chiba, T.; Igarashi, K. & Yamamoto, M. (2004). Oxidative Stress Sensor Keap1 Functions As an Adaptor for Cul3-based E3 Ligase to Regulate Proteasomal Degradation of Nrf2. *Molecular and Cellular Biol*ogy, Vol.24, No.16, (August), pp. 7130-7139, ISSN 0270-7306 (Print)

Kobayashi, A.; Kang, M.I.; Watai, Y.; Tong, K.I.; Shibata, T.; Uchida, K. & Yamamoto, M. (2006). Oxidative and Electrophilic Stresses Activate Nrf2 Through Inhibition of Ubiquitination Activity of Keap1. *Molecular and Cellular Biol*ogy, Vol.26, No.1, (January), pp. 221-229, ISSN 0270-7306 (Print)

Kobayashi, M. & Yamamoto, M. (2006). Nrf2-Keap1 Regulation of Cellular Defense Mechanisms Against Electrophiles and Reactive Oxygen Species. *Advances in Enzyme Regulation*, Vol.46, pp. 113–140, ISSN 0065-2571 (Print)

Kodera, Y.; Suzuki, A.; Imada, O.; Kasuga, S.; Sumioka, I.; Kanezawa, A.; Taru, N.; Fujikawa, M.; Nagae, S.; Masamoto, K.; Maeshige, K. & Ono, K. (2002). Physical, Chemical, and Biological Properties of S-Allylcysteine, an Amino Acid Derived From Garlic. *Journal of Agricultural and Food Chemistry*, Vol.50, No.3, (January), pp. 622-632, ISSN 0021-8561

Kraft, A.D.; Johnson, D.A. & Johnson, J.A. (2004). Nuclear Factor E2-Related Factor 2-Dependent Antioxidant Response Element Activation by Tert-butylhydroquinone and Sulforaphane Occurring Preferentially in Astrocytes Conditions Neurons Against Oxidative Insult. *Journal of Neuroscience*, Vol.24, No.5, (February), pp. 1101-1112, ISSN 0270-6474 (Print)

Kuroda, S. & Siesjo, B.K. (1997). Reperfusion Damage Following Focal Ischemia: Pathophysiology and Therapeutic Windows. *Clinical Neuroscience (New York, N.Y.)*, Vol.4, No.4, pp. 199–212, ISSN 1065-6766 (Print)

Läer, S.; Block, F.; Huether, G.; Heim, C. & Sontag, K.H. (1993). Effect of Transient Reduction of Cerebral Blood Flow in Normotensive Rats on Striatal Dopamine-Release. *Journal of Neural Transmission. General Section*, Vol.92, No.2-3, pp. 203-211, ISSN 0300-9564 (Print)

Lapchak, P.A. (2001). Neuroprotective and Neurotrophic Curcuminoids to Treat Stroke: a Translational Perspective. *Expert Opinion on Investigational Drugs*, Vol.20, No.1, (January), pp. 13-22, ISSN 1354-3784 (Print)

Lawson, L.D. (1998). Garlic: a Review of Its Medicinal Effects and Indicated Active Compounds, In: *Phytomedicines of Europe: Chemistry and Biological Activity*, L.D. Lawson, & R. Bauer, (Ed.), 176-209, ACS symposium series 691, American Chemical Society, ISBN13 9780841235595, Washington, United States

Lee, J.M.; Calkins, M.J.; Chan, K.; Kan, Y.W. & Johnson, J.A. (2003a). Identification of the NF-E2-Related Factor-2-Dependent Genes Conferring Protection Against Oxidative Stress in Primary Cortical Astrocytes Using Oligonucleotide Microarray Analysis. *The Journal of Biological Chemistry*, Vol.278, No.14, (April), pp. 12029-12038, ISSN 0021-9258 (Print)

Lee, J.M.; Shih, A.Y.; Murphy, T.H. & Johnson, J.A. (2003b). NF-E2-Related Factor-2 Mediates Neuroprotection Against Mitochondrial Complex I Inhibitors and Increased Concentrations of Intracellular Calcium in Primary Cortical Neurons. *The Journal of Biological Chemistry*, Vol.278, No.39, (September), pp. 37948–37956, ISSN 0021-9258 (Print)

Lee, J.M. & Johnson, J.A. (2004). An Important Role of Nrf2-ARE Pathway in the Cellular Defense Mechanism. *Journal of Biochemistry and Molecular Biology*, Vol.37, No.2, (March), pp. 139-143, ISSN 1225-8687 (Print)

Lee, J.M.; Li, J.; Johnson, D.A.; Stein, T.D.; Kraft, A.D.; Calkins, M.J.; Jakel, R.J. & Johnson, J.A. (2005). Nrf2, a Multi-Organ Protector? *The FASEB Journal: official Publication of the Federation of American Societies for Experimental Biology*, Vol.19, No.9, (July), pp. 1061-1066, ISSN 0892-6638 (Print)

Li, J.; Lee, J.M. & Johnson, J.A. (2002). Microarray Analysis Reveals an Antioxidant Responsive Element-Driven Gene Set Involved in Conferring Protection From an Oxidative Stress-Induced Apoptosis in IMR-32 Cells. *The Journal of Biological Chemistry*, Vol.277, No.1, (January), pp. 388-394, ISSN 0021-9258 (Print)

Li, W. & Kong, A.N. (2009). Molecular Mechanisms of Nrf2-Mediated Antioxidant Response. *Molecular Carcino*genesis, Vol.48, No.2, (February), pp. 91-104, ISSN 0899-1987 (Print)

Li, M.; Zhang, X.; Cui, L.; Yang, R.; Wang, L.; Liu, L. & Du, W. (2011). The Neuroprotection of Oxymatrine in Cerebral Ischemia/Reperfusion is Related to Nuclear Factor Erythroid 2-Related Factor 2 (Nrf2)-Mediated Antioxidant Response: Role of Nrf2 and Hemeoxygenase-1 Expression. *Biological & Pharmaceutical Bulletin*, Vol.34, No.5, pp. 595-601, ISSN 0918-6158 (Print)

Liu, S.; Liu, M.; Peterson, S.; Miyake, M.; Vallyathan, V. & Liu, K.J. (2003). Hydroxyl Radical Formation is Greater in Striatal Core Than in Penumbra in a Rat Model of Ischemic Stroke. *Journal of Neuroscience Research*, Vol.71, No.6, (March), pp. 882-888, ISSN 0077-7846 (Print)

Liverman, C.S.; Cui, L.; Yong, C.; Choudhuri, R.; Klein, R.M.; Welch, K.M. & Berman, N.E. (2004). Response of the Brain to Oligemia: Gene Expression, c-Fos, and Nrf2 Localization. *Brain Research. Molecular Brain Research*, Vol.126, No.1, (July), pp. 57-66, ISSN 0169-328X (Print)

Lo, S.C. & Hannink; M. (2006). PGAM5, a Bcl-XL-Interacting Protein, is a Novel Substrate for the Redox-Regulated Keap1-Dependent Ubiquitin Ligase Complex. *The Journal of Biological Chemistry*, Vol.281, No.49, (December), pp. 37893-37903, ISSN 0021-9258 (Print)

Lo, S.C. & Hannink, M. (2008). PGAM5 Tethers a Ternary Complex Containing Keap1 and Nrf2 to Mitochondria. *Experimental Cell Research*, Vol.314, No.8, (May), pp. 1789-17803, ISSN 0014-4827 (Print)

Loh, K.P.; Huang, S.H.; De Silva, R.; Tan, B.K. & Zhu, Y.Z. (2006). Oxidative Stress: Apoptosis in Neuronal Injury. *Current Alzheimer Research*, Vol.3, No.4, (September), pp. 327–337, ISSN 1567-2050 (Print)

Longa, E.Z.; Weinstein, P.R.; Carlson, S. & Cummins, R. (1989). Reversible Middle Cerebral Artery Occlusion Without Craniectomy in Rats. *Stroke*, Vol.20, No.1, (January), pp. 84–91, ISSN 0039-2499 (Print)

Maldonado, P.D.; Limón, D.; Galván-Arzate, S.; Santamaria, A. & Pedraza-Chaverri, J. (2009). Medicinal Properties of Garlic: Importance of Its Antioxidant Activity, In: *Garlic Consumption and Health*, M. Pãcurar, & G. Krejci, (Ed.), 61-116, Nova Science Publisher, ISBN 978-1-60741-642-5, New York, United States

Mathew, B.C. & Biju, R.S. (2008). Neuroprotective Effects of Garlic a Review. *The Libyan Journal of Medicine*, Vol.3, No.1, (March), pp. 23-33, ISSN 1993-2820 (Print)

Margaill, I.; Plotkine, M. & Lerouet, D. (2005). Antioxidant Strategies in the Treatment of Stroke. *Free Radical Biology & Medicine*, Vol.39, No.4, (August), pp. 429-443, ISSN 0891-5849 (Print)

McMahon, M.; Itoh, K.; Yamamoto, M. & Hayes, J.D. (2003). Keap1-Dependent Proteasomal Degradation of Transcription Factor Nrf2 Contributes to the Negative Regulation of Antioxidant Response Element-Driven Gene Expression. *The Journal of Biological Chemistry*, Vol.278, No.24, (June), pp. 21592-21600, ISSN 0021-9258 (Print)

McMahon, M.; Thomas, N.; Itoh, K.; Yamamoto, M. & Hayes J.D. (2004). Redox-Regulated Turnover of Nrf2 is Determined by at Least Two Separate Protein Domains, the Redox-Sensitive Neh2 Degron and the Redox-Insensitive Neh6 Degron. *The Journal of Biological Chemistry*, Vol.279, No.30, (July), pp. 31556-31567, ISSN 0021-9258 (Print)

McMahon, M.; Thomas, N.; Itoh, K.; Yamamoto, M. & Hayes, J.D. (2006). Dimerization of Substrate Adaptors Can Facilitate Cullin-Mediated Ubiquitylation of Proteins by a "Tethering" Mechanism: a Two-Site Interaction Model for the Nrf2-Keap1 Complex. *The Journal of Biological Chemistry*, Vol.281, No.34, (August), pp. 24756-24768, ISSN 0021-9258 (Print)

Moi, P.; Chan, K.; Asunis, I.; Cao, A. & Kan, Y.W. (1994). Isolation of NF-E2-Related Factor 2 (Nrf2), a NF-E2-Like Basic Leucine Zipper Transcriptional Activator That Binds to the Tandem NF-E2/AP1 Repeat of the Beta-Globin Locus Control Region. *Proceedings of the National Academy of Sciences of the United States of America*, Vol.91, No.21, (October), pp. 9926-9930, ISSN 0027-8424 (Print)

Moro, M.A.; Almeida, A.; Bolaños, J.P. & Lizasoain, I. (2005). Mitochondrial Respiratory Chain and Free Radical Generation in Stroke. *Free Radical Biology & Medicine*, Vol.39, No.10, (November), pp. 1291-1304, ISSN 0891-5849 (Print)

Motohashi, H.; O'Connor, T.; Katsuoka, F.; Engel, J.D. & Yamamoto, M. (2002). Integration and Diversity of the Regulatory Network Composed of Maf and CNC Families of Transcription Factors. *Gene*, Vol.294, No.1-2, (July), pp. 1-12, ISSN 0378-1119 (Print)

Motohashi, H. & Yamamoto, M. (2004). Nrf2-Keap1 Defines a Physiologically Important Stress Response Mechanism. *Trends Molecular Medicine*, Vol.10, No.11, (November), pp. 549–557, ISSN 1471-4914 (Print)

Murphy, T.H.; De Long, M.J. & Coyle, J.T. (1991). Enhanced NAD(P)H:quinone Reductase Activity Prevents Glutamate Toxicity Produced by Oxidative Stress. *Journal of Neurochemistry*, Vol.56, No.3, (March), pp. 990–995, ISSN 0022-3042 (Print)

Nagae, S.; Ushijima, M.; Hatono, S.; Imai, J.; Fasuga, S.; Matsuura, H.; Iyakura, Y. & Higashi, Y. (1994). Pharmacokinetics of the Garlic Compound S-Allylcysteine. *Planta Medica*, Vol.60, No.3, (June), pp. 214-217, ISSN 0032-0943

National Toxicology Program. (1997). NTP toxicology and carcinogenesis studies of t-butylhydroquinone (CAS no. 1948 -33-0) in F344/N rats and B6C3F(1) mice (feed studies). Natl Toxicol Program Tech Rep Ser 459:1–326

Nguyen, T.; Sherratt, P.J.; Huang, H.C.; Yang, C.S. & Pickett, C.B. (2003). Increased Protein Stability as a Mechanism That Enhances Nrf2-Mediated Transcriptional Activation of the Antioxidant Response Element. Degradation of Nrf2 by the 26 S Proteasome. *The Journal of Biological Chemistry*. Vol.278, No.7, (February), pp. 4536-4541, ISSN 0021-9258 (Print)

Nguyen, T.; Yang, C.S. & Pickett, C.B. (2004). The Pathways and Molecular Mechanisms Regulating Nrf2 Activation in Response to Chemical Stress. *Free Radical Biology & Medicine*, Vol.37, No.4, (August), pp. 433-441, ISSN 0891-5849 (Print)

Nioi, P.; Nguyen, T.; Sherratt, P.J. & Pickett, C.B. (2005). The Carboxy-Terminal Neh3 Domain of Nrf2 is Required for Transcriptional Activation. *Molecular and Cellular Biol*ogy, Vol.25, No.24, (December), pp. 10895-10906, ISSN 0270-7306 (Print)

Numagami, Y.; Sato, S. & Ohnishi, S.T. (1996). Attenuation of Rat Ischemic Brain Damage by Aged Garlic Extracts: a Possible Protecting Mechanism as Antioxidants. *Neurochemistry International*, Vol.29, No.2, (August), pp. 135-143, ISSN 0197-0186 (Print)

Numagami, Y. & Ohnishi, S.T. (2001). S-Allylcysteine Inhibits Free Radical Production, Lipid Peroxidation and Neuronal Damage in Rat Brain Ischemia *Journal of Nutrition*, Vol.131, No.3s, (March), pp. 1100S-1105S, ISSN 0022-3166 (Print)

Orino, K.; Lehman, L.; Tsuji, Y.; Ayaki, H.; Torti, S.V. & Torti, F.M. (2001). Ferritin and the Response to Oxidative Stress. *The Biochemical Journal*, Vol.357, No.Pt1, (July), pp. 241-247, ISSN 0264-6021 (Print)

Peters, O.; Back, T.; Lindauer, U.; Busch, C.; Megow, D.; Dreier, J. & Dirnagl, U. (1998). Increased Formation of Reactive Oxygen Species After Permanent and Reversible Middle Cerebral Artery Occlusion in the Rat. *Journal of Cerebral Blood Flow and Metabolism*, Vol.18, No.2, (February), pp. 196–205, ISSN 0271-678X (Print)

Ping, Z.; Liu, W.; Kang, Z.; Cai, J.; Wang, Q.; Cheng, N.; Wang, S.; Wang, S.; Zhang, J.H. & Sun, X. (2010). Sulforaphane Protects Brains Against Hypoxic-Ischemic Injury Through Induction of Nrf2-Dependent Phase 2 Enzyme. *Brain Research*, Vol.1343, (July), pp. 178-185, ISSN 0006-8993 (Print)

Ramos-Gomez, M.; Kwak, M.K.; Dolan, P.M.; Itoh, K.; Yamamoto, M.; Talalay, P. & Kensler, T.W. (2001). Sensitivity to Carcinogenesis is Increased and Chemoprotective Efficacy of Enzyme Inducers is Lost in Nrf2 Transcription Factor-Deficient Mice. *Proceedings of the National Academy of Sciences of the United States of America*, Vol.98, No.6, (March), pp. 3410-3415, ISSN 0027-8424 (Print)

Rodrigo, J.; Fernandez, A.P.; Serrano, J.; Peinado, M.A. & Martinez, A. (2005). The Role of Free Radicals in Cerebral Hypoxia and Ischemia. *Free Radical Biology & Medicine*, Vol.39, No.1, (July), pp. 26–50, ISSN 0891-5849 (Print)

Rushmore, T.H.; Morton, M.R. & Pickett, C.B. (1991). The Antioxidant Responsive Element. Activation by Oxidative Stress and Identification of the DNA Consensus Sequence

Required for Functional Activity. *The Journal of Biological Chemistry*, Vol.266, No.18, (June), pp. 11632-11639, ISSN 0021-9258 (Print)

Saleem, S.; Ahmad, M.; Ahmad, A.S.; Yousuf, S.; Ansari, M.A.; Khan, M.B.; Ishrat, T. & Islam, F. (2006). Behavioral and Histologic Neuroprotection of Aqueous Garlic Extract After Reversible Focal Cerebral Ischemia. *Journal of Medicinal Food*, Vol.9, No.4, (Winter), pp. 537-544, ISSN 1096-620X (Print)

Sener, G.; Sakarcan, A. & Yegen, B.C. (2007). Role of Garlic in the Prevention of Ischemia Reperfusion Injury. *Molecular Nutrition & Food Research*, Vol.51, No.11, (November), pp. 1345-1352, ISSN 1613-4125 (Print)

Shah, Z.A.; Li, R.C.; Thimmulappa, R.K.; Kensler, T.W.; Yamamoto, M.; Biswal, S. & Doré, S. (2007). Role of Reactive Oxygen Species in Modulation of Nrf2 Following Ischemic Reperfusion Injury. *Neuroscience*, Vol.147, No.1, (June), pp. 53-59, ISSN 0306-4522 (Print)

Shah, Z.A.; Li, R.C.; Ahmad, A.S.; Kensler, T.W.; Yamamoto, M.; Biswal, S. & Doré, S. (2010). The Flavanol (-)-Epicatechin Prevents Stroke Damage Through the Nrf2/HO1 Pathway. *Journal of Cerebral Blood Flow and Metabolism*, Vol.30, No.12, (December), pp. 1951-1961, ISSN 0271-678X (Print)

Shih, A.Y.; Johnson, D.A.; Wong, G.; Kraft, A.D.; Jiang, L.; Erb, H.; Johnson, J.A. & Murphy, T.H. (2003). Coordinate Regulation of Glutathione Biosynthesis and Release by Nrf2-Expressing Glia Potently Protects Neurons From Oxidative Stress. *Journal of Neuroscience*, Vol.23, No.8, (April), pp. 3394–3406, ISSN 0270-6474 (Print)

Shih, A.Y.; Li, P. & Murphy, T.H. (2005). A Small-Molecule-Inducible Nrf2-Mediated Antioxidant Response Provides Effective Prophylaxis Against Cerebral Ischemia in Vivo. *Journal of Neuroscience*, Vol.25, No.44, (November), pp. 10321-10335, ISSN 0270-6474 (Print)

Simonyi, A.; Wang, Q.; Miller, R.L.; Yusof, M.; Shelat, P.B.; Sun, A.Y. & Sun, G.Y. (2005). Polyphenols in Cerebral Ischemia: Novel Targets for Neuroprotection. *Molecular Neurobiology*, Vol.31, No.1-3, pp. 135–148, ISSN 0893-7648 (Print)

Soane, L.; Li Dai, W.; Fiskum, G. & Bambrick, L.L. (2010). Sulforaphane Protects Immature Hippocampal Neurons Against Death Caused by Exposure to Hemin or to Oxygen and Glucose Deprivation. *Journal of Neuroscience Research*, Vol.88, No.6, (May), pp. 1355-1363, ISSN 0360-4012 (Print)

Sun, A.Y.; Wang, Q.; Simonyi, A. & Sun, G.Y. (2008). Botanical Phenolics and Brain Health. *Neuromolecular Medicine*, Vol.10, No.4, pp. 259-274, ISSN 1535-1084 (Print)

Surh, Y.J. & Chun, K.S. (2007). Cancer Chemopreventive Effects of Curcumin. *Advances in Experimental Medicine and Biology*, Vol.595, pp. 149–172, ISSN 0065-2598 (Print)

Surh, Y.J.; Kundu, J.K. & Na, H.K. (2008). Nrf2 as a Master Redox Switch in Turning on the Cellular Signaling Involved in the Induction of Cytoprotective Genes by Some Chemopreventive Phytochemicals. *Planta Medica*, Vol.74, No.13, (Octuber), pp. 1526-1539, ISSN 0032-0943

Sykiotis, G.P. & Bohmann, D. (2010). Stress-Activated Cap'n'collar Transcription Factors in Aging and Human Disease. *Science Signaling*, Vol.3, No.112 (March), pp. re3, ISSN 1937-9145 (Electronic)

Talalay, P. (2000). Chemoprotection Against Cancer by Induction of Phase 2 Enzymes. *Biofactors*, Vol.12, No.1-4, pp. 5–11, ISSN 0951-6433 (Print)

Talalay, P.; Fahey, J.W.; Healy, Z.R.; Wehage, S.L.; Benedict, A.L.; Min, C. & Dinkova-Kostova, A.T. (2007). Sulforaphane Mobilizes Cellular Defenses that Protect Skin Against Damage by UV Radiation. *Proceedings of the National Academy of Sciences of the United States of America*, Vol.104, No.44, (Octuber), pp. 17500–17505, ISSN 0027-8424 (Print)

Tanaka, N.; Ikeda, Y.; Ohta, Y.; Deguchi, K.; Tian, F.; Shang, J.; Matsuura, T. & Abe, K. (2011). Expression of Keap1-Nrf2 System and Antioxidative Proteins in Mouse Brain After Transient Middle Cerebral Artery Occlusion. *Brain Research*, Vol.1370, (January), pp. 246-253, ISSN 0006-8993 (Print)

Thangapazham, R.L.; Sharma, A. & Maheshwari, R.K. (2006). Multiple Molecular Targets in Cancer Chemoprevention by Curcumin. *The AAPS Journal*, Vol.8, No.3, (July), pp. E443–E449, ISSN 1550-7416

Tong, K.I.; Kobayashi, A.; Katsuoka, F. & Yamamoto, M. (2006a). Two-Site Substrate Recognition Model for the Keap1-Nrf2 System: a Hinge and Latch Mechanism. *Biological Chemistry*, Vol.387, No.10-11, (Octuber-November), pp. 1311-1320, ISSN 1431-6730 (Print)

Tong, K.I.; Katoh, Y.; Kusunoki, H.; Itoh, K.; Tanaka, T. & Yamamoto, M. (2006b). Keap1 Recruits Neh2 Through Binding to ETGE and DLG Motifs: Characterization of the Two-Site Molecular Recognition Model. *Molecular and Cellular Biology*, Vol.26, No.8, (April), pp. 2887-2900, ISSN 0270-7306 (Print)

Van Muiswinkel, F.L. & Kuiperij, H.B. (2005). The Nrf2-ARE Signalling Pathway: Promising Drug Target to Combat Oxidative Stress in Neurodegenerative Disorders. *Current Drug Targets. CNS Neurological Disorders*, Vol.4, No.3, (June), pp. 267-281, ISSN 1568-007X (Print)

Van Ommen, B.; Koster, A.; Verhagen, H. & vanBladeren, P.J. (1992). The Glutathione Conjugates of Tert-Butyl Hydroquinone as Potent Redox Cycling Agents and Possible Reactive Agents Underlying the Toxicity of Butylated Hydroxyanisole. *Biochemical and Biophysical Research Communications*, Vol.189, No.1, (November), pp. 309-314, ISSN 0006-291X (Print)

Wakabayashi, N.; Dinkova-Kostova, A.T.; Holtzclaw, W.D.; Kang, M.I.; Kobayashi, A.; Yamamoto, M.; Kensler, T.W. & Talalay, P. (2004). Protection Against Electrophile and Oxidant Stress by Induction of the Phase 2 Response: Fate of Cysteines of the Keap1 Sensor Modified by Inducers. *Proceedings of the National Academy of Sciences of the United States of America*, Vol.101, No.7, (February), pp. 2040—2045, ISSN 0027-8424 (Print)

WHO. (2005). Preventing chronic diseases: a vital investment. Geneva: World Health Organization.

Wong, C.H. & Crack, P.J. (2008). Modulation of Neuro-Inflammation and Vascular Response by Oxidative Stress Following Cerebral Ischemia-Reperfusion Injury. *Current Medicinal Chemistry*, Vol.15, No.1, pp. 1-14, ISSN 0929-8673 (Print)

Wu, C.C.; Sheen, L.Y.; Chen, H.W.; Kuo, W.W.; Tsai, S.J. & Lii, C.K. (2002). Differential Effects of Garlic Oil and its Three Major Organosulfur Components on the Hepatic Detoxification System in Rats. *Journal of Agricultural and Food Chemistry*, Vol.50, No.2, (January), pp. 378- 383, ISSN 0021-8561 (Print)

Yan, C.K. & Zeng, F.D. (2005). Pharmacokinetics and Tissue Distribution of S-Allylcysteine in Rats. *Asian Journal of Drug Metabolism and Pharmacokinetics*, 5, pp. 61-69

Yang, C.; Zhang, X.; Fan, H. & Liu, Y. (2009). Curcumin Upregulates Transcription Factor Nrf2, HO-1 Expression and Protects Rat Brains Against Focal Ischemia. *Brain Research*, Vol.1282, (July), pp. 133-141, ISSN 0006-8993 (Print)

Zhang, Y.; Talalay, P.; Cho, C-G. & Posner, G.H. (1992). A Major Inducer of Anticarcinogenic Protective Enzymes From Broccoli: Isolation and Elucidation of Structure. *Proceedings of the National Academy of Sciences of the United States of America*, Vol.89, No.6, (March), pp. 2399–2403, ISSN 0027-8424 (Print)

Zhang, D.D. & Hannink, M. (2003). Distinct Cysteine Residues in Keap1 are Required for Keap1-Dependent Ubiquitination of Nrf2 and for Stabilization of Nrf2 by Chemopreventive Agents and Oxidative Stress. *Molecular and Cellular Biology*, Vol.23, No.22, (November), pp. 8137-8151, ISSN 0270-7306 (Print)

Zhang, D.D.; Lo, S.C.; Cross, J.V.; Templeton, D.J. & Hannink M. (2004). Keap1 is a Redox-Regulated Substrate Adaptor Protein for a Cul3-Dependent Ubiquitin Ligase Complex. *Molecular and Cellular Biology*, Vol.24, No.24, (December), pp. 10941-10953, ISSN 0270-7306 (Print)

Zhao, J.; Kobori, N.; Aronowski, J. & Dash, P.K. (2006). Sulforaphane Reduces Infarct Volume Following Focal Cerebral Ischemia in Rodents. *Neuroscience Letters*, Vol.393, No.2-3, (January), pp. 108-112, ISSN 0304-3940 (Print)

16

Preconditioning and Postconditioning

Joseph T. McCabe[1], Michael W. Bentley[2] and Joseph C. O'Sullivan[2]
[1]*Department of Anatomy, Physiology & Genetics, and*
The Center for Neuroscience & Regenerative Medicine,
Uniformed Services University of the Health Sciences, Bethesda, Maryland
[2]*U.S. Army Graduate School of Anesthesia Nursing, Graduate School,*
AMEDD Center and School, Academy of Health Sciences,
Fort Sam Houston, San Antonio, Texas
USA

1. Introduction

Cerebral ischemic events from trauma, stroke, hemorrhagic shock, or other cerebral perfusion deficit, initiate a cascade of detrimental processes leading to long lasting tissue injury and poor neurological outcome. Correction of the perfusion deficit is vital. However, no interventions have been identified that protect compromised cerebral tissue during the resolution of the ischemic event.

This chapter reviews two emerging concepts: *preconditioning*, which may have therapeutic utility for the protection of patients for *planned* treatments such as surgical intervention, and *postconditioning*, which may have benefits for amelioration of deficits from ischemic events, vascular injury and accidents. Preconditioning (described below) was first described from maneuvers that induced cytoprotection by temporarily occluding vessels serving the tissue or region of interest. There are inherent risks in performing such a maneuver, so that pharmacological agents—particularly for *delayed preconditioning* (described later) – affecting the aforementioned signal transduction and genomic pathways, are a safer, more realistic area of study. Conditioning is still primarily an experimental phenomenon. However, investigators have made considerable strides in uncovering the multiple, albeit complex signal transduction pathways that mediate conditioning effects. This knowledge may help clinicians one day develop schemes for neuroprotection.

2. Ischemic preconditioning: Origins in cardiology

The preconditioning concept has roots in cardiovascular research. Ischemic preconditioning was originally described in a landmark 1986 study by Murry and associates (Murry, et al., 1986). Using a cardiac dog model, these investigators found that multiple, brief ischemic episodes protected the heart from a subsequent sustained ischemic insult. An experimental group of dogs experienced circumflex artery occlusion for 5-minute intervals with 5-minute reperfusions. This cycle was repeated a total of four times—clamping for 5 minutes and unclamping for 5 minutes. The circumflex artery was then clamped for 40 minutes. The control group of dogs had their circumflex artery occluded for 40 minutes. Surprisingly, despite the additional 20 minutes of ischemia in the preconditioned animals, cardiac damage, measured by infarct size, was significantly reduced to just ¼th of the infarct observed in the hearts of dogs in the control group. This paper was the first to demonstrate and coin the term, *ischemic preconditioning*.

2.1 Preconditioning

Preconditioning has been demonstrated in all species studied to date (rat, mouse, rabbit, dog, human, chicken, sheep, pig and including cell lines), and in all organs studied thus far, including skeletal muscle, brain, kidney, small intestine, heart, and liver (Peralta, et al., 1996; Glazier, et al., 1994; Pang, et al., 1995). Other preconditioning manipulations, such as global hypoxia (Emerson, et al., 1999) and thermal injury (Marber, et al., 1993), are also effective in protection from lasting insult. Prior to this 1986 discovery, the best pharmacological treatments (with varying reproducible results) for the protection of cardiac muscle from infarction only preserved 10-20% of tissue compared to the 75% protection afforded by preconditioning (Yellon & Downey, 2003).

Research has determined that ischemic preconditioning can be subdivided into two distinctive types; *classical* and *delayed*. In *classical* preconditioning, the protective effects of ischemia/perfusion cycles are evident within minutes after the insult and persist for 2-3 hours (Ishida, et al., 1997). Classical preconditioning is independent of protein synthesis, and is therefore dependent upon existing cellular pathways. It involves the direct modulation of energy supplies, pH regulation, Na^+ and Ca^{2+} homeostasis and caspase inactivation (Carini, & Albano, 2003). Investigations have shown many triggers can activate classical ischemic preconditioning, including agonists of G protein-coupled receptors [bradykinin (Goto, et al., 1995), opioids (Schultz, et al., 1998), norepinephrine (Hu & Nattel, 1995), adenosine (Liu, et al., 1991), potassium ATP channel (K_{ATP}) openers, such as diazoxide, pinacidil (Legtenberg, et al., 2002), succinate dehydrogenase inhibitors, such as 3-nitropropionic acid (Ockaili, et al., 2001), and volatile anesthetics, such as sevoflurane and isoflurane (Zaugg, et al., 2002)].

With classic preconditioning, a trigger event, such as brief ischemia, activates a number of intracellular pathways that lead to the protected cell phenotype. The actual sequence of these pathways has not been determined, but some components of the cascade have been identified. G-coupled receptors, for example, activate the epsilon (ε) isoform of protein kinase C (PKC-ε; Mitchell, et al., 1995; Kilts, et al., 2005), which has been implicated as the key PKC subtype involved in preconditioning. Also important is the upstream signaling molecule, phosphatidylinositol-3-kinase (PI3K; Tong, et al., 2000), and mitogen-activated protein kinases (MAPKs; Armstrong, 2004). PI3K activates the serine/threonine kinase, Akt, which inactivates the pro-apoptotic kinase glycogen synthase kinase-3 (GSK-3) via phosphorylation (Tong, et al., 2002). Phosphorylation of GSK-3, in turn, inhibits the opening of the mitochondrial permeability transition pore (mPTP). Cell apoptosis or necrosis often occurs during reperfusion due to opening of the mPTP, a large nonselective pore traversing both inner and outer membranes of mitochondria. Cytochrome c and apoptotic-inducing factor (AIF) are both released through the mPTP during ischemic reperfusion, leading to the activation of caspase and caspase-independent apoptotic pathways (Kadenbach, et al., 2011; Penninger, & Kroemer, 2003). K_{ATP} channels are key intracellular triggers of early ischemic preconditioning. This channel will be described in more detail later in this chapter.

Although not as effective as classical preconditioning, *delayed* or *late* preconditioning becomes apparent approximately 24 hours after initial preconditioning and it can persist for up to 72 hours (Ishida, et al., 1997). The most significant difference between classical and delayed preconditioning is the latter's requirement of the manufacture of new proteins needed to obtain protection; inhibition of new protein synthesis attenuates the protection derived from delayed preconditioning (Rizvi, et al., 1999).

The triggers for delayed preconditioning are similar to classical preconditioning. These include cellular stress factors (sub-lethal ischemia, heat stress, cardiac pacing), which release factors such as reactive oxygen species, adenosine, and endogenous nitric oxide (NO). NO has been determined to have no effect on classical preconditioning and is a trigger specific only for delayed preconditioning (Bolli, 2000). Endogenous preconditioning agents also initiate delayed preconditioning and include adenosine agonists, bradykinin, opioids, NO donors, acetylcholine and norepinephrine (Bolli, 2000). Exogenous agents that activate the preconditioning pathways include, diazoxide, nicorandil, some hypercholesterolemic agents, and volatile anesthetics (Gross, 2005).

Kinase intracellular pathways play a central role in delayed preconditioning, with activation of the PKC-ε isoform being particularly essential. Downstream to PKC-ε, tyrosine kinases and other kinases then activate the important transcription factor, NF-κB, which leads to the upregulation of many protective proteins in the nucleus. Some key proteins identified thus far include: inducible NO synthase (iNOS) (Takano, et al., 1998, cyclooxygenase (COX-2) (Shinmura, et al., 2000), the antioxidant enzyme superoxide dismutase (SOD) (Hoshida, et al., 2002), and heat shock proteins, HSP70, HSP25, and HSP32 (Bolli, 2000). Delayed preconditioning also reduces apoptosis by upregulating the anti-apoptotic protein, Bcl-2, which has been shown to inhibit opening of the mPTP, leading to cell survival (Maulik, et al., 1999). Mitochondrial K_{ATP} (mK_{ATP}) channel opening seems to be the final common pathway for these signaling pathways but it is not yet clear how the opening of these channels affords protection. Delayed preconditioning requires the opening of the mK_{ATP} channels during the ischemic event; its role after 24 hours, when delayed preconditioning occurs, is less clear (Takano, et al., 2000).

By 1993, an appreciable number of studies had confirmed that the direct application of various stimuli (hypoxia, ischemia, triggering agents) resulted in tissue and organ protection. In that year, however, Przyklenk and colleagues made a startling discovery. Using a canine model in which the circumflex artery was occluded (as in Murry's 1986 study), Przyklenk and colleagues observed that cardiac muscle supplied by the descending left coronary artery was also protected from ischemic insult, indicating that the preconditioning stimulus offered protection that was not confined to one area of an organ (Przyklenk, et al., 1993). Further experiments have shown *remote* classical ischemic preconditioning also is effective in other organs. A preconditioning trigger in one area of an organ offers protection to a different region of that same organ or to a different organ. For example, one group demonstrated that intermittent tourniquet application to a hind limb (ischemic preconditioning) implemented protection in other skeletal muscles (Addison, et al., 2003). Remote classical preconditioning of the heart was also obtained via transient ischemia of the small intestine (Liem, et al., 2005; Patel, et al., 2002) or the kidney (Gho, et al., 1996). Other studies have demonstrated remote delayed preconditioning. Induction of small intestine ischemia, for example, engenders myocardial protection 24-72 hours later (Wang, et al., 2001; Xiao, et al., 2001).

The precise mechanism of remote ischemic preconditioning is unknown, but putative factors have been identified. Protection from kidney or intestinal preconditioning on cardiac muscle was eliminated with application of the ganglionic blocker, hexamethonium, suggesting involvement of a neuronal pathway (Gho, et al., 1996). However, stronger evidence exists that a humoral factor may play a more important role. Effluent from a preconditioned heart, transferred by whole blood transfusion, protected a non-conditioned heart from ischemic insult (Dickson, et al., 1999a; 1999b). Remote preconditioning was not activated by adenosine or bradykinin, but was found to be attenuated by the opioid antagonist, naloxone, suggesting opioid receptor involvement (Dickson, et al., 2001).

2.2 Postconditioning

One promising approach for neuroprotective therapies may be derived from *postconditioning,* where supportive measures are employed following an injury. Postconditioning is very similar to preconditioning with the exception of the temporal relationship of the protective maneuver in respect to the prolonged period of ischemia. Preconditioning is an intervention that occurs *prior to* injury while postconditioning interventions occur *after* an injury has occurred and thus may be more clinically relevant. The origin of postconditioning stems from the work of Okamoto and colleagues (Okamoto, et al., 1986). Okamoto's group established that post-ischemic damage could be limited by the use of timely low-pressure reperfusion. Following a period of ischemia, dog hearts were reperfused either with the sudden release of a coronary occlusion, or by low-pressure (40 to 50 mm Hg) coronary reperfusion with normal blood for 20 minutes before completely removing the coronary occlusion. This maneuver focused on the initial stage of reperfusion and established the basis for novel postconditioning approaches to resuscitation. Years later, Mizumura et al. (1995) first demonstrated pharmacological postconditioning. Mizumura's group used the K_{ATP} channel opener, bimakalin. Bimakalin markedly reduced cardiac infarct size in dogs when given 10 minutes before and during the 60-minute coronary reperfusion period following a set time of occlusive hypoxia. Collectively, these initial findings firmly established the concept of postconditioning and emphasized a critical factor that altering the initial moments of reperfusion was beneficial.

In 2003, Zhao and colleagues (2003) first used the term *postconditioning*. They found in a model of occlusive hypoxia in dogs that short, repeated (or stuttered) periods of arterial occlusion and release of previously occluded coronary arteries (three occlusions of 30 seconds each) prior to restoration of perfusion reduced infarct area by 44% as compared to controls. This was an example of a mechanical postconditioning intervention and implied that the first minute of reperfusion is critical in thwarting cellular demise. These findings were further validated by Kin et al. (2004). Kin and colleagues stated that the first minute of reperfusion in the rat was crucial for postconditioning. Three cycles of 10 seconds of coronary occlusion and 10 seconds of coronary release, preceding a full coronary occlusion release, decreased cardiac infarct size by 23%. In the broadest sense, the cellular processes activated by postconditioning are analogous to those activated by preconditioning, and the sole difference between the two interventions is the timing related to the prolonged period of ischemia.

3. Signaling processes linked to preconditioning and postconditioning

Many studies have investigated the mechanism of postconditioning with the aspiration to utilize this powerful protective system in the clinical setting. Recent observations from the employment of mechanical and pharmacological postconditioning suggest the activation of mitochondrial K_{ATP} (mK_{ATP}) channels initiates a series of events that close the mitochondrial permeability transition pore (mPTP) and converge onto the Reperfusion Injury Survival Kinase (RISK) Pathway.

3.1 K_{ATP} channels

K_{ATP} channels were first discovered in 1983 by A. Noma in a patch clamp study using cardiac muscle membrane preparations (Noma, 1983). There are cell surface K_{ATP} (sK_{ATP}) and mitochondrial K_{ATP} (mK_{ATP}) forms. Pharmacologically, these are different channels, but their opening (via PKC or pharmacological agents) leads to increased cell survival. One hypothesis is that activation of K_{ATP} channels hyperpolarizes the cell membrane thereby protecting the cell from detrimental depolarization (Kirino, 2002). In 1997, Garlid and coworkers presented evidence that mK_{ATP} channels have a cardioprotectve role in ischemia and reperfusion, and were a component in the mechanism for preconditioning (Garlid, et al., 1997). A prototypical mK_{ATP} channel, as reviewed by Aguilar-Bryan and Bryan (1999), is an octameric structure consisting of four sulfonylurea receptor (SUR1 or SUR2) subunits and four K^+ inward-rectifying (Kir6.1 or Kir6.2) subunits. Attached to the SUR subunits are two nucleotide binding domains (NBD). The mK_{ATP} channel is activated in low energy states by ADP, binding to NBDs, allowing the influx of K^+ into the mitochondrial inner matrix. Conversely, the mK_{ATP} channel is inhibited in high energy states when ATP closes the Kir channel. In the brain, it appears the predominant subtypes are SUR2 and Kir6.2, although the SUR1 and Kir6.1 subunits are present in smaller amounts (Lacza, et al., 2003). The mK_{ATP} channel may trigger preconditioning or postconditioning via mechanisms dependent on matrix volume stabilization, respiratory inhibition, controlled production of reactive oxygen species (ROS), and the closure of the mPTP.

The physiological functions of mK_{ATP} channels have been debated. The activities of the mK_{ATP} channel and the K^+/H^+ exchanger are believed to maintain K^+ homeostasis within mitochondria by controlling mitochondrial volume and moderating the outer-to-inner pH gradient needed to drive ATP synthesis. In the presence of hypoxia, whole cell pH decreases and ATP production declines. This causes a switch to anaerobic metabolism. A decrease in pH combined with an increase in the AMP/ADP ratio secondary to ATP metabolism causes the mK_{ATP} channel to open allowing the influx of K^+ into the inner matrix. This, in turn, activates the K^+(out)/H^+(in) exchanger decreasing the hydrogen gradient between the outer membrane and inner matrix (Szewczyk & Marbán, 1999). By doing so, the proton motive forces driving ATP production are attenuated and mitochondria energetics slow. During this time, the mPTP is closed as membrane stability and electrical potential are better maintained by the simultaneous activity of the mK_{ATP} channel and the K^+/H^+ exchanger. In addition, reactive oxygen species (ROS) generation is proportional to the availability of oxygen and activation of mK_{ATP} channel appears to moderate ROS production (Ferranti, et al., 2003; Saitoh, et al., 2006). However, this effect is only protective to a limited extent. For example, a moderate or controlled production of ROS signals promote prosurvival signaling while excessive ROS production promotes apoptotic signaling.

As anaerobic metabolism continues in response to an extended period of severe hypoxia, ATP hydrolysis exceeds ATP generation causing a dramatic rise in H^+ within the cell and mitochondrial inner matrix. At some point H^+ entry becomes lethal as it exceeds the outward pumping capacity of the mitochondrial electron transport chain already hindered by anaerobic metabolism. This results in a total loss of proton motive force driving ATP production. If prolonged, this loss results in osmotic matrix swelling, mitochondrial degradation, and release of apoptotic proteins such as cytochrome C.

Upon resolution of a perfusion defect, abrupt reperfusion following prolonged ischemia results in a substantial amount of ROS generation. Following restoration of flow to intact but vulnerable cells, ATP levels begin to rise, mK_{ATP} channels close and K^+ transport into the mitochondrial matrix declines. This indirectly decreases the activity of the K^+/H^+ exchanger. As H^+ ions are rapidly removed from the matrix during mitochondrial respiration, the inner matrix quickly alkalinizes, causing the mPTP to open (Vinten-Johansen, et al., 2007). Opening the mPTP rapidly elevates inner matrix osmotic pressure leading to matrix distension and if allowed to remain open, mitochondrial rupture.

In total, mK_{ATP} channel closure associated with abrupt reperfusion cand result in the significant elevation of ROS and increase the mitochondrial inner matrix osmotic pressure, causing the mitochondria to quickly swell or rupture, releasing apoptotic factors such as cytochrome C (Armstrong, 2004). It is reasonable to suggest that maintaining the patency of the mK_{ATP} channel would be beneficial during reperfusion. Allowing the mK_{ATP} channel to remain open during reperfusion could: 1) moderate the generation of ROS, 2) reduce osmotic force within the matrix by promoting ion exchange, and 3) reduce the activity of the mPTP thereby providing a protective effect.

Activation of mK_{ATP} channels have been shown to be protective during reperfusion in cardiac and brain tissue (Obal, et al., 2005; O'Sullivan, et al., 2007; Penna, et al., 2007; Wu, et al., 2006). Obal and colleagues (2005), for example, demonstrated the utility of inhaling volatile anesthetics as a postconditioning trigger through mK_{ATP} channel activation. In rats subjected to cardiac ischemia, postconditioning was invoked by administering 1 minimum alveolar concentration (MAC) of sevoflurane for 2 minutes with the onset of reperfusion. This resulted in a significant decrease in cardiac infarct size. Penna et al. (2007, isolated rat hearts and exposed them to an ischemic period followed by reperfusion. Their results suggested that postconditioning mechanisms are activated by a bradykinin or a diazoxide mechanism resulting in the upregulation of protein kinase G (PKG). This upregulation was dependent on early ROS generation triggered by mK_{ATP} channel activation. They emphasized that their results were different from mechanical manipulations by showing that pharmacological agents, such as bradykinin or diazoxide, administered during the reperfusion period could induce protection. ROS also regulate the activity of heat shock proteins (HSPs). Using an *in vitro* vascular smooth muscle preparation, Madamanchi and colleagues (2001) discovered that the application of H_2O_2 significantly upregulated HSP70.

3.2 mPTPs

As previously mentioned, the mPTP is inhibited with the activation of mK_{ATP}. The existence of the mPTP was confirmed in 1992 in rat liver mitoblast membranes (Szabó & Zoratti, 1992). The primary components of the mPTP are the voltage-dependent anion channel in the outer membrane, the adenine nucleotide translocator, and the cyclophilin D protein within the matrix (Lin & Lechleiter, 2002). In general, it is thought that the opening of the mPTP occurs with a decrease in the inner matrix potential, decreased AMP and ADP levels, increased matrix Ca^{2+}, with alkalinization, or during oxidative stress (Gateau-Roesch, et al., 2006). mPTP opening blocks ATP formation and allows for the equilibration of small molecules (Gateau-Roesch, et al., 2006; Halestrap, 2004). mPTP opening increases osmotic forces within the mitochondria inner matrix and leads to degradation of the matrix membrane, causing the release of apoptotic factors, especially cytochrome C (Honda, et al., 2005). Also, as the mitochondrial membrane potential is perturbed, ATP synthase reverses its primary function and serves as an ATPase; further depleting cellular ATP concentrations and increasing H^+ levels.

Feng and colleagues (2005) determined that volatile anesthesia-induced postconditioning prevented the opening of the mPTP by inhibiting glycogen synthase kinase 3β (GSKβ). This inactivation was a result of PI3K-AKT signaling pathway inactivation with the resulting phosphorylation and inactivation of GSKβ, which protected against reperfusion damage. Argaud et al. (2005) found that mechanical postconditioning decreased cellular Ca^{2+} and protected *in vivo* rabbit hearts, suggesting that the mPTP could be inhibited by the PI3K-AKT-eNOS cascade. Bopassa et al. (2006), using a rat heart preparation undergoing postconditioning, concluded that PI3K signaling regulates the closure of mPTP. In addition, Cohen, Yan, and Downey (2007) observed that postconditioning prevented mPTP opening as a result of inhaled CO_2-induced acidosis during the first minutes of reperfusion. They suggested that low cellular pH inhibits the opening of mPTP in heart tissue, but as the cellular pH normalizes, the inhibition of mPTP is lost. They hypothesized that by maintaining the cellular pH at a lower level while introducing oxygen during reperfusion, it was possible to keep the mPTP closed allowing the redox signaling necessary to trigger preconditioning-like protection. Cohen, Yan, and Downey further suggest that moderate acidosis during reperfusion might be protective. This hypothesis was addressed through the use of sodium bicarbonate ($NaHCO_3$) during postconditioning. In isolated rabbit hearts, acidic CO_2 perfusate at the time of reperfusion mimicked postconditioning while an alkaline $NaHCO_3$ perfusate blocked that effect. They hypothesized that an acidic environment inhibited mPTP opening while an alkaline environment favored mPTP opening. Fujita and colleagues (2007) also hypothesized that $NaHCO_3$ would blunt the protective properties of postconditioning. Using *in vivo* dog hearts that underwent ischemia, the administration of $NaHCO_3$ during four intermittent cycles of one-minute reperfusion with one-minute reocclusion of a coronary vessel completely abolished the postconditioning effects. Their results suggested that postconditioning leads to the opening of mK_{ATP} channels as a result of decreased pH, leading to the attenuation of cardiac infarct size.

3.3 Reperfusion Survival Kinase Pathway

The Reperfusion Injury Survival Kinase (RISK) pathway begins with the activation of PI3K and ERK to promote cell survival. RISK can be activated by insulin, urocortin, atorvastatin, adenosine, bradykinin, opioid agonists, volatile anesthetics, or diazoxide (Bell & Yellon, 2003a,b; Chiari, et al., 2005; Gross, et al., 2004; Jonassen, et al., 2001; Schulman, et al., 2002; Wang, et al., 2004; Yang, et al., 2004). The RISK pathway promotes pro-survival signaling while inhibiting pathways associated with apoptosis. In 2004, Tsang and colleagues (2004) reported that in isolated rat hearts, which had undergone mechanical postconditioning following a period of ischemia, postconditioning is mediated by the PI3K-AKT-eNOS/p70s6K pathway. They also suggested MEK 1/2-ERK 1/2 pathways were indirectly involved. Zhu and coworkers (2006) followed by finding that cardioprotection from postconditioning in the remodeled rat myocardium is regulated through PI3K-AKT signaling. The role of ERK 1/2 was addressed by Darling et al. (2005) and Krolikowski et al. (2006). Darling and colleagues utilized mechanical postconditioning in isolated rabbit hearts and found ERK1/2 but not PI3K activity provided cardiac protection. Krolikowski and colleagues exposed rabbits to isoflurane before and during early reperfusion and suggested a central role of ERK1/2, p70s6k, and eNOS in anesthetic-induced postconditioning. Downstream in the RISK pathway, phosphorylation of AKT occurs with the subsequent phosphorylation of protein kinase C (PKC) and GSKβ. When PKC is phosphorylated it is stimulated while the phosphorylation of GSKβ inhibits its activity. In a rabbit model, Philipp and colleagues (2006) demonstrated through inhibitor studies that adenosine, PKC, and PI3K mediated the effects of mechanical postconditioning. In their investigation, they concluded that protection was conferred through the activation of adenosine receptors by endogenous adenosine, a cellular metabolite. This, in turn, activated the PI3K component of the RISK pathway resulting in activation of PKC. In regards to GSKβ, Feng and colleagues (2005), using isoflurane as a postconditioning trigger along with an AKT inhibitor, showed that when inhaled early in reperfusion, isoflurane phosphorylated AKT and GSKβ. Phosphorylated GSKβ was inhibited and could not promote the opening of mPTP. They also determined that while the PI3K-AKT signal was strong, the ERK1/2-p38 MAPK was not altered. This suggests a primary role of PI3K-AKT in the RISK pathway and in mPTP closure. Recently, in human tissue, it has been found that the cytoprotective proteins, HSP25 and HSP70, are upregulated by the PI3K-AKT pathway (Dickson, et al., 2001).

3.4 The heat shock response

Both preconditioning and postconditioning upregulate proteins identified as Heat Shock Proteins (HSPs), specifically HSP25 and HSP70. The heat shock response was discovered in 1962. *Drosophilia* larvae, when heated, developed puffing patterns in certain chromosomal regions. This suggested a change in the synthetic activity of the chromosomal bands concerned (Ritossa, 1962). Sixteen years later, the RNA for *Drosophilia* exposed to a thermal stimulus was coded using hybrid-arrested translation and indicated that proteins of 83, 72, 70, 68, 28, 26, 23 and 22 kilodaltons were upregulated (Livak, et al., 1978). Over the following decades, the investigation of the heat shock response has confirmed that a family of highly conserved HSPs is upregulated following a variety of sublethal stressors, possibly as a result of non-native proteins accumulating in a stressed cell (Voellmy & Boellmann, 2007). These proteins are subcategorized by their molecular weight and are either inherently present or can be induced following sublethal stress (O'Sullivan, et al., 2008). In particular, HSP25 and HSP70 have been thoroughly investigated with the consensus being they are protective when upregulated following stress (Beere, et al., 2000; Garrido, et al., 2006; Takayama, et al., 2003).

3.4.1 Heat Shock Protein 25/27

HSP25 is the rodent equivalent of the primate HSP27 and often the terms are used interchangeably. HSP27 confers protection at different levels as it can interact with several proteins implicated in cell death based upon its phosphorylation and oligomerization condition and not upon ATP. The main mechanisms for how HSP27 confers cytoprotection appear to be: molecular chaperoning, interference with cell death pathways, signaling of antiapoptotic pathways, stabilization of the cytoskeleton, and antioxidant activities. Serving as a chaperone, HSP27 can bind folded intermediate non-native proteins, inhibiting their aggregation, and in the presence of HSP70 these HSP27-bound proteins can be reactivated (Ehrnsperger, et al., 1997). Within the cytosol, HSP27 can sequester cytochrome C;

interfering with the formation of the apoptotic protease activating factor-1 (APAF-1)-cytochrome c multimeric apoptosome and the activation of procaspase 9 (Bruey, et al., 2000; Concannon, et al., 2001; Garrido, et al., 1999). HSP27 also directly interacts with procaspase-3, decreasing the activity of activated caspase-3 (Concannon, et al., 2001). HSP27 serves as a signaling messenger by causing the activation of serine/threonine kinase Akt thereby inhibiting Bcl-2 and caspase-9 (Cardone, et al., 1998). HSP25/27 has other actions. Phosphorylated HSP27 can stabilize F-actin and increase the number of cells retaining microfilament organization thus stabilizing membrane structure (Lavoie, et al., 1995). Additionally, HSP27 is able to increase glutathione levels, thereby reducing levels of ROS (Kretz-Remy, et al., 1996).

3.4.2 Heat Shock Protein 70

Over the last three decades, HSP70 has become the most thoroughly investigated protein of the HSP family of proteins. Like HSP25, HSP70 can inhibit cell death at various sites within the cell. However, unlike HSP25, HSP70 function is "ATP-dependent." HSP70 is typically found *in vivo* bound by ATP and HSP70 function is typically based upon the hydrolysis of the attached ATP molecule. HSP70 serves as a chaperone protein, inhibits stress signaling, prevents mitochondrial membrane permeabilization, and inhibits apoptotic pathways. HSP70 may chaperone kinases by binding to an unfolded carboxyl terminus, preventing aggregation, and allowing re-autophosphorylation of the kinase enzyme; thus stabilizing the enzyme and restoring function (Gao & Newton, 2002). HSP70 also binds the death receptors, DR4 and DR5, inhibiting Apo-2L/TRAIL-induced cell death (Guo, et al., (2005), and HSP70 blocks Bax translocation into the mitochondrial outer membrane. The latter effect prevents the permeabilization of the mitochondrial membrane and subsequent release of apoptosis-inducing factor (AIF) and cytochrome C (Stankiewicz , et al., 2005). HSP70 binds AIF within the cytosol; inhibiting its nuclear translocation and limiting nuclear condensation (Ruchalski, et al., 2006). Similar to HSP25, HSP70 prevents cell death by binding to Apaf-1 and interfering in the formation of the apoptosome complex and subsequent recruitment of procaspase-9 (Beere, et al., 2000). Lastly, HSP70 suppresses apoptotic signaling by binding precursor forms of caspase-3 and caspase-7; preventing their cleavage and activation (Komarova, et al., 2004).

3.5 Cleaved caspase 3

Both HSP25 and HSP70 inhibit the cleavage of caspase-3 (Concannon, et al., 2001; Komarova, et al., 2004). Cleaved caspase-3 (CC3) is a primary executioner of apoptosis as it is responsible for the total or partial proteolytic cleavage of numerous key cellular survival proteins (Fernandes-Alnemri , et al., 1994). One of those proteins being the abundant nuclear enzyme polymerase, which functions in DNA repair and protein modification during oxidative stress (Smith, 2001). Thus, induction of HSP25 and HSP70 may alleviate cerebral ischemic injury and resuscitation injury that results from the mitochondrial release of cytochrome C with subsequent cleavage of caspase-3.

4. Evidence of preconditioning and postconditioning in the brain

Wu and colleagues (Wu, et al., 2006) directly examined the roles of mPTP and the mK_{ATP} channel in preconditioning and postconditioning in a rat model of cerebral stroke. These investigators activated the mK_{ATP} channel with diazoxide 20 minutes before middle cerebral artery occlusion followed by reperfusion, or inhibited the mPTP by infusion of cyclosporin A 15 minutes before reperfusion. It was discovered that both measures significantly increased functional performance scores and reduced infarction volumes. Importantly, both of these effects were abolished by blocking the adenine nucleotide port located on the mPTP. Their results strongly suggested that the mK_{ATP} channel and mPTP activity during reperfusion share a common protective pathway; the Reperfusion Survival Kinase Pathway (RISK). More recently, Feng, Rhodes, and Bhatt (2010) discovered that hypoxic preconditioning could invoke neuroprotection through the activation of AKT, a kinase that is part of the aforementioned RISK pathway. These investigators subjected newborn rats to 3 hours of 8% oxygen followed by 24 hours of reoxygenation. Following reoxygenation, the right carotid artery was permanently ligated and again the rats were subjected to 8% oxygen but for 140 minutes instead of 3 hours. Compared to rats subjected to normoxia prior to carotid ligation, preconditioned rats had a significant reduction in cerebral injury. It was found that preconditioning preserved RISK pathway signaling and attenuated caspase-3 activity.

Acute models of postconditioning have emphasized the benefit of cerebral reperfusion under controlled conditions. For example, several groups have shown that carefully controlled periods of reperfusion, before the full return of cerebral circulation, results in reduced injury. Zhao and colleagues (2006) employed permanent middle cerebral artery occlusion in combination with transient common carotid artery occlusions. Shorter periods of repeated common carotid occlusion resulted in a reduction in infarct size. Pignataro, et al. (2008) also employed middle cerebral artery occlusion for 100 minutes. Reperfusion of the artery that included a 10-minute period of occlusion was found to be the most effective, although intermittent occlusions were also beneficial. Gao, Ren and Zhao (2008) found that three cycles of reperfusion of the common carotid artery, in conjunction with permanent middle artery occlusion, reduced infarct size, while ten cycles was not effective. These publications, as well as numerous reports with cardiac models, emphasis the criticality of the duration of cerebral ischemia (longer periods of ischemia result in more cerebral damage, including irreversibility), as well as the essential specifics of the timing, duration, number of cycles, and inter-reperfusion intervals for effective postconditioning.

As well, recent work has shown the benefit of pharmacological postconditioning in cerebral ischemia. O'Sullivan and colleagues (2007) employed a rat model of combined hemorrhagic shock and permanent unilateral common carotid artery occlusion. The administration of diazoxide at the time of hemorrhagic resuscitation significantly increased the expression of heat shock proteins in the cerebral cortex and hippocampus. Robin and colleagues (2011), using a middle cerebral artery occlusion model, found that in Wistar strain rats ischemic postconditioning decreased infarct size by 40% and improved neurological outcomes. Specifically, pharmacological postconditioning by diazoxide administration decreased cerebral infarct by 60%. In addition, these beneficial effects in both ischemic postconditioning and diazoxide postconditioning were blocked through the use of the K_{ATP} blocker, 5-hydroxydecanoate (5-HD), which blocked the inhibition of the mPTP opening caused by ischemic postconditioning and diazoxide.

In 2011, Wang and colleagues discovered that selective delta opioid peptide [D-Ala2, D-Leu5] enkephalin (DADLE) provided a postconditioning effect by protecting hippocampal CA1 neurons in a model of forebrain ischemia. In this investigation, DADLE triggered postconditioning neuroprotection for hippocampal CA1 neurons and improved spatial learning and memory in rats. This protection was dependent upon DADLE-induced activation of the PI3K/Akt signaling.

5. Conclusion

As reviewed, the majority of research related to pre- and post-conditioning has not been performed in studies related to cerebral ischemia. As recently stated by Keep and colleagues (2010), the question remains—"Is there a place for cerebral preconditioning in the clinic?" The clinical utility of cerebral conditioning is potentially limited by issues of safety, the relatively narrow therapeutic window, and the need to present the stimulus before the injury.

Brief periods of ischemia can enact classical and delayed conditioning. These momentary periods of ischemia have been shown to protect neuronal cells *in vitro* and to reduce injury *in vivo* in several experiment models and species (Koch, 2010). Since safety issues prevent deliberately inducing conditioning by cerebrovascular occlusion, research has focused on pharmacological agents, including volatile anesthetics, inhibitors of cellular metabolism, K_{ATP} channel activators, and inflammatory mediators (Keep, et al., 2010). Other agents that have been effective in producing conditioning are hyperbaric oxygen, cooling and hyperthermia, and acupuncture (Keep, et al., 2010). Recent research has also given credence to remote conditioning where ischemia to a hindlimb (e.g., by application of a tourniquet) protects the brain from later middle cerebral artery occlusion. Remote preconditioning or ischemia probably has the most practical use for clinical utilization. However, currently there are no clinical data to strongly support the use of any type of conditioning for brain protection.

From a clinical standpoint, a major problem with the application of conditioning is timing. With the exception of a planned neurosurgical intervention, classically employed technique such as vascular clamping is impractible as a pretreatment. Pharmacological agents, then. Given at the time of reperfusion may hold promise. Agents such as $MgSO_4$, erythropoietin, anti-hypertension drugs, anticoagulants, and statins all given to patients at risk for stroke have shown limited damage from a stroke should it occur (Keep, et al., 2010).

In addition, there is still little *clinical* evidence from basic research regarding the use of preconditioning for neuroprotection. Research models currently in use have at least four important limitations. First, experiments are routinely conducted on young, disease-free animals (Koch, 2010). The majority of patients who suffer cerebral ischemic events are older, and may have artherosclerosis, cardiac or kidney disease, or other co-morbidities, such as obesity, hypertension, diabetes, as well as additional risk factors such as sedentary lifestyle, and tobacco, alcohol, or illicit drug abuse. The 'chronic' ischemic state of these patients, with a chronic conditioning compensatory state, may not allow further conditioning protection with interventions. Secondly, both Keep, et al. (2010) and Koch (2010) noted that the effect of medications used by patients has a potential to interfere with preconditioning effects. Do certain prescribed medications or self-administered substances such as herbal products interfere with the conditioning signaling pathways? Third, the neuroprotective cascade might be very specific to gender, diet, genetic background, and age (Dirnagl, et al., 2009). Lastly, major issues to be resolved include determination of doses of preconditioning drugs that are safe and whether premorbid conditions, for example intermittent transient ischemic events, act as a conditioning stimulus event (Dirnagl, et al., 2009; Keep, et al., 2010; Koch, 2010).

Finally, optimal neuroprotection may be a combination of physiological manipulations (e.g., body temperature regulation) and pharmacological treatment(s). Gidday (2010) provides an excellent overview of the current state of pharmacological approaches for neuroprotection. Related to the present review, the translational possibilities require continued bench science to characterize the signal transduction pathways mediating neuroprotection, and whether or not they have potential clinical applicability. There are many "gaps" in understanding the mechanisms of action of the >20 drugs presently known to be beneficial (Gidday, 2010), and we must determine how best to employ these agents.

The landmark study by Murry and colleagues on cardiac tissue heralded new and exciting research regarding classic and delayed and remote preconditioning as well as the more clinically important postconditioning effect. Research continues with pharmacological or physical manipulations that can mimic pre- or post- conditioning and this could eventually have significant clinical ramifications. Further work is needed that considers the aforementioned limitations. Reducing the long-term effect of stroke or traumatic brain injury by preserving ischemic tissue can vastly improve the quality of life for patients. Likewise, billions of dollars saved from long-term care requirements, lost wages, family care-giver issues, and the reduced burden on our health care system will all stand to benefit from progress in this critical field of study.

6. Acknowledgments

The views expressed in this work are those of the authors and do not reflect those of the United States Army, Department of Defense, or the United States Governmental Institution.

7. References

Addison, P. D., Neligan, P. C., Ashrafpour, H., Khan, A., Zhong, A., Moses, M., Forrest, C. R. & Pang, C. Y. (2003). Noninvasive remote ischemic preconditioning for global protection of skeletal muscle against infarction. *Am J Physiol Heart Circ Physiol*, Vol. 285, No. 4, pp. H1435-H1443

Aguilar-Bryan, L. & Bryan, J. (1999). Molecular biology of adenosine triphosphate-sensitive potassium channels. *Endocr Rev*, Vol. 20, No. 2, pp. 101-135

Argaud, L., Gateau-Roesch, O., Muntean, D., Chalabreysse, L., Loufouat, J., Robert, D. & Ovize, M. (2005). Specific inhibition of the mitochondrial permeability transition prevents lethal reperfusion injury. *J Mol Cell Cardiol*, Vol. 38, No. 2, pp. 367-374

Armstrong, S. C. (2004). Protein kinase activation and myocardial ischemia/reperfusion injury. *Cardiovasc Res*, Vol. 61, No. 3, pp. 427-436

Beere, H. M., Wolf, B. B., Cain, K., Mosser, D. D., Mahboubi, A., Kuwana, T., Tailor, P., Morimoto, R. I., Cohen, G. M. & Green, D. R. (2000). Heat-shock protein 70 inhibits apoptosis by preventing recruitment of procaspase-9 to the Apaf-1 apoptosome. *Nat Cell Biol*, Vol. 2, No. 8, pp. 469-475

Bell, R. M. & Yellon, D. M. (2003a). Atorvastatin, administered at the onset of reperfusion, and independent of lipid lowering, protects the myocardium by up-regulating a pro-survival pathway. *J Am Coll Cardiol*, Vol. 41, No. 3, pp. 508-515

Bell, R. M. & Yellon, D. M. (2003b). Bradykinin limits infarction when administered as an adjunct to reperfusion in mouse heart: the role of PI3K, Akt and eNOS. *J Mol Cell Cardiol*, Vol. 35, No. 2, pp. 185-193

Bolli, R. (2000). The late phase of preconditioning. *Circ Res*, Vol. 87, No. 11, pp. 972-983

Bopassa, J.-C., Ferrera, R., Gateau-Roesch, O., Couture-Lepetit, E. & Ovize, M. (2006). PI 3-kinase regulates the mitochondrial transition pore in controlled reperfusion and postconditioning. *Cardiovasc Res*, Vol. 69, No. 1, pp. 178-185

Bruey, J. M., Ducasse, C., Bonniaud, P., Ravagnan, L., Susin, S. A., Diaz-Latoud, C., Gurbuxani, S., Arrigo, A. P., Kroemer, G., Solary, E. & Garrido, C. (2000). Hsp27 negatively regulates cell death by interacting with cytochrome c. *Nat Cell Biol*, Vol. 2, No. 9, pp. 645-652

Cardone, M. H., Roy, N., Stennicke, H. R., Salvesen, G. S., Franke, T. F., Stanbridge, E., Frisch, S. & Reed, J. C. (1998). Regulation of cell death protease caspase-9 by phosphorylation. *Science*, Vol. 282, No. 5392, pp. 1318-1321

Carini, R. & Albano, E. (2003). Recent insights on the mechanisms of liver preconditioning. *Gastroenterology*, Vol. 125, No. 5, pp. 1480-1491

Chiari, P. C., Bienengraeber, M. W., Pagel, P. S., Krolikowski, J. G., Kersten, J. R. & Warltier, D. C. (2005). Isoflurane protects against myocardial infarction during early reperfusion by activation of phosphatidylinositol-3-kinase signal transduction: evidence for anesthetic-induced postconditioning in rabbits. *Anesthesiology*, Vol. 102, No. 1, pp. 102-109

Cohen, M. V., Yang, X.-M. & Downey, J. M. (2007). The pH hypothesis of postconditioning: staccato reperfusion reintroduces oxygen and perpetuates myocardial acidosis. *Circulation*, Vol. 115, No. 14, pp. 1895-1903

Concannon, C. G., Orrenius, S. & Samali, A. (2001). Hsp27 inhibits cytochrome c-mediated caspase activation by sequestering both pro-caspase-3 and cytochrome c. *Gene Expr*, Vol. 9, No. 4-5, pp. 195-201

Darling, C. E., Jiang, R., Maynard, M., Whittaker, P., Vinten-Johansen, J. & Przyklenk, K. (2005). Postconditioning via stuttering reperfusion limits myocardial infarct size in rabbit hearts: role of ERK1/2. *Am J Physiol Heart Circ Physiol*, Vol. 289, No. 4, pp. H1618-H1626

Dickson, E. W., Blehar, D. J., Carraway, R. E., Heard, S. O., Steinberg, G. & Przyklenk, K. (2001). Naloxone blocks transferred preconditioning in isolated rabbit hearts. *J Mol Cell Cardiol*, Vol. 33, No. 9, pp. 1751-1756

Dickson, E. W., Lorbar, M., Porcaro, W. A., Fenton, R. A., Reinhardt, C. P., Gysembergh, A. & Przyklenk, K. (1999a). Rabbit heart can be "preconditioned" via transfer of coronary effluent. *Am J Physiol*, Vol. 277, No. 6 Pt 2, pp. H2451-H2457

Dickson, E. W., Reinhardt, C. P., Renzi, F. P., Becker, R. C., Porcaro, W. A. & Heard, S. O. (1999b). Ischemic preconditioning may be transferable via whole blood transfusion: preliminary evidence. *J Thromb Thrombolysis*, Vol. 8, No. 2, pp. 123-129

Dirnagl, U., K. Becker, &A. Meisel (2009). Preconditioning and tolerance against cerebral ischaemia: from experimental strategies to clinical use. *Lancet Neurol*, Vol. 8, No. 4, pp. 398-412

Ehrnsperger, M., Gräber, S., Gaestel, M. & Buchner, J. (1997). Binding of non-native protein to Hsp25 during heat shock creates a reservoir of folding intermediates for reactivation. *EMBO J*, Vol. 16, No. 2, pp. 221-229

Emerson, M. R., Nelson, S. R., Samson, F. E. & Pazdernik, T. L. (1999). Hypoxia preconditioning attenuates brain edema associated with kainic acid-induced status epilepticus in rats. *Brain Res*, Vol. 825, No. 1-2, pp. 189-193

Feng, J., Lucchinetti, E., Ahuja, P., Pasch, T., Perriard, J.-C. & Zaugg, M. (2005). Isoflurane postconditioning prevents opening of the mitochondrial permeability transition pore through inhibition of glycogen synthase kinase 3beta. *Anesthesiology*, Vol. 103, No. 5, pp. 987-995

Feng, Y., Rhodes, P. G. & Bhatt, A. J. (2010). Hypoxic preconditioning provides neuroprotection and increases vascular endothelial growth factor A, preserves the phosphorylation of Akt-Ser-473 and diminishes the increase in caspase-3 activity in neonatal rat hypoxic-ischemic model. *Brain Res*, Vol. 1325, 1-9

Fernandes-Alnemri, T., Litwack, G. & Alnemri, E. S. (1994). CPP32, a novel human apoptotic protein with homology to *Caenorhabditis elegans* cell death protein Ced-3 and mammalian interleukin-1 beta-converting enzyme. *J Biol Chem*, Vol. 269, No. 49, pp. 30761-30764

Ferranti, R., da Silva, M. M. & Kowaltowski, A. J. (2003). Mitochondrial ATP-sensitive K^+ channel opening decreases reactive oxygen species generation. *FEBS Lett*, Vol. 536, No. 1-3, pp. 51-55

Fujita, M., Asanuma, H., Hirata, A., Wakeno, M., Takahama, H., Sasaki, H., Kim, J., Takashima, S., Tsukamoto, O., Minamino, T., Shinozaki, Y., Tomoike, H., Hori, M. & Kitakaze, M. (2007). Prolonged transient acidosis during early reperfusion contributes to the cardioprotective effects of postconditioning. *Am J Physiol Heart Circ Physiol*, Vol. 292, No. 4, pp. H2004-H2008

Gao, T. & Newton, A. C. (2002). The turn motif is a phosphorylation switch that egulates the binding of Hsp70 to protein kinase C. *J Biol Chem*, Vol. 277, No. 35, pp. 31585-31592

Gao, X., Ren, C. & Zhao, H. (2008). Protective effects of ischemic postconditioning compared with gradual reperfusion or preconditioning. *J Neurosci Res*, Vol. 86, No. 11, pp. 2505-2511

Garlid, K. D., Paucek, P., Yarov-Yarovoy, V., Murray, H. N., Darbenzio, R. B., D'Alonzo, A. J., Lodge, N. J., Smith, M. A. & Grover, G. J. (1997). Cardioprotective effect of diazoxide and its interaction with mitochondrial ATP-sensitive K^+ channels. Possible mechanism of cardioprotection. *Circ Res*, Vol. 81, No. 6, pp. 1072-1082

Garrido, C., Bruey, J. M., Fromentin, A., Hammann, A., Arrigo, A. P. & Solary, E. (1999). HSP27 inhibits cytochrome c-dependent activation of procaspase-9. *FASEB J*, Vol. 13, No. 14, pp. 2061-2070

Garrido, C., Brunet, M., Didelot, C., Zermati, Y., Schmitt, E. & Kroemer, G. (2006). Heat shock proteins 27 and 70: anti-apoptotic proteins with tumorigenic properties. *Cell Cycle*, Vol. 5, No. 22, pp. 2592-2601

Gateau-Roesch, O., Argaud, L. & Ovize, M. (2006). Mitochondrial permeability transition pore and postconditioning. *Cardiovasc Res*, Vol. 70, No. 2, pp. 264-273

Gho, B. C., Schoemaker, R. G., van den Doel, M. A., Duncker, D. J. & Verdouw, P. D. (1996). Myocardial protection by brief ischemia in noncardiac tissue. *Circulation*, Vol. 94, No. 9, pp. 2193-2200

Gidday, J.M. (2010). Pharmacologic preconditioning: Translating the promise. *Transl Stroke Res*, Vol. 1, No. 1, pp. 19-30

Glazier, S. S., O'Rourke, D. M., Graham, D. I. & Welsh, F. A. (1994). Induction of ischemic tolerance following brief focal ischemia in rat brain. *J Cereb Blood Flow Metab*, Vol. 14, No. 4, pp. 545--553

Goto, M., Liu, Y., Yang, X. M., Ardell, J. L., Cohen, M. V. & Downey, J. M. (1995). Role of bradykinin in protection of ischemic preconditioning in rabbit hearts. *Circ Res*, Vol. 77, No. 3, pp. 611-621

Gross, E. R., Hsu, A. K. & Gross, G. J. (2004). Opioid-induced cardioprotection occurs via glycogen synthase kinase beta inhibition during reperfusion in intact rat hearts. *Circ Res*, Vol. 94, No. 7, pp. 960-966

Gross, G. J. (2005). Pharmacological preconditioning: Potential new treatment modalities for the ischemic myocardium. *Vascul Pharmacol*, Vol. 42, No. 5-6, pp. 199

Guo, F., Sigua, C., Bali, P., George, P., Fiskus, W., Scuto, A., Annavarapu, S., Mouttaki, A., Sondarva, G., Wei, S., Wu, J., Djeu, J., & Bhalla, K. (2005). Mechanistic role of heat shock protein 70 in Bcr-Abl-mediated resistance to apoptosis in human acute leukemia cells. *Blood*, Vol. 105, No. 3, pp. 1246-55

Halestrap, A. P. (2004). Does the mitochondrial permeability transition have a role in preconditioning?. *Circulation*, Vol. 110, No. 11, pp. e303

Honda, H. M., Korge, P. & Weiss, J. N. (2005). Mitochondria and ischemia/reperfusion injury. *Ann N Y Acad Sci*, Vol. 1047, 248-258

Hoshida, S., Yamashita, N., Otsu, K. & Hori, M. (2002). The importance of manganese superoxide dismutase in delayed preconditioning: involvement of reactive oxygen species and cytokines. *Cardiovasc Res*, Vol. 55, No. 3, pp. 495-505

Hu, K. & Nattel, S. (1995). Mechanisms of ischemic preconditioning in rat hearts. Involvement of alpha 1B-adrenoceptors, pertussis toxin-sensitive G proteins, and protein kinase C. *Circulation*, Vol. 92, No. 8, pp. 2259-2265

Ishida, T., Yarimizu, K., Gute, D. C. & Korthuis, R. J. (1997). Mechanisms of ischemic preconditioning. *Shock*, Vol. 8, No. 2, pp. 86-94

Jonassen, A. K., Sack, M. N., Mjøs, O. D. & Yellon, D. M. (2001). Myocardial protection by insulin at reperfusion requires early administration and is mediated via Akt and p70s6 kinase cell-survival signaling. *Circ Res*, Vol. 89, No. 12, pp. 1191-1198

Kadenbach, B., Ramzan, R., Moosdorf, R. & Vogt, S. (2011) The role of mitochondrial membrane potential in ischemic heart failure. *Mitochondrion*, Vol. 11, No. 5, pp. 700-706

Keep, R. F., Wang, M. M. Xiang, J. Hua, Y. & Xi, G. (2010). Is there a place for cerebral preconditioning in the clinic? *Transl Stroke Res*, Vol. 1, No. 1, pp. 4-18

Kilts, J. D., Grocott, H. P. & Kwatra, M. M., (2005). G alpha(q)-coupled receptors in human atrium function through protein kinase C epsilon and delta. *J Mol Cell Cardiol*, Vol. 38, No. 2, pp. 267-276

Kin, H., Zhao, Z.-Q., Sun, H.-Y., Wang, N.-P., Corvera, J. S., Halkos, M. E., Kerendi, F., Guyton, R. A. & Vinten-Johansen, J. (2004). Postconditioning attenuates myocardial ischemia-reperfusion injury by inhibiting events in the early minutes of reperfusion. *Cardiovasc Res*, Vol. 62, No. 1, pp. 74-85

Kirino, T. (2002). Ischemic tolerance. *J Cereb Blood Flow Metab* 22, Vol., No. 11, pp. 1283-1296

Koch, S. (2010). Preconditioning the human brain: Practical considerations for proving cerebral protection. *Transl Stroke Res*, Vol. 1, No. 3, pp. 161-169

Komarova, E. Y., Afanasyeva, E. A., Bulatova, M. M., Cheetham, M. E., Margulis, B. A. & Guzhova, I. V. (2004). Downstream caspases are novel targets for the antiapoptotic activity of the molecular chaperone hsp70. *Cell Stress Chaperones*, Vol. 9, No. 3, pp. 265-275

Kretz-Remy, C., Mehlen, P., Mirault, M. E. & Arrigo, A. P. (1996). Inhibition of I kappa B-alpha phosphorylation and degradation and subsequent NF-kappa B activation by glutathione peroxidase overexpression. *J Cell Biol*, Vol. 133, No. 5, pp. 1083-1093

Krolikowski, J. G., Weihrauch, D., Bienengraeber, M., Kersten, J. R., Warltier, D. C. & Pagel, P. S. (2006). Role of Erk1/2, p70s6K, and eNOS in isoflurane-induced cardioprotection during early reperfusion in vivo. *Can J Anaesth*, Vol. 53, No. 2, pp. 174-182

Lacza, Z., Snipes, J. A., Kis, B., Szabó, C., Grover, G. & Busija, D. W. (2003). Investigation of the subunit composition and the pharmacology of the mitochondrial ATP-dependent K^+ channel in the brain. *Brain Res*, Vol. 994, No. 1, pp. 27-36

Lavoie, J. N., Lambert, H., Hickey, E., Weber, L. A. & Landry, J. (1995). Modulation of cellular thermoresistance and actin filament stability accompanies phosphorylation-induced changes in the oligomeric structure of heat shock protein 27. *Mol Cell Biol*, Vol. 15, No. 1, pp. 505-516

Legtenberg, R. J., Rongen, G. A., Houston, R. J. E., Oeseburg, B. & Smits, P. (2002). The role of myocardial K_{ATP}-channel blockade in the protective effects of glibenclamide against ischaemia in the rat heart. *Pharmacol Toxicol*, Vol. 91, No. 2, pp. 51-56

Liem, D. A., te Lintel Hekkert, M., Manintveld, O. C., Boomsma, F., Verdouw, P. D. & Duncker, D. J. (2005). Myocardium tolerant to an adenosine-dependent ischemic preconditioning stimulus can still be protected by stimuli that employ alternative signaling pathways. *Am J Physiol Heart Circ Physiol*, Vol. 288, No. 3, pp. H1165-H1172

Lin, D.-T. & Lechleiter, J. D. (2002). Mitochondrial targeted cyclophilin D protects cells from cell death by peptidyl prolyl isomerization. *J Biol Chem*, Vol. 277, No. 34, pp. 31134-31141

Liu, G. S., Thornton, J., Winkle, D. M. V., Stanley, A. W., Olsson, R. A. & Downey, J. M. (1991). Protection against infarction afforded by preconditioning is mediated by A1 adenosine receptors in rabbit heart. *Circulation*, Vol. 84, No. 1, pp. 350-356

Livak, K. J., Freund, R., Schweber, M., Wensink, P. C. & Meselson, M. (1978). Sequence organization and transcription at two heat shock loci in *Drosophila*. *Proc Natl Acad Sci USA*, Vol. 75, No. 11, pp. 5613-5617

Madamanchi, N. R., Li, S., Patterson, C. & Runge, M. S. (2001). Reactive oxygen species regulate heat-shock protein 70 via the JAK/STAT pathway. *Arterioscler Thromb Vasc Biol*, Vol. 21, No. 3, pp. 321-326

Marber, M. S., Latchman, D. S., Walker, J. M. & Yellon, D. M. (1993). Cardiac stress protein elevation 24 hours after brief ischemia or heat stress is associated with resistance to myocardial infarction. *Circulation*, Vol. 88, No. 3, pp. 1264-1272

Maulik, N., Engelman, R. M., Rousou, J. A., Flack, J. E., Deaton, D. & Das, D. K. (1999). Ischemic preconditioning reduces apoptosis by upregulating anti-death gene Bcl-2. *Circulation*, Vol. 100, No. 19 Suppl, pp. II369-II375

Mitchell, M. B., Meng, X., Ao, L., Brown, J. M., Harken, A. H. & Banerjee, A. (1995). Preconditioning of isolated rat heart is mediated by protein kinase C. *Circ Res*, Vol. 76, No. 1, pp. 73-81

Mizumura, T., Nithipatikom, K. & Gross, G. J. (1995). Bimakalim, an ATP-sensitive potassium channel opener, mimics the effects of ischemic preconditioning to reduce infarct size, adenosine release, and neutrophil function in dogs. *Circulation*, Vol. 92, No. 5, pp. 1236-1245

Murry, C. E., Jennings, R. B. & Reimer, K. A. (1986). Preconditioning with ischemia: a delay of lethal cell injury in ischemic myocardium. *Circulation*, Vol. 74, No. 5, pp. 1124--1136

Noma, A. (1983). ATP-regulated K^+ channels in cardiac muscle. *Nature*, Vol. 305, No. 5930, pp. 147-148

Obal, D., Dettwiler, S., Favoccia, C., Scharbatke, H., Preckel, B. & Schlack, W. (2005). The influence of mitochondrial K_{ATP}-channels in the cardioprotection of preconditioning and postconditioning by sevoflurane in the rat *in vivo*. *Anesth Analg*, Vol. 101, No. 5, pp. 1252-1260

Ockaili, R. A., Bhargava, P. & Kukreja, R. C. (2001). Chemical preconditioning with 3-nitropropionic acid in hearts: role of mitochondrial K_{ATP} channel. *Am J Physiol Heart Circ Physiol*, Vol. 280, No. 5, pp. H2406-H2411

Okamoto, F., Allen, B. S., Buckberg, G. D., Bugyi, H. & Leaf, J. (1986). Reperfusion conditions: importance of ensuring gentle versus sudden reperfusion during relief of coronary occlusion. *J Thorac Cardiovasc Surg*, Vol. 92, No. 3 Pt 2, pp. 613-620

O'Sullivan J., Fu D., Alam H.B., & McCabe J.T. (2008). Diazoxide increases liver and kidney HSP25 and HSP70 after shock and stroke. *J Surg Res*, Vol. 49, No. 1, pp. 120-130

O'Sullivan, J. C., Yao, X.-L., Alam, H. & McCabe, J. T. (2007). Diazoxide, as a postconditioning and delayed preconditioning trigger, increases HSP25 and HSP70 in the central nervous system following combined cerebral stroke and hemorrhagic shock. *J Neurotrauma*, Vol. 24, No. 3, pp. 532-546

Pang, C. Y., Yang, R. Z., Zhong, A., Xu, N., Boyd, B. & Forrest, C. R. (1995). Acute ischaemic preconditioning protects against skeletal muscle infarction in the pig.. *Cardiovasc Res, Vol.* 29, No. 6, pp. 782-788

Patel, H. H., Moore, J., Hsu, A. K. & Gross, G. J. (2002). Cardioprotection at a distance: mesenteric artery occlusion protects the myocardium via an opioid sensitive mechanism. *J Mol Cell Cardiol*, Vol. 34, No. 10, pp. 1317-1323

Penna, C., Mancardi, D., Rastaldo, R., Losano, G. & Pagliaro, P. (2007). Intermittent activation of bradykinin B2 receptors and mitochondrial K_{ATP} channels trigger cardiac postconditioning through redox signaling. *Cardiovasc Res*, Vol. 75, No. 1, pp. 168-177

Penninger, J. M. & Kroemer, G. (2003). Mitochondria, AIF and caspases–rivaling for cell death execution. *Nat Cell Biol*, Vol. 5, No. 2, pp. 97-99

Peralta, C., Closa, D., Hotter, G., Gelpí, E., Prats, N. & Roselló-Catafau, J. (1996). Liver ischemic preconditioning is mediated by the inhibitory action of nitric oxide on endothelin. *Biochem Biophys Res Commun*, Vol. 229, No. 1, pp. 264--270

Philipp, S., Yang, X.-M., Cui, L., Davis, A. M., Downey, J. M. & Cohen, M. V. (2006). Postconditioning protects rabbit hearts through a protein kinase C-adenosine A2b receptor cascade. *Cardiovasc Res*, Vol. 70, No. 2, pp. 308-314

Pignataro, G., Meller, R., Inoue, K., Ordonez, A.N., Ashley, M.D., Xiong, Z. & Simon, R.P. (2008). *In vivo* and *in vitro* characterization of a novel neuroprotective strategy for stroke: ischemic postconditioning. J Cereb Blood Flow Metab, Vol. 28, No. 2, pp. 232-241

Przyklenk, K., Bauer, B., Ovize, M., Kloner, R. A. & Whittaker, P. (1993). Regional ischemic 'preconditioning' protects remote virgin myocardium from subsequent sustained coronary occlusion. *Circulation*, Vol. 87, No. 3, pp. 893-899

Ritossa, F. (1962). A new puffing pattern induced by heat shock and DNP in *Drosophilia*. *Experentia*, Vol. 18, No. 86, pp. 571-573

Rizvi, A., Tang, X. L., Qiu, Y., Xuan, Y. T., Takano, H., Jadoon, A. K. & Bolli, R. (1999). Increased protein synthesis is necessary for the development of late preconditioning against myocardial stunning. *Am J Physiol*, Vol. 277, No. 3 Pt 2, pp. H874-H884

Robin, E., Simerabet, M., Hassoun, S. M., Adamczyk, S., Tavernier, B., Vallet, B., Bordet, R. & Lebuffe, G. (2011). Postconditioning in focal cerebral ischemia: role of the mitochondrial ATP-dependent potassium channel. *Brain Res*, Vol. 1375, 137-146

Ruchalski, K., Mao, H., Li, Z., Wang, Z., Gillers, S., Wang, Y., Mosser, D. D., Gabai, V., Schwartz, J. H. & Borkan, S. C. (2006). Distinct hsp70 domains mediate apoptosis-inducing factor release and nuclear accumulation. *J Biol Chem*, Vol. 281, No. 12, pp. 7873-7880

Saitoh, S., Zhang, C., Tune, J. D., Potter, B., Kiyooka, T., Rogers, P. A., Knudson, J. D., Dick, G. M., Swafford, A. & Chilian, W. M. (2006). Hydrogen peroxide: a feed-forward dilator that couples myocardial metabolism to coronary blood flow. *Arterioscler Thromb Vasc Biol*, Vol. 26, No. 12, pp. 2614-2621

Schulman, D., Latchman, D. S. & Yellon, D. M. (2002). Urocortin protects the heart from reperfusion injury via upregulation of p42/p44 MAPK signaling pathway. *Am J Physiol Heart Circ Physiol*, Vol. 283, No. 4, pp. H1481-H1488

Schultz, J. E., Hsu, A. K. & Gross, G. J. (1998). Ischemic preconditioning in the intact rat heart is mediated by delta1- but not mu- or kappa-opioid receptors. *Circulation*, Vol. 97, No. 13, pp. 1282-1289

Shinmura, K., Tang, X. L., Wang, Y., Xuan, Y. T., Liu, S. Q., Takano, H., Bhatnagar, A. & Bolli, R. (2000). Cyclooxygenase-2 mediates the cardioprotective effects of the late phase of ischemic preconditioning in conscious rabbits. *Proc Natl Acad Sci U S A*, Vol. 97, No. 18, pp. 10197-10202

Smith, S. (2001). The world according to PARP. *Trends Biochem Sci*, Vol. 26, No. 3, pp. 174-179

Stankiewicz, A. R., Lachapelle, G., Foo, C. P. Z., Radicioni, S. M. & Mosser, D. D. (2005). Hsp70 inhibits heat-induced apoptosis upstream of mitochondria by preventing Bax translocation. *J Biol Chem*, Vol. 280, No. 46, pp. 38729-38739

Szabó, I. & Zoratti, M. (1992). The mitochondrial megachannel is the permeability transition pore. *J Bioenerg Biom*embr, Vol. 24, No. 1, pp. 111-117

Szewczyk, A. & Marbán, E. (1999). Mitochondria: a new target for K channel openers? *Trends Pharmacol Sci*, Vol. 20, No. 4, pp. 157-161

Takano, H., Manchikalapudi, S., Tang, X. L., Qiu, Y., Rizvi, A., Jadoon, A. K., Zhang, Q. & Bolli, R. (1998). Nitric oxide synthase is the mediator of late preconditioning against myocardial infarction in conscious rabbits. *Circulation*, Vol. 98, No. 5, pp. 441-449

Takano, H., Tang, X. L. & Bolli, R. (2000). Differential role of K_{ATP} channels in late preconditioning against myocardial stunning and infarction in rabbits. *Am J Physiol Heart Circ Physiol*, Vol. 279, No. 5, pp. H2350-H2359

Takayama, S., Reed, J. C. & Homma, S. (2003). Heat-shock proteins as regulators of apoptosis. *Oncogene*, Vol. 22, No. 56, pp. 9041-9047

Tong, H., Chen, W., Steenbergen, C. & Murphy, E. (2000). Ischemic preconditioning activates phosphatidylinositol-3-kinase upstream of protein kinase C. *Circ Res*, Vol. 87, No. 4, pp. 309-315

Tong, H., Imahashi, K., Steenbergen, C. & Murphy, E. (2002). Phosphorylation of glycogen synthase kinase-3beta during preconditioning through a phosphatidylinositol-3-kinase–dependent pathway is cardioprotective. *Circ Res*, Vol. 90, No. 4, pp. 377-379

Tsang, A., Hausenloy, D. J., Mocanu, M. M. & Yellon, D. M. (2004). Postconditioning: a form of "modified reperfusion" protects the myocardium by activating the phosphatidylinositol 3-kinase-Akt pathway. *Circ Res*, Vol. 95, No. 3, pp. 230-232

Vinten-Johansen, J., Jiang, R., Reeves, J. G., Mykytenko, J., Deneve, J. & Jobe, L. J. (2007). Inflammation, proinflammatory mediators and myocardial ischemia-reperfusion Injury. *Hematol Oncol Clin North Am*, Vol. 21, No. 1, pp. 123-145

Voellmy, R. & Boellmann, F. (2007). Chaperone regulation of the heat shock protein response. *Adv Exp Med Biol*, Vol. 594, 89-99

Wang, S., Duan, Y., Su, D., Li, W., Tan, J., Yang, D., Wang, W., Zhao, Z. & Wang, X., No. 2011). Delta opioid peptide [D-Ala2, D-Leu5] enkephalin (DADLE) triggers postconditioning against transient forebrain ischemia. *Eur J Pharmacol*, Vol. 658, No. 2-3, pp. 140-144

Wang, Y., Ahmad, N., Kudo, M. & Ashraf, M. (2004). Contribution of Akt and endothelial nitric oxide synthase to diazoxide-induced late preconditioning. *Am J Physiol Heart Circ Physiol*, Vol. 287, No. 3, pp. H1125-H1131

Wang, Y., Xu, H., Mizoguchi, K., Oe, M. & Maeta, H. (2001). Intestinal ischemia induces late preconditioning against myocardial infarction: a role for inducible nitric oxide synthase. *Cardiovasc Res*, Vol. 49, No. 2, pp. 391-398

Wu, L., Shen, F., Lin, L., Zhang, X., Bruce, I. C. & Xia, Q. (2006). The neuroprotection conferred by activating the mitochondrial ATP-sensitive K^+ channel is mediated by inhibiting the mitochondrial permeability transition pore. *Neurosci Lett*, Vol. 402, No. 1-2, pp. 184-189

Xiao, L., Lu, R., Hu, C. P., Deng, H. W. & Li, Y. J. (2001). Delayed cardioprotection by intestinal preconditioning is mediated by calcitonin gene-related peptide. *Eur J Pharmacol*, Vol. 427, No. 2, pp. 131-135

Yang, X.-M., Proctor, J. B., Cui, L., Krieg, T., Downey, J. M. & Cohen, M. V. (2004). Multiple, brief coronary occlusions during early reperfusion protect rabbit hearts by targeting cell signaling pathways. *J Am Coll Cardiol*, Vol. 44, No. 5, pp. 1103-1110

Yellon, D. M. & Downey, J. M. (2003). Preconditioning the myocardium: from cellular physiology to clinical cardiology. *Physiol Rev*, Vol. 83, No. 4, pp. 1113-1151

Zaugg, M., Lucchinetti, E., Spahn, D. R., Pasch, T. & Schaub, M. C. (2002). Volatile anesthetics mimic cardiac preconditioning by priming the activation of mitochondrial K_{ATP} channels via multiple signaling pathways. *Anesthesiology*, Vol. 97, No. 1, pp. 4-14

Zhao, H., Sapolsky, R.M. & Steinberg, G.K. (2006). Interrupting reperfusion as a stroke therapy: ischemic postconditioning reduces infarct size after focal ischemia in rats. *J Cereb Blood Flow Metab*, Vol. 26, No. 9, pp. 1114-1121

Zhao, Z.-Q., Corvera, J. S., Halkos, M. E., Kerendi, F., Wang, N.-P., Guyton, R. A. & Vinten-Johansen, J. (2003). Inhibition of myocardial injury by ischemic postconditioning during reperfusion: comparison with ischemic preconditioning. *Am J Physiol Heart Circ Physiol*, Vol. 285, No. 2, pp. H579-H588

Zhu, M., Feng, J., Lucchinetti, E., Fischer, G., Xu, L., Pedrazzini, T., Schaub, M. C. & Zaugg, M. (2006). Ischemic postconditioning protects remodeled myocardium via the PI3K-PKB/Akt reperfusion injury salvage kinase pathway. *Cardiovasc Res*, Vol. 72, No. 1, pp. 152-162

17

Could Mannitol-Induced Delay of Anoxic Depolarization be Relevant in Stroke Patients?

Maurizio Balestrino*, Enrico Adriano and Patrizia Garbati
Department of Neuroscience, Ophtalmology and Genetics, University of Genova, Italy

1. Introduction

The use of hyperosmotic agents in stroke is still a matter of debate, since their usefulness has repeatedely been suggested but not conclusively demonstrated (Righetti E et al., 2002). Better understanding of the possible mechanism of protection by hyperosmotic agents may help identifying clinical situations where they may be more useful. It is generally assumed that their effect in stroke is due to their capacity to reduce brain edema. However, increasing extracellular osmolarity has direct effects on neuronal electrical function (Osehobo and Andrew, 1993; Rudehill et al., 1993), and one of us has previously reported that adding mannitol to the perfusing medium of brain slices delays anoxic depolarization (AD) (Balestrino, 1995a; Balestrino, 1995b). Since the latter is a factor in causing neuronal damage in anoxia and ischemia (Balestrino and Somjen, 1986; Jarvis et al., 2001; Kaminogo et al., 1998; Somjen et al., 1990), this may be another mechanism of brain protection by hyperosmotic agents in stroke. This study investigates whether or not this delay occurs at values of hyperosmolarity that may be obtained in clinical practice. We first carried out a survey of the literature on osmolarity changes after administration of hyperosmotic agents in vivo, under both clinical and experimental conditions. Then, we did a dose-response study of mannitol-induced delay of AD. Finally we compared the two sets of data to gauge whether or not mannitol-induced delay of AD occurs in the range of hyperosmolarity that might be obtained in clinical practice.

2. Materials and methods

Sprague-Dawley female rats (155-190g.) were anaesthetised with ether and decapitated. The left hippocampus was dissected free and cut in 600 µm thick transversal slices. Slices were immediately transferred into an "interface" recording chamber (Fine Science Tools, Vancouver B. C. Canada) and incubated at 35±1°C. They were bathed by Artificial CerebroSpinal Fluid (ACSF) flowing at 2 ml/min and having the following composition: NaCl 130 mM, KCl 3.5 mM, NaH_2PO_4 1.25 mM, $NaHCO_3$ 24 mM, $CaCl_2$ 2.4 mM, $MgSO_4$ 1.2 mM, glucose 10 mM. This medium was continuously bubbled with 95% O_2 / 5% CO_2, resulting in a pH of 7.35-7.40. The same warmed, humidified 95% O_2 / 5% CO_2 mixture aerated the slices representing the gas phase. Anoxia was induced by replacing oxygen with

* Corresponding Author

nitrogen in the gas phase. The DC-coupled, ground-referenced extracellular potential of the tissue was constantly monitored in the cell body layer of CA1. As soon as the sudden fall in this potential that is the hallmark of AD was observed, oxygen flow was restored. A cross-over study design was observed, with the same slice being subjected to anoxia, at 30′ intervals, both in the presence and in the absence of mannitol. Each slice was subjected to two anoxic episodes. The sequence of treatments (mannitol first, or control ACSF first) was alternated in consecutive experiments, to minimize the bias due to possible effects of repeated anoxia *per se* on AD latency. In two experiments, the same slice was subjected to three anoxic episodes the first one in mannitol, the second in control ACSF, the third one in mannitol again. For statistical analysis, in each experiment the difference in latency between AD in mannitol and AD in control ACSF was computed, and used as a gauge of mannitol efficacy in that experiment.

3. Results

3.1 Literature search on serum osmolarity changes in vivo

Results are summarized in figure 1 and in Table 1.

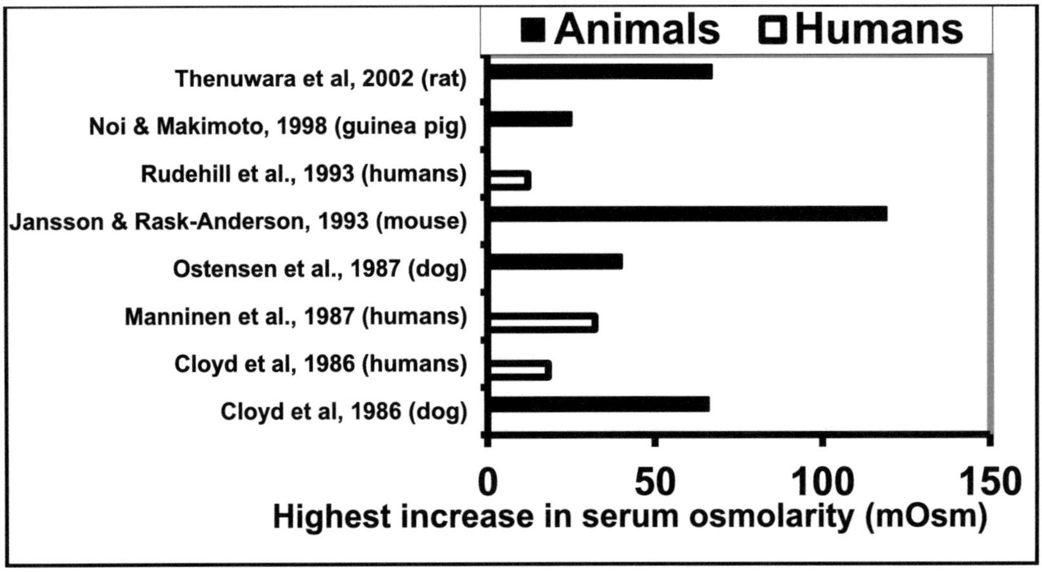

Fig. 1. **Increases in serum osmolarity reported in the literature:** This figure depicts the highest increase in serum osmolarity reported in each of the papers listed in Table 1. It refers to papers quoted in the Reference List. This figure is meant to graphically visualize the highest reported increases. Refer to Table I and to text for further information.

In human patients, use of mannitol at the dose of 0.5-2 g/Kg body weight is reported (Cloyd et al., 1986; Newman, 1979; Rudehill et al., 1993). Such a dose leads, still in human patients, to a maximum increase in serum osmolarity of about 10-32 mOsm (Cloyd et al., 1986; Manninen et al., 1987; Rudehill et al., 1993). When experimental animals are considered, administration of 1 g/Kg body weight to rats yelded a serum osmolarity increase of 4 mOsm (Thenuwara et al., 2002). In dogs, mannitol administration of 0.5, 1 or 1.5 g/Kg lead to a peak increase (mean±SD) of 43±18, 66±18 and 52±23 mOsm, respectively, during the brief time of the infusion, and to the

Paper	Animal species	Osmotic agent infused	Dose	Serum osmolarity increase
(Cloyd et al., 1986)	Humans	Mannitol	0.5, 0.7 g/Kg	10 - 18 mOsm
(Cloyd et al., 1986)	Dog	Mannitol	0.5, 1, 1.5 g/Kg	43-66 mOsm
(Jansson and Rask-Anderson, 1993)	Mice	Glycerol	1.3, 2.6 and 5.2 g /kg	12-119 mOsm
(Manninen et al., 1987)	Humans	Mannitol	1, 2 g/Kg	32 mOsm
(Newman, 1979)	Humans	Mannitol	2 g/Kg	Not reported
(Noi and Makimoto, 1998)	Guinea pig	Glycerol	30-min infusion of 50% glycerol	6 mOsm
(Noi and Makimoto, 1998)	Guinea pig	Urographin®	30-min infusion of 76% Urographin®	25 mOsm
(Ostensen et al., 1987)	Dog	Mannitol		40 mOsm
(Rudehill et al., 1993)	Humans	Mannitol	1 g/Kg	12 mOsm.
(Thenuwara et al., 2002)	Rat	Mannitol	1, 4, 8 g/Kg, with or without furosemide	4-67 mOsm

Table 1. **Literature data on changes in serum osmolarity after i.v. infusion of osmotic agents.** The table summarizes available literature data on changes in serum osmolarity after i.v. infusion of osmotic agents. When different changes in osmolarity are reported following different doses of osmotic agent, in the table the range of increases is given. The values given in the table are either the numbers provided by the Authors or those obtained by measuring graphs in their papers. In the latter case, the value is obviously less precise. When the Authors reported mean±SD for pre- and post-infusion osmolarity, in the table the corresponding difference between means is given.

lower increase of 10 mOsm or less afterwards (Rudehill et al., 1993). Higher doses of mannitol (4 g/Kg and 8 g/Kg, with or without the addition of furosemide) lead, in rats, to a rather high serum osmolarity increase, reaching an average as high as 67 mOsm (Thenuwara et al., 2002). Under experimental conditions in vivo, glycerol infusion leads to average increases in serum osmolarity of 6 mOsm in guinea pigs (Noi and Makimoto, 1998) and of up to 119 mOsm in dogs (Jansson and Rask-Anderson, 1993). Using Urografin® infusion, a 25 mOsm increase in serum osmolarity was obtained in guinea pigs (Noi and Makimoto, 1998).

3.2 Effects of increasing mannitol in vitro

The previously shown robust effect of mannitol in delaying AD was first confirmed in double wash-out experiments, where the same slice was subjected to transient anoxia in the presence of mannitol, then in control ACSF, then again in the presence of mannitol. These experiments are illustrated in figure 2. Mannitol concentrations of 100 and 500 mM were used in these experiments, as they were those that had been previously shown to most reliably delay AD (Balestrino, 1995).

The effects of mannitol where then investigated at different concentrations. Fig. 3 summarizes these results. As it can be seen, 1 and 10 mM were not effective in delaying AD. Twenty-five mM significantly delayed AD, while 50 mM did not show a statistically significant effect. The quite high concentrations of 100 and 500 mM significantly increased the latency of AD.

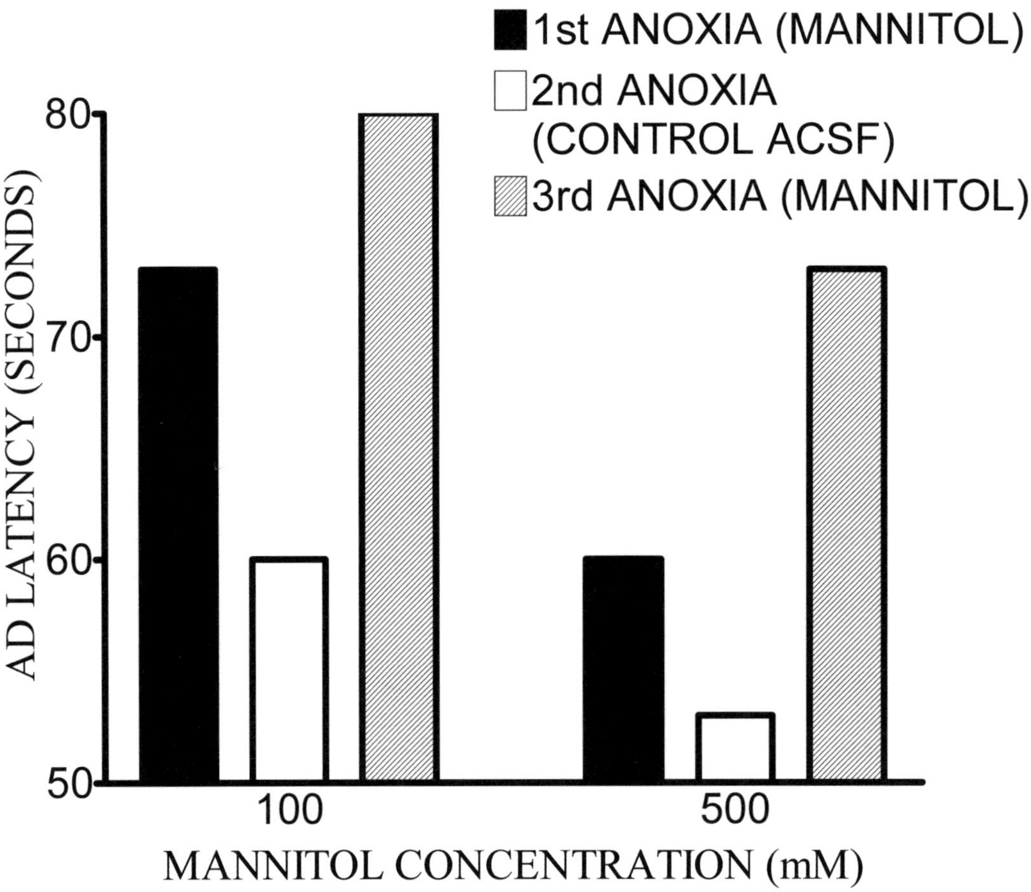

Fig. 2. **Double wash-out experiments showing mannitol effectiveness in delaying anoxic depolarization.** In two different slices, anoxia was induced in mannitol-fortified Artificial CerebroSpinal Fluid (ACSF), then in control ACSF, then again in ACSF with added mannitol. In one experiment (set of bars at left) 100 mM mannitol were used, in the other (set of bars at right) 500 mM mannitol were used. Bars represent latency of AD in each anoxia episode. Control ACSF reversibly decreased AD latency, thus confirming the previously published efficacy of mannitol in increasing AD latency.

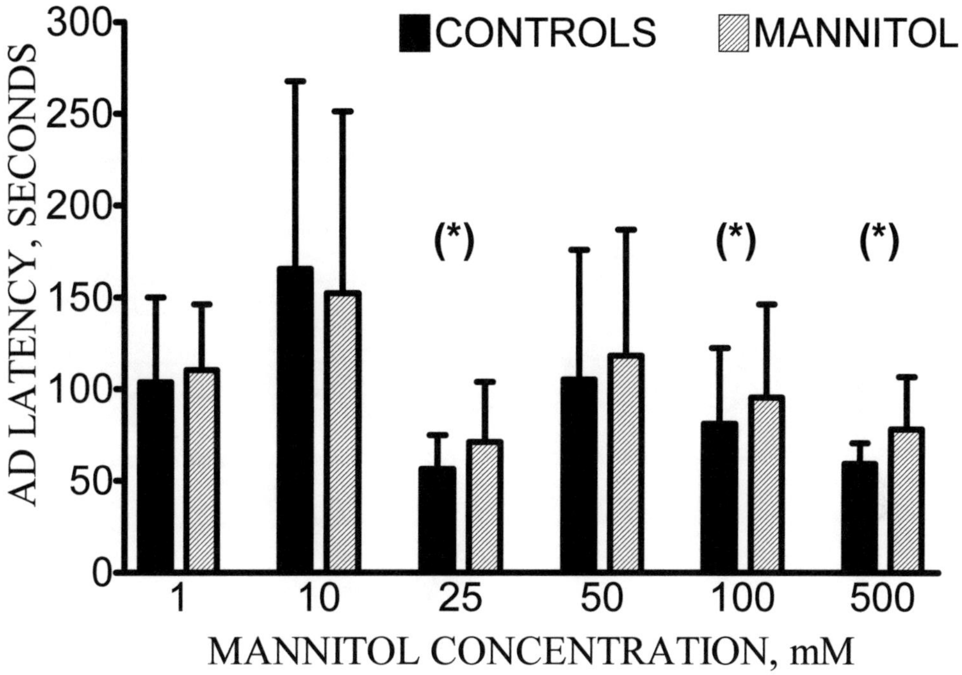

Fig. 3. **Effects of different mannitol concentrations in delaying anoxic depolarization.** The bars show latency of AD (mean± SD)in both control and mannitol-fortified ACSF for different mannitol concentrations. Asterisks mark the groups in which the difference is statistically significant ($p<0.03$, t-test for paired data). N=3 for 1mM, N=4 for 10 mM, N=8 for 25 mM, N=7 for 50 mM, N=6 for 100 mM, N=6 for 500 mM. See text for experiment design.

Figure 4 shows an example of AD delay by mannitol.

In a further analysis, we calculated for each slice the difference between the latency of AD in mannitol and the latency of AD in control ACSF. Such a difference was used as a gauge of mannitol effectiveness in that particular slice. If the difference had been positive, it would have indicated that latency in mannitol was longer that in control (i.e., AD occurred later), thus showing protection by mannitol and quantifying its degree. The opposite would have been true for a negative difference. Results are shown in Figure 5. As it can be seen, above 10 mM all concentrations of mannitol delay AD to a comparable extent. Such a finding has already been reported, from our laboratory, for AD delay by creatine (Balestrino, 1995).

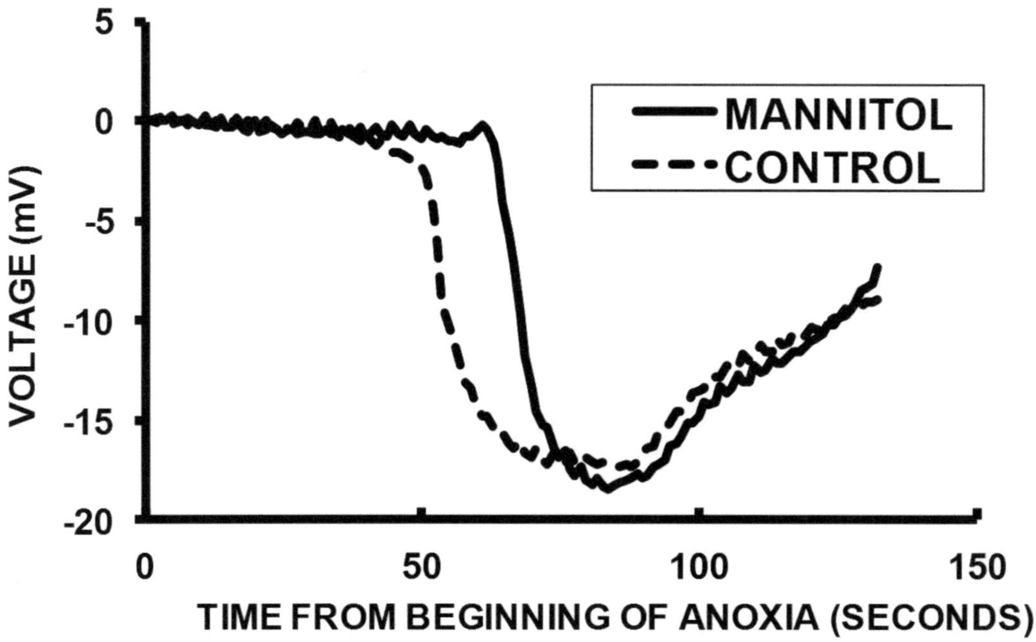

Fig. 4. **Sample anoxic depolarization in control and mannitol-treated ACSF.** Two different anoxic episodes in the same slice. The dotted line represents DC tracing (showing anoxic depolarization) during anoxia in control ACSF, the solid line represents the same tracing during anoxia in ACSF with added mannitol. AD occurs later in mannitol-fortified ACSF.

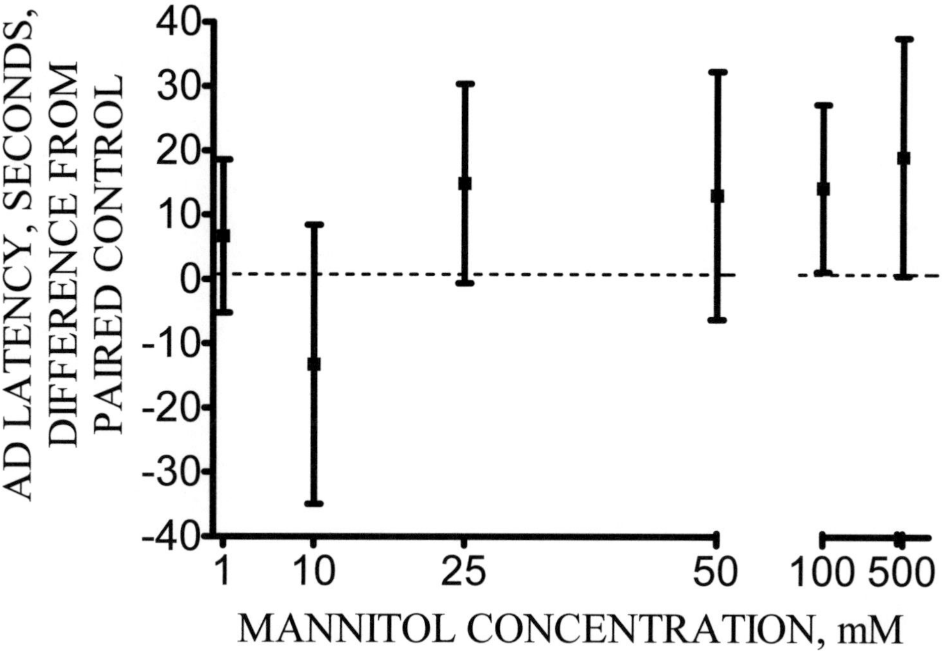

Fig. 5. **Measure of AD delay in different mannitol concentrations.** Same experiments as in figure 3. This figure depicts more precisely the increase in AD latency determined by mannitol at each concentration. For each slice, the difference (AD latency in ACSF with mannitol) - (AD latency in control ACSF) was computed. A positive difference means that AD latency was longer in mannitol (i.e., AD occurred later), the opposite is true for a negative difference. Data were grouped for mannitol concentration. For each concentration, mean±SD is provided. Number of experiments as in figure 3. Concentrations of 25 mM mannitol and higher all delay AD to the same extent.

4. Discussion

The effectiveness of hyperosmolarity in delaying AD was confirmed by these findings. Delay of AD may be relevant to neuroprotection in stroke, because AD is a factor in the generation of anoxic damage, and its delay has been associated with better outcome under experimental conditions (Balestrino and Somjen, 1986; Jarvis et al., 2001; Kaminogo et al., 1998; Somjen et al., 1990). The present study indicates that significant delay of AD is obtained at mannitol concentrations greater than 10 mM, 25 mM being the lowest effective dose among those tested. An overview of the literature showed that in human patients serum osmolarity increases, under common clinical settings, by 10-32 mOsm after administration of 1 g/Kg mannitol (Table 1 and fig. 1). This is equivalent to adding 10-32 mM mannitol to in vitro slices[1]. At the lower end of this range, such an

[1] Since the molecule of mannitol does not split in acqueous solutions, the molarity of mannitol in solution (here expressed in mM) corresponds to the consequent increase in osmolarity (1mM=1mOsm).

increase would be insufficient (10 mM (Cloyd et al., 1986; Rudehill et al., 1993)) or perhaps barely sufficient (18 mM (Cloyd et al., 1986)) to afford delay of AD. In the upper end, a 32 mM increase (Manninen et al., 1987) would probably be somehow effective in delaying AD. In fact, we showed that in vitro the addition of 25 mM mannitol (increasing osmolarity by 25 mOsm) significantly delays AD. The delay in AD was not significant after addition of 50 mM (increasing osmolarity by 50 mOsm), indicating that these osmolarity increases (25-50 mOsm) are of borderline efficacy. However, much higher increases, up to 100 mOsm and more, were reliably effective in vitro, and have been reported under experimental conditions in laboratory animals, apparently without severe adverse effects (Table 1 and figure 1). The latter increases would be in a range that does cause AD delay (compare figure 5 with figure 1). If further studies suggested that a comparable increase in serum osmolarity can be safely obtained in human patients, it might be useful not only by decreasing brain edema, but also by having a direct effect on tissue depolarization.

Two more considerations are in order.

First, in human stroke mannitol or other hyperosmotic agents would be adiminstered when AD has already occurred. In fact, AD is an event that occurs in the core of an infarction soon after ischemia. Nevertheless, under experimental conditions continuous or repeated depolarizations have been demonstrated in the hours following stroke (Chen et al., 1993; Ohta et al., 1997). Their reduction has been associated with better outcome (Chen et al., 1993). Given the striking similarity of these events with "classical" AD, it is very likely that hyperosmolarity can delay or suppress these waveforms as well, thus providing protection.

Second, the changes reported in the literature are in serum, not in the interstitial space of the brain. To the best of our knowledge, no study has yet measured increases in osmolarity in the interstitial space of the brain, probably due to the technical difficulty of this investigation. However, it is reasonable to assume that an increase in osmotic pressure in the serum draws water from the brain interstitial space, thus increasing its osmolarity to a comparable degree. Therefore, increase in serum osmolarity should be comparable, at least to an extent, to increase in osmolarity of the brain interstitial space.

Finally, it should be noted that future clinical studies on hyperosmotic agents in stroke should take into account the increase in serum osmolarity that was obtained in the single patients. In fact, our data indicate that the latter is a critical variable in determining whether the hyperosmotic therapy will be effective or not.

Summing up, we conclude that the increase in serum osmolarity that is commonly obtained in clinical practice is not sufficient to delay AD. Larger increases in serum osmolarity have been, however, reported in animal experiments. If further studies indicated that such increases were safe in humans as well as in animals, they might provide brain protection by decreasing AD and AD-like depolarizations. Future clinical studies on hyperosmotic agents in stroke should measure and take into account the degree of changes that were obtained in serum osmolarity.

5. Acknowledgment

We thank Prof. Aroldo Cupello for his useful comments on the manuscript.

6. References

Balestrino M. (1995) Studies on anoxic depolarization. In: Brain Slices in Basic and Clinical Research (A.Schurr, B.M.Rigor, eds), pp 273-293 Boca Raton, Florida: CRC Press.

Balestrino M (Pathophysiology of anoxic depolarization: new findings and a working hypothesis. J Neurosci Methods 59:99-103.1995).

Balestrino M, Somjen GG (Chlorpromazine protects brain tissue in hypoxia by delaying spreading depression-mediated calcium influx. Brain Res 385:219-226.1986).

Chen Q, Chopp M, Bodzin G, Chen H (Temperature modulation of cerebral depolarization during focal cerebral ischemia in rats: correlation with ischemic injury. J Cereb Blood Flow Metab 13:389-394.1993).

Cloyd JC, Snyder BD, Cleeremans B, Bundlie SR, Blomquist CH, Lakatua DJ (Mannitol pharmacokinetics and serum osmolality in dogs and humans. J Pharmacol Exp Ther 236:301-306.1986).

Jansson B, Rask-Anderson H (Correlations between serum osmolality and endolymphatic sac response using hypertonic glycerol. ORL J Otorhinolaryngol Relat Spec 55:185-192.1993).

Jarvis CR, Anderson TR, Andrew RD (Anoxic Depolarization Mediates Acute Damage Independent of Glutamate in Neocortical Brain Slices. Cerebral Cortex 11:249-259.2001).

Kaminogo M, Suyama K, Ichikura A, Onizuka M, Shibata S (Anoxic depolarization determines ischemic brain injury. Neurol Res 20:343-348.1998).

Manninen P, Lam A, Gelb A, Brown S (The effect of high-dose mannitol on serum and urine electrolytes and osmolality in neurosurgical patients. Canadian Journal of Anesthesia / Journal canadien d'anesthésie 34:442-446.1987).

Newman SL (Monitoring serum osmolality in mannitol treatment of Reye's syndrome. N Engl J Med 301:945-946.1979).

Noi O, Makimoto K (Comparative effects of glycerol and Urografin on cochlear blood flow and serum osmolarity. Hear Res 123:55-60.1998).

Ohta K, Graf R, Rosner G, Heiss WD (Profiles of cortical tissue depolarization in cat focal cerebral ischemia in relation to calcium ion homeostasis and nitric oxide production. J Cereb Blood Flow Metab 17:1170-1181.1997).

Osehobo EP, Andrew RD (Osmotic effects upon the theta rhythm, a natural brain oscillation in the hippocampal slice. Exp Neurol 124:192-199.1993).

Ostensen J, Bugge JF, Stokke ES, Langberg H, Kiil F (Mechanism of osmotic diuresis studied by infusion of NaHCO3 and mannitol in dogs. Acta Physiol Scand 131:397-409.1987).

Righetti E, Celani MG, Cantisani T, Sterzi R, Boysen G, Ricci S (2002) Glycerol for acute stroke (Cochrane Review). In: The Cochrane Library, Issue 2 2002 Oxford: Update Software.

Rudehill A, Gordon E, Ohman G, Lindqvist C, Andersson P (Pharmacokinetics and effects of mannitol on hemodynamics, blood and cerebrospinal fluid electrolytes, and osmolality during intracranial surgery. J Neurosurg Anesthesiol 5:12.1993).

Somjen GG, Aitken PG, Balestrino M, Herreras O, Kawasaki K (Spreading depression-like depolarization and selective vulnerability of neurons. A brief review. Stroke 21:III179-III183.1990).

Thenuwara K, Todd MM, Brian JE, Jr. (Effect of mannitol and furosemide on plasma osmolality and brain water. Anesthesiology 96:416-421.2002).

Fasudil (a Rho Kinase Inhibitor) Specifically Increases Cerebral Blood Flow in Area of Vasospasm After Subarachnoid Hemorrhage

Masato Shibuya, Kenko Meda and Akira Ikeda
Department of Neurosurgery, Chukyo Hospital, Nagoya, Japan

1. Introduction

Subarachnoid hemorrhage due to a rupture of cerebral aneurysm is a severe disease with morbidity and mortality. Although, if patients' conditions are fair before surgery, they are rather safely operated by either clipping or coiling, vasospasm remains as a major complication of this disease. There are still many patients who suffer from vasospasm causing neurological deficits. Both strong vasoconstriction and inflammation are involved in the pathphysiological mechanism of vasospasm. In 1992 we had reported specific effects of a vasodilating drug "fasudil" in the treatment of vasospasm, but mechanisms how fasudil ameliorated vasospasm had not been clearly understood as it is today.

RhoA/Rho kinase had been found in 1996 and was revealed to act as molecular on-off switches that control multiple signaling pathways. Upregulated Rho kinase is known to be involved in various diseases from vascular disease to cancer. In cerebral vasospasm, upregulated Rho kinase was found to be involved in many aspects, such as increased calcium sensitivity, reduced production of nitric oxide, migration of inflammatory cells and their production of superoxide anions and increased blood viscosity. Interestingly, fasudil was found to specifically increase cerebral blood flow in the area with vasospasm. In the present paper pathophysiological mechanism of vasospasm and effects of fasudil are reviewed and mechanisms why fasudil increases cerebral blood flow in the area with vasospasm without so much changing that of normal flow area will be discussed.

2. Cerebral vasospasm following subarachnoid hemorrhage

Cerebral infarction due to delayed vasospasm is still the leading cause of a poor postoperative outcome of patients with a ruptured cerebral aneurysm especially if we consider deficits in higher neurological functions such as cognitive functions. Several days after a subarachnoid hemorrhage (SAH), blood vessels begin to be contracted by substances eluted from the blood clot such as oxyhemoglobin, endothelin, amines and many other chemical substances. Most of the patients show contraction of the blood vessels (angiographic spasm). In about one third of the patients, signs of neurological deficits appear (symptomatic spasm) on an average of day 7 after the hemorrhage (Bederson et al., 2009, Shibuya et al., 1992). Patients may even die of severe spasm, especially due to vasospasm of arteries supplying basal part of the brain: hypothalamus and brainstem. A representative case of a patient with severe vasospasm is shown in Fig. 1.

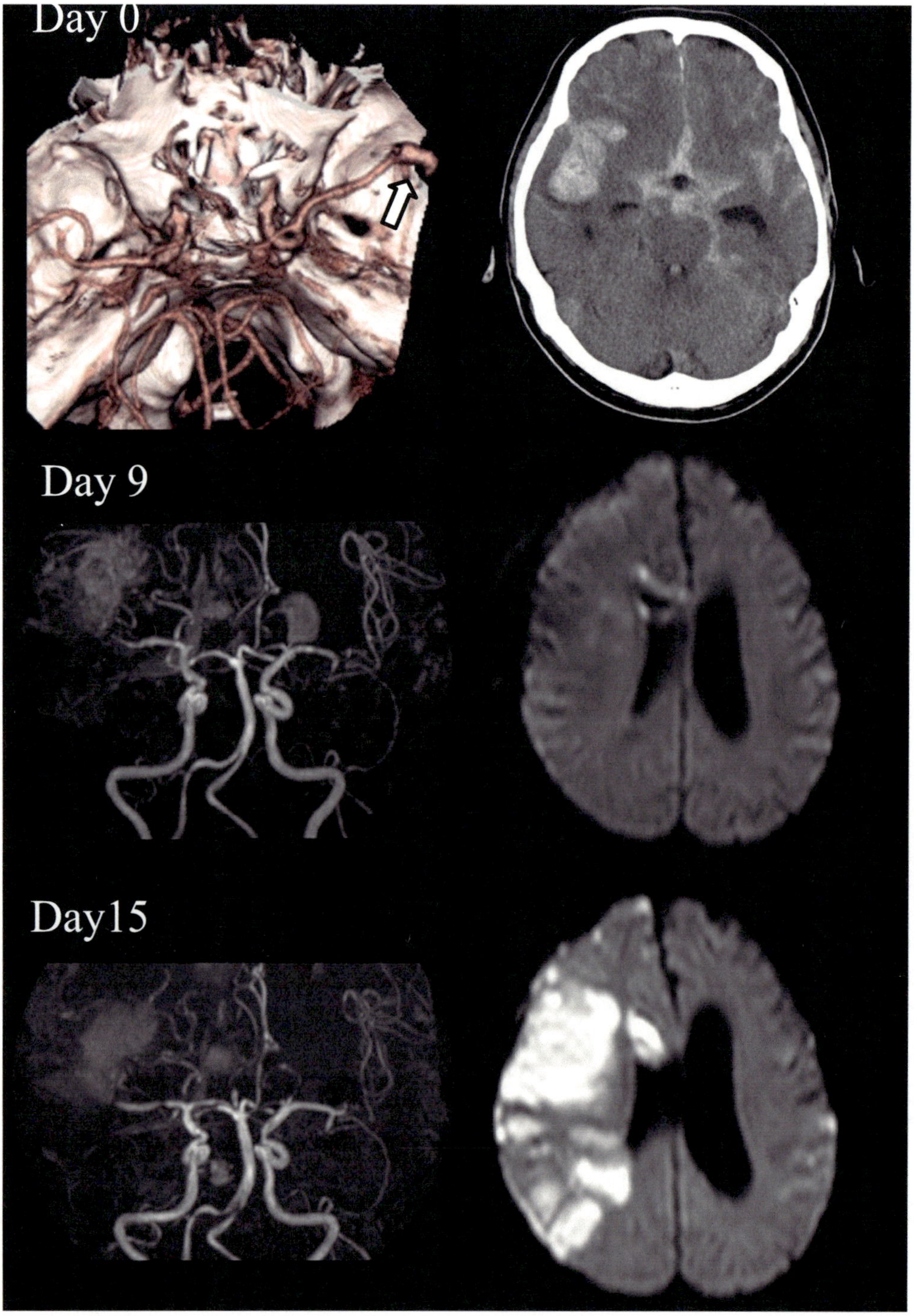

Fig. 1. Representative case of a patient with severe vasospasm.
Patient is a 70y/o male with a past history of prostatic cancer, hypertension and diabetes mellitus. He had a sudden onset of severe headache and lost consciousness two times at

home. He was slightly drowsy and disoriented (Hunt & Hess grade III) with mild weakness in the left arm and leg. A head computed tomography (CT) (upper right) showed a diffuse subarachnoid hemorrhage and a large hematoma in the right Sylvian fissure. A 3-D CT angiogram (upper left) showed a 10mm long aneurysm at the bifurcation of the right middle cerebral artery (MCA) (arrow). The aneurysm was clipped and subarachnoid space was washed with urokinase on the same day. He smoothly recovered from surgery and he was treated routinely postoperatively to prevent vasospasm with careful management of blood pressure, water and electrolytes balance. Fasudil 30mg (i.v./30min, t.i.d.) was started on day 1. His postoperative course was smooth with clear consciousness and a mild left hemiparesis.

A routine checkup, on day 9, by a magnetic resonance angiography (MRA, middle left) showed a moderately severe vasospasm in the right MCA, a segmental vasospasm in the left MCA and proximal portion of the right anterior cerebral artery (ACA). Diffusion weighted magnetic resonance image (DWI) showed no abnormality (middle right). His blood pressure was elevated with dopamine and daily dose of fasudil was increased to 60mg (i.v., t.i.d.) to prevent development of further neurological deficits.

However, the next day (day 10), his left hemiparesis deteriorated and he became drowsy. MRA on day 15 showed that vasospasm in bilateral MCAs progressed. Especially, distal branches of the right MCA were hardly seen. Segmental vasospasm appeared in the proximal portion of the right MCA, left ACA and distal portion of the vertebral arteries (lower left). However, vasospasm in the proximal portion of the right ACA improved. DWI on the same day showed an infarction in the right MCA territory (lower right). In spite of deterioration of vasospasm on MRI and MRA on day 15, he began to recover his consciousness the same day. Although he was communicable and could eat by himself, his left hemiplegia did not improve and he was discharged to a rehabilitation hospital. Now, two years after the onset, he is bed ridden and taken care at his home.

Vasospasm is not a simple contraction of blood vessels but it is complex pathological phenomena consisting of abnormal contraction of blood vessels which is not easily relaxed by usual calcium antagonists and inflammation. Tissue damage is seen in vascular endothelium and smooth muscle cells in the medial wall caused by free radicals released from inflammatory cells. Decreased production of nitric oxide (NO) is also contributing to both contraction and tissue damage. Rho kinase has been found to be deeply implicated in the pathophysiology of vasospasm (Miyagi et al., 2000; Sato et al., 2000) and use of a Rho kinase inhibitor: fasudil dramatically improved patients' outcome (Shibuya et al., 1992)

3. Effects of Fasudil, a Rho kinase inhibitor on cerebral vasospasm

Fasudil HCl: (hexahydro-1-5-isoquinolinesulfonyl)-1H-1.4-diazepine HCl, (also called HA1077, AT877, or Eril@) is originally considered to be an intracellular calcium antagonist. By experimental studies in dogs we had found that fasudil dilated spastic arteries without causing systemic hypotension, which could not been shown by any of the previously presented drugs (Takayasu et al., 1986). The effectiveness was also confirmed in patients by a double blind trial (Shibuya et al., 1992). Fasudil showed stronger brain protection from ischemic damage than dilatation of the spastic artery itself, suggesting its possible effects in patients with cerebral infarction as well. Fasudil is now routinely used in Japan for patients with SAH. Zhao et al. (2007) in China showed by a randomized trial that fasudil was significantly better for vasospasm than nimodipine which was most commonly used in the western countries.

After Rho kinase was found (Kimura et al., 1996), it became clear that upregulated Rho kinase worked unfavorably to the host in many vascular diseases and effects of fasudil on vasospasm mainly depended on its inhibition of Rho kinase. Fasudil was found to inhibit Rho kinase most strongly than any other protein kinases such as protein kinases C, A, and G (Hidaka et al., 2005). Fasudil is metabolized in human to hydroxyfasudil. Both fasudil and hydroxyfasudil are strong inhibitors of Rho kinase, however biological half-life of fasudil and hydroxyfasudil after an intravenous infusion of fasudil in human are 18 min and 6 hours, respectively. Thus major effect is considered to depend on hydroxyfasudil rather than fasudil itself.

Upregulated Rho kinase inhibits relaxation of the contracted blood vessels by inhibiting dephosphorylation of phosphorylated myosin light chain (MLC) either directly or through inhibition of endothelial NO synthase (eNOS). In an experimental model of vasospasm induced by $PGF_2\alpha$, double phosphorylation of MLC, at Thr18 in addition to Ser19, was found. This is considered to be the underlying mechanism of the strong contraction or increased sensitivity to Ca^{++}. Furthermore, fasudil was found to inhibit the second (pathological) phosphorylation at Thr18 of MLC more strongly (IC50: 0.3uM) than the first phosphorylation at Ser19 (IC50: 3uM) (Seto et al., 1991).

4. Fasudil specifically increases rCBF in area with vasospasm

Specific effect of fasudil on cerebral vasospasm has been suggested to depend on its inhibition of the abnormal phosphorylation of MLC. On the other hand, under normal situation, increased intracellular calcium phosphorylates MLC by activating calmodulin and myosin light chain kinase (MLCK) which is relaxed by dephosphorylation of MLC by phosphatase.

In a two hemorrhage canine model of SAH, basilar artery diameter is decreased to about 60% on day 7. Intravenous administration of a calcium antagonist nicardipine (0.1mg/kg, i.v./30min) did not dilate the spastic basilar artery but caused systemic hypotension. While fasudil (HA1077) (0.5~3mg/kg, i.v. /30min) significantly dilated the spastic artery without causing hypotension (Takayasu et al., 1986). It can be explained by specific inhibition of Rho kinase by fasudil. In other words, fasudil dilated spastic artery more specifically than normal or non-spastic arteries.

Specific vasodilating effect of fasudil has been shown by measuring regional cerebral blood flow (rCBF). In patients who had been operated on their ruptured aneurysms, Ueda (2000) compared the effects of fasudil on rCBF using 99mTc-HMPAO with that of nicardipine. Nicardipine (2mg, i.v.) decreased BP and increased pulse rate. It decreased rCBF in the low flow (spastic) area (to -10%, $P<0.05$) without changing rCBF of the normal flow area, suggesting a loss of autoregulation in the spastic area. On the other hand, fasudil (15 mg, i.v.) increased rCBF in the low flow area by 16% ($P<0.05$) without changing that of normal flow area.

Using CT perfusion method in patients with SAH, Ono et al. (2005) have examined changes in the cerebral blood perfusion (CBP) by fasudil (30mg, i.v./30min) in both normal (>40ml/100g/min) and low flow (<40ml) regions due to vasospasm. The mean CBP in the low flow area (34.4±4.7ml) was significantly increased (to 41.0±8.2 ml, $P<0.05$, $n=43$), whereas the mean CBP of the normal flow region (51.8±7.6ml) did not change after fasudil

(50.4±8.4ml, n=125). We also have shown by using 99mTc-HMPAO that fasudil (30-60mg/i.v./30 min) significantly increased rCBF in the operated side of the brain in patients showing ischemic signs of vasospasm. Such difference was not found in patients without vasospasm (Shibuya et al., 2008).

These data suggest that upregulated Rho kinase is involved in the decrease of rCBF in patients with vasospasm which was specifically improved by a Rho kinase inhibitor fasudil. On the other hand calcium antagonist dilated normal arteries more than spastic arteries leading to a systemic hypotension and a steal phenomenon, a steal of blood from a spastic region to a normal region.

5. Effects of fasudil on cerebral infarction

Rho kinase is also up-regulated in patients with cerebral infarction, both in ischemic brain and in migrated WBCs. It is involved in many aspects of ischemic brain damage caused by migration of inflammatory cells to the ischemic site and their production of free radicals by activated NADPH oxidase. Rho kinase elevates blood viscosity by producing the tissue factor (also called factor III, thrombokinase, or CD142) which triggers the coagulation cascade. Blood viscosity is also elevated by reduced plasticity of RBCs due to polymerization of actin fibers which is induced by activated Rho kinase and protein kinase C (Arai et al., 1993; Brabeck et al., 2003; Feske et al., 2009; Satoh et al., 2010). Effectiveness of fasudil on cerebral infarction has been shown both by experimental (Tsuchiya et al., 1993) and clinical studies (Shibuya et al., 2005). After specific effects of fasudil on cerebral vasospasm and infarction had been shown, it has been tried and showed effectiveness in various kinds of vascular diseases such as coronary ischemia, glaucoma, pulmonary hypertension, chronic kidney disease and so on (Dong et al., 2010, Schmandke et al., 2007).

6. Discussion

6.1 Rho kinase

Rho kinase is the immediate downstream target of RhoA, a small GTP binding protein belonging to Ras, Rho, Rab and Ran subfamilies and acts as molecular on-off switches that control multiple signaling pathways. Inactive form of Rho-GDP is activated by guanine nucleotide exchange factors (GEFs) and Guanine dissociation inhibitors (GDIs) through stimulation by lysophosphatidic acid (LPA) and sphyngosine-1-phosphate (S1P). Active form (GTP and membrane-bound) RhoA is inactivated by GTPase activating proteins (GAPs) to GDP bound form in cytosole. Rho kinase is a serine-threonine protein kinase that are involved in diverse cellular functions including vascular smooth muscle cell (SMC) contraction such as cerebral and coronary vasospasm, atherosclerosis, actin cytoskelton arrangement, cell adhesion, motility and gene expression (Noma et al., 2006).

6.2 Upregulated Rho kinase and increased sensitivity to calcium in vasospasm

Miyagi et al. (2000) showed that RhoA and mRNA of Rho kinase was increased in the basilar artery of SAH rats. Sato et al. (2000) clearly showed, in a two hemorrhage dog model, that Rho kinase was up-regulated with the decrease in basilar artery diameter and with the increase of phosphorylation of myosin binding subunit (MBS) of myosin phosphatase of the basilar artery, all of which were inhibited by a Rho kinase inhibitor Y27632. Activated Rho kinase inhibits MLC phosphatase by phosphorylating its component MBS at Thr697 (Feng et al., 1999) either directly or through activation of protein kinase C (PKC). PKC activated protein kinase C-potentiated inhibitory protein-17 (CPI-17) by phosphorylating at Thr38 (Koyama et al., 2000). In vasospastic condition, contraction force is increased without changes in intracellular concentration of Ca^{++}. Thus double (sometimes triple) phosphorylation of MLC by upregulated Rho kinase is considered to be the mechanism of so called increased sensitivity to Ca^{++}.

6.3 Involvement of inflammation in vasospasm

Inflammatory cells migrate to vasospasm or infarction sites and cause tissue injury by producing free radicals. When human WBCs were incubated in a Boyden chamber, WBCs migrated through a millipore filter by adding a chemoattractant such as formyl-methionyl-leucyl-phenylalanine (fMLP) to one side of the chamber. This migration was dose dependently inhibited by fasudil (Satoh et al., 1999). When WBCs were incubated with phorbol myristate acetate (PMA), a protein kinase C activator, they produced superoxide anion (O_2^{-}) by NADPH oxidase, which also was dose dependently inhibited by fasudil (Arai et al., 1993). Free radicals such as O_2^- are known to cause structural damage in endothelial cells and SMCs, leading to a decreased production of nitric oxide (NO) by endothelial NO synthase (eNOS).

6.4 Inhibition of NO synthase (eNOS) by Rho kinase

Nitric oxide (NO) plays an important role in the regulation of vascular tone, inhibition of platelet aggregation, suppression of SMC proliferation and prevention of leukocyte recruitment to the vessel wall. Activity of eNOS is controlled by a variety of signals surrounding blood vessels. Laminar shear stress, O_2 tension and transforming growth factor (TGF)β1 can regulate eNOS expression at the transcriptional level. Chronic hypoxia, tissue necrosis factor (TNF)α, thrombin, oxidized low density lipoprotein (LDL) and cellular proliferation are known to regulate eNOS expression at postscriptional level. Shear stress and vascular endothelial growth factor (VEGF) rapidly activated eNOS by phosphorylating at Ser1177. Hypoxia is known to upregulate Rho kinase which inhibits eNOS by phosphorylating at Thr495 (Flemming et al., 2001; Noma et al., 2006; Sugimoto et al., 2007). On the other hand, inhibition of Rho kinase by hydroxyfasudil increased phosphorylation of protein kinase Akt Ser473 and production of NO (Wolfrum et al., 2004). NO relaxes blood vessels by activating guanylate cyclase (which produced cyclic GMP) and protein kinase G, which activated MLC phosphatase by phosphorylating its component MBS at Ser695 (Nakamura & Ikebe, 2007, see also Fig. 2).

Pulmonary hypertension is a fatal disease in which eNOS activity is decreased. When human vascular endothelium was incuvated under hypoxic state of 3% O_2, both expression of mRNA of eNOS and eNOS activity were suppressed. The suppression was ameliorated by Rho kinase inhibitors, botulinus C3 transferase and fasudil (Takemoto et al., 2002). Actually, fasudil showed good results in patients with pulmonary hypertension (Fukumoto et al., 2005).

6.5 Increased blood viscosity in cerebral vasospasm and infarction

Blood viscosity is elevated in patients with acute cerebral infarction (Coull et al., 1991). However, it is not clear if this reflects a pre-existing risk factor or an acute phase response to the stroke itself or both. In rats model of temporary ischemia, by passing a nylon thread through the carotid artery for one hour and then removed, blood viscosity measured 24 hours later by a cone-plated discometer (at 37.5 rpm), was elevated from a control of 5.31 centipoise (cP) to 6.05 cP. Fasudil (1~10mg/kg) dose dependently inhibited the elevation of blood viscosity (Hitomi et al., 2000). Both production of the tissue factor (Zhang et al., 2007) and Rho kinase-activated polymerization of f-actin are considered to be involved in the increase of blood viscosity which were ameliorated by fasudil (Feske et al., 2009, Nagata et al., 20022Satoh et al., 2010).

RhoA/Rho kinase pathway has been shown to be involved in many other vascular diseases such as angiogenesis, atherosclerosis, cerebral and coronary spasm and infarction, glomerulosclerosis, hypertension, ischemia-reperfusion injury, neointimal proliferation, bronchial asthma, glaucoma and so on. Our current concepts about the Rho-kinase related mechanisms and effects of a Rho kinase inhibitor fasudil in cerebral vasospasm and infarction are shown in Fig. 2.

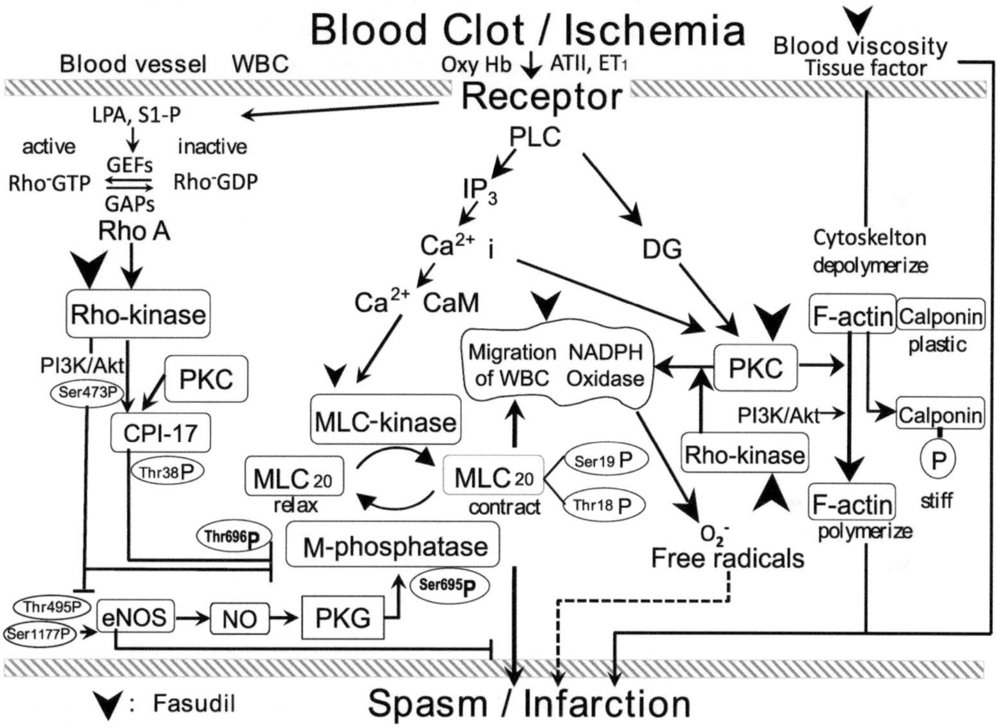

Fig. 2. Rho kinase related mechanisms and effects of fasudil in cerebral vasospasm and infarction

Chemical ligands eluted from subarachnoid blood clot or from ischemic brain such as oxyhemoglobin, angiotensin II and endothelin increase intracellular lysophosphatidic acid (LPA) and sphyngosine-1-phosphate (S1-P) which activate RhoA through activation of guanine nucleotide exchange factors (GEFs) from an inactive GDP-Rho in the cytosole to an active and membrane bound GTP-Rho. Activated Rho kinase contracts blood vessels by inhibiting myosin light chain (MLC) phosphatase by phosphorylating its component myosin binding subunit (MBS) at Thr696 through activation of protein kinase C-potentiated inhibitory protein-17 (CPI-17). Rho kinase also inhibits relaxation of contracted blood vessels by inhibiting endothelial nitric oxide synthase (eNOS) through inhibition of phosphatidylinositol-3kinase (PI3K)/protein kinase Akt. On the other hand, eNOS is activated by dephosphorylation at Thr495 or phosphorylation at Ser1177 when Rho kinase is inhibited. NO relaxes blood vessels by activating guanylate cyclase and protein kinase G (PKG). PKG activates MLC phosphatase by phosphorylating its component myosin binding subunit (MBS) at Ser695.

On the other hand, migration of inflammatory cells like WBCs and their production of free radicals by NADPH oxidase are stimulated by upregulated Rho kinase and protein kinase C. Rho kinase also increases blood viscosity by producing the tissue factor which triggers the coagulation cascade and also by decreasing plasticity of RBCs. Plasticity of RBCs is decreased when f-actin, consisting cytoskeleton, is polymerized by Rho kinase and protein kinase C.

These adverse phenomena: abnormal contraction of blood vessels, migration of inflammatory cells and their production of free radicals, increase of blood viscosity had all been ameliorated by a Rho kinase inhibitor fasudil which showed in turn that upregulated Rho kinase is involved in each of these sites (see text for references). Arrow head indicates acting points of fasudil.

7. Conclusion

Upregulated Rho kinase is deeply implicated in the complex mechanisms of delayed cerebral vasospasm after a subarachnoid hemorrhage, in both vasoconstriction and inflammation. Double phosphorylation of myosin light chain leading to pathological contraction, suppression of eNOS, production of free radicals are all induced by upregulated Rho kinase. Fasudil improved these situations by mainly inhibiting upregulated Rho kinase, which can explain why fasudil specifically increased cerebral blood flow in the area with vasospasm.

8. References

Arai, M., Sasaki, Y. & Nozawa, R. (1993) Inhibition by the protein kinase inhibitor HA1077 of the activation of NADPH oxidase in human neutrophils. *Biochem Pharmacol* 46:1487-1490

Bederson, J.B., Connolly, E.S.Jr, Batjer, H.H. et al. (2009) American Heart Association. Guidelines for the management of aneurysmal subarachnoid hemorrhage. Stroke 40:994-1025

Brabeck, C., Mittelbronn, M., Bekure, K. et al. (2003) Effect of cerebral infarctions on regional RhoA and RhoB expression. *Arch Neurol* 60:1245-1249

Coull, B.M., Beamer, N., de Garmo, P. et al. (1991) Chronic blood hyperviscosity in subjects with acute stroke, transient ischemic attack, and risk factors for stroke. *Stroke* 22:162-168

Dong, M., Yan, B.P., Liao J.K. et al. (2010) Rho-kinase inhibition: a novel therapeutic target for the treatment of cardiovascular diseases. Drug Discovery Today 15:622-629.

Feng, J., Ito, M., Ichikawa, K. et al. (1999) Inhibitory phosphorylation site for rho-associated kinase on smooth muscle myosin phosphatase. *J Biol Chem* 274:3744-3752

Feske, S.K., Sorond, F.A., Henderson, G.V. et al. (2009) Increased leukocyte ROCK activity in patients after ischemic attack. *Brain Res* 1257:89-93

Flemming, I., Fisslthaler, B., Dimmeler, S. et al. (2001) Phosphorylation of Thr 495 regulates Ca2+/calmodulin-dependent endothelial nitric oxide synthase activity. *Circ Res* 88:E68-E75.

Fukumoto, Y., Matoba, T., Ito, A. et al. (2005) Acute vasodilator effects of a Rho-kinase inhibitor fasudil in patients with severe pulmonary hypertension. *Heart* 91:391-392

Hidaka, H., Shibuya, M., Suzuki, Y. et al. (2005) Isoquinolinesulfonamide: A specific inhibitor of Rho-kinase and the clinical aspect of anti-Rho-kinase therapy. *HEP* 167:411-432

Hitomi, A., Satoh, S., Ikegaki, I. et al. (2000) Hemorrheological abnormalities in experimental cerebral ischemia and effects of protein kinase inhibitor on blood fluidity. *Life Sci* 67:1929-1939

Kimura, K., Ito, M., Amano, M. et al. (1996) Regulation of myosin phosphatase by Rho and Rho-associated kinase (Rho-kinase). *Science* 273:245-258

Koyama, M., Ito, M., Feng, J. et al. (2000) Phosphorylation of CPI-17, an inhibitory phosphoprotein of smooth muscle myosin phosphatase, by rho-kinse. *FEBS Let* 475:197-200

Miyagi, Y., Carpenter, R.C., Meguro, T. et al. (2000) Upregulation of RhoA and Rho kinase RNAs in the basilar artery of a rat model of subarachnoid hemorrhage. *J Neurosurg* 93:471-476

Nagata, K., Ishibashi, T., Sakamoto, T. et al. (2002) Rho/Rho-kinase is involved in the synthesis of tissue factor in human monocytes. *Atherosclerosis* 163:39-47

Nakamura, K. & Ikebe, M. (2007) cGMP-dependent relaxation of smooth muscle is coupled with the change in the phosphorylation of myosin phosphatase. *Circ Res* 101: 712-722

Noma, K., Oyama, N. & Liao, J.K. (2006) Physiological role of ROCKs in the cardiovascular system. *Am J physiol* 290:C661-C668

Ono, K., Shirotani, T., Yuba, K. et al. (2005) Cerebral circulation dynamics following fasudil intravenous infusion: a CT perfusion study. *Brain Nerve (Tokyo)* 57:779-783.

Sato, M., Tani, E., Fujikawa, H. et al. (2000) Involvement of Rho kinase mediated phosphorylation of myosin light chain in enhancement of cerebral vasospasm. *Circ Res* 87:195-200

Satoh, S., Hitomi, A., Ikegaki, I. et al. (2010) Amelioration of endothelial damage /dysfunction is a possible mechanism for neuroprotecive effects of Rho-kinase inhibitors against ischemic brain damage. *Brain Res Bull* 81:191-195

Satoh, S., Kobayashi, T., Hitomi, A. et al. (1999) Inhibition of neutrophil migration by a protein kinase inhibitor for the treatment of ischemic brain infarction. *Jpn J Pharmacol* 80:41-48

Schmandke, A., Schmandke, A. & Strittmatter, S.M. (2007) ROCK and Rho: Biochemistry and neuronal functions of Rho-associated protein kinases. Neuroscientist 13:454-469.

Seto, M., Sasaki, Y., Sasaki, Y. et al. (1991) Effect of HA1077, a protein kinase inhibitor, on myosin phosphorylation and a tension in smooth muscle. *Eur J Pharmacol 195:267-272*

Shibuya, M., Suzuki, Y., Sugita, K. et al. (1992) Effect of AT877 on cerebral vasospasm after aneurysmal subarachnoid hemorrhage. *J Neurosurg* 76: 571-577

Shibuya, M., Hirai, S, Seto, M. et al. (2005) Effects of fasudil in ischemic stroke: results of a prospective placebo-controlled double blind trial. *J Neurol Sci* 238:31-39

Shibuya, M, Ikeda, A., Ohsuka, K. et al. (2008) Fasudil (a rho kinase inhibitor) may specifically increase rCBF in spastic area. *Acta Neurochir Suppl* 104:275-278

Sugimoto, M., Nakayama, M., Gotoh, T.M. et al. (2007) Rho-kinase phosphorylates eNOS at threonine 495 in endothelial cells. *BBRC* 361:462-467

Takayasu, M., Suzuki, Y., Shibuya, M. et al. (1986) The effects of HA compound calcium antagonists on delayed cerebral vasospasm in dogs. *J Neurosurg* 65:80-85

Takemoto, M., Sun, J., Hiroki, J. et al. (2002) Rho-kinase mediates hypoxia-induced downregulation of endothelial nitric oxide synthase. *Circulation* 106:57-62

Tsuchiya, T., Sako, K., Yonemasu, Y. et al. (1993) The effects of HA1077, a novel protein kinase inhibitor, on reductions of cerebral blood flow and glucose metabolism following acute and/or chronic bilateral carotid ligation in Wistar rats. *Exp Brain Res* 97:233-238

Ueda, T. (2000) Effect on increase of cerebral blood flow with cerebral vasospasm by fasudil hydrochloride. *Med Pharmacy (Tokyo)* 42:753-759.

Wolfrum, S., Dendorfer, A., Rikitake, Y. et al (2004) Inhibition of Rho-kinase leads to rapid activation of phosphatidylinositol 3 kinase/protein kinase Akt and cardiovascular protection. *Atheroscler thromb Vasc Biol* 24:1842-1847

Zhao, J., Zhou, D., Guo, J. et al. (2006) Effect of fasudil hydrochloride, a protein kinase inhibitor, on cerebral vasospasm after aneurysmal subarachnoid hemorrhage. Results of a randomized trial of fasudil hydrochloride versus nimodipine. *Neurol Med Chir (Tokyo)* 46:421-428

Zhang, X.P., Hu, Y., Hong, M., et al., (2007) Plasma thrombomodulin, fibrinogen, and activity of tissue factor as risk factors for acute cerebral infarction. *Am J Clin Pathol* 128:287-292

19

Endogenous Agents That Contribute to Generate or Prevent Ischemic Damage

Ornella Piazza[1] and Giuliana Scarpati[2]
[1]*Anestesiologia e Rianimazione, Università Degli Studi di Salerno*
[2]*Anestesiologia e Rianimazione, Università Degli Studi di Napoli Federico II*
Italy

1. Introduction

From single to multicellular organisms, protective mechanisms have evolved against endogenous and exogenous noxious stimuli. Over the past decades numerous signaling pathways by which the brain senses and reacts to such insults as neurotoxins, substrate deprivation and inflammation have been discovered. Research on preconditioning is aimed at understanding endogenous neuroprotection to boost it or to supplement its effectors therapeutically once damage to the brain has occurred, such as after stroke or brain trauma. Another goal of establishing preconditioning protocols is to induce endogenous neuroprotection in anticipation of incipient brain damage. Currently several endogenous neuroprotectants are being investigated in controlled clinical trials. There is consensus that many of the neuroprotectants, which were highly effective in animal models of stroke, but failed in clinical trials, were unsuccessful because of side effects, which in many cases led to premature termination of the trial. Nowadays research aims to overcome this problem by developing compounds which induce, mimic, or boost endogenous protective responses and thus do not interfere with physiological neurotransmission. In the present review we will give a short overview on the signals, sensors, transducers, and effectors of endogenous neuroprotection. We will first focus on common mechanisms, on which pathways of endogenous neuroprotection converge. We will then discuss various applications of endogenous neuroprotectors and explore the prospects of endogenous neuroprotective therapeutic approaches.

2. Phisiopatology of cerebral ischemia

Development of stroke prophylaxis involves the understanding of the mechanisms of damage following cerebral ischemia and elucidation of the endogenous mechanisms that combat further brain injury (FIGURE 1).

The binding of glutamate to its receptors and the activation of voltage-gated $Ca2^{+}$ channels (VGCC) causes calcium to influx into the cell. Calcium is among the mediators that initiate the genomic response to cerebral ischemia. The superoxide dismutase (SOD) gene is upregulated to neutralize the reactive oxygen species (ROS). The generation of nitrous oxide (NO) in the neuron is cytotoxic. The interaction between antiapoptotic genes, such as Bcl-2, and proapoptotic genes, such as Bax, determines whether cytochrome c will be translocated from the mitochondria to the cytosol. In the cytosol, cytochrome c combines with Apaf-1 to activate the caspases. Proinflammatory cytokines, such as interleukin-1 (IL-1) and tumor necrosis factor-a (TNF-a), are generated. Survival pathways involving growth factors (GFs), immediate early genes (IEGs), and heat shock proteins (Hsps) are also stimulated. Ultimately, the activation of these genetic pathways determines the fate of the ischemic cell.

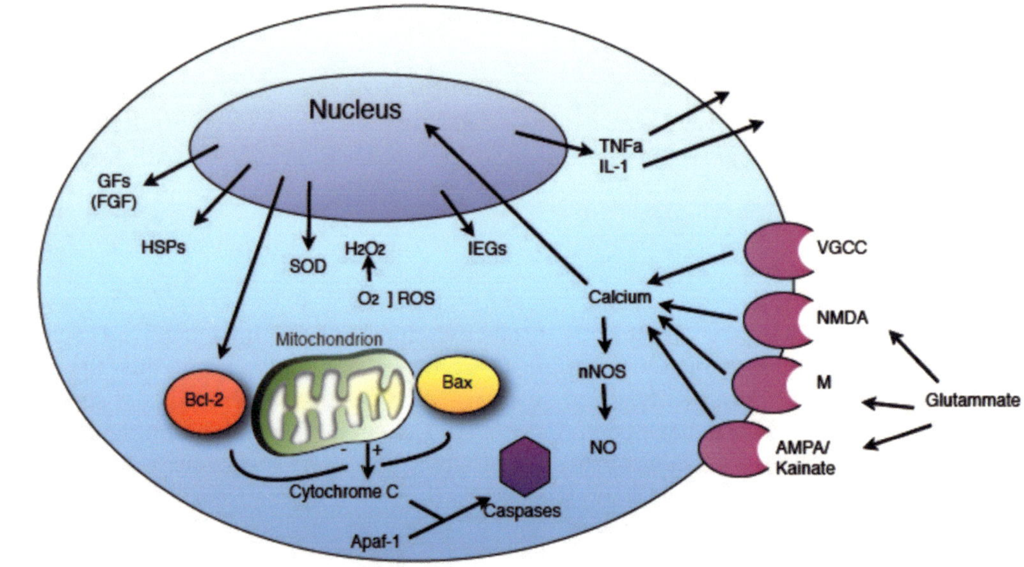

Fig. 1. Phisiopatology of cerebral ischemia

2.1 Excitotoxicity and calcium

Although the brain represents only 2% of body weight, it uses an astonishing 20% of the body's oxygen in adults. The innumerable cells of the brain require an almost continuous flow of oxygen and glucose, making them exquisitely sensitive to any interruption in energy supply. Energy depletion and reduced levels of adenosine triphosphate initiate a series of events that cause cells to die. Glutamate, the main excitatory neurotransmitter of the central nervous system, is a trigger of neuronal loss during stroke. During ischemia, an excess of glutamate is released into the extracellular space. The mechanism to clear glutamate is energy dependent; glutamate quickly builds to toxic levels when energy is depleted. Glutamate causes ionic shifts; Na^+ enters the cell and K^+ exits. Water passively follows the influx of Na^+ leading to cellular swelling and edema. The membrane potential is lost and the cell depolarizes. In the ischemic core, cells undergo anoxic depolarization and never repolarize. However, cells in the penumbra initially retain the ability to repolarize so that they may depolarize again. As cells in the penumbra undergo these peri-infarct depolarizations the energy supply and ionic homeostasis are further compromised, resulting in an increase in the size of the ischemic lesion. Glutamate activates three main families of receptors: N-methyl-d-aspartate (NMDA), a-amino-3-hydroxy-5 methylisoxazole/kainate, and metabotropic glutamate receptors. Activation of these receptors leads to a buildup of Ca^{2+} within the cell. Ischemia therefore triggers glutamate receptor-mediated excitotoxicity and Ca^{2+} overload within the cell. Originally, neuronal death from excitotoxicity was believed to result from depletion of cellular energy stores from overexcited neurons. However, the influx of Ca^{2+} seems to be the major pathogenic event contributing to cell death. This translocation of Ca^{2+} is accomplished through glutamate, particularly through the NMDA receptor, as well as through voltage-gated Ca^{2+} channels that open after cell depolarization. Calcium channel antagonists have displayed neural protection in animal models but have not shown benefit in clinical trials partially because they were administered too late after stroke onset or in insufficient quantity. However, it appears that Ca^{2+} influx into the cell is only the initial step in a complex biochemical cascade.

2.2 Free radicals

Reactive oxygen species are produced after the induction of ischemia and upon reperfusion. The oxidative stress produced by the reactive oxygen species destroys the cell through lipid peroxidation, protein oxidation, and DNA damage. Certain endogenous antioxidants scavenge and neutralize the reactive oxygen species. In particular, the antioxidant superoxide dismutase detoxifies the superoxide ($O2^-$) free radical by converting it to hydrogen peroxide (H2O2). Glutathione peroxidase can then convert H2O2 into oxygen and water. During times of oxidative stress, the superoxide dismutase gene is upregulated. Neural protection strategies have included both the administration of exogenous superoxide dismutase and manipulation of the superoxide dismutase gene family. Nitric oxide (NO) is another free radical that is increased during ischemia due to an increase in intracellular Ca^{2+}. The formation of NO is catalyzed by the enzyme NO synthase (NOS). NOS has several isoforms—a neuronal type (nNOS) located in neurons and an endothelial type (eNOS) in the vascular endothelium. NO is also generated in microglia, astrocytes and invading macrophages after the induction of an inducible isoform (iNOS). Initially after ischemia, the formation of NO in the vascular endothelium by eNOS may improve CBF through vasodilatation offering neuroprotection. However, synthesis of NO by nNOS and iNOS is cytotoxic, leading to an inhibition of mitochondrial respiration, glycolysis, and DNA synthesis. Because of the dual role of NO in cerebral ischemia, neuronal protection strategies need to target the specific isoform of NOS. For instance, deletion of the nNOS or iNOS gene in animal models has provided neuronal protection.

2.3 Apoptosis

After an ischemic event, cells in the penumbra may initiate a program of autodestruction known as apoptosis. Apoptosis occurs in the developing brain. More than half of progenitor neurons undergo this process of programmed cell death while forming neural circuits. During ischemia, cells in the ischemic core undergo necrosis while cells in the ischemic penumbra may actually self destruct through this process of apoptosis. The mitochondria is regarded as the apoptotic headquarters of the cell. One of the key events in apoptosis is the translocation of cytochrome c from the intermembrane of the mitochondria into the cytosol. In the cytosol, cytochrome c combines then with apoptotic activating factor (Apaf-1) to activate a set of proteases known as caspases. These caspases actually dismantle the cell during apoptosis. A family of death-promoting genes, known as the Bcl-2 family, determines whether a cell will undergo apoptosis. The Bcl-2 gene is antiapoptotic and prevents the translocation of cytochrome c and activation of caspases. However, the Bax gene (one of the members of the Bcl-2 family) is proapoptotic, facilitating the translocation of cytochrome c and apoptosis. During ischemia, proapoptotic genes such as Bax are activated, resulting in the autodestruction of the cell. Thus, neuronal protection may be gained through blocking these death-promoting genes. Other strategies include giving caspase antagonists or preventing the translocation of cytochrome c from the mitochondria. Preventing apoptosis in the penumbra is another effective technique in animal models for neuronal protection.

2.4 Inflammation

The inflammatory response may be an important part of the ischemic cascade. Soon after the onset of stroke, leukocytes invade the ischemic zone. The mechanisms by which these inflammatory cells contribute to the evolution of ischemia include microvascular occlusion by adherence to the endothelium, producing cytotoxic enzymes and generating injurious free radicals. Cytokines are intracellular messengers that mediate the recruitment of the leukocytes and the induction of adhesion molecules. The two main proinflammatory cytokines are interleukin-1 (IL-1) and tumor necrosis factor-a (TNF-a). The adhesion molecules that facilitate the movement of leukocytes along the surface of the endothelium are the E and P selectins, whereas intracellular adhesion molecules attach the leukocytes to the endothelium so that they may leave the vascular space and enter the site of injury. Research has been focusing on the manipulation of these proinflammatory cytokines and adhesion molecules to provide neuronal protection.

2.4.1 Survival pathways

The cytokines that are activated during ischemia also include growth factors that actually promote neuronal survival and, in some cases, neuronal outgrowth and synapse formation. Fibroblast growth factor is the most extensively studied growth factor. Although the exact mechanism of neuroprotection of fibroblast growth factor is not fully understood, it includes upregulation of free radical scavenging enzymes and Ca^{2+} binding proteins, downregulation of the NMDA receptor and vasodilatation. The administration of growth factors has provided cerebral protection in animal models. Because they exert both protective and trophic influences on neurons, growth factors remain an exciting prospect in drug development for stroke. Other gene families and proteins are activated during ischemia. Immediate early genes, such as those of the Fos and Jun families, are activated soon after ischemia. It is believed that Ca^{2+} and reactive oxygen species are involved in the expression of immediate early genes. Although the exact role of each of the immediate early genes in ischemia is not yet understood, they are known to participate in apoptosis. Some immediate early genes may even afford neuronal protection. Ischemia also induces the expression of molecular chaperones known as heat shock proteins, which maintain protein function and assist in protein transport in response to injury. Increasing the expression of heat shock proteins to combat ischemia has been attempted.

3. Erythropoietin

The hormone erythropoietin (Epo) is a 165-amino acid (~30 kDa) glycoprotein that belongs to the cytokine type I superfamily. Originally, it was believed that the only role of Epo was the regulation of erythropoiesis. This role is attributed to the ability of Epo to inhibit programmed cell death (apoptosis) in erythroid cells and thus allow the maturation of erythrocytes. Since blood oxygen availability is the main regulator of erythropoiesis, hypoxia induces the gene expression of Epo in the kidney, the main site for Epo production, and in the liver (Cotena et al, 2008) in a negative feedback system between the kidney and the bone marrow. Research performed in the last decade has shown that Epo and its receptor (EpoR) are expressed in tissues other than those involved in erythropoiesis. These include the brain, the reproductive tract (Kobayashi et al, 2002; Marti et al, 1996; Masuda et al, 2000), the lung, the spleen, and the heart (Fandrey and Bunn, 1993). Accordingly, a novel cytoprotective effect of Epo was established in several organs. For example, Epo reduced injury and dysfunction after ischemia-reperfusion in the mouse kidney (Patel et al, 2004), and it showed protection in various myocardial ischemia models (Bogoyevith,2004; Cai et al, 2003; Parsa et al, 2003).

3.1 Epo/EpoR expression and regulation

Epo is mainly produced in the interstitial fibroblasts in the adult kidney and the hepatocytes of the fetus, whereas EpoR is normally expressed in erythroid precursor cells in the bone marrow (Marti, 2004). However, recent data have shown that the expression of Epo and its receptor, EpoR (both mRNA and protein), coincides in the same organ and even within the same cell. Epo and EpoR expression are widely distributed in the mammalian brain (Genc *et al*, 2004; Marti, 2004), albeit at lower levels than in the kidney (Brines and Cerami, 2005). Epo thus has to be added to the growing list of hematopoietic growth factors found to be expressed and act in the central nervous system (CNS).

3.2 Expression of Epo/EpoR in the brain

Epo/EpoR mRNA and protein were detected is several regions of the murine and primate brain, including cortex, hippocampus and amygdale, cerebellum, hypothalamus, and caudate nucleus (Siren et al, 2001). With respect to the type of cells in the brain that express Epo, astrocytes are the main source of Epo in the brain (Masuda et al, 1994). Moreover, it has been shown in vitro and in vivo that neurons express Epo (Bernaudin et al, 1999, 2000). Similarly, EpoR is expressed on neurons and astrocytes. In addition, primary cultures of human neurons, astrocytes, and microglia express EpoR mRNA (Nagai et al, 2001), and EpoR expression was also detected in primary cultures of rat oligodendrocytes (Genc et al, 2006). In addition to neurons, oligodendrocytes, and glial cells, a strong immunoreactivity for EpoR was found to be associated with brain vascular endothelial cells, showing that these cells also express EpoR (Brines et al, 2000). These findings implicate a broad spectrum of actions of Epo in the brain.

3.3 Regulation of Epo/EpoR expression

As mentioned above, Epo is upregulated in response to hypoxia. As, for many of the hypoxic adaptation processes in the body, the regulation of Epo expression is based on the transcriptional regulation of two hypoxia-inducible factors HIF-1 and HIF-2 (Wenger, 2000). HIFs are heterodimers composed of an α- and a β -subunit. Two forms of the oxygen-labile α exist, 1α and 2α. The α-subunit is stabilized under hypoxic conditions leading to the binding of the heterodimer HIF-1 or HIF-2 to specific DNA sequences located in the hypoxia response elements of target genes such as Epo or vascular endothelial growth factor (VEGF) (Wenger, 2002). Although HIF-1α was originally identified as the transcription factor responsible for Epo expression (Semenza et al, 1991), more recent evidence suggests that Epo is a target of HIF-2 (Eckardt and Kurtz, 2005). The stability of HIF-α is regulated by enzymatic hydroxylation of specific amino acids on the α subunit by a group of oxygenases (FIGURE 2). Under normoxic conditions, a specific prolyl hydroxylation within the oxygen-dependent degradation domain of HIF-α takes place. This prolyl hydroxylation allows binding of the von Hippel-Lindau protein (pVHL), leading to ubiquitylation and proteasomal degradation of the HIF-α subunit (Ivan et al, 2001; Jaakkola et al, 2001). The enzymes responsible for this hydroxylation are termed prolyl hydroxylase domain enzymes (PHD1-3) (Bruick and McKnight, 2001; Epstein et al, 2001) and are widely expressed. Furthermore, in the presence of oxygen, another hydroxylation reaction takes place on an asparaginyl group in the COOH-terminal transactivation domain of HIF-α, blocking its binding to the transcriptional coactivators (Lando et al, 2002a). This process is governed by a specific asparaginyl hydroxylase termed factor-inhibiting HIF (FIH) (Hewitson et al, 2002; Lando et al, 2002b). So, under normoxia, FIH and PHD(s) are active, leading to transcriptional inactivation and degradation of HIF-α, whereas under hypoxic conditions both enzymes are inactive. HIF is then stabilized and able to induce the expression of target genes, including Epo.

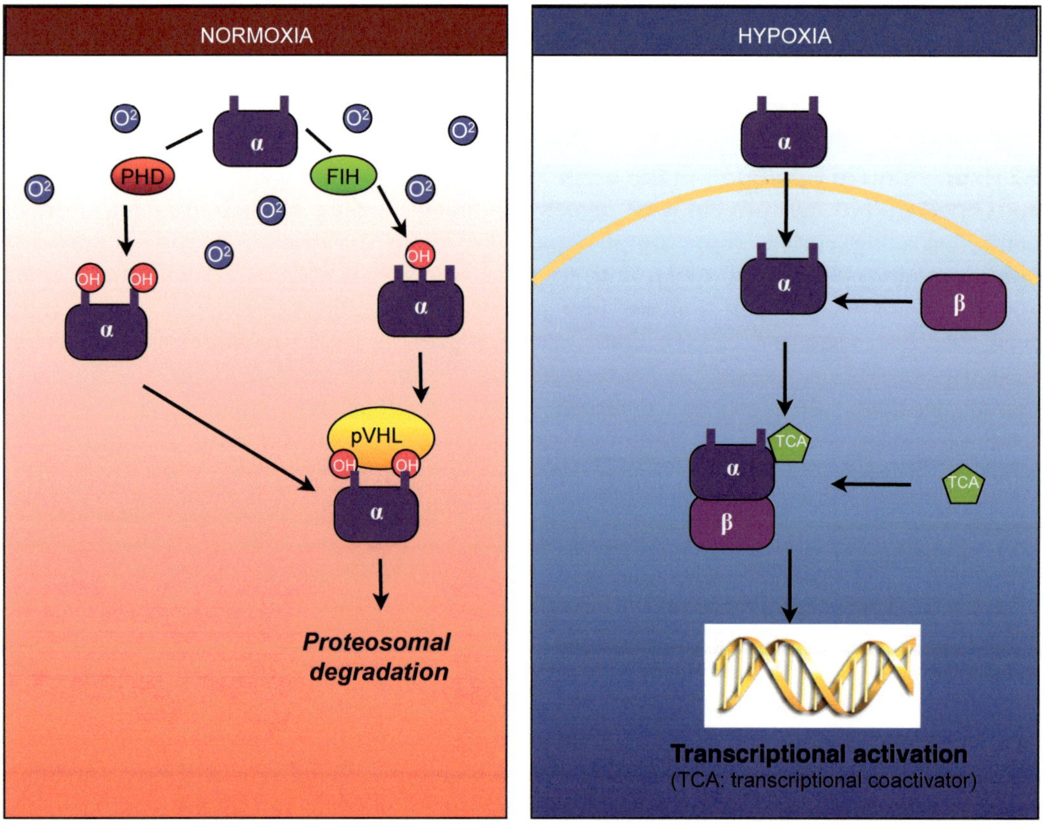

Fig. 2. Under normoxic conditions, specific prolyl hydroxylation within the oxygen-dependent degradation domain of HIF- α takes place. By contrast, under hypoxic conditions, FIH and PHD(s) are both inactive, and HIF is stabilized and able to induce the expression of target genes including Epo.

This basic mechanism of regulation seems to be of relevance for brain-expressed Epo, since in several experimental systems Epo was upregulated under hypoxic conditions in the brain of several mammalian species including mouse, rat, monkey, and human (Marti et al, 1996, 2000; Siren et al, 2001). However, depending on the severity of hypoxia, Epo mRNA level can increase 3- to 20-fold in the brain in contrast to 200-fold in the kidney. Moreover, although the increase in Epo expression in the kidney seems to be transient with a decrease after 8 h of continuous hypoxia, the level of Epo in the brain remains high for at least 24 h (Chikuma et al, 2000). This indicates a tissue-specific degree of regulation. Indeed, although HIF-1α levels in the kidney under systemic hypoxia peak after 1 h and again reach basal levels 4 h thereafter, in the brain the HIF-1α peak level is reached after only 5 h and returns to the basal level not before 12 h (Stroka et al, 2001). A possible explanation for the different time course in the brain might be an altered composition of the various PHD forms. It has to be noted that hypoxia is not the only factor activating HIF. Several studies have shown that pro-inflammatory mediators such as tumor necrosis factor-α (TNF-α), interleukin-1β (IL-1β) or lipopolysaccharide (LPS) induce the expression of HIF (Frede et al, 2007). With regard to the EpoR, it is regulated by pro-inflammatory cytokines (Nagai et al, 2001), such as TNF-α, IL-1β, and Epo itself (Chin et al, 2000). The role of hypoxia in the regulation of EpoR expression is controversial. Whereas we did not observe hypoxic induction of EpoR expression in neurons or astrocytes (Bernaudin et al, 2000), anemic stress induced EpoR expression in the brain of human EpoR transgenic mice (Chin et al, 2000). Moreover, in the same study, hypoxia increased EpoR expression in neuronal cells in vitro. The mechanism of hypoxic EpoR regulation remains to be established, since EpoR has not been identified as HIF target gene so far.

3.4 Epo signaling

Epo promotes cell survival through inhibiting apoptosis (FIGURE 3).

In erythroid cells, after binding of Epo to its receptor (EpoR), Janus tyrosine kinase 2 (JAK2) is phosphorylated and thus activated. This leads to engaging secondary signaling molecules such as signal transducer and activator of transcription 5 (STAT5), followed by the activation of Ras mitogen-activated protein kinase (MAPK), ERK-1/-2, and PI3K/Akt (22). Moreover, Epo induced the upregulation of the anti-apoptotic protein BCL-XL (Kilic et al, 2005). The functional significance of these signaling molecules in erythropoiesis is not absolutely clear though. For instance, whereas in one study STAT5 knockout adult mice were largely unaffected in their erythroid lineage (Teglund et al, 1998), in another study STAT5 knockout embryos suffered from severe anemia, showed a reduced number of erythroid progenitors cells, and had higher numbers of apoptotic cells (Socolovsky et al, 1999). Most of these pathways seem also to be functional in the brain (Brines and Cerami, 2005; Kilic et al, 2005). In vitro, inhibition of MAPK and PI3K blocked Epo-mediated protection of rat hippocampal neurons against hypoxia (Siren et al, 2001b). Moreover, using ERK-1/-2 and Akt inhibitors, Kilic et al. showed that activation of these proteins is essential for Epo-mediated neuroprotection in an animal model of focal cerebral ischemia. The role of STAT5 in Epo-induced neuroprotection is, however, controversial. STAT5 phosphorylation has been shown to occur in hippocampal CA1 neurons after transient global cerebral ischemia in rats (Zhang et al, 2007). Therefore, the authors concluded that STAT5 plays a role in Epo-mediated neuroprotection. However, in a very recent study, in an in vitro model of glutamate toxicity using hippocampal neuronal culture from STAT5 knockout mouse fetuses, STAT5 was not required for Epo-mediated neuroprotection (Byts et al, 2008). However, STAT5 was indispensable for the neurotrophic function of Epo. A unique pathway for the brain seems to be that activation of EpoR induces nuclear factor- κB (NF-κB) translocation into the nucleus and that this effect is important for Epo-mediated neuroprotection (Digicaylioglu and Lipton, 2001). Interestingly, Epo-induced NF-κB translocation was observed only in neuronal cells and not in astrocytes. Thus it appears likely that NF-κB, in the nucleus, induces the expression of neuroprotective and anti-apoptotic proteins. However, some differences exist between the signaling cascade activated by Epo in the CNS and in erythroid cells. For instance, in one study, BCL-XL has been found to be important in Epo-mediated protection of erythroid but not neuronal cells (Rischer et al, 2002). Additionally, Epo has been found to activate phospholipase C-gamma (PLCγ) (Marreo et al, 1998) and thus can directly influence neuronal activity (Koshimura et al, 1999) and neurotransmitter release (Kawakami et al, 2000) by modulating intracellular calcium concentrations in neurons.

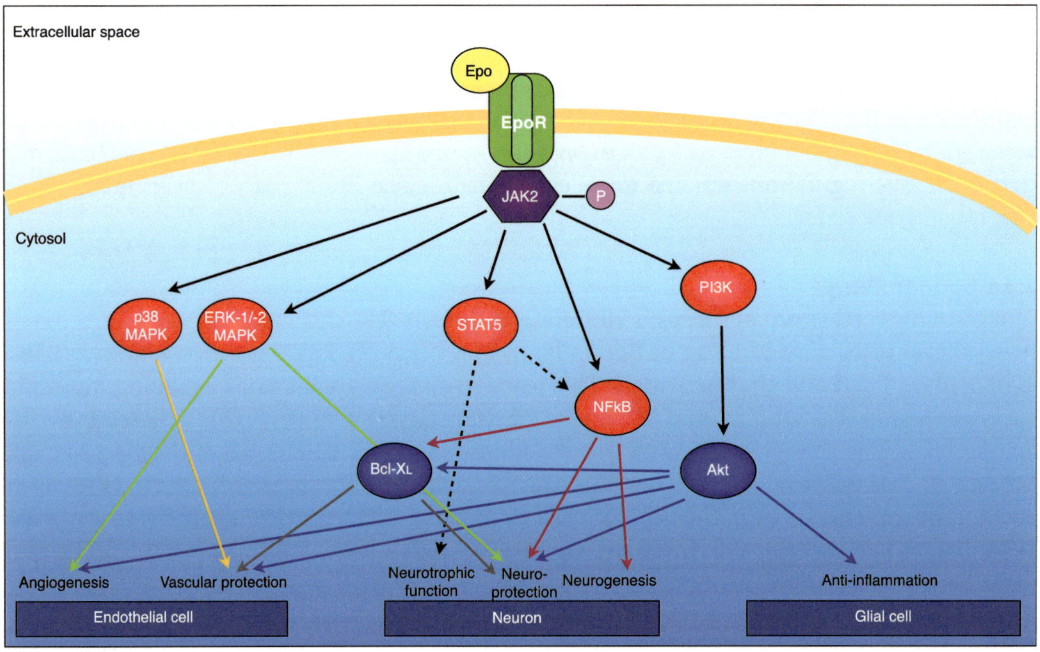

Fig. 3. Epo Signaling

3.5 Epo function in the CNS

For almost a century, Epo was thought to be involved in the process of erythropoiesis only. Through its antiapoptotic action, it enables committed erythroid progenitor cells to survive and mature (Jelkmann, 1992). However, during the last decade, it became evident that Epo is implicated in other processes such as neuroprotection, neurogenesis, and angiogenesis, and plays an important role as neurotrophic as well as immunomodulatory factor. The important role of Epo in the CNS is also evident from studies with EpoR knockout mice. As a result of EpoR deficiency, these mice show massive apoptosis and a reduction in the number of neuronal progenitor cells (Yu et al, 2002). A comprehensive description of the role of the Epo/EpoR system in development is found elsewhere (Arcasoy, 2008; Dame et al, 2001).

3.5.1 Neuroprotection

For a long time, Epo has been used clinically in patients suffering from anemia due to end-stage renal failure. In addition to the correction of anemia, these patients showed improved cognitive abilities (Siren and Ehrenreich, 2001). Initially, since it was believed that systemic Epo cannot pass through the blood-brain-barrier due to its large size (Recny et al, 1987) and brain-derived Epo production and expression of EpoR in the CNS were not yet discovered, the positive effect on cognition was attributed to the improved oxygen-carrying capacity of the blood after Epo-induced erythropoiesis. However, since later studies have shown that both Epo and its receptor are expressed in different regions of the brain by different cell types (Genc et al, 2004; Marti, 2004), the hypothesis was established that locally produced as well as exogenously added Epo could directly influence cognitive function. Interestingly, the expression level of Epo and EpoR is especially high in regions of the brain known to be particularly sensitive to acute hypoxia (Lipton, 1999), the hippocampus and the telencephalon (Digicaylioglu et al, 1995), suggesting that Epo might act as a protective agent against hypoxia. Indeed, infusion of soluble EpoR (capable of binding with endogenous EPO, thus sequestering it) into the brain of gerbils, which were subjected to a mild form of ischemia that normally does not cause neuronal damage, resulted in neuronal death in the hippocampus, clearly showing that endogenous Epo has a neuroprotective effect (Sakanaka et al, 1998).

3.5.2 Neurotrophic function and neurogenesis

Besides neuroprotection under hypoxic conditions, Epo also has a neurotrophic function in normoxic neurons. This was first demonstrated by Konishi and co-workers showing that Epo augments the activity of choline acetyltransferase in primary cultured mouse septal neurons (Konishi et al, 1993). Epo promoted the regeneration of septal cholinergic neurons in adult rats that had undergone fimbria-fornix transections. In addition and similar to its anti-apoptotic role in erythropoiesis, Epo promoted the survival and differentiation of dopaminergic precursor neurons in vitro (Studer et al, 2000). Moreover, hypoxia-induced Epo production appeared to directly act on neuronal stem cells in the forebrain, showing that Epo plays a direct role in neurogenesis after hypoxia (Shingo et al, 2001). In addition, Epo also acts indirectly by inducing brain-derived neurotrophic factor (BDNF) expression (Wang et al, 2004), which in turn augmented the effect of Epo on neurogenesis. These data show that Epo is not only involved in neuroprotection, but also in neuronal survival, differentiation, and neurogenesis.

3.5.3 Angiogenesis and vascular permeability

Besides its direct effects on neurons, Epo-induced neuroprotection may be attributed to an improvement in brain perfusion by promoting new vessel growth. Anagnostou et al demonstrated mitogenic and chemotactic effects of Epo on human umbilical vein and bovine adrenal capillary endothelial cells (Anagnostou et al, 1990). Moreover, Epo stimulated vessel outgrowth of rat aortic rings (Carlini et al, 1995), suggesting that Epo has angiogenic effects. This was further supported by the observation that Epo injection into the mouse uterine cavity stimulated neovascularization in the endometrium (Yasuda et al, 1998). Similarly, neovascularization was stimulated in the chick embryo chorioallantonic membrane upon Epo administration (Ribatti et al, 1999a). The angiogenic effect of Epo was also found in the brain, since capillary endothelial cells express two forms of EpoR mRNA and Epo showed a dose-dependent mitogenic activity on brain capillary endothelial cells (Yamaji et al, 1996). This angiogenic effect was finally confirmed in mice genetically engineered to lack either Epo or its receptor (EpoR) where mutant embryos suffer from severe defects in angiogenesis (Kertesz et al, 2004). In addition to its angiogenic effect, Epo is involved in the regulation of vascular permeability. In an in vitro model of the blood-brain barrier (BBB), Epo treatment protected bovine brain endothelial cells against VEGF-induced increase in vascular permeability (Martinez-Estrada et al, 2003). This suggests that the protective effect of Epo on the brain could be mediated by stimulating angiogenesis as well as by protecting the BBB.

3.5.4 Anti-inflammation

Inflammatory processes play a major role in the pathogenesis of cerebral ischemia, where Epo is protective. Inflammation results in influx of leukocytes from the blood into the brain and in activation of resident microglial cells (Dirnagl et al, 1999). These cells produce inflammatory mediators and cytokines leading to barrier damage, microvascular occlusion, and thus the aggravation of the injury (Witko-Sarsat et al, 2000). In an animal model of cerebral ischemia, administration of Epo resulted in the reduction of the local production of TNF, IL-6, and the chemokine MCP-1, all markers of inflammation, subsequently leading to a marked reduction of infarct size. These results indicate that Epo has an anti-inflammatory effect that contributes to its direct neuroprotective effect during cerebral ischemia (Villa et al, 2003). Since Epo did not reduce cytokine production in response to LPS applied directly in vivo and in vitro, the authors concluded that the observed antiinflammatory effect is due to inhibiting neuronal apoptosis and not to a direct effect on inflammatory cells. Epo might reduce leukocyte transmigration through endothelial cells, since Epo enhances the resistance of endothelial cells toward ischemia (Chong et al, 2002). The protective effect of Epo on oligodendrocytes against cytotoxicity induced by inflammatory stimuli (Genc et al, 2006) could explain the beneficial effect of Epo in case of MS where oligodendrocytes play a crucial role in the pathogenesis of the disease.

3.5.5 Transport through BBB

An important prerequisite for considering Epo as a therapeutic agent in CNS diseases is to answer the question as of whether Epo, administered systemically, is able to cross the BBB. Brines et al. (Brines et al, 2000) injected mice with biotinylated Epo and subsequently visualized brain section with peroxidase-labeled streptavidin. Indeed, a signal for biotin was detected in a region surrounding the capillaries extending into brain parenchyma. The authors concluded that Epo crosses the BBB. However, biotin might not be an ideal tool to study BBB permeability since it is rapidly transported across the BBB (Shi et al, 1993; Spector and Mock, 1987), and, therefore, even a small amount of free biotin in the blood will cross the BBB leading to false results. Since the authors detected EpoR in the brain capillaries, they attributed Epo transport through BBB to transcytosis. This hypothesis was later challenged by the observation that radiolabeled Epo and albumin crossed the BBB and entered the brain parenchyma in similar kinetics, showing that the transport of Epo across BBB is rather mediated by the extracellular pathways (Banks et al, 2004). However, variations in physiological serum Epo level may not result in significant changes of Epo levels within the brain, since no correlation between serum and liquor Epo concentrations was found when the BBB is intact (Marti et al, 1997). In summary, one can conclude that endogenously produced Epo (by kidney or liver) has only a marginal influence on brain Epo availability, whereas high dosages of therapeutically administered r-hu Epo can penetrate even the intact BBB (Marti et al, 1997). Accordingly, many studies are currently ongoing to test the therapeutic potential of Epo in many CNS diseases.

3.6 Epo in stroke

The first hint came from the observation that the expression of Epo and its receptor in the brain is upregulated upon cerebral ischemia (Bernaudin et al, 1999; Siren et al, 2001). Several in vivo experiments confirmed this hypothesis. Intracerebroventricular injection of Epo 24 h before permanent occlusion of the MCA in mice reduced infarct volume significantly. Similarly, infusion of Epo in the lateral ventricles of gerbils in a global ischemia model rescued hippocampal CA1 neurons and increased the number of synapses in the same region (Sakanaka et al, 1998). Moreover, in another experimental rodent model of cerebral ischemia where the MCA is transiently occluded, systemic administration of Epo also reduced the infarct size (Brines et al, 2000). Significantly, this protective effect of Epo was retained even when Epo was applied 6 h after the onset of the cerebral ischemia. In addition, brain-specific overexpression of Epo reduced infarct size in mice subjected to transient cerebral ischemia (Kilic et al, 2005). Other studies, where the functional outcome of Epo treatment was investigated, have shown that Epo not only reduces infarct volume but also improves the learning ability in gerbils and reduces the navigation disability in rats (Sadamoto et al, 1998; Sakanaka et al, 1998). Epo has also been shown to be protective in models of hemorrhagic stroke where the interruption of the cerebral blood flow is due to subarachnoid or cerebral hemorrhage (Alafaci et al, 2000; Grasso et al, 2002). The above-mentioned studies prompted the initiation of clinical trials in stroke patients. The safety and proof-of-concept phases of the Göttingen-Epo-Stroke Study have shown Epo to be safe and to improve the patient functional outcome after stroke (Ehrenreich et al, 2002). Although good evidence for direct neuroprotection exists, the observed brain-protective effect of Epo could also be attributed to its effect on astrocytes. Astrocytes protect neurons from oxidative stress by neutralizing reactive oxygen species (Dringen and Hirrlinger, 2003). It has been reported that activated astrocytes in ischemic human brain express increased levels of EpoR (Siren et al, 2001). Since Epo enhances brain glutathione peroxidase activity (Kumral et al, 2005), Epo, by binding to EpoR on the surface of activated astrocytes, might contribute to the astrocyte-mediated neuroprotective effect against ischemia-induced free-radical formation.

3.7 Safety concerns with the clinical use of EPO

Clinical studies are ongoing to test the safety and efficacy of EPO for the treatment of different neurological diseases. In the recent multicenter Epo stroke trial (Ehreich et al, 2009), adult stroke patients receiving Epo after tissue-plasminogen activator (t-PA)-induced thrombolysis reported increased mortality, intra-cerebral hemorrhage, brain edema, and thromboembolic events. The increased death rate in the rtPA population is still unexplained and may result from a combinant of factors and/or potential rtPA-EPO interactions. In contrast, in non rtPA population, the tendency toward a higher death rate in the EPO group might be explained by higher stroke severity of dead patients on inclusion (before any study medication was applied). Moreover, the mechanism of action of EPO is different from the clot-dissolving strategy pursued by thrombolysis. It would, therefore, have been most attractive to see that the neuroprotective approach using EPO, aimed at salvaging potentially viable brain tissue from spreading of death signals, and thrombolysis, targeting reopening of the feeding artery, had provided additive beneficial outcome. However, the unexpected observation that a combination of EPO and rtPA is not advantageous, and can even be detrimental, poses at present a contraindication for acute EPO treatment in patients receiving rtPA.

4. Albumin

Albumin is the most abundant plasma protein synthesized mainly in the liver. Albumin is also a major component of most extracellular fluids including cerebrospinal fluid (CSF), interstitial fluid (ISF) and lymph. It is a non-glycosylated and negatively charged protein with high ligand binding and transport capacity. It has multifunctional properties which include the maintenance of colloid osmotic pressure of plasma, transportation of hormones, fatty acids, drugs and metabolites, regulation of microvascular permeability, antioxidant activity, anti-thrombotic activity and anti-inflammatory activity (Evans, 2002; Garcovich et al, 2009). Owing to its multifunctional properties it has been widely used in therapeutics related to hepatology. The volumeexpanding property of albumin, in combination with other therapeutic approaches, has been used for the clinical benefit of patients with liver cirrhosis. Also, human serum albumin (HSA) as an iso-oncotic (4-5%) solution has been used to combat blood volume deficits and as a hyperoncotic (20-25%) solution has been used for restoration of oncotic deficits (Arroyo, 2002; Garcovich et al, 2009). Albumin has been shown to play a crucial role in the microcirculation of many organs including brain. Owing to its strong hemodynamic and binding capacity, it has been implicated in physiological and many disease conditions of the brain. Albumin has been implicated in neurological diseases such as ischemic stroke, Alzheimer's disease and epilepsy. High-dose human albumin is robustly neuroprotective in preclinical ischemia models and it is currently in Phase III clinical trials for acute ischemic stroke (Ginsberg, 2008). Albumin also has the potential to produce direct neuroprotective action on neuronal and glial cells.

4.1 Albumin synthesis and distribution

Albumin protein contains a single polypeptide chain of 585 amino acids with a molecular mass of approximately 67 kDa.

In the mouse liver, the albumin gene becomes active during early foetal stages and the transcript levels gradually increase after birth until high levels are reached in the adult animal (Tilghman and Belayew, 1982). Albumin is synthesized as preproalbumin in the liver, which has an N-terminal peptide that is removed before the nascent protein is released from the rough endoplasmic reticulum. The product, proalbumin, is in turn cleaved in the Golgi vesicles to produce albumin. Albumin synthesis predominantly occurs in the liver at the rate of 10-15 g/day. In healthy human adults, total albumin content is approximately 250-300 g/70 kg of the body weight and the majority of synthesized albumin (40-45 %) is maintained in the plasma. A very small amount of albumin is stored in liver (< 2 g) and the remaining amount is located in the muscle and skin (Quinlan et al, 2005). Albumin synthesis is regulated at both the transcriptional and post-transcriptional levels and this regulation is important to meet the demands of plasma, because albumin is not stored in the liver in large amounts. The rate of albumin transcription is affected by several conditions such as trauma, sepsis, hepatic diseases, diabetes and fasting. The change in interstitial colloid oncotic pressure is thought to be the predominant factor for regulation of albumin synthesis. Albumin homeostasis is maintained by balanced catabolism occurring in all tissues but most of the albumin (40-60 %) is degraded in the muscle and skin. However, the liver (15 %), kidney (10 %) and gastro-intestinal tract (10 %) are also responsible for albumin degradation. Albumin leaks from plasma at a rate of 5 % per hour and is returned to the vascular space at an equivalent rate through the lymphatic system. Albumin is also diffused into CSF and ISF compartments of the central nervous system (CNS) from blood circulation of the brain (Nicholson et al, 2000). Blood derived albumin in CSF and interstitial fluid (ISF is implicated in normal as well as many pathophysiological conditions of the brain.

4.2 Albumin in the CSF

CSF originates from choroid plexus in the ventricles. CSF flows through cisternae and subarachnoid space and finally drains through the arachnoid villi into venous blood. CSF has several important functions; it mainly helps to provide mechanical support for the brain. CSF also acts as a drainage pathway for the brain, by providing a ' sink ' into which products of metabolism or synaptic activity are diluted and subsequently removed. Also, it acts as a route of communication within the CNS, i.e., it carries hormones, nutrients and transmitters between different areas of the brain. CSF albumin is predominantly a blood derived protein and it is mainly entered from the leptomeningeal blood CSF barrier (BCSFB) or from choroid plexus BCSFB (Johanson et al, 2008). The albumin quotient (Q alb) in the CSF is approximately 30-80 % of the total protein. The altered Albumin CSF/serum ratio (QAlb) is the indicator of the dysfunction of the BCSFB. CSF serum Q alb, along with other blood derived proteins in CSF, is widely used in the diagnosis of neurological diseases (Reiber, 1998, 2003; Reiber and Peter, 2001). The exact role of albumin in CSF is not fully known, but it is proposed that albumin could be involved in the maintenance of CSF oncotic pressure, delivery of a wide range of molecules that are important for normal brain function and in the removal of some of the harmful molecules from the brain. The exact roles of albumin in CSF and in the brain function are not fully understood. However, many recent studies indicate that albumin might have a neuroprotective role via multiple mechanisms in different pathophysiological conditions.

4.3 Albumin induced neuroprotection in experimental stroke

Ischemic stroke is an acute cerebrovascular disease resulting from a transient or permanent reduction in the cerebral blood flow (CBF). It mainly occurs due to blockade of the major cerebral blood vessels by a local thrombus or an embolus. Ischemia causes reduction in the oxygen and nutrient supply to the brain areas which leads to neuronal cell damage or cell death. It can cause long-term disabilities such as muscle paralysis, cognitive deficits, language deficits, emotional deficits and even coma or death. Stroke is the third leading cause of death worldwide after coronary heart disease and cancer (Lloyd-Jones et al, 2009) and ischemic stroke comprises approximately 87 % of all types of brain strokes. The only approved treatment with intravenous fibrinolytic such as tissue plasminogen activator (tPA) within 3 h of stroke onset yields reperfusion and clinical benefits (rt -PA Stroke Study

Group, 1995; Hacke et al, 2004; Juttler et al, 2006). However, the goal is to discover a neuroprotective drug which can inhibit reperfusion injury and provide neuroprotection within a wide therapeutic window. Hemodilution is an old approach which has been investigated for many decades as a potential therapy for ischemic stroke. Infusion of dextran has been shown to increase CBF of both the normal and ischemic brain, either by decreasing blood viscosity or by vasodilation in response to diminished oxygen delivery (Wood and Kee, 1985; Korosue and Heros, 1992). Despite neuroprotective benefi ts in experimental set-ups, several clinical trials of hemodilution in ischemic stroke have nonetheless proven negative or inconclusive (Scandinavian Stroke Study Group, 1987; Italian Acute Stroke Study Group, 1988; The Hemodilution in Stroke Study Group,1989). Subsequently, albumin has emerged as an alternative hemodiluting agent to dextran owing to its volume expanding properties (Sundt et al, 1967; Little et al, 1981; Emerson, 1989). However, only recently it has been rigorously evaluated for its anti-ischemic neuroprotective efficacy. Transient focal cerebral ischemia induced by middle cerebral artery occlusion (MCAO) is the most widely used model to study molecular mechanisms of cerebral ischemia-reperfusion injury and to screen neuroprotective drugs. It is less invasive with a low rate of mortality and a low coefficient of variation in lesion size (Longa et al, 1989; Belayev et al, 1997b). In the rat MCAO model, Cole et al. reported that 5 % albumin administration at the onset of ischemia reduced ischemic brain injury as evidenced by reduced hematocrit, infarct volume and cerebral edema (Cole et al, 1990). In another study, administration of concentrated (20%) HSA (1% body weight, intravenously) to rats at the onset of recirculation induced substantial diminution of infarct volume together with a marked reduction of brain edema. Thus, it is proposed that albumin might modify water homeostasis and ultimately reduce edema of the ischemic brain (Belayev et al, 1997a). These two initial studies suggested that albumin therapy at the onset of ischemia or reperfusion induces neuroprotection.In a detailed study using magnetic resonance imaging, by means of diffusion-weighted magnetic resonance imaging (DWI), 25% Human Serum Albumin (HSA) solution (1% by body weight) administered immediately after reperfusion was associated with DWI normalization and a mitigation of pannecrotic changes within zones of residual injury at 24 h of injury. Albumin therapy lowered the hematocrit on average by 37% and raised plasma colloid oncotic pressure by 56%, improved the neurological score and reduced brain swelling throughout the 3-day survival period (Belayev et al, 1998). Similar treatment also improved local CBF as measured autoradiographically with 14C-iodoantipyrine after 1 h of recirculation (Huh et al, 1998). Using laser scanning confocal microscopy and laser Doppler perfusion imaging, it was found that a beneficial effect of albumin therapy was attributed to reversal of stagnation, thrombosis and corpuscular adherence within cortical venules in the reperfusion phase after focal ischemia (Belayev et al, 2002). It was also reported that after 1 h of reperfusion, 1.25 g/kg intravenous HSA administration increased replenishment of polyunsaturated fatty acid (PUFA) lost from cellular membranes during ischemia (Rodriguez de Turco et al, 2002). These studies collectively indicate that albumin induced neuroprotection is attributed to properties such as reversal of thrombosis, improvement in microvascular blood perfusion, reduction in brain swelling and replenishment of PUFA in brain. All these actions could indicate that actions of albumin are confined in vascular space. However, it has been shown that treatment with human albumin following 2 h of MCAO also leads to albumin extravasations and subsequently cellular uptake. It has been observed that cortical neurons with preserved structural features had taken up human albumin. Thus, it is reasonable to speculate that treatment with human albumin could also provide direct neuronal protection (Remmers et al, 1999). For the effective treatment of ischemic stroke, treatment should be started within a narrow therapeutic window of 3 h. Moderate-dose albumin therapy (1.25 g/kg intravenously) markedly provides neuroprotection even when treatment is delayed up to 4 h after onset of ischemia (Belayev et al, 2001). Albumin treatment has also been found to be neuroprotective in other models of focal ischemia. Prompt albumin therapy improved neurological function and blood-brain barrier integrity after acute intracortical hematoma (ICH) (Belayev et al, 2005). In a model of laser-induced cortical arteriolar thrombosis, high-dose albumin therapy induced a prompt, sustained improvement in microvascular hemodynamics distal to a cortical arteriolar thrombosis (Nimmagadda et al, 2008). In acute ischemic stroke, albumin combination therapy can attenuate the deleterious effects of tPA (Tang et al, 2009). Furthermore, albumin (1.25 g/kg) treatment maintains serum albumin at a higher level and attenuates cortex and hippocampus vascular endothelial growth factor (VEGF) expression at 6 h and 1 day after MCAO. This could partially contribute to the protective effects of albumin on reduction of brain edema and infarct size in the early stage of ischemia (Yao et al, 2010). The above mentioned studies prove that in experimental transient ischemia albumin provides neuroprotection via different indirect and direct mechanisms. Albumin has been found to be effective in other models of stroke such as permanent MCAO, global ischemia induced by bilateral common carotid occlusion (BCCO) and traumatic brain injury (TBI). In permanent MCAO, rats treated with 2 g/kg/day concentrated (25%) albumin begun after 30 min of ischemia showed diminished brain edema and infarct volume up to 6 days (Matsui et al, 1993). Furthermore, albumin (1.25 and 2.5 g/kg) significantly reduced cortical and striatal infarct areas and increased cortical perfusion in the permanent ischemia model (Liu et al, 2001). In transient global ischemia, HSA-treated rats showed signifi cantly improved neurological deficits throughout a 7-day survival period along with increases in numbers of surviving CA1 hippocampal pyramidal neurons compared to saline-treated animals (Belayev et al, 1999b). In TBI, 15 min after trauma, HSA administration signifi cantly improved neurological defi cits and also significantly reduced total contusion area (Belayev et al, 1999a). These experimental trials altogether indicated significant neuroprotective roles of albumin in different models of ischemic stroke and encouraged the further development of this important molecule for possible treatment of ischemic stroke in humans.

4.4 Albumin in clinical trials for ischemic stroke

The Albumin In Acute Stroke (ALIAS) Pilot Clinical Trial was conducted during 2001 – 2005 at two clinical sites (Universities of Calgary and Miami). This study was designed to investigate the safety and tolerability of albumin therapy in acute ischemic stroke. The ALIAS Pilot Clinical Trial used a multiple-tier, open-label, dose-escalation design. Human albumin (25%) in doses ranging up to 2.05 g/kg was well tolerated by patients with acute ischemic stroke without major dose-limiting complications. Concurrent tPA therapy did not affect the safety profile of albumin (Ginsberg et al, 2006a). Also, in this pilot trial the neuroprotective efficacy of albumin was evaluated and was found to be neuroprotective after ischemic stroke (Palesch et al, 2006). Based on the encouraging results of pilot trials of albumin, the National Institutes of Health has funded a randomized multicenter placebo-controlled effi cacy trial - the ALIAS Phase III Trial. A randomised, multicenter, double-blind, placebo controlled trial (ALIAS Phase III Trial, www.clinicaltrials. gov; NCT00235495) is currently being conducted at approximately 70 clinical sites in North America (Ginsberg et al, 2006b; Hill et al, 2011).

4.5 Direct neuroprotection by albumin: Mechanisms

The neuroprotective mechanisms of albumin in ischemic stroke and AD are largely attributed to its hemodynamic properties and binding properties. However, in different in vitro systems, albumin has been reported to possess several direct neuroprotective actions. (Figure 4)

Albumin could produce various neuroprotective actions in the intravascular compartment, cerebrospinal fluid-interstitial fluid compartment and intracellular compartment.

HSA and its N-terminal tetrapeptide DAHK can block oxidant-driven cultured neuronal injury produced by hydrogen peroxide and copper/ascorbic acid (Gum et al, 2004). Furthermore, bovine serum albumin has been found to be neuroprotective by reducing both the DNA damage and apoptosis rates in cultured cortical neurons and these effects are probably due to its antioxidant activity (Baltanas et al, 2009). Albumin has been reported to play an important role in astrocyte functions. It is shown that albumin affects metabolism of cultured astrocytes (Tabernero et al, 1999). Albumin up on transcytosis into cultured astrocytes stimulates the synthesis of neurotrophic factor oleic acid which promotes neuronal differentiation (Tabernero et al, 2002). Megalin is a receptor for albumin in astrocytes and is required for the synthesis of the neurotrophic factor oleic acid (Bento - Abreu et al, 2008). Also, this megalin induced albumin transcytosis and synthesis of

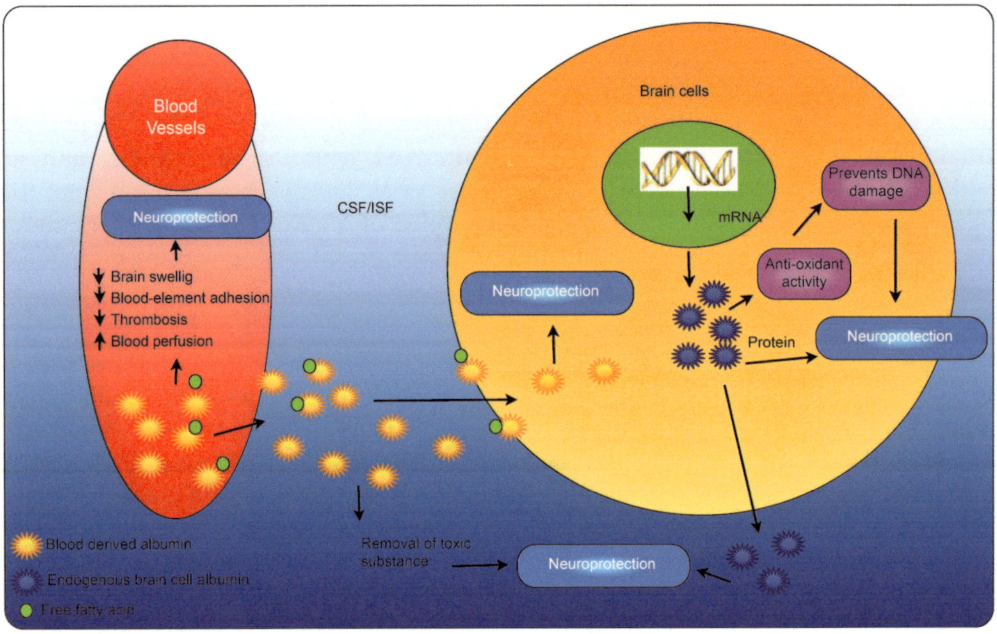

Fig. 4. Overview of possible neuroprotective mechanisms of albumin.

neurotrophic factor is dependent on caveola and the adaptor protein cytosolic adaptor protein disabled (Dab-1) in cultured astrocytes (Bento -Abreu et al, 2009). These studies indicate that albumin could play a role in neuronal differentiation and development. Albumin also induces calcium mobilisation in cultured as well as brain astrocytes (Manning and Sontheimer, 1997; Nadal et al, 1998; Hooper et al, 2005). Albumin elicits calcium entry in the microglia which promotes proliferation of the microglia (Hooper et al, 2005). Astrocyte calcium signalling caused by albumin could have important physiological and pathophysiological consequences when the blood-brain barrier breaks down and allows albumin to enter the CNS. It is reported that albumin leakage induced by blood-brain barrier breaks is followed by albumin uptake into astrocytes which is responsible for epileptogenesis in rats (Ivens et al, 2007; van Vliet et al, 2007). Albumin causes downregulation of Kir current which results in the abnormal accumulation of $[K^{+}]$ o and consequent NMDA-receptor dependent pathological plasticity which isresponsible for epileptogenesis (Ivens et al, 2007). Recently, it was shown that albumin activates astrocytes and microglia producing infl ammatory responses via the mitogen-activated protein kinase pathway and these effects could be involved both in the mechanism of cellular injury and repair (Ralay Ranaivo and Wainwright, 2010). Altogether these fi ndings suggest that the majority of the effects of albumin on astrocytes, microglia and neuronal cells seem to be benefi cial; however, at augmented levels it could contribute towards astrocyte dysfunction. The direct effects of albumin on neuronal and glial cells necessitate further detailed investigation in individual pathological conditions.

4.6 Endogenous albumin and neuroprotection: possible new paradigm

Although albumin is mainly synthesized in the liver, mRNA expression level of albumin has been found in many non-hepatic rat tissues such as lungs, heart, kidney and pancreas, but not in the brain (Nahon et al, 1988). Also, non-hepatic albumin expression at the protein level is rarely confirmed. A recent study suggests that human brain microglia cells can express albumin both at mRNA and protein levels; furthermore, this expression is increased by amyloid beta (Aβ) and lipopolysaccharide treatment (Ahn et al, 2008). It is suggested that enhanced levels of albumin and subsequent secretion by microglia could be implicated in A β removal from the brain (Ahn et al, 2008). We have also found upregulation of albumin at both mRNA and protein levels in ischemic rat brain. Upregulation of albumin in ischemic brain could play a neuroprotective role against altered brain functions (Prajapati et al, 2010). These results indicate that de novo synthesis of albumin also occurs in the brain tissue. However, possible intracellular and extracellular neuroprotective actions of endogenously synthesized albumin is an unexplored area and warrants further investigations.

5. Antithrombin III

Antithrombin III (ATIII) is a single-chain glycoprotein in plasma and belongs to the family of the serpins. It is synthesized in liver parenchymal cells, and it plays a central role in regulating haemostasis. When bound to glycosaminoglycans, it is an important inhibitor of several serine protease, including factors Xa, IXa, XIa, and thrombin (Bauer and Rosenberg, 1991), wich are involved in blood coagulation. Equimolar, irreversible complexes are formed between ATIII and the enzymes. Heparin and heparan sulfate glycoproteins (HSPGs) bind to multiple sites of the ATIII molecule resulting in a steric reconfiguration, thereby increasing the interaction between ATIII and the activated enzymes. It is believed that much of the physiological inactivation of enzymes by ATIII occurs in the endothelium, mediated by heparan sulfate (Figure 5) (Mammen, 1998).

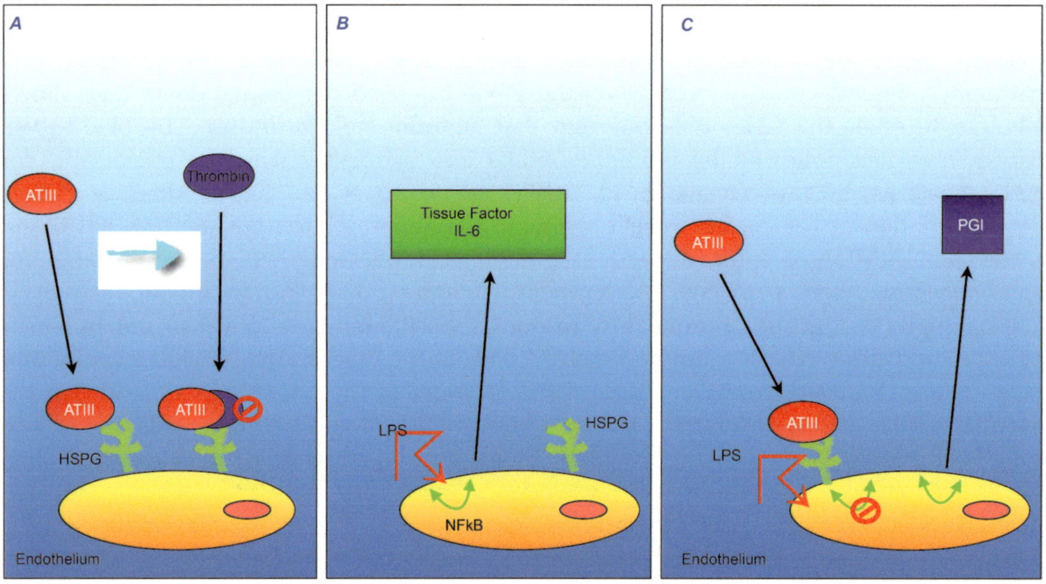

Fig. 5. Role of heparan sulfate proteoglycan (HSPG) in inhibition of thrombin, in induction of prostacyclin, and inhibition of cytokine and tissue factor release from endothelial cells by antithrombin III.

A large number of recent studies have shown that ATIII has anti-inflammatory actions, (Cuomo et al, 2007) which are independent of its effects on coagulation. These effects include the heterologous deactivation of activated leukocytes and the interaction with the endothelium, thereby reducing vessel wall transmigration and subsequent tissue and organ damage. Thus, ATIII may have two distinct and indipendent actions in patients with cerebral ischemia: (1) interference with pathologic coagulation, and (2) inhibition of inflammation.

5.1 Effects of ATIII on abnormal coagulation

The prothrombotic, proinflammatory state of stroke results in a promotion of thrombin formation and fibrin deposition at the vascular wall, as well as in the formetion of platelet-leukocyte coaggregates, leading to severe disturbance of the microcirculation, capillary leakage and tissue damage (Piazza et al, 2010). Many of the events involved in this proinflammatory state have been shown to be inhibited by ATIII. The inhibition of factor Xa by ATIII may be particularly important for protection against, and treatment of, inflammation. This activated clotting factor has a number of proinflammatory effects, including stimulation if the production of IL-6, IL-8, MCP-1, E-selectin, and the soluble adhesion molecules ICAM-1 and vascular cell adhesion molecule (VCAM)-1, wich can be experimentally blocked by ATIII (Senden et al, 1998). The proinflammatory functions of thrombin include stimulation of neutrophil/monocyte adhesion, action as a chemotactic factor for polymorphonuclear leukocytes (Esmon, 2000), and increased expression of the recently discovered inhibitor of fibrinolysis, thrombin-activable fibrinolysis inhibitor (TAFI) (Opal, 2000). Thrombin also stimulates the increased expression of IL-8 and plays an important role in ischemia-induced leukocyte rolling and adhesion (Kaur et al, 2001; Ludwicka-Bradley et al, 2000; Rabiet et al, 1994). Thus, the ability of ATIII to inhibit the actions of both factor Xa and thrombin gives it the potential to block, in part or fully, a wide range of proinflammatory events (Seegers, 1978).

5.2 Coagulation-indipendent anti-inflammatory effects of ATIII

In the late 1980s, initial publications reported on the property of ATIII to stimulate prostacyclin release from endothelial cells independent of thrombin interaction. Although some recent studies question such a mechanism, at least in vitro, a number of papers make an in vivo contribution of prostacyclin release as part of the ATIII anti-inflammatory properties likely (Uchiba and Okajima, 2001). Independent of ATIII's anticoagulatory activities at multiple points of action, a variety of studies provide evidence for a potent anti-inflammatory ATIII effect, wich can only be induced by high ATIII plasma activities in the range of 150%-200% (Harada et al, 1999; Hoffmann et al, 2000; Okajiama and Uchiba, 1998; Uchiba et al, 1996, 1998). These anti-inflammatory ATIII actions may be mainly mediated by an interaction of ATIII with the endothelium (Hoffmann et al, 2002), thereby producing a profound increase in endothelial prostacyclin production (Figure 5C) (Yamauchi et al, 1989).

5.3 Effects of ATIII on leukocyte-endothelium interactions

ATIII expresses the ability to inhibit leukocyte rolling and adhesion, wich are hallmarks of inflammatory reactions, and have explored the mechanisms underlying these effects. Ostrovsky et al (Ostrovsky et al, 1997) showed that ATIII administration significantly reduced neutrophil rolling and adhesion to pretreatment levels in a feline mesentery ischaemia-reperfusion model. Nevière et al (Nevière et al, 2001) and Hoffmann et al (Hoffmann et al, 2000) showed that the beneficial effects resulting from ATIII's blocking of leukocyte-endothelium interactions were eliminated when indomethacin, a cyclo-oxygenase inhibitor that blocks prostacyclin production, was added to the treatment. The administration of recombinant hirudin did not result in comparable beneficial effects, supporting the thrombin-indipendent mode of action of ATIII. As a consequence of the limited activated leukocyte-endothelium interaction, the severity of subsequent capillary leakage, disturbance of microcirculation, and organ damage were significantly reduced. A report by Yamashiro et al (Yamashiro et al, 2001) suggests direct affects of ATIII on leukocytes and endothelium by demonstrating the downmodulation of P-selectin by ATIII in the LPS-stimulated endothelium, thereby diminishing leukocyte rolling and subsequent transmigration. Support of this hypothesis has also been provided by the work of Souter et al (Souter et al, 2001) showing that the addition of ATIII to LPS-treated whole blood, HUVEC, and mononuclear cells inhibited production of both IL-6 and tissue factor; recombinant hirudin, a specific thrombin inhibitor, did not reduce the production of IL-6 or tissue factor, again suggesting that the observed inhibition by ATIII was not due solely to its ability ti inhibit thrombin (figure 5B and C).

5.4 Direct effect of ATIII on leukocytes

Dunzendorfer et al (Dunzendorfer et al, 2000, 2001) have uncovered a second mechanism by which ATIII may inhibit neutrophil migration and adhesion to the endothelium; namely, heterologous deactivation of activated leukocytes by ATIII. These investigators noted that signaling in ATIII-induced neutrophil chemotaxis mimics an IL-8-induced response, ATIII inhibited migration of neutrophils towards IL-8, GRO-alpha, and fMLP; staurosporine, bisindolylmaleimide I, pertussis toxin, and an anti-CXCR1 monoclonal antibody all blocked ATIII-induced neutrophil chemotaxis. However, additional assays did not reveal binding of ATIII to CXCR1. Thus, the results of these studies are generally consistent with the conclusion that the effect of ATIII in neutrophil migration appear to involve a CXCR1-related signaling pathway, its G-proteins, and protein kinase C. Recent findings have shown that the signalling pathway activated by ATIII in leukocytes are different in neutrophils, monocytes, and lymphocytes (Dunzendorfer et al, 2001; Kaneider et al, 2001, 2002). All togheter, these experiments led to the conclusion that ATIII in circulation protects leukocytes from premature activation.

5.5 ATIII and nuclear factor-kappaB

Oelschager et al (Oelshager et al, 2001) showed that ATIII produces a dose-dependent reduction in both LPS and tissue necrosis factor (TNF)-α activation of nuclear factor-kappaB (NF-κB) in cultured monocytes and endothelial cells. Results reported by this working group and by Iampietro et al (Iampietro et al, 2000) indicate that these actions of ATIII block the increase in IL-6, IL-8, TNF, and tissue factor mRNA expression (figure 5B and C). Beyond control of coagulation, ATIII displays anti-inflammatory properties through an interaction with cells, reducing the synthesis and release of proinflammatory mediators, thereby modulating leukocyte activation and their interaction with the vessel wall. As a consequence, tissue damage and organ failure are reduced.

6. Toll-like receptors

The TLRs, so-called because of their homology to the Drosophila Toll receptor, were first characterized in mammals by their ability to recognize pathogen-associated molecular patterns such as those found in the bacterial cell wall components peptidoglycan (TLR2) and lipopolysaccharide (LPS) (TLR4), as well as viral dsRNA (TLR3), ssRNA (TLR7), and nonmethylated cytosine-guanine (CpG) DNA (TLR9). Recently it has been found that in addition to their role in pathogen detection and defense, TLRs act as sentinels of tissue damage and mediate inflammatory responses to aseptic tissue injury. Surfactant, HSP60, components of the extracellular matrix, and fibrinogen have all been shown to activate TLR4, while host HMGB1 and host mRNA and DNA are endogenous ligands of TLR2 (and TLR4), TLR3 and TLR9, respectively. TLRs, upon activation by either pathogen- or host-derived ligands, induce downstream signals that lead to cytokine and chemokine production and thereby initiate inflammatory responses. TLRs are located on antigen presenting cells such as B cells, dendritic cells, monocytes/macrophages and microglia. In addition, these receptors can be expressed by the cerebral endothelium and by cells within the brain parenchyma such as astrocytes, oligodendrocytes, and neurons (Bsibsi et al., 2002; Singh and Jiang, 2004; Jack et al., 2005; Bsibsi et al., 2006). The TLRs signal through common intracellular pathways leading to transcription factor activation and the generation of cytokines and chemokines (Figure 6) (Vogel et al., 2003; Takeda and Akira, 2005). Each TLR family member, with the exception of TLR3, initiates intracellular signaling via recruitment of the intracellular Toll-interleukin 1 receptor (TIR)-domain-containing adaptor MyD88. When recruited to plasma membrane-associated TLRs, either directly (TLRs 5 and 11) or via the TIRAP adaptor (TLRs 1, 2, 4, 6), MyD88 enlists members of the IRAK family, including IRAK1, IRAK2, and IRAK4, to begin a process of auto- and cross-phosphorylation among the IRAK molecules. Once phosphorylated, IRAKs dissociate from MyD88 and bind TRAF6, an E3 ligase. TRAF6 in turn activates TAK1 which itself activates the IKK complex and MAPKKs. The IKK complex, composed of IKKα, IKKβ and the regulatory subunit IKKγ/NEMO, phosphorylates IκB proteins. This phosphorylation is necessary for the ubiquitination and proteosomal degradation of IκBs and the subsequent nuclear translocation of the transcription factor NFκB. Members of the MAPK family phosphorylate and activate components of the transcription factor AP-1. Together, these transcription factors induce inflammatory cytokine production (e.g. TNFα, IL1). MyD88 is also recruited to the endosomal receptors TLR7 and TLR9 again enlisting members of the IRAK family. Due to the endosomal location of the complex, the phosphorylated IRAKs are able to bind TRAF3 in addition to TRAF6. Activation of TRAF3 leads to phosphorylation, dimerization, and nuclear localization of the transcription factors IRF3, IRF5, and IRF7 with resultant type I interferon (IFN) production. Hence these endosomal TLRs are capable of signaling to NFκB, AP-1 and IRFs, resulting in a diverse genomic response. Endosomal TLR3 is unique among the TLRs because it does not signal through MyD88 but signals instead via recruitment of the Toll-interleukin 1 receptor domain-containing adaptor inducing interferon β (TRIF). TRIF enlists the non-canonical IKKs, TBK1 and IKKε, which activate IRF3. Further, TRIF recruits TRAF6 and RIP-1, which results in activation of MAPK and IKKα/β. Hence TLR3, like the other endosomal receptors, is capable of activating NFκB, AP-1 and IRFs. Of all the TLRs, only TLR4 can recruit either MyD88 (via TIRAP) or TRIF (via TRAM) and can thus induce either the pro-inflammatory cytokines TNFα and IL1 via NFκB or the anti-viral IFNβ via IRF3. The complement of TLR family members expressed by a cell depends on its identity and its activation status. Constitutive expression of TLRs within the brain occurs in microglia and astrocytes and is largely restricted to the circumventricular organs and meninges—areas with direct access to the circulation (Laflamme and Rivest, 2001; Laflamme et al., 2001; Chakravarty and Herkenham, 2005). Human and murine microglia express TLRs 1–9 and generate cytokine profiles specifically tailored by the TLR stimulated (Bsibsi et al., 2002; Olson and Miller, 2004; Jack et al., 2005). Similarly, human and murine astrocytes express multiple TLRs, with particularly prominent TLR3 expression (Bsibsi et al., 2002, 2006; Carpentier et al., 2005; Jack et al., 2005; McKimmie and Fazakerley, 2005). Microglia and astrocytes respond differently to specific TLR engagement reflective of their distinct roles in the brain. Microglia initiate robust cytokine and chemokine responses to stimulation of TLR2 (TNFα, IL-6, IL-10), TLR3 (TNFα, IL-6, IL-10, IL-12, CXCL-10, IFNβ), and TLR4 (TNFα, IL-6, IL-10, CXCL-10, IFNβ), yet astrocytes initiate only minor IL-6 responses to all but TLR3 stimulation (Jack et al., 2005). Microglia express TLR3 and TLR4 at the cell surface while astrocytes express these receptors intracellularly (Bsibsi et al., 2002). The cellular location of TLRs affects their downstream signaling cascades (Kagan et al., 2008), which may explain the different responses of these cells to TLR stimulation. The

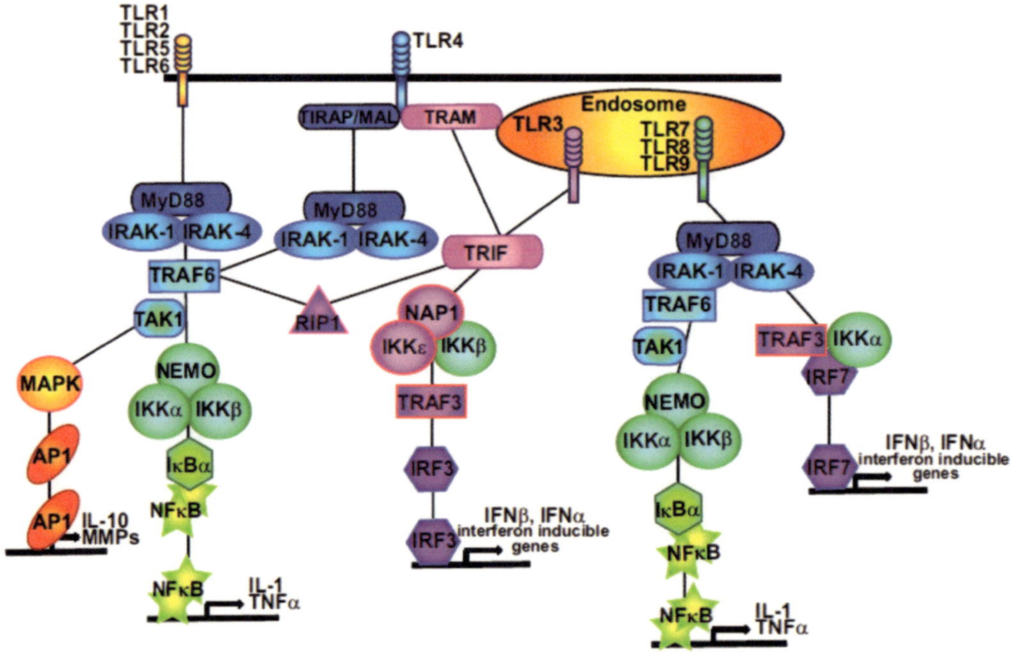

Fig. 6. TLRs signaling

inflammatory milieu also plays a critical role in regulating TLR expression. Microglia stimulated with CpG specifically up-regulate TLR9, whereas those stimulated with a synthetic TLR3 ligand suppress all TLRs except TLR3 (Olson and Miller, 2004). Similarly, astrocytes stimulated with LPS up-regulate TLRs 2 and 3 but suppress TLR4, while astrocytes exposed to RNA viruses up-regulate TLR3 and TLR9 (McKimmie and Fazakerley, 2005). Thus microglia and astrocytes initiate a layered and multifaceted response to TLR engagement. Oligodendrocytes and endothelial cells express a relatively limited repertoire of TLRs. Oligodendrocytes express TLRs 2 and 3 (Bsibsi et al., 2002), while cerebral endothelial cells constitutively express TLRs 2, 4, and 9 (Constantin et al., 2004) and increase their expression of these TLRs in response to stressful stimuli, including systemic LPS and cerebral ischemia (Singh and Jiang, 2004; Zhou et al., 2007; Ziegler et al., 2007). In response to LPS, endothelial cells up-regulate E-selectin, an NFκB-dependent molecule, and IFNβ, an IRF3-dependent molecule, indicating that these cells utilize the TLR–NFκB and the TLR–IRF3 signaling pathways (Lloyd-Jones et al., 2008). Neurons express TLR3 and generate inflammatory cytokines (TNFα, IL-6), chemokines (CCL5, CXCL10) and antiviral molecules (IFNβ) in response to dsRNA (Lafon et al., 2006; Prehaud et al., 2005). Neurons also employ TLRs in their development and differentiation. TLRs 3 and 8 are expressed on murine neurons early in development and inhibit neurite outgrowth in a MyD88- and NFκB-independent manner (Ma et al., 2006). TLR2 and TLR4 have been found on adult neural progenitor cells where they appear to elicit opposing effects. While TLR2 activation stimulates neuronal differentiation of these cells, TLR4 activation decreases proliferation and neuronal differentiation, driving these cells toward an astrocytic fate (Rolls et al., 2007). Curiously, both TLRs exert these endogenous effects in a MyD88-dependent manner, suggesting that these molecules utilize MyD88 in distinct ways. Hence even minor alterations of these fine-tuned endogenous pathways can have profound effects on cellular responses to TLR engagement. Studies with TLR knockout mice illustrate the endogenous function of TLRs in health and disease. TLR2 and TLR4 have been shown to play detrimental roles in the development of congestive heart failure and cardiac hypertrophy, respectively, by signaling through MyD88 and NFκB (Shishido et al., 2003; Ha et al., 2005). TLR2 has additionally been found to be proatherogenic in hyperlipidemic mice (Tobias and Curtiss, 2007), and TLR4 has been shown to produce inflammatory reactions in adipose tissue and thereby mediates obesity and insulin resistance (Tsukumo et al., 2007; Davis et al., 2008). Conversely, TLR2 and TLR4 activation by hyaluronic acid protects lung tissue from non-infectious injury (Jiang et al., 2006), and TLR4 has been shown to help maintain lung integrity, and prevent the development of emphysema, by modulating oxidant generation (Zhang et al., 2006). The effects of endogenous TLR stimulation are clearly varied, depending on the cell and tissue type in which the receptors are found and on the disease process in which they are involved. The overwhelming and generally damaging inflammatory response of TLRs to aseptic tissue injury may be a consequence of TLR evolution in response to pathogens. In the setting of pathogen invasion, an inflammatory deluge may be the most effective means to clear microorganisms. The activation and influx of leukocytes, with the concomitant release of free radicals and tissue-destroying enzymes, assails not only the invading pathogen but any host cells that harbor the pathogen. However, when this same powerful response is co-opted by the host to clear and resolve tissue damage, it can destroy the very cells it is meant to save. This damage promoting characteristic is prominently observed following brain ischemia, where inflammation plays a critical role in both injury progression and resolution.

6.1 TLRS and ischemic damage

A significant portion of the damage associated with stroke injury is due to the resultant inflammatory response. This aspect of the innate immune response is exemplified by the fact that some anti-inflammatory strategies have been shown to ameliorate ischemic damage (Relton et al., 1996; Hara et al., 1997; Spera et al., 1998). The inflammatory response to stroke is initiated by the detection of injury associated molecules by local cells such as microglia and astrocytes. The response is further promoted by infiltrating neutrophils and macrophages, resulting in the production of inflammatory cytokines, proteolytic enzymes, and other cytotoxic mediators. In the mouse, leukocytes and brain cells (microglia, astrocytes and neurons) express TLRs (Zarember and Godowski, 2002; Olson and Miller, 2004). Hence, injury-associated molecules such as HSP60 and HMGB1 may act as endogenous ligands for TLRs, thereby initiating the damaging inflammatory response to stroke. It is increasingly clear that TLRs do in fact play a role in ischemic damage (Fig.). The pathogenic role of TLRs in ischemic processes was first demonstrated in a mouse model myocardial ischemia/reperfusion injury, because mice lacking functional TLR4 incur less damage than wild type mice (Oyama et al., 2004). Since then, TLR2 has also been shown to cause dysfunction following cardiac ischemia and both have been shown to exacerbate renal ischemic damage, in a MyD88-dependent and a MyD88-independent manner (Sakata et al., 2007; Shigeoka et al., 2007). However, the particular pathway responsible for the damaging effects of TLR activation may differ depending on the cell type or organ affected as TLR4 worsens ischemic damage following liver transplant in a MyD88-independent, IRF3 dependent fashion (Zhai et al., 2004; Shen et al., 2005). Importantly, TLR2 and TLR4 have been shown to play a role in cerebral ischemic damage. Mice lacking either functional TLR2 or TLR4 are less susceptible to transient focal cerebral ischemia/reperfusion damage, demonstrating smaller infarcts than wild type controls (Cao et al., 2007; Lehnardt et al., 2007; Ziegler et al., 2007). Further, mice lacking TLR4 incur less damage following global cerebral ischemia and permanent focal ischemia (Caso et al., 2007; Hua et al., 2007). The TLR endogenous ligands HSP 60, HSP70 and HMGB1 are found in the brain following injury (Kinouchi et al., 1993; Faraco et al., 2007; Lehnardt et al., 2008). Hence these molecules may activate TLR2 and TLR4 within the brain itself, leading to the generation of inflammatory mediators such as TNFα, IL1, IL6, and iNOS, all known to be associated with stroke damage.

6.2 TLRS and neuroprotection

In contrast to the detrimental role of TLRs in response to ischemia, stimulation of these receptors prior to ischemia provides robust neuroprotection. TLR4-induced tolerance to cerebral ischemia was first demonstrated with low dose systemic administration of LPS (endotoxin), a cell wall component of gram-negative bacteria, which caused spontaneously hypertensive rats to become tolerant to subsequent ischemic brain damage induced by middle cerebral artery occlusion (MCAO) (Tasaki et al., 1997). Since then, LPS-induced tolerance to brain ischemia has been demonstrated in a mouse model of stroke and in a porcine model of deep hypothermic circulatory arrest (Rosenzweig et al., 2004; Hickey et al., 2007) (for additional information on the dual effects of neuro-immune crosstalk, please refer to Kerschensteiner et al., in this issue). Neuroprotection induced by LPS is time and dose dependent. Tolerance appears by 24 h after LPS administration and extends out to 7 days but is gone by 14 days (Rosenzweig et al., 2007). Protective doses of LPS appear to depend on the animal model of stroke and the route of systemic administration, ranging from 0.02–1 mg/kg (Tasaki et al., 1997; Ahmed et al., 2000; Bordet et al., 2000; Furuya et al., 2005; Hickey et al., 2007; Kunz et al., 2007; Rosenzweig et al., 2007). Tolerance induction has been shown to require new protein synthesis and a modest inflammatory response, as it can be blocked by prior administration of cycloheximide or dexamethasone (Bordet et al., 2000). Specifically, TNFα has been implicated as a mediator of LPS-induced ischemic tolerance because inhibition of TNFα systemically (Tasaki et al., 1997) or within the brain (Rosenzweig et al., 2007) blocks neuroprotection, and mice lacking TNFα fail to be protected by LPS preconditioning (Rosenzweig et al., 2007). In addition to its neuroprotective effects, LPS preconditioning has vasculoprotective efficacy. Nitric oxide appears to play a critical role in the protective effects of LPS. Mice lacking iNOS expression fail to be protected by LPS pretreatment (Kunz et al., 2007), and eNOS expression within the brain is directly correlated to the time window of LPS-induced neuroprotection (Furuya et al., 2005). LPS pretreatment has further been shown to prevent the impairment of endothelial and smooth muscle relaxation normally induced by ischemia/reperfusion injury (Bastide et al., 2003), resulting in normalization of cerebral blood flow in peri-infarct regions lasting out to 24 h after MCAO (Dawson et al., 1999; Furuya et al., 2005). LPS-induced ischemic protection requires an inflammatory response prior to the ischemic event, yet protection occurs through modulation of the inflammatory response following ischemia. Rosenzweig et al. (2004) have shown that LPS preconditioning changes the response of circulating leukocytes to stroke, attenuating stroke-induced neutrophilia, lymphopenia, and monocyte activation. This altered inflammatory response extends into the brain itself. LPS preconditioning attenuates activation of microglia after stroke and reduces neutrophil infiltration into the ischemic hemisphere. Hence, LPS-induced preservation of microvascular function following MCAO may be due to suppressed lymphocyte adhesion to activated endothelium, either by TNFα-induced suppression of endothelial activation and adhesion molecules (Ginis et al., 1999; Ahmed et al., 2000) or by prevention of cellular inflammatory responses to ischemia (Rosenzweig et al., 2004). One hallmark of LPS preconditioning is suppression of cytotoxic TNFα signaling following stroke. Mice that have been preconditioned with LPS prior to ischemia display a pronounced suppression of the TNFα pathway following stroke, as evinced by reduced TNFα in the serum, decreased levels of cellular TNFR1, and enhanced levels of neutralizing soluble-TNFR1. These mice are thus protected from the cytotoxic effects of TNFα after cerebral ischemia (Rosenzweig et al., 2007). Collectively, these mechanisms lead to a muted TNFα response to ischemic injury and increased cell survival. Recently a new TLR ligand has been shown to induce tolerance to brain ischemia. As with TLR4 and LPS, stimulation of TLR9 by systemically administered CpG oligodeoxynucleotides induces robust protection against brain ischemia in a time and dose dependent manner. CpG pretreatment protects neurons in both in vivo and in vitro models of stroke (Stevens et al., 2008). Notably, the protection afforded by CpG depends on TNFα, as systemic CpG administration acutely and significantly increases serum TNFα, and TNFα knockout mice fail to be protected by CpG preconditioning. Similarities among the known TLR signaling pathways and their shared ability to induce TNFα, itself a potent preconditioning stimulus, suggest that stimulation of TLR4 and TLR9 may induce ischemic tolerance by similar means. The neuroprotective potential of other TLRs has yet to be explored, but this family of molecules may be a rich source of therapeutic targets. The finding that TLRs are mediators of ischemic injury provides insight into the potential mechanisms of LPS- and CpG-induced neuroprotection. In fact, TLR-induced tolerance to subsequent ischemia may occur by the same mechanisms that govern a very similar phenomenon—that of LPS-induced tolerance to subsequent LPS exposure. The latter phenomenon is known as "endotoxin tolerance" and occurs when pretreatment with a low dose of LPS renders cells or whole animals tolerant to the normally detrimental effects of a second, higher dose of LPS. Cells that are tolerant to LPS are defined by their inability to generate TNFα in response to TLR4 activation. Upon TLR4 ligation, LPS tolerant cells, unlike naive cells, do not recruit MyD88 to TLR4, and fail to activate IRAK-1 and NFκB (Medvedev et al., 2002). The TLR4–NFκB signaling axis becomes decommissioned following a primary exposure to LPS via an elaborate negative feedback loop that involves known inhibitors of TLR signaling. Among those inhibitors are Ship-1, which prevents TLR4-MyD88 interaction, IRAK-M, a non-functional IRAK decoy, and TRIM30α, which destabilized the TAK1 complex (Kobayashi et al., 2002; Sly et al., 2004; Shi et al., 2008). Thus, subsequent signaling of TLR4 to NFκB is blocked and inflammatory cytokine production is suppressed. Conversely, secondary exposure causes enhanced IFNβ release, suggesting increased signaling via the TLR4-IRF3 axis (Broad et al., 2007). Thus, pretreatment with LPS causes cells to switch their transcriptional response to TLR4 stimulation by enhancing the IRF3- induced cytokine IFNβ and suppressing the NFκB-induced cytokine TNFα. Similar to endotoxin tolerance, priming TLR9 with its ligand, CpG, induces a state of hypo-responsiveness to subsequent challenge with CpGs (Dalpke et al., 2005). Interestingly, cross-tolerance between the two receptors has also been reported, as ligands for TLR9 induce tolerance against a subsequent challenge with a TLR4 ligand (Bagchi et al., 2007; Broad et al., 2007). CpG-pretreated cells not only produce less TNFα when secondarily challenged with LPS, they also produce significantly higher levels of IFNβ (Broad et al., 2007). Together, the aforementioned studies suggest the intriguing possibility that TLR stimulation prior to stroke may reprogram ischemia-induced TLR activation (Fig.). Specifically, administration of LPS or CpG may activate TLR4 and TLR9, respectively, causing a small inflammatory response, with an initial rise in TNFα. Cells would then regulate their inflammatory response through expression of negative feedback inhibitors of the TLR4–NFκB signaling axis that remain present when cells are subsequently exposed to endogenous TLR ligands generated from ischemia-injured tissue. Within this new cellular environment, stimulated TLRs such as TLR2 and TLR4 would be unable to activate NFκB-inducing pathways. Because of this, stroke-induced TLR2 signaling may be blocked completely leading to reduced injury, and stroke-induced TLR4 signaling would shift from NFκB induction to IRF3 induction (Fig.). Suppression of NFκB induction would be expected to protect the brain, as mice lacking the p50 subunit of NFκB suffer less cerebral ischemic damage than wild type mice (Schneider et al., 1999). Enhancement of IRF signaling would also be expected to protect the brain, as IFNβ, a downstream product of IRF3 induction, has been shown to act as an acute neuroprotectant (Liu et al., 2002; Veldhuis et al., 2003a). IFNβ, best known for its anti-viral effects, has potent anti-inflammatory activities as well. Several studies have shown that IFNβ can stabilize the blood–brain barrier, potentially by reducing matrix metalloprotease production by activated glia (Veldhuis et al., 2003b; Kraus et al., 2004; Liuzzi et al., 2004). Similarly, it has been shown to inhibit monocyte migration across human brainderived endothelial cells (Seguin et al., 2003) and reduce cellular infiltration into damaged brain regions (Veldhuis et al., 2003b). On a cellular level, IFNβ has been shown to reduce reactive oxygen species (Lopez-Collazo et al., 1998; Stewart et al., 1998; Hua et al., 2002), suppress inflammatory cytokine production and induce IL-1Ra (Bosca et al., 2000; Palmer et al., 2004), promote nerve growth factor production by astrocytes (Boutros et al., 1997) and protect neurons from toxicity induced by activated microglia (Jin et al., 2007). In addition, systemic administration of IFNβ has been shown to reduce infarct damage in rat and rabbit models of ischemic stroke (Liu et al., 2002; Veldhuis et al., 2003a). Therefore, in the setting of LPS preconditioning, upregulation of this cytokine following stroke would be expected to contribute to neuroprotection. IFNβ may not be the only neuroprotective molecule downstream of IRF signaling. TLR3 signals exclusively through the TRIF-dependent pathway and stimulation of TLR3 in human astrocyte cultures induces the expression of several neuroprotective molecules such as brainderived neurotrophic factor, neurotrophin 4, pleiotrophin, and TGFβ2 (Bsibsi et al., 2006), all of which have been implicated in endogenous neuroprotection (Yeh et al., 1998; Endres et al., 2000; Zhang et al., 2005). Astrocytic TLR3 stimulation also results in production of the anti-inflammatory cytokine IL-10 (Bsibsi et al., 2006). Conditioned media from these cultures enhance neuronal survival and suppress astrocyte growth in slice cultures. Interestingly, LPS stimulation of macrophages has been shown to upregulate TLR3 expression (Nhu et al., 2006), inviting the possibility that LPS preconditioning may upregulate TLR3 in the brain, further enhancing stroke-induced IRF signaling. We suggest that pretreatment with TLR ligands reprograms the brain's response to ischemia and alters endogenous stroke-induced TLR signaling by suppression of the NFκB-inducing pathway and upregulation of the IRF-inducing pathway. Reprogramming causes a finely controlled shift in the balance of proinflammatory and antiinflammatory cytokines, and represents an endogenously orchestrated mechanism that protects the organism from additional damage. We further suggest that reprogramming of endogenous TLR signaling, with the subsequent generation of neuroprotective type I IFNs, is a unifying property of the neuroprotected phenotype. The brain has evolved numerous mechanisms that allow it to withstand the shortage of energy and the oxidative stress caused by ischemia. This tolerant state can be induced by prior exposure to LPS or CpG, or by prior exposure to other non-damaging (i.e. sub-threshold) noxious stimuli. For example, mild exposure to ischemia, excitotoxic stimuli, or inflammatory mediators can precondition the brain to better tolerate a subsequent injurious ischemic event. These mild preconditioning exposures herald impending danger and, as such, induce endogenous protective strategies in anticipation of injury. Though the final outcome of tolerance induction is the same—protection of brain tissue from ischemic injury—the effector mechanisms employed by the brain are as diverse as the preconditioning stimuli that induced them. In fact, the phenotype of neuroprotection may be specifically tailored by the nature of the preconditioning stimulus (Stenzel-Poore et al., 2007). For example, preconditioning events that deprive the brain of oxygen or glucose for a short time lead to conservation of energy regulation and mitochondrial integrity during the injurious ischemic episode (Stenzel-Poore et al., 2003; McFalls et al., 2006). Further, as we have described above, preconditioning events that invoke a small inflammatory response lead to altered inflammatory responses to damaging ischemia (Rosenzweig et al., 2004, 2007). It should be emphasized that although significant overlap exists in the cellular processes induced by these diverse stimuli, the pathways that dominate each response are distinct. The first demonstration that a short period of oxygen deprivation could protect the brain from a subsequent extended period of hypoxia occurred in 1943 (Noble, 1943). Since then, hundreds of studies have been undertaken to better understand the underlying mechanisms of "ischemic preconditioning." Though several endogenously protective pathways are induced by the initiating ischemic event, one particular theme is emerging—that of mitochondrial maintenance and energy conservation (Dirnagl and Meisel, 2008). The priming ischemic episode appears to induce cellular pathways that protect mitochondria against stroke induced deficits in the electron transport chain (Dave et al., 2001). These pathways protect mitochondrial membrane potential (Wu et al., 2004), preserve mitochondrial cytochrome c (Zhan et al., 2002), increase mitochondrial sequestration of Ca^+ and increase Ca^+-ATPase activity. In addition, ischemic preconditioning appears to suppress molecules that regulate ion channels, leading to channel arrest—i.e. reduction in ion permeability through the plasma membrane—which has been shown to reduce the amount of ATP required to maintain ionic homeostasis (Buck and Hochachka, 1993; Stenzel-Poore et al., 2003). Finally, a decrease in the overall cellular metabolic rate limits the stressful effects of oxygen deprivation. The pre preconditioning stimulus suppresses the expression of genes involved in protein turnover, proteasomal degradation, and energy metabolism (Stenzel-Poore et al., 2003). Although ischemic preconditioning has also been shown to help maintain protein structure and function and to suppress the damaging inflammatory response to stroke, it is increasingly clear that sustaining mitochondrial integrity and conserving energy are important mechanisms driving endogenous ischemic tolerance. Several studies have shown that the priming ischemic event induces HSP70 within the brain (Truettner et al., 2002). In addition to its role in stabilizing protein structure, HSP70 acts as an endogenous ligand of TLR4. In fact, extracellular HSP70 has been shown to induce endotoxin tolerance (Aneja et al., 2006). Hence TLRs may be stimulated in the course of ischemic preconditioning, resulting in a reprogrammed TLR response to subsequent injurious ischemia. One of the molecular consequences of reprogrammed TLR signaling is an increase in IFNβ. Notably, IFNβ has been shown to aid in the maintenance of mitochondrial integrity. For example, treatment of astrocytes with IFNβ prevents neuronal mitochondrial respiratory chain damage (Stewart et al., 1998) and reduce IFNβ induced nitric oxide synthase (Stewart et al., 1997). Thus reprogrammed TLR signaling may help shape the phenotype of ischemia-induced tolerance The phenomenon of inflammation-induced cross-tolerance to ischemia is not limited to LPS, but extends to TNFα as well. Nawashiro et al. (1997) were the first to demonstrate that intracisternal administration of TNFα protects the brain from subsequent ischemic challenge. This protection is correlated to a decrease in CD11b immunoreactivity, suggesting a decrease in the inflammatory response to ischemia in the setting of preconditioning. Consistent with this observation, TNFα pretreatment of astrocytes and endothelial cells, through its signaling intermediate ceramide, produces a state of hypo-responsiveness as pretreated cells fail to upregulate ICAM-1 during subsequent hypoxia (Ginis et al., 2002). The decrease in ICAM-1 does not reflect global cellular suppression, but instead signifies a reprogrammed genomic response to stroke, as the hypoxiainduced expression of cytoprotective MnSOD is not affected by preconditioning. Evidence for a reprogrammed genomic response to ischemia is supported by the observation that TNFα preconditioning prevents hypoxia-induced phosphorylation of the proinflammatory transcription factor component NFκBp65, thereby preventing its interaction with the transcriptional activator p300. Taken together, these data indicate that pretreatment with TNFα reprograms the cellular environment and hence alters inflammatory reactions in response to ischemia. Just as TNFα can induce tolerance to subsequent ischemic exposure, it can induce tolerance to subsequent LPS exposure (Porter et al., 1998; Ferlito et al., 2001; Murphey and Traber, 2001). Hence TNFα preconditioning has the potential to induce a state of cross-tolerance to TLR ligands, and thereby reprogram the TLR response to stroke. IFNβ has been shown to cause many of the effects observed in TNFα-induced ischemic tolerance, such as suppression of inflammatory cytokine production, including TNFα itself, and reduction of cellular infiltration into ischemic brain regions (Veldhuis et al., 2003a). Together, these studies suggest that multiple preconditioning stimuli may cause a reprogrammed TLR response to stroke. IFNβ, produced secondary to this reprogrammed response, may aid in maintaining mitochondrial stability and in dampening the inflammatory responses to injurious ischemia.

7. The receptor for Advanced Glycation End Products (RAGE)

Advanced glycation end products (AGEs) are nonenzymatical adducts of proteins, lipids, and nucleic acids which form in a time-dependent manner in a pro-oxidant environment, especially when target molecules turnover slowly and the level of aldoses is elevated

(Schmidt et al, 1995; Vlassara et al, 1994; Bierhaus et al, 1998; Baynes, 2003; Thornalley, 1998; Brownlee, 2000). Glycation of macromolecules was originally thought to mark senescent proteins for subsequent degradation by macrophages. Receptors binding AGEs were regarded as scavenger receptors involved in AGE disposal and cell regeneration, and defective clearance of such modified proteins was believed to be important in aging and diseases with accelerated AGE-formation, such as diabetes or atherosclerosis (Vlassara et al,1994, 1985). However, when the receptor for AGEs (RAGE) was cloned and first characterized (Neeper et al,1992; Schmidt et al,1992, 1994) it turned out that binding of AGEs to RAGE did not accelerate their clearance and degradation. Rather, ligand–receptor interaction induced sustained post-receptor signaling, including activation of p21ras, MAP kinases, and the NF-κB pathway (Lander et al, 1997; Basta et al, 2002; Bucciarelli et al, 2002). Thus, the concept of RAGE as a scavenger/clearance receptor has to be revised and extended.

7.1 RAGE: Structure and ligand recognition

RAGE is a member of the immunoglobulin superfamily of cell surface molecules (Schmidt et al, 1993; Sugaya, 1994). The gene is localized on chromosome 6 near the HLA locus in the vicinity of the MHCIII complex in humans and mice, in close proximity to the homeobox gene HOX12 and the human counterpart of the mouse mammary tumor gene int-3 (Malherbe et al, 1999). The receptor is composed of three immunoglobulin-like regions: one "V"- type domain and two "C"-type-domains, a short transmembrane domain, and a 43-amino acid cytoplasmic tail (Neeper et al, 1992; Schmidt et al, 1994; Lander et al, 1997). While the "V-type" domain confers ligand binding, the cytoplasmic tail is critical for intracellular signaling. Shortly after RAGE was recognized as a receptor for AGEs, it became evident that a number of other ligands also interacted with the receptor (Bucciarelli et al, 2002; Schmidt et al, 2001; Du Yan et al, 1997; Yan et al, 1996, 2000). Structural analysis of ligand–RAGE interaction revealed that the receptor recognized three-dimensional structures, such as β-sheets and fibrils, rather than specific amino acid sequences (i.e., primary structure) (Bucciarelli et al, 2002; Schmidt et al, 2001). In addition to AGEs, RAGE binds amyloid-β peptide (accumulating in Alzheimer's disease) (Du Yan et al, 1997; Yan et al, 2000) and amyloid A (accumulating in systemic amyloidosis). Further, ligands of RAGE are S100/calgranulins, a family of closely related calcium-binding polypeptides that accumulate extracellularly at sites of chronic inflammation (Hofmann et al, 1999; Marenholz et al, 2004). Another proinflammatory ligand of RAGE is the DNA binding protein HMGB1 (amphoterin), which is released by cells undergoing necrosis (Hori et al, 1995; Wang et al, 1999; Anderson and Tracey, 2003; Treutiger et al, 2003). Besides binding ligands actively participating in chronic inflammatory and immune responses, RAGE also interacts with surface molecules on bacteria (Chapman et al, 2002), prions (Sasaki et al, 2002), and leukocytes (Chavakis et al, 2003). Thus, RAGE is much more than a receptor for AGEs; it has a broad repertoire of ligands, which share the propensity to accumulate in tissues during aging, chronic degenerative diseases, inflammation and the host response (Tretiger et al,2003). Therefore, RAGE should be considered a pattern recognition receptor (PRR) (Schmidt et al, 2001; Chavakis et al, 2003; Liliensiek et al, 2004; Gordon, 2002), and potential similarities to members of the family of Toll-like receptors should be considered (Akira et al, 2001).

7.2 RAGE-mediated NF-κB activation

Engagement of RAGE results in intracellular signaling which leads to activation of the proinflammatory transcription factor NF-κB, the latter rapidly activated as part of the first line of cellular defense (Bierhaus et al, 2001). In resting cells, NF-κB resides in the cytoplasm in its inactive form bound to the inhibitor molecule IκBα (Barnes and Karin, 1997). Upon activation, IκBα is rapidly phosphorylated and degraded, resulting in release and translocation of NF-κB (preferentially the NF-κB-heterodimer p50/p65) into the nucleus. Subsequent to nuclear translocation, NF-κB binds to decameric DNA sequences and activates transcription of NF-κB regulated target genes, such as cytokines, adhesion molecules, prothrombotic and vasoconstrictive gene products, RAGE itself, and IκBα (Barnes and Karin, 1997; Li and Schmidt, 1997; Bierhaus et al, 2000). A number of anti-apoptotic genes, including Bcl-XL, Bcl-2, and the Bcl-2 homologues A1, are also under control of NF-κB. NF-κB activation therefore provides a rapid and sensitive cellular response in the absence of new protein synthesis, which promotes cellular survival. One unique feature of RAGE-mediated NF-κB activation is the prolonged time course which appears to overwhelm endogenous autoregulatory feedback inhibition loops (Bierhaus et al, 2001). NF-κB activation subsequent to ligation of RAGE is initiated by the degradation of IκBα and IκBβ, followed by new synthesis of NF-κBp65 in the presence of newly synthesized IκBβ. De novo synthesis of p65 mRNA results in a constantly growing pool of excess transcriptionally active NF-κBp65. In contrast, the amount of newly synthesized IκBα is not sufficient to retain NF-κBp65 in the cytoplasm. In addition, newly synthesized IκBβ has been shown to be hyperphosphorylated, thereby sequestering newly synthesized NF-κB from IκBα (Thompson et al, 1995; Johnson et al, 1996)? Thus, new synthesis of IκBβ might further promote RAGEdependent sustained NF-κB activation. Since, in turn, RAGE expression is induced by NF-κB (Li and Schmidt, 1997), sustained activation of NF-κB results in upregulation of the receptor and further ensures maintenance and amplification of the signal.

7.3 AGEs and RAGE affect cellular defense mechanisms

Besides activating proinflammatory responses, RAGE downregulates cellular defense mechanisms. Ligation of RAGE by AGEs results in the suppression of reduced glutathione (GSH) and ascorbic acid levels and thereby contributes to increased intracellular oxidant stress (Lander et al, 1997; Bierhaus et al, 1997). Depletion of glutathione accounts for diminished glyoxalase-1 recycling and decreased in situ activity of glyoxalase-1 (Thornalley,1998). Glyoxalase-1, in turn, is required to catalyze the conversion of reactive, acyclic alpha-oxoaldehydes into the corresponding alpha-hydroxyacids (Degenhard 1998; Thornalley et al,1999). Since alpha-oxoaldehydes, such as methylglyoxal, represent the largest pool of reactive intracellular AGEs, glyoxalase-1 has an important role in reduction of the cellular AGE load. Consistent with this concept, in vitro experiments with cultivated endothelial cells have demonstrated that glyoxalase-1 overexpression prevents intracellular AGE formation (Shinohara et al,1998). Studies in the model organism Caenorhabditis elegans have recently confirmed that overexpression of glyoxalase-1 not only prevents AGE formation, but also protects the animals from deleterious effects of oxidant stress, as evidenced by increased longevity (Morcos et al,2004). These observations imply that engagement of RAGE not only results in increased cellular activation, but also in reduction of AGE detoxifying mechanisms.

7.4 RAGE and neuroprotection

RAGE transcription is controlled by several transcription factors, including SP-1, AP-2, NF-κB, and NF-IL6 (Li and Schmidt, 1997). RAGE expression occurs in both a constitutive and inducible manner, depending on the cell type and developmental stage (Hori et al,1995; Brett et al,1993). Whereas RAGE is constitutively expressed during embryonic development, its expression is downregulated in adult life. However, known exceptions are skin and lung, which constitutively express RAGE throughout life. Most other cells, including monocytes/macrophages, endothelial cells, smooth musclecells, fibroblasts, and neuronal cells, do not express significant amounts of RAGE under physiological conditions but can be induced to express RAGE in situations where either ligands accumulate and/or transcription factors regulating RAGE are activated (Basta et al, 2002; Bucciarelli et al, 2002; Hanford et al, 2004; Akira et al, 2001; Li et al,2004; Sorci et al, 2004a, 2004b; Cortizo et al, 2003; Shanmugam et al, 2003; Ishihara et al, 2003). Due to its ability to sustain cellular activation, RAGE has the potential to function as a master switch capable of converting a transient proinflammatory response, evoked by an inflammatory stimulus into sustained cellular dysfunction (Schmidt et al, 2001; Bierhaus et al, 2001). The majority of cellular stressors induce both the formation of reactive oxygen species (ROS) and transient activation of NF-κB (Yeh et al, 2001; Taguchi et al, 2000; Huttunen et al, 19999; Huang et al, 2001; Wautier et al, 2001). In addition, inflammatory cells directly release RAGE ligands, such as S100/calgranulins and HMGB-1 (Kokkola et al, 2005). The myeloperoxidase system of human phagocytes generates N" -(carboxymethyl)lysine, a highly reactive AGE and RAGE-ligand, at sites of inflammation (Anderson et al, 1999; Kislinger et al, 1999). High glucose concentrations promote AGE formation inside and outside cells (Brownlee, 2000; Schiekofer et al, 2003). Such time-dependent formation of AGE might also play a role in the expression of binding sites for amyloid peptides (Yan et al, 2000). In turn, RAGE has been shown to mediate transport of pathophysiologically relevant concentrations of amyloid-β peptide into the CNS (Mackic et al, 1998). Thus, stimuli initially inducing oxidant stress and NF-κB activation have the potential to activate RAGE and thereby sustain NF-κB-dependent gene expression. Activation of NF-κB results in increased RAGE expression and increases the number of ligand binding sites, thereby prolonging NF-κB activation (Schmidt et al, 2001; Bierhaus et al, 2001). Frequently, the biology of RAGE coincides with settings in which ligands of the receptor accumulate, especially in a proinflammatory environment such as diabetes mellitus, atherosclerosis, neurodegenerative disorders, rheumatoid arthritis, chronic renal disease, and inflammatory bowl disease (Basta et al, 2002; Schmidt et al, 2001; Lalla et al, 2001; Wendt et al, 2003; Bierhaus et al, 2004; Sakaguchi et al, 2003; Kislinger et al, 2001; Drinda et al, 2004; Chen et al, 2004; Goosa et al, 2001). To better understand the role of RAGE in these pathophysiological situations, interaction of ligands with cell surface RAGE was intercepted using soluble RAGE (sRAGE). Soluble RAGE is a truncated form of the receptor comprising the extracellular domain and thereby functions as a decoy that prevents ligands from interacting with cell surface receptor. Application of sRAGE in vitro and in vivo resulted in an effective blockade of RAGE, according to a decoy mechanism, in a range of animal models (Hudson et al, 2003; Lue et al, 2001; Arancio et al, 2004; Constien et al, 2001). sRAGE prevented development of micro- and macrovascular diseases in rodents, suggesting a key role for RAGE in the development of chronic vascular disorders. Moreover, sRAGE efficiently reduced late complications of experimental diabetes in both autoimmune (Chen et al, 2004) and streptozotocin induced diabetes (Wendt et al, 2003; Bierhaus et al,

2004), restored delayed wound healing (Goosa et al, 2001), protected rodent from tumor metastases and growth of primary tumors (Taguchi et al, 2000), and improved the outcome of experimental colitis (Hofmann et al, 1999). sRAGE and anti-RAGE F(ab')2-fragments suppressed abnormal findings associated with Alzheimer's-like pathology in transgenic rodent models (Lue et al, 2001; Arancio et al, 2004) and reduced the transport of amyloid-β-peptide across the blood-brain barrier (Mackic et al, 1998) . Since most of the data obtained with sRAGE were confirmed by application of neutralizing antibodies to the receptor and/or transfection with plasmids overexpressing dominant negative RAGE, the receptor has been suggested as a potentially effective therapeutic target (Hudson et al, 2003). At the same time, it seemed unlikely that RAGE could mediate so many deleterious effects in such diverse models of disease. Since RAGE has properties of a PRR, binding to a variety of ligands, the promising effects observed with sRAGE might not only result from intercepting the interaction of ligands with cell surface RAGE, but possibly with other receptors. For example, S100 proteins and HMGB1 certainly do not exclusively bind to RAGE. These ligands also recognize other cellular structures (Robinson et al, 2002; Erlandsson et al, 2004). In order to test the potential impact of RAGE blockade and to further define a potential role of RAGE in diabetic complications and chronic inflammatory disease, homozygous RAGE-deficient mice (RAGE−/− mice) and mice with tissue-specific RAGE expression (tie2-RAGE and tie2-RAGE°−RAGE−/−) have been made (Constien et al, 2001). These mice are viable and display normal reproductive fitness without any striking phenotype (Wendt et al, 2003; Bierhaus et al, 2004; Sakaguchi et al, 2003). Induction of diabetes in these mice confirmed that RAGE contributes, at least in part, to the development of diabetic complications. Diabetic nephropathy, characterized by renal enlargement, glomerular hypertrophy, albuminuria, and mesangial expansion, was significantly increased in diabetic mice overexpressing RAGE in the vasculature, but was reduced in RAGE−/−mice (Yamamoto et al, 2001). Similar changes were observed in diabetic neuropathy. Whereas diabetic mice overexpressing RAGE showed an increase in functional deficits, such as delayed motor nerve conduction velocity (Yajima et al, 2004), RAGE−/− mice were partially protected from diabetes-induced loss of neural function (Bierhaus et al, 2004). Neointimal expansion in RAGE−/− mice was significantly suppressed compared with that observed in wildtype littermates using a femoral artery denudation protocol to induce arterial injury (Sakaguchi et al, 2003). Remarkably, in each of these models (diabetic nephropathy, neuropathy, arterial restenosis, etc.), protection from development of pathology was more profound in wild-type mice treated with sRAGE than in RAGE−/− mice. In diabetic neuropathy, for example, administration of sRAGE to diabetic wild-type animals completely restored pain perception, whereas diabetic RAGE−/− mice were only partly protected from loss of pain perception. These observations suggest that ligands sequestered by sRAGE are likely to interact with cellular structures different from RAGE and are also involved in perturbation of pain perception. The absence of a developmental phenotype in RAGE−/− mice and the possibility that RAGE might impact on multiple chronic disease states have largely focussed attention away from physiologic roles of the receptor. So far, only a few reports have suggested that RAGE expression might contribute to developmental paradigms, based on in vitro studies. For example, in axonal sprouting which accompanies neuronal development, RAGE-HMGB1 interaction may contribute (Fages et al, 2000; Hittinen et al, 2000). Huttunen et al. further demonstrated that activation of RAGE by HMGB1 (amphoterin) and S100B can promote cell survival through increased expression of the anti-apoptotic protein Bcl-2. However, whereas nanomolar concentrations of S100B induced trophic effects in RAGEexpressing cells, micromolar concentrations caused apoptosis in a manner that appeared to depend on oxidant stress. For both of these outcomes, the cytoplasmic domain of RAGE was required, as cells expressing a dominant-negative mutant (i.e., lacking the cytosolic tail) are unresponsive to these stimuli. The neurite outgrowth-promoting role of RAGE was recently confirmed in vivo in a unilateral sciatic nerve crush model, in which blockade of RAGE, either by sRAGE or by blocking F(ab')2 fragments of antibodies (raised to either RAGE or to S100/calgranulins or amphoterin) reduced functional regeneration of the peripheral nerve (Rong et al, 2004a). Similar results were observed in transgenic mice overexpressing dominant negative RAGE (Rong et al, 2004b). However, RAGE−/− mice demonstrate neither obvious neuronal deficits nor overt behavior abnormalities, indicating that RAGE may contribute to neuronal development, but that there are redundant systems that substitute for this receptor in its absence. Furthermore, it will be interesting to see if future experiments in RAGE−/− mice confirm a role for RAGE in the repair of peripheral nerve injury. In terms of a contribution for RAGE in development, expression of the receptor in vivo appears to mirror developmental processes. After being highly expressed during embryonic development, RAGE is downregulated in most organs during normal life (Kokkola et al, 2005). Upon aging, RAGE expression increases again, although it is not known whether this is due to accumulation of RAGE ligands (which upregulate receptor expression) or whether this represents a compensatory mechanism protecting aging cells from cell death. Another line of evidence for a role of RAGE in the regulation of differentiation comes from recently published studies showing that non-small cell lung carcinomas are characterized by downregulation of RAGE (Bartling et al, 2004). One reason for this might be that loss of HMGB1(amphoterin)/RAGE-mediated regulation of tumor cell migration and invasive processes results in more aggressive tumor behavior (Huttunen et al, 2002). A COOH-terminal motif in HMGB1 (amino acids 150–183) has recently been identified as responsible for RAGE binding. This portion of HMGB1 efficiently inhibits RAGE-mediated extension of cellular processes and transendothelial migration of tumor cells. This observation leads us to propose that loss of RAGE might promote tumor growth, at least in settings affecting the lung, one of the few tissues in which RAGE is constitutively expressed at high levels. Since this observation contrasts with a previous finding in which sRAGE suppressed tumor growth and metastasis (Taguchi et al, 2000), the latter observations might be due to the ability of sRAGE to intercept the interaction of RAGE ligands with other receptors.

8. Conclusion and prospective

Cell death from ischemia involves a complex biological cascade. Initially, energy failure is followed by glutamate overload and Ca^{2+} influx into the cell. These processes initiate a series of events, including the generation of free radicals, apoptosis, an inflammatory response and generation of growth factors. Many of these processes are the direct result of the up- or downregulation of specific gene families. Thus, a desirable neuroprotectant would, in theory, be one that antagonises multiple injury mechanisms. The studies described above demonstrate an emerging role for endogenous neuroprotectant in ischemic damage and ischemic prophylaxis. Among these, erythropoietin (Epo), has a dominant role for neuroprotection, neurogenesis and act as a neurotrophic factor in the central nervous system. These functions make erythropoietin a good candidate for treating disease associated with neuronal cell death. However, our understanding of the underlying mechanisms is far from being complete and a number of open questions remain to be answered: 1) What is the exact route and mechanism through which Epo passes through the BBB? 2) Which cellular mechanisms govern the immunomodulatory effects of Epo in glial cells? 3) Does Epo activate the same or diverse intracellular signaling pathways in the different cells that express EpoR in the brain, neurons, glial, and endothelial cells? Nevertheless, since the discovery of Epo expression in the brain less than 15 years ago, a tremendous achievement in the understanding of its action in the CNS has been accomplished. Today, Epo is a prominent member of a growing list of hematopoietic and angiogenic factors found to be expressed and acting as protective factors in the CNS. Because of the observed increased death rate, rtPA-treated patients should be excluded from acute poststroke EPO application. In cerebral ischemia, albumin is mainly involved in the improvement of blood microcirculation; however, direct neuroprotection cannot be overlooked. Different in vitro and in vivo studies indicate that albumin has direct neuroprotective effects by acting on astrocytes, microglia and neurons. Altogether albumin can alter brain function by many direct and indirect mechanisms and detailed study of these actions will reveal the role of this multifunctional protein in brain functions. Furthermore, the evidence of de novo synthesis of albumin in microglial cells could encourage the neurologist to investigate newer roles of this multifunctional protein in many neurodegenerative diseases. The prothrombotic, proinflammatory state of stroke results in a promotion of thrombin formation and fibrin deposition at the vascular wall, as well as in the formation of platelet-leukocyte coaggregates, leading to severe disturbance of the microcirculation, capillary leakage and tissue damage. The ability of ATIII to inhibit the actions of both factor Xa and thrombin gives it the potential to block, in part or fully, a wide rage of proinflammatory events. Heparin and heparan sulfate glycoproteins (HSPGs) appear to function as receptors for ATIII on endothelium and leukocytes and can lead to the reduced expression of procoagulatory tissue factor and proinflammatory cytokines as well as heterologous receptor regulatory processes. ATIII has been shown in vitro to increase prostacyclin responses and to inhibit a variety of cell responses including endotoxin-induced nuclear translocation of NF-kB, a key step in the generation of the inflammatory response.

Here, we also discussed the critical role of Toll-like receptors in mediating cerebral ischemic injury and suggested endogenous mechanisms that, when induced, redirect this role from detrimental to beneficial. In fact, many diverse neuroprotective paradigms may redirect TLR signaling as one mechanism of endogenous protection. Paradoxically, TLR ligands administered systemically induce a state of tolerance to subsequent ischemic injury. Herein we suggest that stimulation of TLRs prior to ischemia reprograms TLR signaling that occurs following ischemic injury. Such reprogramming leads to suppressed expression of pro-inflammatory molecules and enhanced expression of numerous anti-inflammatory mediators that collectively confer robust neuroprotection. Research findings indicate that numerous preconditioning stimuli lead to TLR activation, an event that occurs prior to ischemia and ultimately leads to TLR reprogramming. Thus genomic reprogramming of

TLR signaling may be a unifying principle of tolerance to cerebral ischemia. Recent studies have also demonstrated an increased expression of the cell-surface RAGE in dying neurons after hypoxic-ischemic insults and human cerebral ischemia, and suggested that the RAGE-ligand interaction causes neuronal cytotoxicity. RAGE also has a circulating truncated variant isoform, soluble RAGE (sRAGE), which corresponds to its extracellular domain only. Exogenously administered sRAGE has been successfully used to antagonize advanced glycation end products (AGE)-RAGE-mediated vascular damage. Accordingly, sRAGE may compete with cell-surface RAGE for the ligand, thus functioning as a decoy and possibly exerting a cytoprotective effect. Most of the data available so far point to the RAGE/NF-κB axis as an attractive target for future clinical interventions in several chronic disease states. However, until physiologic properties of RAGE have been clearly deciphered, it is most prudent to adopt a cautious approach when future therapeutic strategies involving long-term blockade of RAGE or its ligands are considered. Another important issue to be addressed concerns how studies performed in rodent models will translate to human disease. Alternatively, if RAGE antagonists are eventually used in humans, it will be fascinating to understand the impact of long-term blockade of RAGE in critically ill patients, in view of the likely complex role of RAGE, and other receptors interacting with RAGE ligands, in regulating physiologic and pathophysiologic processes in a wide range of situations.

9. References

Ahmed S, He Y, Nassief A, Xu J, Xu X, Hsu C (2000) Effects of lipopolysaccharide priming on acute ischemic brain injury. Stroke 31:193–199.

Ahn, S.M., Byun, K., Cho, K., Kim, J.Y., Yoo, J.S., Kim, D., Paek, S.H., Kim, S.U., Simpson, R.J., and Lee, B. (2008). Human microglial cells synthesize albumin in brain. PLoS One *3* , e2829.

Akira S, Takeda K, Kaisho T (2001) Toll-like receptors: critical proteins linking innate and acquired immunity. Nat Immunol 1:675–680

Alafaci C, Salpietro F, Grasso G, Sfacteria A, Passalacqua M, Morabito A, Tripodo E, Calapai G, Buemi M, Tomasello F. Effect of recombinant human erythropoietin on cerebral ischemia following experimental subarachnoid hemorrhage. *Eur J Pharmacol* 406: 219–225, 2000.

Anagnostou A, Lee ES, Kessimian N, Levinson R, Steiner M. Erythropoietin has a mitogenic and positive chemotactic effect on endothelial cells. *Proc Natl Acad Sci USA* 87: 5978–5982, 1990.

Anderson MM, Requena JR, Crowley JR, Thorpe SR, Heinecke JW (1999) The myeloperoxidase system of human phagocytes generates Nepsilon-(carboxymethyl)lysine on proteins: a mechanism for producing advanced glycated endproduts at sites of inflammation. J Clin Invest 104:103–113

Andersson U, Tracey KJ (2003) HMGB1 in sepsis. Scand J Infect Dis 35:577–584

Aneja R, Odoms K, Dunsmore K, Shanley TP, Wong HR (2006) Extracellular heat shock protein-70 induces endotoxin tolerance in THP-1 cells. J Immunol 177:7184–7192.

Arancio O, Zhang HP, Chen X, Lin C, Trinchese F, Puzzo D, Liu S, Hegde A, Yan SF, Stern A, Luddy JS, Lue LF, Walker DG, Roher A, Buttini M, Mucke L, Li W, Schmidt AM, Kindy M, Hyslop PA, Stern DM, Du Yan SS (2004) RAGE potentiates Abeta-induced perturbation of neuronal function in transgenic mice. EMBO J 23:4096–4105

Arcasoy MO. The non-haematopoietic biological effects of erythropoietin. *Br J Haematol* 141: 14–31, 2008.

Arroyo, V. (2002). Review article: albumin in the treatment of liver diseases - new features of a classical treatment. Aliment Pharmacol. Ther. *16* (Suppl. 5), 1 - 5.

Bagchi A, Herrup EA, Warren HS, Trigilio J, Shin HS, Valentine C, Hellman J (2007) MyD88-dependent and MyD88- independent pathways in synergy, priming, and tolerance between TLR agonists. J Immunol 178:1164–1171.

Baltanas, F.C., Weruaga, E., Valero, J., Recio, J.S., and Alonso, J.R. (2009). Albumin attenuates DNA damage in primary- cultured neurons. Neurosci. Lett. *450* , 23 - 26.

Banks WA, Jumbe NL, Farrell CL, Niehoff ML, Heatherington AC. Passage of erythropoietic agents across the blood- brain barrier: a comparison of human and murine erythropoietin and the analog darbepoetin alfa. *Eur J Pharmacol* 505: 93–101, 2004

Barnes PJ, Karin M (1997) Nuclear factor-κB-a pivotal transcription factor in chronic inflammatory diseases. N Engl J Med 336:1066–1071

Bartling B, Hofmann HS, Weigle B, Silber RE, Simm A (2004) Down-regulation of the receptor for advanced glycation endproducts (RAGE) supports non-small cell lung carcinoma. Carcinogenesis [Epub ahead of print]

Basta G, Lazzerini G, Massaro M, Simoncini T, Tanganelli P, Fu C, Kislinger T, Stern DM, Schmidt AM, De Caterina R (2002) Advanced glycation end products activate endothelium through signal-transduction receptor RAGE: a mechanism for amplification of inflammatory responses. Circulation 105:816–822

Bastide M, Gele P, Petrault O, Pu Q, Caliz A, Robin E, Deplanque D, Duriez P, Bordet R (2003) Delayed cerebrovascular protective effect of lipopolysaccharide in parallel to brain ischemic tolerance. J Cereb Blood Flow Metab 23:399- 405.

Bauer KA, Rosenberg RD: Role of antithrombin III as a regulator of in vivo coagulation. Semin Hematol 1991;28:10-18.

Baynes JW (2003) Chemical modification of proteins by lipids in diabetes. Clin Chem Lab Med 41:1159–1165

Belayev, L., Alonso, O.F., Huh, P.W., Zhao, W., Busto, R., and Ginsberg, M.D. (1999a). Posttreatment with high-dose albumin reduces histopathological damage and improves neurological deficit following fl uid percussion brain injury in rats. J. Neurotrauma *16* , 445 - 453.

Belayev, L., Busto, R., Zhao, W., Clemens, J.A., and Ginsberg, M.D. (1997a). Effect of delayed albumin hemodilution on infarction volume and brain edema after transient middle cerebral artery occlusion in rats. J. Neurosurg. *87* , 595 - 601.

Belayev, L., Liu, Y., Zhao, W., Busto, R., and Ginsberg, M.D. (2001). Human albumin therapy of acute ischemic stroke: marked neuroprotective efficacy at moderate doses and with a broad therapeutic window. Stroke *32* , 553 - 560.

Belayev, L., Pinard, E., Nallet, H., Seylaz, J., Liu, Y., Riyamongkol, P., Zhao, W., Busto, R., and Ginsberg, M.D. (2002). Albumin therapy of transient focal cerebral ischemia: in vivo analysis of dynamic microvascular responses. Stroke *33* , 1077 - 1084.

Belayev, L., Saul, I., Busto, R., Danielyan, K., Vigdorchik, A., Khoutorova, L., and Ginsberg, M.D. (2005). Albumin treatment reduces neurological defi cit and protects blood-brain barrier integrity after acute intracortical hematoma in the rat. Stroke *36* , 326 - 331.

Belayev, L., Saul, I., Huh, P.W., Finotti, N., Zhao, W., Busto, R., and Ginsberg, M.D. (1999b). Neuroprotective effect of highdose albumin therapy against global ischemic brain injury in rats. Brain Res. *845* , 107 - 111.

Belayev, L., Zhao, W., Busto, R., and Ginsberg, M.D. (1997b). Transient middle cerebral artery occlusion by intraluminal suture: I. Three-dimensional autoradiographic image-analysis of local cerebral glucose metabolism-blood flow interrelationships during ischemia and early recirculation. J. Cereb. Blood Flow Metab. *17* , 1266 - 1280.

Belayev, L., Zhao, W., Pattany, P.M., Weaver, R.G., Huh, P.W., Lin, B., Busto, R., and Ginsberg, M.D. (1998). Diffusion- weighted magnetic resonance imaging confi rms marked neuroprotective efficacy of albumin therapy in focal cerebral ischemia. Stroke *29* , 2587 - 2599.

Bento-Abreu, A., Velasco, A., Polo-Hernandez, E., Lillo, C., Kozyraki, R., Tabernero, A., and Medina, J.M. (2009). Albumin endocytosis via megalin in astrocytes is caveola- and Dab-1 dependent and is required for the synthesis of the neurotrophic factor oleic acid. J. Neurochem. *111* , 49 - 60.

Bento-Abreu, A., Velasco, A., Polo-Hernandez, E., Perez-Reyes, P.L., Tabernero, A., and Medina, J.M. (2008). Megalin is a receptor for albumin in astrocytes and is required for the synthesis of the neurotrophic factor oleic acid. J. Neurochem. *106* , 1149 - 1159.

Bernaudin M, Bellail A, Marti HH, Yvon A, Vivien D, Duchatelle I, MacKenzie ET, Petit E. Neurons and astrocytes express EPO mRNA: oxygen-sensing mechanisms that involve the redox-state of the brain. *Glia* 30: 271–278, 2000.

Bernaudin M, Marti HH, Roussel S, Divoux D, Nouvelot A, MacKenzie ET, Petit E. A potential role for erythropoietin in focal permanent cerebral ischemia in mice. *J Cereb Blood Flow Metab* 19: 643–651, 1999.

Biere, A.L., Ostaszewski, B., Stimson, E.R., Hyman, B.T., Maggio, J.E., and Selkoe, D.J. (1996). Amyloid beta-peptide is transported on lipoproteins and albumin in human plasma. J. Biol. Chem. *271* , 32916 - 32922.

Bierhaus A, Chen J, Liliensiek B, Nawroth PP (2000) LPS and cytokine activated endothelium. In: Nawroth PP (ed) Seminars in Thrombosis and Hemostasis, vol. 26, pp 571–588

Bierhaus A, Chevion S, Chevion M, Hofmann M, Quehenberger P, Illmer T, Luther T, Wahl P, Tritschler H, Müller M, Ziegler R, Nawroth PP (1997) Advanced glycation endproduct (AGEs) induced activation of NF-κB is suppressed by α-lipoic acid in cultured endothelial cells. Diabetes 46:1481–1490

Bierhaus A, Haslbeck KM, Humpert PM, Liliensiek B, Dehmer T, Morcos M, Sayed AA, Andrassy M, Schiekofer S, Schneider J, Schulz J, Heuss D, Neundörfer B, Dierl S, Huber J, Tritschler H, Schmidt AM, Schwaninger M, Häring HU, Schleicher E, Stern DM, Kasper M, Arnold B, Nawroth PP (2004) Loss of pain perception in diabetic neuropathy is dependent on a receptor of the immune globulin superfamily. J Clin Invest 114:1741–1751

Bierhaus A, Hofmann MA, Ziegler R, Nawroth PP (1998) The AGE/RAGE pathway in vascular disease and diabetes mellitus. Part I: the AGE-concept. Cardiovasc Res 37:586–600

Bierhaus A, Schiekofer S, Schwaninger M, Andrassy M, Humpert P, Chen J, Hong M, Luther T, Henle T, Klöting I, biphasic activation of NF-κB. Cell 80:573–582

Boada, M., Ortiz, P., Anaya, F., Hernandez, I., Munoz, J., Nunez, L., Olazaran, J., Roca, I., Cuberas, G., Tarraga, L., et al. (2009). Amyloid-targeted therapeutics in Alzheimer ' s disease: use of human albumin in plasma exchange as a novel approach for Abeta mobilization. Drug News Perspect. *22* , 325 - 339.

Bogoyevitch MA. An update on the cardiac effects of erythropoietin cardioprotection by erythropoietin and the lessons learnt from studies in neuroprotection. *Cardiovasc Res* 63: 208–216, 2004.

Bohrmann, B., Tjernberg, L., Kuner, P., Poli, S., Levet-Trafi t, B., Naslund, J., Richards, G., Huber, W., Dobeli, H., and Nordstedt, C. (1999). Endogenous proteins controlling amyloid beta-peptide polymerization. Possible implications for beta-amyloid formation in the central nervous system and in peripheral tissues. J. Biol. Chem. *274* , 15990 - 15995.

Bond R, Rerkasem K, Shearman CP, Rothwell PM (2004) Time trends in the published risks of stroke and death due to endarterectomy for symptomatic carotid stenosis. Cerebrovasc Dis 18:37–46.

Bordet R, Deplanque D, Maboudou P, Puisieux F, Pu Q, Robin E, Martin A, Bastide M, Leys D, Lhermitte M, Dupuis B (2000) Increase in endogenous brain superoxide dismutase as a potential mechanism of lipopolysaccharide- induced brain ischemic tolerance. J Cereb Blood Flow Metab 20:1190–1196.

Bosca L, Bodelon OG, Hortelano S, Casellas A, Bosch F (2000) Anti-inflammatory action of type I interferons deduced from mice expressing interferon beta. Gene Ther 7:817–825.

Boutros T, Croze E, Yong VW (1997) Interferon-beta is a potent promoter of nerve growth factor production by astrocytes. J Neurochem 69:939–946.

Brett J, Schmidt AM, Yan SD, Zhou YS, Weidmann E, Pinsky D, Nowygrod R, Neeper M, Przysiecki C, Dhaw A, Migheli A, Stern DM (1993) Survey of the distribution of a newly characterized receptor for advanced glycation end products in tissue. Am J Pathol 143:1699–1712

Brines M, Cerami A. Emerging biological roles for erythropoietin in the nervous system. *Nat Rev Neurosci* 6: 484–494, 2005.

Brines ML, Ghezzi P, Keenan S, Agnello D, de Lanerolle NC, Cerami C, Itri LM, Cerami A. Erythropoietin crosses the blood-brain barrier to protect against experimental brain injury. *Proc Natl Acad Sci USA* 97: 10526–10531, 2000.

Broad A, Kirby JA, Jones DE (2007) Toll-like receptor interactions: tolerance of MyD88-dependent cytokines but enhancement of MyD88-independent interferon-beta production. Immunology 120:103–111.

Brownlee M (2000) Negative consequences of glycation. Metabolism 49:9–13

Bruick RK, McKnight SL. A conserved family of prolyl-4- hydroxylases that modify HIF. *Science* 294: 1337-1340, 2001.

Bsibsi M, Persoon-Deen C, Verwer RW, Meeuwsen S, Ravid R, Van Noort JM (2006) Toll-like receptor 3 on adult human astrocytes triggers production of neuroprotective mediators. Glia 53:688–695.

Bsibsi M, Ravid R, Gveric D, van Noort JM (2002) Broad expression of Toll-like receptors in the human central nervous system. J Neuropathol Exp Neurol 61:1013–1021.

Bucciarelli LG, Wendt T, Rong L, Lalla E, Hofmann MA, Goova MT, Taguchi A, Yan SF, Yan SD, Stern DM, Schmidt AM (2002) RAGE is a multiligand receptor of the immunoglobulin superfamily: implications for homeostasis and chronic disease.Cell Mol Life Sci 59:1117–1128

Bucerius J, Gummert JF, Borger MA, Walther T, Doll N, Onnasch JF, Metz S, Falk V, Mohr FW (2003) Stroke after cardiac surgery: a risk factor analysis of 16,184 consecutive adult patients. Ann Thorac Surg 75:472–478.

Buck LT, Hochachka PW (1993) Anoxic suppression of Na^{+}-K^{+}-ATPase and constant membrane potential in hepatocytes: support for channel arrest. Am J Physiol 265:R1020–R1025.

Byts N, Samoylenko A, Fasshauer T, Ivanisevic M, Hennighausen L, Ehrenreich H, Siren AL. Essential role for Stat5 in the neurotrophic but not in the neuroprotective effect of erythropoietin. *Cell Death Differ* 15: 783–792, 2008.

Cai Z, Manalo DJ, Wei G, Rodriguez ER, Fox-Talbot K, Lu H, Zweier JL, Semenza GL. Hearts from rodents exposed to intermittent hypoxia or erythropoietin are protected against ischemiareperfusion injury. *Circulation* 108: 79–85, 2003.

Candelario-Jalil E, Yang Y, Rosenberg GA (2009) Diverse roles of matrix metalloproteinases and tissue inhibitors of metalloproteinases in neuroinflammation and cerebral ischemia. Neuroscience 158:983–994.

Cao CX, Yang QW, Lv FL, Cui J, Fu HB, Wang JZ (2007) Reduced cerebral ischemia-reperfusion injury in Toll-like receptor 4 deficient mice. Biochem Biophys Res Comm 353:509–514.

Carlini RG, Reyes AA, Rothstein M. Recombinant human erythropoietin stimulates angiogenesis in vitro. *Kidney Int* 47: 740–745, 1995.

Carpentier PA, Begolka WS, Olson JK, Elhofy A, Karpus WJ, Miller SD (2005) Differential activation of astrocytes by innate and adaptive immune stimuli. Glia 49:360–374.

Caso JR, Pradillo JM, Hurtado O, Lorenzo P, Moro MA, Lizasoain I (2007) Toll-like receptor 4 is involved in brain damage and inflammation after experimental stroke. Circulation 115:1599–1608.

Chakravarty S, Herkenham M (2005) Toll-like receptor 4 on nonhematopoietic cells sustains CNS inflammation during endotoxemia, independent of systemic cytokines. J Neurosci 25:1788–1796.

Chapman MR, Robinson LS, Pinkner JS, Roth R, Heuser J, Hammar M, Normark S, Hultgren SJ (2002) Role of Escherichia coli curli operons in directing amyloid fiber formation. Science 5556:851–855

Chavakis T, Bierhaus A, Schneider D, Linn T, Nagashima K, Arnold B, Preissner KT, Nawroth PP (2003) The pattern recognition receptor (RAGE) is a counter receptor for leukocyte integrins: a novel pathway for inflammatory cell recruitment. J Exp Med 198:1507–1515

Chen Y, Yan SS, Colgan J, Zhang HP, Luban J, Schmidt AM, Stern D, Herold KC (2004) Blockade of late stages of autoimmune diabetes by inhibition of the receptor for advanced glycation end products. J Immunol 173:1399- 1405

Chikuma M, Masuda S, Kobayashi T, Nagao M, Sasaki R. Tissue-specific regulation of erythropoietin production in the murine kidney, brain, and uterus. *Am J Physiol Endocrinol Metab* 279: E1242–E1248, 2000.

Chin K, Yu X, Beleslin-Cokic B, Liu C, Shen K, Mohrenweiser HW, Noguchi CT. Production and processing of erythropoietin receptor transcripts in brain. *Brain Res Mol Brain Res* 81: 29–42, 2000.

Chong ZZ, Kang JQ, Maiese K. Erythropoietin is a novel vascular protectant through activation of Akt1 and mitochondrial modulation of cysteine proteases. *Circulation* 106: 2973–2979, 2002.

Cole, D.J., Drummond, J.C., Osborne, T.N., and Matsumura, J. (1990). Hypertension and hemodilution during cerebral ischemia reduce brain injury and edema. Am. J. Physiol. *259* , H211 - H217.

Constantin D, Cordenier A, Robinson K, Ala'Aldeen DA, Murphy S (2004) Neisseria meningitidis-induced death of cerebrovascular endothelium: mechanisms triggering transcriptional activation of inducible nitric oxide synthase. J Neurochem 89:1166–1174.

Constien R, Forde A, Liliensiek B, Grone HJ, Nawroth PP, Hammerling G, Arnold B (2001) Characterization of a novel EGFP reporter mouse to monitor Cre recombination as demonstrated by a Tie2 Cre mouse line. Genesis 30:36- 44

Cortizo AM, Lettieri MG, Barrio DA, Mercer N, Etcheverry SB, McCarthy AD (2003) Advanced glycation end-products (AGEs) induce concerted changes in the osteoblastic expression of their receptor RAGE and in the activation of extracellular signal-regulated kinases (ERK). Mol Cell Biochem 250:1–10

Cotena S, Piazza O, Tufano R: The use of erythtropoietin in cerebral diseases. Panminerva Medica 2008;50(2):185-92.

Cuomo O, Pignataro G, Gala R, Scorziello A, Gravino E, Piazza O, Tufano R, Di Renzo G, Annunziato L. Antithrombin reduces ischemic volume, ameliorates neurologic deficits, and prolongs animal survival in both transient and permanent focal ischemia. Stroke. 2007 Dec;38(12):3272-9. Epub 2007 Nov 1.

Dalpke AH, Lehner MD, Hartung T, Heeg K (2005) Differential effects of CpG-DNA in Toll-like receptor-2/-4/-9 tolerance and cross-tolerance. Immunology 116:203-212.

Dame C, Juul SE, Christensen RD. The biology of erythropoietin in the central nervous system and its neurotrophic and neuroprotective potential. *Biol Neonate* 79: 228–235, 2001.

Dave KR, Saul I, Busto R, Ginsberg MD, Sick TJ, Perez-Pinzon MA (2001) Ischemic preconditioning preserves mitochondrial function after global cerebral ischemia in rat hippocampus. J Cereb Blood Flow Metab 21:1401- 1410.

Davis JE, Gabler NK, Walker-Daniels J, Spurlock ME (2008) Tlr-4 deficiency selectively protects against obesity induced by diets high in saturated fat. Obesity 16:1248-1255.

Dawson DA, Furuya K, Gotoh J, Nakao Y, Hallenbeck JM (1999) Cerebrovascular hemodynamics and ischemic tolerance: lipopolysaccharide-induced resistance to focal cerebral ischemia is not due to changes in severity of the initial ischemic insult, but is associated with preservation of microvascular perfusion. J Cereb Blood Flow Metab 19:616–623.

Degenhard TP, Thorpe SR, Baynes J (1988) Chemical modification of proteins by methylglyoxal. Cell Mol Biol (Noisy- legrand) 44:1139–1145

Digicaylioglu M, Bichet S, Marti HH, Wenger RH, Rivas LA, Bauer C, Gassmann M. Localization of specific erythropoietin binding sites in defined areas of the mouse brain. *Proc Natl Acad Sci USA* 92: 3717–3720, 1995.

Digicaylioglu M, Lipton SA. Erythropoietin-mediated neuroprotection involves cross-talk between Jak2 and NF-kappaB signalling cascades. *Nature* 412: 641–647, 2001.

Dirnagl U, Iadecola C, Moskowitz MA. Pathobiology of ischaemic stroke: an integrated view. *Trends Neurosci* 22: 391- 397, 1999.

Dirnagl U, Meisel A (2008) Endogenous neuroprotection: mitochondria as gateways to cerebral preconditioning? Neuropharmacology 55:334–344.

Drinda S, Franke S, Ruster M, Petrow P, Pullig O, Stein G, Hein G (2004) Identification of the receptor for advanced glycation end products in synovial tissue of patients with rheumatoid arthritis. Rheumatol Int [Epub ahead of print]

Dringen R, Hirrlinger J. Glutathione pathways in the brain. *Biol Chem* 384: 505–516, 2003.

Du Yan S, Zhu H, Fu J, Yan SF, Roher A, Tourtellotte WW, Rajavashisth T, Chen X, Godman GC, Stern D, Schmidt A (1997) Amyloid-beta peptide-receptor for advanced glycation endproduct interaction elicits neuronal expression of macrophage-colony stimulating factor: a proinflammatory pathway in Alzheimer disease. Proc Natl Acad Sci U S A 94:5296–5301

Dunzendorfer S, Kaneider N, Rabensteiner A, Meierhofer C, Reinisch C, Romisch J, Wiedermann CJ: Cell-surface heparan sulfate proteoglycan-mediated regulation of neutrophil migration by the serpin antithrombin III. Blood 2001;97:1079-1085.

Dunzendorfer S, Rabensteiner A, Kaneider N, Meierhofer C, Romisch J, Wiedermann CJ: Involvement of CXC-receptor-1 in antithrombin-induced neutrophil migration. In: Faist E (ed): Proceedings of the 5th World Congress on Trauma, Shock, Inflammation and Sepsis, Munich, Germany, 29 February-4 March 2000. Monduzzi Editore, Italy, 2000, pp 703-706.

Eckardt KU, Kurtz A. Regulation of erythropoietin production. *Eur J Clin Invest* 35, *Suppl* 3: 13–19, 2005.

Ehrenreich H, Hasselblatt M, Dembowski C, Cepek L, Lewczuk P, Stiefel M, Rustenbeck HH, Breiter N, Jacob S, Knerlich F, Bohn M, Poser W, Ruther E, Kochen M, Gefeller O, Gleiter C, Wessel TC, De Ryck M, Itri L, Prange H, Cerami A, Brines M, Siren AL. Erythropoietin therapy for acute stroke is both safe and beneficial. *Mol Med* 8: 495–505, 2002.

Ehrenreich H, Weissenborn K, Prage H et al: Epo Stroke Trial Group. Recombinant human erythropoietin in the treatment of acute ischemic stroke. Stroke.2009 Dec;40(12):e647-56.

Ekdahl CT, Kokaia Z, Lindvall O (2009) Brain inflammation and adult neurogenesis: the dual role of microglia. Neuroscience 158: 1021–1029.

Emerson, T.E., Jr. (1989). Unique features of albumin: a brief review. Crit. Care Med. *17* , 690 - 694.

Endres M, Fan G, Hirt L, Fujii M, Matsushita K, Liu X, Jaenisch R, Moskowitz MA (2000) Ischemic brain damage in mice after selectively modifying BDNF or NT4 gene expression. J Cereb Blood Flow Metab 20:139–144.

Epstein AC, Gleadle JM, McNeill LA, Hewitson KS, O'Rourke J, Mole DR, Mukherji M, Metzen E, Wilson MI, Dhanda A, Tian YM, Masson N, Hamilton DL, Jaakkola P, Barstead R, Hodgkin J, Maxwell PH, Pugh CW, Schofield CJ, Ratcliffe PJ. *C. elegans* EGL-9 and mammalian homologs define a family of dioxygenases that regulate HIF by prolyl hydroxylation. *Cell* 107: 43–54, 2001.

Erlandsson Harris H, Andersson U (2004) Mini-review: the nuclear protein HMGB1 as a proinflammatory mediator. Eur J Immunol 34:1503–1512

Esmon C: The protein C pathway. Crit Care Med 2000;28(Suppl):44-48.

Evans, T.W. (2002). Review article: albumin as a drug - biological effects of albumin unrelated to oncotic pressure. Aliment Pharmacol. Ther. *16* (Suppl. 5), 6 - 11.

Fages C, Nolo R, Huttunen HJ, Eskelinen E, Rauvala H (2000) Regulation of cell migration by amphoterin. J Cell Sci 113:611–620

Fandrey J, Bunn HF. In vivo and in vitro regulation of erythropoietin mRNA: measurement by competitive polymerase chain reaction. *Blood* 81: 617–623, 1993.

Faraco G, Fossati S, Bianchi ME, Patrone M, Pedrazzi M, Sparatore B, Moroni F, Chiarugi A (2007) High mobility group box 1 protein is released by neural cells upon different stresses and worsens ischemic neurodegeneration in vitro and in vivo. J Neurochem 103:590–603.

Ferlito M, Romanenko OG, Ashton S, Squadrito F, Halushka PV, Cook JA (2001) Effect of cross-tolerance between endotoxin and TNFalpha or IL-1beta on cellular signaling and mediator production. J Leukoc Biol 70:821–829.

Frede S, Berchner-Pfannschmidt U, Fandrey J. Regulation of hypoxia-inducible factors during inflammation. *Methods Enzymol* 435: 405–419, 2007.

Furuya K, Zhu L, Kawahara N, Abe O, Kirino T (2005) Differences in infarct evolution between lipopolysaccharide- induced tolerant and nontolerant conditions to focal cerebral ischemia. J Neurosurg 103:715–723.

Garcovich, M., Zocco, M.A., and Gasbarrini, A. (2009). Clinical use of albumin in hepatology. Blood Transfus. *7* , 268 - 277.

Genc K, Genc S, Baskin H, Semin I. Erythropoietin decreases cytotoxicity and nitric oxide formation induced by inflammatory stimuli in rat oligodendrocytes. *Physiol Res* 55: 33–38, 2006.

Genc S, Koroglu TF, Genc K. Erythropoietin and the nervous system. *Brain Res* 1000: 19–31, 2004.

Ginis I, Jaiswal R, Klimanis D, Liu J, Greenspon J, Hallenbeck J (2002) TNFa induced tolerance to ischemic injury involves differential control of NF-kB transactivation: the role of NF-kB association with p300 adaptor. J Cereb Blood Flow Metab 22:142–152.

Ginis I, Schweizer U, Brenner M, Liu J, Azzam N, Spatz M, Hallenbeck J (1999) TNF-alpha pretreatment prevents subsequent activation of cultured brain cells with TNF-alpha and hypoxia via ceramide. Am J Physiol 276:C1171.

Ginsberg, M.D. (2008). Neuroprotection for ischemic stroke: past, present and future. Neuropharmacology *55* , 363 - 389.

Ginsberg, M.D., Hill, M.D., Palesch, Y.Y., Ryckborst, K.J., and Tamariz, D. (2006a). The ALIAS Pilot Trial: a dose escalation and safety study of albumin therapy for acute ischemic stroke- I: Physiological responses and safety results. Stroke *37* , 2100 - 2106.

Ginsberg, M.D., Palesch, Y.Y., and Hill, M.D. (2006b). The ALIAS (ALbumin In Acute Stroke) Phase III randomized multicentre clinical trial: design and progress report. Biochem. Soc. Trans. *34* , 1323 - 1326.

Ginsberg, M.D., Palesch, Y.Y., Martin, R.H., Hill, M.D., Moy, C.S., Waldman, B.D., Yeatts, S.D., Tamariz, D., and Ryckborst, K. (2011). The Albumin In Acute Stroke (ALIAS) Multicenter Clinical Trial: safety analysis of part 1 and rationale and design of part 2. Stroke *42* , 119 - 127.

Goosa MT, Li J, Kislinger T, Qu W, Lu Y, Bucciarelli LG, Nowgrod S, Wolf BM, Calistle X, Yan SD, Stern DM, Schmidt AM (2001) Blockade of receptor for Advanced Glycation Endproducts restores effective wound healing in diabetic mice. Am J Pathol 159:513–525

Gordon S (2002) Pattern recognition receptors: doubling up for the innate immune response. Cell 111:927–930

Grasso G, Buemi M, Alafaci C, Sfacteria A, Passalacqua M, Sturiale A, Calapai G, De Vico G, Piedimonte G, Salpietro FM, Tomasello F. Beneficial effects of systemic administration of recombinant human erythropoietin in rabbits subjected to subarachnoid hemorrhage. *Proc Natl Acad Sci USA* 99: 5627–5631, 2002.

Gum, E.T., Swanson, R.A., Alano, C., Liu, J., Hong, S., Weinstein, P.R., and Panter, S.S. (2004). Human serum albumin and its N-terminal tetrapeptide (DAHK) block oxidant-induced neuronal death. Stroke *35* , 590 - 595.

Ha T, Li Y, Hua F, Ma J, Gao X, Kelley J, Zhao A, Haddad GE, Williams DL, William Browder I, Kao RL, Li C (2005) Reduced cardiac hypertrophy in toll-like receptor 4-deficient mice following pressure overload. Cardiovasc Res 68:224–234.

Hacke, W., Donnan, G., Fieschi, C., Kaste, M., von Kummer, R., Broderick, J.P., Brott, T., Frankel, M., Grotta, J.C., Haley, E.C., Jr., et al. (2004). Association of outcome with early stroke treatment: pooled analysis of ATLANTIS, ECASS, and NINDS rt-PA stroke trials. Lancet *363* , 768 - 774.

Hanford LE, Enghild JJ, Valnickova Z, Petersen SV, Schaefer LM, Schaefer TM, Reinhart TA, Oury TD (2004) Purification and characterization of mouse soluble Receptor for Advanced Glycation End Products (sRAGE). J Biol Chem 279:50019–50024

Hara H, Friedlander RM, Gagliardini V, Ayata C, Fink K, Huang Z, Shimizu-Sasamata M, Yuan J, Moskowitz MA (1997) Inhibition of interleukin 1beta converting enzyme family proteases reduces ischemic and excitotoxic neuronal damage. Proc Natl Acad Sci U S A 94:2007–2012.

Harada N, Okajima K, Kushimoto S, Isobe H, Tanaka K: Antithrombin reduces ischemia/reperfusion injury of rat liver by increasing the hepatic level of prostacyclin. Blood 1999;93:157-164.

Hasselblatt M, Ehrenreich H, Siren AL. The brain erythropoietin system and its potential for therapeutic exploitation in brain disease. *J Neurosurg Anesthesiol* 18: 132–138, 2006.

Hewitson KS, McNeill LA, Riordan MV, Tian YM, Bullock AN, Welford RW, Elkins JM, Oldham NJ, Bhattacharya S, Gleadle JM, Ratcliffe PJ, Pugh CW, Schofield CJ. Hypoxia-inducible factor (HIF) asparagine hydroxylase is identical to factor inhibiting HIF (FIH) and is related to the cupin structural family. *J Biol Chem* 277: 26351- 26355, 2002.

Hickey EJ, You X, Kaimaktchiev V, Stenzel-Poore M, Ungerleider RM (2007) Lipopolysaccharide preconditioning induces robust protection against brain injury resulting from deep hypothermic circulatory arrest. J Thorac Cardiovasc Surg 133:1588–1596.

Hill MD, Martin RH, Palesh YY, Tamariz D, Waldman BD, Ryckborst KJ, May CS, Barsan WG, Ginsberg MD; ALIAS Investigators; Neurological Emergencies Treatment trials Network. The Albumin in acute Stroke Part 1 Trial: an exploratory efficacy analysis. Stroke 2001Jun;42(6):1621-5.

Hoffmann JN, Vollmar B, Roemisch J, Inthorn D, Schildberg FW, Menger MD: Antithrombin effects on endotoxin- induced microcirculatory disorders are mainly mediated by its interaction with microvascular endothelium. Crit Care Med, Jan 2002-30(1):218-225.

Hofmann MA, Drury S, Fu C, Wu Q, Taguchi A, Lu Y, Avila C, Kambham N, Slattery T, Beach D, McClary J, Nagashima M, Morser J, Bierhaus A, Neurath M, Nawroth P, Stern D, Schmidt AM (1999) RAGE mediates a novel proinflammatory axis: the cell surface receptor for S100/calgranulin polypeptides. Cell 97:889–901

Hooper, C., Taylor, D.L., and Pocock, J.M. (2005). Pure albumin is a potent trigger of calcium signalling and proliferation in microglia but not macrophages or astrocytes. J. Neurochem. *92* , 1363 - 1376.

Hori O, Brett J, Slattery T, Cao R, Zhang J, Chen JX, Nagashima M, Lundh ER, Vijay S, Nitecki D, Morser J, Stern D, Schmidt AM (1995) The receptor for advanced glycation end products (RAGE) is a cellular binding site for amphoterin. Mediation of neurite outgrowth and co-expression of rage and amphoterin in the developing nervous system. J Biol Chem 270:25752–25761

Hua F, Ma J, Ha T, Xia Y, Kelley J, Williams DL, Kao RL, Browder IW, Schweitzer JB, Kalbfleisch JH, Li C (2007) Activation of Toll-like receptor 4 signaling contributes to hippocampal neuronal death following global cerebral ischemia/reperfusion. J Neuroimmunol 190:101–111.

Hua L, Kim M, Brosnan C, Lee S (2002) Modulation of astrocyte inducible nitric oxide synthase and cytokine expression by interferon beta is associated with induction and inhibition of interferon gamma-activated sequence binding activity. J Neurochem 83:1120–1128.

Huang JS, Guh JY, Chen HC, Hung WC, Lai YH, Chuang LY (2001) Role of receptor for advanced glycation end-product (RAGE) and the JAK/STAT-signaling pathway in AGE-induced collagen production in NRK-49F cells. J Cell Biochem 81:102–113

Hudson BI, Bucciarelli LG, Wendt T et al (2003) Blockade of receptor for advanced glycation endproducs: a new target for therapeutic intervention in diabetic complications and inflammatory disorders. Arch Biochem Biophys 419:80–88

Huh, P.W., Belayev, L., Zhao, W., Busto, R., Saul, I., and Ginsberg, M.D. (1998). The effect of high-dose albumin therapy on local cerebral perfusion after transient focal cerebral ischemia in rats. Brain Res. *804* , 105 - 113.

Huttunen HJ, Fages C, Kuja-Panula J, Ridley AJ, Rauvala H (2002) Receptor for advanced glycation end products- binding COOH-terminal motif of amphoterin inhibits invasive migration and metastasis. Cancer Res 62:4805- 4811

Huttunen HJ, Fages C, Rauvala H (1999) Receptor for advanced glycation end products (RAGE)-mediated neurite outgrowth and activation of NF-kappaB require the cytoplasmic domain of the receptor but different downstream signaling pathways. J Biol Chem 274:19919–19924

Huttunen HJ, Kuja-Panula J, Sorci G, Agneletti AL, Donato R, Rauvala H (2000) Coregulation of neurite outgrowth and cell survival by amphoterin and S100 proteins through receptor for advanced glycation end products (RAGE) activation. J Biol Chem 275:40096–40105

Iampietro R, Souter P, Romisch J, Poole S, Gray E: Antithrombin inhibits in vitro lipopolysaccharide induced interleukin- 6 production by suppression of mRNA. Intensive Care Med 2000;26(Suppl 3):302.

Ishihara K, Tsutsumi K, Kawane S, Nakajima M, Kasaoka T (2003) The receptor for advanced glycation end-products (RAGE) directly binds to ERK by a D-domain-like docking site. FEBS Lett 550:107–113

Italian Acute Stroke Study Group. (1988). Haemodilution in acute stroke: results of the Italian Haemodilution Trial. Lancet *i* , 318 - 321.

Ivan M, Kondo K, Yang H, Kim W, Valiando J, Ohh M, Salic A, Asara JM, Lane WS, Kaelin, WG Jr. HIFalpha targeted for VHL-mediated destruction by proline hydroxylation: implications for O2 sensing. *Science* 292: 464–468, 2001.

Ivens, S., Kaufer, D., Flores, L.P., Bechmann, I., Zumsteg, D., Tomkins, O., Seiffert, E., Heinemann, U., and Friedman, A. (2007). TGF-beta receptor-mediated albumin uptake into astrocytes is involved in neocortical epileptogenesis. Brain *130* , 535 - 547.

Jaakkola P, Mole DR, Tian YM, Wilson MI, Gielbert J, Gaskell SJ, Kriegsheim A, Hebestreit HF, Mukherji M, Schofield CJ, Maxwell PH, Pugh CW, Ratcliffe PJ. Targeting of HIF-alpha to the von Hippel-Lindau ubiquitylation complex by O2-regulated prolyl hydroxylation. *Science* 292: 468–472, 2001.

Jack CS, Arbour N, Manusow J, Montgrain V, Blain M, McCrea E, Shapiro A, Antel JP (2005) TLR signaling tailors innate immune responses in human microglia and astrocytes. J Immunol 175: 4320–4330.

Jelkmann W. Erythropoietin: structure, control of production, and function. *Physiol Rev* 72: 449–489, 1992.

Jiang D, Liang J, Li Y, Noble PW (2006) The role of Toll-like receptors in non-infectious lung injury. Cell Res 16:693–701.

Jin S, Kawanokuchi J, Mizuno T, Wang J, Sonobe Y, Takeuchi H, Suzumura A (2007) Interferon-beta is neuroprotective against the toxicity induced by activated microglia. Brain Res 1179:140–146.

Johanson, C.E., Duncan, J.A., 3rd, Klinge, P.M., Brinker, T., Stopa, E.G., and Silverberg, G.D. (2008). Multiplicity of cerebrospinal fluid functions: new challenges in health and disease. Cerebrospinal Fluid Res. *5* , 10.

Johnson DR, Douglas I, Jahnke A, Ghosh S, Pober JS (1996) A sustained reduction in IκB-β may contribute to persistent NF-κB activation in human endothelial cells. J Biol Chem 271:16317–16322

Juttler, E., Kohrmann, M., and Schellinger, P.D. (2006). Therapy for early reperfusion after stroke. Nat. Clin. Pract. Cardiovasc. Med. *3* , 656 - 663.

Kagan JC, Su T, Horng T, Chow A, Akira S, Medzhitov R (2008) TRAM couples endocytosis of Toll-like receptor 4 to the induction of interferon-beta. Nat Immunol 9:361–368.

Kaneider NC, Egger P, Dunzendorfer S, Wiedermann CJ: Syndecan-4 as antithrombin receptor of human neutrophils. Biochem Biophys Res Commun 2001;287:42-46.

Kaneider NC, Reinisch CM, Dunzendorfer S, Romisch J, Wiedermann CJ: Syndecan-4 on huan peripheral blood lymphocytes and monocytes mediates effects of antithrombin on chemotaxis. J Cell Sci 2002

Kaur J, Woodman RC, Ostrovsky L, Kubes P: Selective recruitment of neutrophils and lymphocytes by thrombin: a role for NF-kappaB. Am J Physiol Heart Circ Physiol 2001; 281:784-795.

Kawakami M, Iwasaki S, Sato K, Takahashi M. Erythropoietin inhibits calcium-induced neurotransmitter release from clonal neuronal cells. *Biochem Biophys Res Commun* 279: 293–297, 2000.

Kerschensteiner M, Meinal E, Hohlfeld R (2009) Neuro-immune crosstalk in CNS diseases. Neuroscience 158:1122–1132.

Kertesz N, Wu J, Chen TH, Sucov HM, Wu H. The role of erythropoietin in regulating angiogenesis. *Dev Biol* 276: 101– 110, 2004.

Kilic E, Kilic U, Soliz J, Bassetti CL, Gassmann M, Hermann DM. Brain-derived erythropoietin protects from focal cerebral ischemia by dual activation of ERK-1/-2 and Akt pathways. *FASEB J* 19: 2026–2028, 2005.

Kinouchi H, Sharp FR, Hill MP, Koistinaho J, Sagar SM, Chan PH (1993) Induction of 70-kDa heat shock protein and hsp70 mRNA following transient focal cerebral ischemia in the rat. J Cereb Blood Flow Metab 13:105–115.

Kislinger T, Fu C, Huber B, Qu W, Taguchi A, Du Yan S, Hofmann M, Yan SF, Pischetsrieder M, Stern D, Schmidt AM (1999) N(epsilon)-(carboxymethyl)lysine adducts of proteins are ligands for receptor for advanced glycation end products that activate cell signaling pathways and modulate gene expression. J Biol Chem 274:31740–31749

Kislinger T, Tanji N, Wendt T, Qu W, Lu Y, Ferran LJ Jr, Taguchi A, Olson K, Bucciarelli L, Goova M, Hofmann MA, Cataldegirmen G, D'Agati V, Pischetsrieder M, Stern DM, Schmidt AM (2001) Receptor for advanced glycation end products mediates inflammation and enhanced expression of tissue factor in vasculature of diabetic apolipoprotein E-Null mice. Arterioscl Thromb Vasc Biol 21:905–910

Kobayashi K, Hernandex L, Galan J, Janeway J, Medzhitov R, Flavell R (2002) IRAK-M is a negative regulator of Toll-like receptor signaling. Cell 110:191–202.

Kobayashi T, Yanase H, Iwanaga T, Sasaki R, Nagao M. Epididymis is a novel site of erythropoietin production in mouse reproductive organs. *Biochem Biophys Res Commun* 296: 145–151, 2002.

Kokkola R, Andersson A, Mullins G, Ostberg T, Treutiger CJ, Arnold B, Nawroth P, Andersson U, Harris RA, Harris HE (2005) RAGE is the major receptor for the proinflammatory activity of HMGB1 in rodent macrophages. Scand J Immunol 61:1–9

Konishi Y, Chui DH, Hirose H, Kunishita T, Tabira T. Trophic effect of erythropoietin and other hematopoietic factors on central cholinergic neurons in vitro and in vivo. *Brain Res* 609: 29–35, 1993.

Korosue, K. and Heros, R.C. (1992). Mechanism of cerebral blood flow augmentation by hemodilution in rabbits. Stroke *23* , 1487 - 1492; discussion 1492 - 1493.

Koshimura K, Murakami Y, Sohmiya M, Tanaka J, Kato Y. Effects of erythropoietin on neuronal activity. *J Neurochem* 72: 2565–2572, 1999.

Kraus J, Ling AK, Hamm S, Voigt K, Oschmann P, Engelhardt B (2004) Interferon-beta stabilizes barrier characteristics of brain endothelial cells in vitro. Ann Neurol 56:192–205.

Kumral A, Gonenc S, Acikgoz O, Sonmez A, Genc K, Yilmaz O, Gokmen N, Duman N, Ozkan H. Erythropoietin increases glutathione peroxidase enzyme activity and decreases lipid peroxidation levels in hypoxic-ischemic brain injury in neonatal rats. *Biol Neonate* 87: 15–18, 2005.

Kunz A, Park L, Abe T, Gallo EF, Anrather J, Zhou P, Iadecola C (2007) Neurovascular protection by ischemic tolerance: role of nitric oxide and reactive oxygen species. J Neurosci 27:7083–7093.

Laflamme N, Rivest S (2001) Toll-like receptor 4: the missing link of the cerebral innate immune response triggered by circulating gramnegative bacterial cell wall components. FASEB J 15:155–163.

Laflamme N, Soucy G, Rivest S (2001) Circulating cell wall components derived from gram-negative, not gram-positive, bacteria cause a profound induction of the gene-encoding Toll-like receptor 2 in the CNS. J Neurochem 79:648- 657.

Lafon M, Megret F, Lafage M, Prehaud C (2006) The innate immune facet of brain: human neurons express TLR-3 and sense viral dsRNA. J Mol Neurosci 29:185–194.

Lalla E, Lamster IB, Stern DM, Schmidt AM (2001) Receptor for advanced glycation end products, inflammation, and accelerated periodontal disease in diabetes: mechanisms and insights into therapeutic modalities. Ann Periodontol 6:113–118

Lander HM, Taurus JM, Ogiste JS, Hori O, Moss RA, Schmidt AM(1997) Activation of the receptor for advanced glycation end products triggers a p21(ras)-dependent mitogen-activated protein kinase pathway regulated by oxidant stress. J Biol Chem 272:17810–17814

Lando D, Peet DJ, Gorman JJ, Whelan DA, Whitelaw ML, Bruick RK. FIH-1 is an asparaginyl hydroxylase enzyme that regulates the transcriptional activity of hypoxia-inducible factor. *Genes Dev* 16: 1466–1471, 2002b.

Lando D, Peet DJ, Whelan DA, Gorman JJ, Whitelaw ML. Asparagine hydroxylation of the HIF transactivation domain a hypoxic switch. *Science* 295: 858–861, 2002a.

Lehnardt S, Lehmann S, Kaul D, Tschimmel K, Hoffmann O, Cho S, Krueger C, Nitsch R, Meisel A, Weber JR (2007) Toll- like receptor 2 mediates CNS injury in focal cerebral ischemia. J Neuroimmunol 190:28–33.

Lehnardt S, Schott E, Trimbuch T, Laubisch D, Krueger C, Wulczyn G, Nitsch R, Weber JR (2008) A vicious cycle involving release of heat shock protein 60 from injured cells and activation of toll-like receptor 4 mediates neurodegeneration in the CNS. J Neurosci 28: 2320–2331.

Li J, Schmidt AM (1997) Characterization and functional analysis of the promoter of RAGE, the receptor for advanced glycation end products. J Biol Chem 272(1):6498–6506

Li JH, Wang W, Huang XR, Oldfield M, Schmidt AM, Cooper ME, Lan HY (2004) Advanced glycation end products induce tubular epithelial-myofibroblast transition through the RAGEERK1/2 MAP kinase signaling pathway. Am J Pathol 164: 1389–1397

Liliensiek B, Weigand MA, Bierhaus A, Nicklas W, Kasper M, Hofer S, Plaschky J, Gröne HJ, Kurschus FJ, Schmidt AM, Yan SD, Martin E, Schleicher E, Stern DM, Hämmerling GJ, Nawroth PP, Arnold B (2004) Receptor for advanced glycation end products (RAGE) regulates sepsis, but not the adaptive immune response. J Clin Invest 113:1641–1650

Lipton P. Ischemic cell death in brain neurons. *Physiol Rev* 79: 1431–1568, 1999.

Little, J.R., Slugg, R.M., Latchaw, J.P., Jr., and Lesser, R.P. (1981). Treatment of acute focal cerebral ischemia with concentrated albumin. Neurosurgery *9* , 552 - 558.

Liu H, Xin L, Chan BPL, Teoh R, Tang BL, Tan YH (2002) Interferon beta administration confers a beneficial outcome in a rabbit model of thromboembolic cerebral ischemia. Neurosci Lett 327:146–148.

Liu, Y., Belayev, L., Zhao, W., Busto, R., Belayev, A., and Ginsberg, M.D. (2001). Neuroprotective effect of treatment with human albumin in permanent focal cerebral ischemia: histopathology and cortical perfusion studies. Eur. J. Pharmacol. *428* , 193 - 201.

Liuzzi GM, Latronico T, Fasano A, Carlone G, Riccio P (2004) Interferon-beta inhibits the expression of metalloproteinases in rat glial cell cultures: implications for multiple sclerosis pathogenesis and treatment. Mult Scler 10:290–297.

Lloyd-Jones KL, Kelly MM, Kubes P (2008) Varying importance of soluble and membrane CD14 in endothelial detection of lipopolysaccharide. J Immunol 181:1446–1453.

Lloyd-Jones, D., Adams, R., Carnethon, M., De Simone, G., Ferguson, T.B., Flegal, K., Ford, E., Furie, K., Go, A., Greenlund, K., et al. (2009). Heart disease and stroke statistics - 2009 update: a report from the American Heart Association Statistics Committee and Stroke Statistics Subcommittee. Circulation *119* , e21 - e181.

Longa, E.Z., Weinstein, P.R., Carlson, S., and Cummins, R. (1989). Reversible middle cerebral artery occlusion without craniectomy in rats. Stroke *20* , 84 - 91.

Lopez-Collazo E, Hortelano S, Rojas A, Bosca L (1998) Triggering of peritoneal macrophages with IFN-alpha/beta attenuates the expression of inducible nitric oxide synthase through a decrease in NF-kappaB activation. J Immunol 160:2889–2895.

Ludwicka-Bradley A, Tourkina E, Suzuki S, Tyson E, Bonner M, Fenton JW II, Hoffman S, Silver RM: Thrombin upregulates interleukin-8 in lung fibroblasts via cleavage of proteolytically activated receptor-I and protein kinase C-gamma activation. Am J Respir Cell Mol Biol 2000;22:235-243.

Lue LF, Walker DG, Brachova L, Beach TG, Rogers J, Schmidt AM, Stern DM, Yan SD (2001) Involvement of microglial receptor for advanced glycation endproducts (RAGE) in Alzheimer's disease: identification of a cellular activation mechanism. Exp Neurol 171:29–45

Ma Y, Li J, Chiu I, Wang Y, Sloane JA, Lu J, Kosaras B, Sidman RL, Volpe JJ, Vartanian T (2006) Toll-like receptor 8 functions as a negative regulator of neurite outgrowth and inducer of neuronal apoptosis. J Cell Biol 175:209– 215.

Mackic JB, Stins M, McComb JG, Calero M, Ghiso J, Kim KS, Yan SD, Stern D, Schmidt AM, Frangione B, Zlokovic BV (1998) Human blood-brain barrier receptors for Alzheimer's amyloid-beta 1–40. Asymmetrical binding, endocytosis, and transcytosis at the apical side of brain microvascular endothelial cell monolayer. J Clin Invest 102:734–743

Malherbe R, Richards JG, Gaillard H, Thompson A, Diener C, Schuler A, Huber G (1999) cDNA cloning of a novel secreted isoform of the human receptor for advanced glycation end products and characterisation of cells co- expresing cell-surface scavenger receptors and Swedish mutant amyloid precursor protein. Mol Brain Res 71:159–170

Mammen EF: Antithrombin: its physiological importance and role in DIC. Semin Thromb Hemost 1998;24:19-25.

Manning, T.J., Jr. and Sontheimer, H. (1997). Bovine serum albumin and lysophosphatidic acid stimulate calcium mobilization and reversal of cAMP-induced stellation in rat spinal cord astrocytes. Glia *20* , 163 - 172.

Marenholz I, Heizmann CW, Fritz G (2004) S100 proteins in mouse and man: from evolution to function and pathology (including an update of the nomenclature). Biochem Biophys Res Commun 322:1111–1122

Marrero MB, Venema RC, Ma H, Ling BN, Eaton DC. Erythropoietin receptor-operated Ca2+ channels: activation by phospholipase C-gamma 1. *Kidney Int* 53: 1259–1268, 1998.

Marti HH, Bernaudin M, Petit E, Bauer C. Neuroprotection and angiogenesis: dual role of erythropoietin in brain ischemia. *News Physiol Sci* 15: 225–229, 2000.

Marti HH, Gassmann M, Wenger RH, Kvietikova I, Morganti-Kossmann MC, Kossmann T, Trentz O, Bauer C. Detection of erythropoietin in human liquor: intrinsic erythropoietin production in the brain. *Kidney Int* 51: 416–418, 1997.

Marti HH, Wenger RH, Rivas LA, Straumann U, Digicaylioglu M, Henn V, Yonekawa Y, Bauer C, Gassmann M. Erythropoietin gene expression in human, monkey and murine brain. *Eur J Neurosci* 8: 666–676, 1996.

Marti HH. Erythropoietin and the hypoxic brain. *J Exp Biol* 207: 3233–3242, 2004.

Martinez-Estrada OM, Rodriguez-Millan E, Gonzalez-De Vicente E, Reina M, Vilaro S, Fabre M. Erythropoietin protects the in vitro blood-brain barrier against VEGF-induced permeability. *Eur J Neurosci* 18: 2538–2544, 2003.

Masuda S, Kobayashi T, Chikuma M, Nagao M, Sasaki R. The oviduct produces erythropoietin in an estrogen- and oxygen-dependent manner. *Am J Physiol Endocrinol Metab* 278: E1038–E1044, 2000.

Masuda S, Okano M, Yamagishi K, Nagao M, Ueda M, Sasaki R. A novel site of erythropoietin production. Oxygen- dependent production in cultured rat astrocytes. *J Biol Chem* 269: 19488–19493, 1994.

Matsui, T., Sinyama, H., and Asano, T. (1993). Benefi cial effect of prolonged administration of albumin on ischemic cerebral edema and infarction after occlusion of middle cerebral artery in rats. Neurosurgery *33* , 293 - 300; comment 300.

McFalls EO, Sluiter W, Schoonderwoerd K, Manintveld OC, Lamers JM, Bezstarosti K, van Beusekom HM, Sikora J, Ward HB, Merkus D, Duncker DJ (2006) Mitochondrial adaptations within chronically ischemic swine myocardium. J Mol Cell Cardiol 41:980–988.

McKhann GM, Grega MA, Borowicz LM Jr, Baumgartner WA, Selnes OA (2006) Stroke and encephalopathy after cardiac surgery: an update. Stroke 37:562–571.

McKimmie CS, Fazakerley JK (2005) In response to pathogens, glial cells dynamically and differentially regulate Toll-like receptor gene expression. J Neuroimmunol 169:116–125.

Medvedev AE, Lentschat A, Wahl LM, Golenbock DT, Vogel SN (2002) Dysregulation of LPS-induced Toll-like receptor 4-MyD88 complex formation and IL-1 receptor-associated kinase1 activation in endotoxin-tolerant cells. J Immunol 169:5209–5216.

Morcos M, Hofmann M, Tritschler H, Weigle B, Kasper M, Smith MA, Perry G, Schmidt AM, Stern DM, Häring HU, Schleicher E, Nawroth PP (2001) Diabetes-associated sustained activation of the transcription factor NF-κB. Diabetes 50:2792–2809

Morcos M, Sayed A, Pfisterer F, Hutter H, Thornalley P, Ahmed N, Miftari N, Mörlen F, Hamann A, Bierhaus A,

Murphey ED, Traber DL (2001) Protective effect of tumor necrosis factor-alpha against subsequent endotoxemia in mice is mediated, in part, by interleukin-10. Crit Care Med 29:1761–1766.

Murphy, M.P. and LeVine, H., 3rd. (2010). Alzheimer ' s disease and the amyloid-beta peptide. J. Alzheimers Dis. *19* , 311 - 323.

Murray CJ, Lopez AD (1997) Alternative projections of mortality and disability by cause 1990–2020: Global Burden of Disease Study. Lancet 349:1498–1504.

Nadal, A., Sul, J.Y., Valdeolmillos, M., and McNaughton, P.A. (1998). Albumin elicits calcium signals from astrocytes in brain slices from neonatal rat cortex. J. Physiol. *509* , 711 - 716.

Nagai A, Nakagawa E, Choi HB, Hatori K, Kobayashi S, Kim SU. Erythropoietin and erythropoietin receptors in human CNS neurons, astrocytes, microglia, and oligodendrocytes grown in culture. *J Neuropathol Exp Neurol* 60: 386– 392, 2001.

Nahon, J.L., Tratner, I., Poliard, A., Presse, F., Poiret, M., Gal, A., Sala-Trepat, J.M., Legres, L., Feldmann, G., and Bernuau, D. (1988). Albumin and alpha-fetoprotein gene expression in various nonhepatic rat tissues. J. Biol. Chem. *263* , 11436 - 11442.

Nawashiro H, Tasaki K, Ruetzler CA, Hallenbeck JM (1997) TNFalpha pretreatment induces protective effects against focal cerebral ischemia in mice. J Cereb Blood Flow Metab 17:483–490.

Nawroth PP (2004) Glyoxalase I als endogener Schutz vor Advanced Glycation Endproducts (AGE)-formation und oxidativem stress in Caenorhabditis elegans. Diab Stoffw 13 (Supplementheft 1):33 V-70

Neeper M, Schmidt AM, Brett J, Yan SD, Wang F, Pa YCE, Elliston K, Stern DM, Shaw A (1992) Cloning and Expression of a cell surface receptor for advanced glycosylation end products of proteins. J Biol Chem 267:14998–15004

Neugroschl, J. and Sano, M. (2010). Current treatment and recent clinical research in Alzheimer ' s disease. Mt. Sinai J. Med. *77* , 3 - 16.

Neviere R, Tournoys A, Mordon S, Marechal X, Song FL, Jourdain M, Fourrier F: Antithrombin reduces mesenteric venular leukocyte interactions and small intestine injury in endotoxemic rats. Shock 2001;15:220-225.

Nhu QM, Cuesta N, Vogel SN (2006) Transcriptional regulation of lipopolysaccharide (LPS)-induced Toll-like receptor (TLR) expression in murine macrophages: role of interferon regulatory factors 1 (IRF-1) and 2 (IRF-2). J Endotoxin Res 12:285–295.

Nicholson, J.P., Wolmarans, M.R., and Park, G.R. (2000). The role of albumin in critical illness. Br. J. Anaesth. *85* , 599 - 610.

Nimmagadda, A., Park, H.P., Prado, R., and Ginsberg, M.D. (2008). Albumin therapy improves local vascular dynamics in a rat model of primary microvascular thrombosis: a two-photon laserscanning microscopy study. Stroke *39* , 198 - 204.

Noble R (1943) The development of resistance by rats and guinea pigs to amounts of trauma usually fatal. Am J Physiol 38:346–351.

Oelschlager C, Leithauser B, Romisch J, Tillmanns H, Holschermann H: Antithrombin inhibits NF-KB signaling pathways in monocytes and endothelial cells in vitro. Ann Hematol 2001;80(Suppl 1):A51.

Okajima K, Uchiba M: The anti-inflammatory properties of antithrombin III:new therapeutic implications. Semin Thromb Hemost 1998;24:27-32.

Olson JK, Miller SD (2004) Microglia initiate central nervous system innate and adaptive immune responses through multiple TLRs. J Immunol 173:3916–3924.

Opal SM: Phylogenetic and functional relationship between coagulation and the innate immune response. Crit Care Med 2000;28(Suppl):77-80.

Ostrovsky L, Woodman RC, Payne D, Teoh D, Kubes P: Antithrombin III prevents and rapidly reverse leukocyte recruitment in ischemia/reperfusion. Circulation 1997;96:2302-2310.

Oyama J, Blais C Jr, Liu X, Pu M, Kobzik L, Kelly RA, Bourcier T (2004) Reduced myocardial ischemia-reperfusion injury in toll-like receptor 4-deficient mice. Circulation 109:784–789.

Palesch, Y.Y., Hill, M.D., Ryckborst, K.J., Tamariz, D., and Ginsberg, M.D. (2006). The ALIAS Pilot Trial: a dose escalation and safety study of albumin therapy for acute ischemic stroke - II: neurologic outcome and effi cacy analysis. Stroke *37* , 2107 - 2114.

Palmer G, Mezin F, Juge-Aubry CE, Plater-Zyberk C, Gabay C, Guerne PA (2004) Interferon beta stimulates interleukin 1 receptor antagonist production in human articular chondrocytes and synovial fibroblasts. Ann Rheum Dis 63:43–49.

Parsa CJ, Matsumoto A, Kim J, Riel RU, Pascal LS, Walton GB, Thompson RB, Petrofski JA, Annex BH, Stamler JS, Koch WJ. A novel protective effect of erythropoietin in the infarcted heart. *J Clin Invest* 112: 999–1007, 2003.

Patel NS, Sharples EJ, Cuzzocrea S, Chatterjee PK, Britti D, Yaqoob MM, Thiemermann C. Pretreatment with EPO reduces the injury and dysfunction caused by ischemia/reperfusion in the mouse kidney in vivo. *Kidney Int* 66: 983–989, 2004.

Piazza O, Scarpati G, Cotena S, Lonardo M, Tufano R:Thrombin antithrombin complex and IL-18 serum levels in stroke patients. Neurol Int. 2010 Jun 21;2(1):e1.

Porter MH, Arnold M, Langhans W (1998) TNF-alpha tolerance blocks LPS-induced hypophagia but LPS tolerance fails to prevent TNFalpha- induced hypophagia. Am J Physiol 274:R741–R745.

Prajapati, K.D., Sharma, S.S., and Roy, N. (2010). Upregulation of albumin expression in focal ischemic rat brain. Brain Res. *1327* , 118 - 124.

Prehaud C, Megret F, Lafage M, Lafon M (2005) Virus infection switches TLR-3-positive human neurons to become strong producers of beta interferon. J Virol 79:12893–12904.

Quinlan, G.J., Martin, G.S., and Evans, T.W. (2005). Albumin: biochemical properties and therapeutic potential. Hepatology *41* , 1211 - 1219.

Rabiet MJ, Plantier JL, Dejana E: Thrombin-induced endothelial cell dysfunction. Br Med Bull 1994;50:936-945.

Ralay Ranaivo, H. and Wainwright, M.S. (2010). Albumin activates astrocytes and microglia through mitogen-activated protein kinase pathways. Brain Res. *1313* , 222 - 231.

Recny MA, Scoble HA, Kim Y. Structural characterization of natural human urinary and recombinant DNA-derived erythropoietin. Identification of des-arginine 166 erythropoietin. *J Biol Chem* 262: 17156–17163, 1987.

Reiber, H. (1998). Cerebrospinal fl uid - physiology, analysis and interpretation of protein patterns for diagnosis of neurological diseases. Mult. Scler. *4* , 99 - 107.

Reiber, H. (2003). Proteins in cerebrospinal fl uid and blood: barriers, CSF fl ow rate and source-related dynamics. Restor. Neurol. Neurosci. *21* , 79 - 96.

Reiber, H. and Peter, J.B. (2001). Cerebrospinal fl uid analysis: disease- related data patterns and evaluation programs. J. Neurol. Sci. *184* , 101 - 122.

Relton JK, Martin D, Thompson RC, Russell DA (1996) Peripheral administration of interleukin-1 receptor antagonist inhibits brain damage after focal cerebral ischemia in the rat. Exp Neurol 138:206–213.

Remmers, M., Schmidt-Kastner, R., Belayev, L., Lin, B., Busto, R., and Ginsberg, M.D. (1999). Protein extravasation and cellular uptake after high-dose human-albumin treatment of transient focal cerebral ischemia in rats. Brain Res. *827* , 237 - 242.

Ribatti D, Presta M, Vacca A, Ria R, Giuliani R, Dell'Era P, Nico B, Roncali L, Dammacco F. Human erythropoietin induces a pro-angiogenic phenotype in cultured endothelial cells and stimulates neovascularization in vivo. *Blood* 93: 2627–2636, 1999.

Robinson MJ, Tessier P, Poulsom R, Hogg N (2002) The S100 family heterodimer, MRP-8/14, binds with high affinity to heparin and heparan sulfate glycosaminoglycans on endothelial cells. J Biol Chem 277:3658–3665

Rodriguez de Turco, E.B., Belayev, L., Liu, Y., Busto, R., Parkins, N., Bazan, N.G., and Ginsberg, M.D. (2002). Systemic fatty acid responses to transient focal cerebral ischemia: infl uence of neuroprotectant therapy with human albumin. J. Neurochem. *83* , 515- 524.

Rolls A, Shechter R, London A, Ziv Y, Ronen A, Levy R, Schwartz M (2007) Toll-like receptors modulate adult hippocampal neurogenesis. Nat Cell Biol 9:1081–1088.

Rong LL, Trojaborg W, Qu W, Kostov K, Yan SD, Gooch C, Szabolcs M, Hays AP, Schmidt AM (2004) Antagonism of RAGE suppresses peripheral nerve regeneration. FASEB J 18: 1812–1817

Rong LL, Yan SF, Wendt T, Hans D, Pachydaki S, Bucciarelli LG, Adebayo A, Qu W, Lu Y, Kostov K, Lalla E, Yan SD, Gooch C, Szabolcs M, Trojaborg W, Hays AP, Schmidt AM (2004) RAGE modulates peripheral nerve regeneration via recruitment of both inflammatory and axonal outgrowth pathways. FASEB J 18:1818–1825

Rosenzweig HL, Lessov NS, Henshall DC, Minami M, Simon RP, Stenzel-Poore MP (2004) Endotoxin preconditioning prevents the cellular inflammatory response during ischemic neuroprotection in mice. Stroke 35:2576–2581.

Rosenzweig HL, Minami M, Lessov NS, Coste SC, Stevens SL, Henshall DC, Meller R, Simon RP, Stenzel-Poore MP (2007) Endotoxin preconditioning protects against the cytotoxic effects of TNFa after stroke: a novel role for TNFa in LPS-ischemic tolerance. J Cereb Blood Flow Metab 27:1663–1674.

rt-PA Stroke Study Group. (1995). Tissue plasminogen activator for acute ischemic stroke. The National Institute of Neurological Disorders and Stroke rt-PA Stroke Study Group. N. Engl. J. Med. *333* , 1581 - 1587.

Ruscher K, Freyer D, Karsch M, Isaev N, Megow D, Sawitzki B, Priller J, Dirnagl U, Meisel A. Erythropoietin is a paracrine mediator of ischemic tolerance in the brain: evidence from an in vitro model. *J Neurosci* 22: 10291- 10301, 2002.

Sadamoto Y, Igase K, Sakanaka M, Sato K, Otsuka H, Sakaki S, Masuda S, Sasaki R. Erythropoietin prevents place navigation disability and cortical infarction in rats with permanent occlusion of the middle cerebral artery. *Biochem Biophys Res Commun* 253: 26–32, 1998.

Sakaguchi T, Yan SF, Yan SD, Belov D, Rong LL, Sousa M, Andrassy M, Marso SP, Duda S, Arnold B, Liliensiek B, Nawroth PP, Stern DM, Schmidt AM, Naka Y (2003) Central role of RAGE-dependent neointimal expansion in arterial restenosis. J Clin Invest 111:959–972

Sakanaka M, Wen TC, Matsuda S, Masuda S, Morishita E, Nagao M, Sasaki R. In vivo evidence that erythropoietin protects neurons from ischemic damage. *Proc Natl Acad Sci USA* 95: 4635–4640, 1998.

Sakata Y, Dong JW, Vallejo JG, Huang CH, Baker JS, Tracey KJ, Tacheuchi O, Akira S, Mann DL (2007) Toll-like receptor 2 modulates left ventricular function following ischemia-reperfusion injury. Am J Physiol Heart Circ Physiol 292:H503–H509.

Sasaki N, Takeuchi M, Chowei H, Kikuchi S, Hayashi Y, Nakano N, Ikeda H, Yamagishi S, Kitamoto T, Saito T, Makita Z (2002) Advanced glycation end products (AGE) and their receptor (RAGE) in the brain of patients with Creutzfeldt-Jakob disease with prion plaques. Neurosci Lett 326:117–120

Scandinavian Stroke Study Group. (1987). Multicenter trial of hemodilution in acute ischemic stroke. I. Results in the total patient population. Stroke *18* , 691 - 699.

Schiekofer S, Andrassy M, Schneider J, Fritsche A, Chen J, Humpert P, Stumvoll M, Schleicher E, Häring HU, Nawroth PP, Bierhaus A (2003) Acute (2 h) hyperglycemic clamp causes intracellular formation of carboxymethyllysine, activation of Ras, p42/p44 MAPK and NF-κB in peripheral blood mononuclear cells. Diabetes 52:621–633

Schmidt AM, Mora R, Cap R, Yan SD, Brett J, Ramakrishnan R, Tsang TC, Simionescu M, Stern D (1994) The endothelial cell binding site for advanced glycation end products consists of a complex: an integral membrane protein and a lactoferrin-like polypeptide. J Biol Chem 269:9882–9888

Schmidt AM, Vianna M, Gerlach M, Brett J, Ryan J, Kao Jm Esposito C, Hegarty H, Hurley W, Clauss M, Wang F, Pan YE, Tsang C, Stern D (1992) Isolation and characterisation of two binding proteins gor advanced glycosylation end products from bovine lung which are present on the endothelial cell surface. J Biol Chem 267:14987–14997

Schmidt AM, Yan SD, Brett J, Mora R, Nowygrod R, Stern D (1993) Regulation of human mononuclear phagocyte migration by cell surface-binding proteins for advanced glycation end products. J Clin Invest 91:2155–2168

Schmidt AM, Yan SD, Stern DM (1995) The dark side of glucose. Nat Med 1:1002–1004

Schmidt AM, Yan SD, Yan SF, Stern DM (2001) The multiligand receptor RAGE is a progression factor amplifying immune and inflammatory responses. J Clin Invest 108:949–955

Schneider A, Martin-Villalba A, Weih F, Vogel J, Wirth T, Schwaninger M (1999) NF-kappaB is activated and promotes cell death in focal cerebral ischemia. Nat Med 5:554–559.

Seegers WH: Antithrombin III: theory and clinical applications: H.P. Smith Memorial Lecture. Am J Clin Pathol 1978;69:299-359.

Seguin R, Moditi Z, Rotondo R, Biernacki K, Wosik K, Prat A, Antel JP (2003) Human brain endothelial cells supply support for monocyte immunoregulatory functions. J Neuroimmunol 135:96–106.

Selkoe, D.J. (1991). The molecular pathology of Alzheimer ' s disease. Neuron *6* , 487 - 498.

Semenza GL, Nejfelt MK, Chi SM, Antonarakis SE. Hypoxia-inducible nuclear factors bind to an enhancer element located 3′ to the human erythropoietin gene. *Proc Natl Acad Sci USA* 88: 5680–5684, 1991.

Senden NH, Jeunhomme TM, Heemskerk JW, Wagen voord R, van't Veer C, Hemker HC, Buurman WA: Factor Xa induces cytokine production and expression of adhesion molecules by human umbilical vein endothelial cells. J Immunol 1998;161:4318-4324.

Shanmugam N, Kim YS, Lanting L, Natarajan R (2003) Regulation of cyclooxygenase-2 expression in monocytes by ligation of the receptor for advanced glycation end products. J Biol Chem 278:34834–34844

Shen XD, Ke B, Zhai Y, Gao F, Busuttil RW, Cheng G, Kupiec- Weglinski JW (2005) Toll-like receptor and heme oxygenase-1 signaling in hepatic ischemia/reperfusion injury. Am J Transplant 5:1793–1800.

Shi F, Bailey C, Malick AW, Audus KL. Biotin uptake and transport across bovine brain microvessel endothelial cell monolayers. *Pharm Res* 10: 282–288, 1993.

Shi M, Deng W, Bi E, Mao K, Ji Y, Lin G, Wu X, Tao Z, Li Z, Cai X, Sun S, Xiang C, Sun B (2008) TRIM30 alpha negatively regulates TLR-mediated NF-kappa B activation by targeting TAB2 and TAB3 for degradation. Nat Immunol 9:369–377.

Shigeoka AA, Holscher TD, King AJ, Hall FW, Kiosses WB, Tobias PS, Mackman N, McKay DB (2007) TLR2 is constitutively expressed within the kidney and participates in ischemic renal injury through both MyD88- dependent and -independent pathways. J Immunol 178:6252–6258.

Shingo T, Sorokan ST, Shimazaki T, Weiss S. Erythropoietin regulates the in vitro and in vivo production of neuronal progenitors by mammalian forebrain neural stem cells. *J Neurosci* 21: 9733–9743, 2001.

Shinohara M, Thornalley PJ, Giardino I, Beisswenger P, Thorpe SR, Onorato J, Brownlee M (1998) Overexpression of glyoxalase-I in bovine endothelial cells inhibits intracellular advanced glycation endproduct formation and prevents hyperglycemia- induced increases in macromolecule endocytosis. J Clin Invest 101:1142–1147

Shishido T, Nozaki N, Yamaguchi S, Shibata Y, Nitobe J, Miyamoto T, Takahashi H, Arimoto T, Maeda K, Yamakawa M, Takeuchi O, Akira S, Takeishi Y, Kubota I (2003) Toll-like receptor-2 modulates ventricular remodeling after myocardial infarction. Circulation 108: 2905–2910.

Singh AK, Jiang Y (2004) How does peripheral lipopolysaccharide induce gene expression in the brain of rats? Toxicology 201: 197–207.

Siren AL, Ehrenreich H. Erythropoietin: a novel concept for neuroprotection. *Eur Arch Psychiatry Clin Neurosci* 251: 179– 184, 2001.

Siren AL, Fratelli M, Brines M, Goemans C, Casagrande S, Lewczuk P, Keenan S, Gleiter C, Pasquali C, Capobianco A, Mennini T, Heumann R, Cerami A, Ehrenreich H,

Ghezzi P. Erythropoietin prevents neuronal apoptosis after cerebral ischemia and metabolic stress. *Proc Natl Acad Sci USA* 98: 4044–4049, 2001b.

Siren AL, Knerlich F, Poser W, Gleiter CH, Bruck W, Ehrenreich H. Erythropoietin and erythropoietin receptor in human ischemic/hypoxic brain. *Acta Neuropathol (Berl)* 101: 271–276, 2001a.

Sly LM, Rauh MJ, Kalesnikoff J, Song CH, Krystal G (2004) LPSinduced upregulation of SHIP is essential for endotoxin tolerance. Immunity 21:227–239.

Socolovsky M, Fallon AE, Wang S, Brugnara C, Lodish HF. Fetal anemia and apoptosis of red cell progenitors in Stat5a- /-5b-/- mice: a direct role for Stat5 in Bcl-X(L) induction. *Cell* 98: 181–191, 1999.

Sorci G, Riuzzi F, Agneletti AL, Marchetti C, Donato R (2004) S100B causes apoptosis in a myoblast cell line in a RAGEindependent manner. J Cell Physiol 199:274–283

Sorci G, Riuzzi F, Arcuri C, Giambanco I, Donato R (2004) Amphoterin stimulates myogenesis and counteracts the antimyogenic factors basic fibroblast growth factor and S100B via RAGE binding. Mol Cell Biol 24:4880–4894

Souter PJ, Thomas S, Hubbard AR, Poole S, Romish J, Gray E: Antithrombin inhibits lipoopolysaccharide-induced tissue factor and interleukin-6 production by mononuclear cells, human umbilical vein endothelial cells, and whole blood. Crit Care Med 2001;29:134-139.

Spector R, Mock D. Biotin transport through the blood-brain barrier. *J Neurochem* 48: 400–404, 1987.

Spera PA, Ellison JA, Feuerstein GZ, Barone FC (1998) IL-10 reduces rat brain injury following focal stroke. Neurosci Lett 251:189–192.

Stenzel-Poore MP, Stevens SL, King JS, Simon RP (2007) Preconditioning reprograms the response to ischemic injury and primes the emergence of unique endogenous neuroprotective phenotypes: a speculative synthesis. Stroke 38:680–685.

Stenzel-Poore MP, Stevens SL, Xiong Z, Lessov NS, Harrington CA, Mori M, Meller R, Rosenzweig HL, Tobar E, Shaw TE, Chu X, Simon RP (2003) Effect of ischemic preconditioning on genomic response to cerebral ischemia: similarity to neuroprotective strategies in hibernation and hypoxia-tolerant states. Lancet 362:1028–1037.

Stevens SL, Ciesielski TM, Marsh BJ, Yang T, Homen DS, Boule JL, Lessov NS, Simon RP, Stenzel-Poore MP (2008) Toll- like receptor 9: a new target of ischemic preconditioning in the brain. J Cereb Blood Flow Metab 28:1040–1047.

Stewart VC, Giovannoni G, Land JM, McDonald WI, Clark JB, Heales SJ (1997) Pretreatment of astrocytes with interferon-alpha/beta impairs interferon-gamma induction of nitric oxide synthase. J Neurochem 68:2547–2551.

Stewart VC, Land JM, Clark JB, Heales SJ (1998) Pretreatment of astrocytes with interferon-alpha/beta prevents neuronal mitochondrial respiratory chain damage. J Neurochem 70:432–434.

Stroka DM, Burkhardt T, Desbaillets I, Wenger RH, Neil DA, Bauer C, Gassmann M, Candinas D. HIF-1 is expressed in normoxic tissue and displays an organ-specific regulation under systemic hypoxia. *FASEB J* 15: 2445–2453, 2001.

Studer L, Csete M, Lee SH, Kabbani N, Walikonis J, Wold B, McKay R. Enhanced proliferation, survival, and dopaminergic differentiation of CNS precursors in lowered oxygen. *J Neurosci* 20: 7377–7383, 2000.

Sugaya K, Fukagawa T, Matsumoto K, Mita K, Takahashi E, Ando A, Inoko H, Ikemura T (1994) Three genes in the human MHC class III region near the junction with the class II: gene for receptor of advanced glycosylation end products, PBX2 homeobox gene and a notch homolog, human counterpart of mouse mammary tumor gene int- 3. Genomics 23:408–419

Sundt, T.M., Jr., Waltz, A.G., and Sayre, G.P. (1967). Experimental cerebral infarction: modifi cation by treatment with hemodiluting, hemoconcentrating, and dehydrating agents. J. Neurosurg. *26* , 46 - 56.

Swerdlow, R.H., Burns, J.M., and Khan, S.M. (2010). The Alzheimer ' s disease mitochondrial cascade hypothesis. J. Alzheimers Dis. *20* (Suppl. 2), S265 - S279.

Tabernero, A., Medina, A., Sanchez-Abarca, L.I., Lavado, E., and Medina, J.M. (1999). The effect of albumin on astrocyte energy metabolism is not brought about through the control of cytosolic Ca2 + concentrations but by free-fatty acid sequestration. Glia *25* , 1 - 9.

Tabernero, A., Velasco, A., Granda, B., Lavado, E.M., and Medina, J.M. (2002). Transcytosis of albumin in astrocytes activates the sterol regulatory element-binding protein-1, which promotes the synthesis of the neurotrophic factor oleic acid. J. Biol. Chem. *277* , 4240 - 4246.

Taguchi A, Blood DC, del Toro G, Canet A, Lee DC, Qu W, Tanji N, Lu Y, Lalla E, Fu C, Hofmann MA, Kislinger T, Ingram M, Lu A, Tanaka H, Hori O, Ogawa S, Stern DM, Schmidt AM (2000) Blockade of RAGE-amphoterin signaling suppresses tumour growth and metastases. Nature 405:354- 360

Takeda K, Akira S (2005) Toll-like receptors in innate immunity. Int Immunol 17:1–14.

Tang, J., Li, Y.J., Mu, J., Li, Q., Yang, D.Y., and Xie, P. (2009). Albumin ameliorates tissue plasminogen activator-mediated blood-brain barrier permeability and ischemic brain injury in rats. Neurol. Res. *31* , 189 - 194.

Tasaki K, Ruetzler CA, Ohtsuki T, Martin D, Nawashiro H, Hallenbeck JM (1997) Lipopolysaccharide pre-treatment induces resistance against subsequent focal cerebral ischemic damage in spontaneously hypertensive rats. Brain Res 748:267-270.

Teglund S, McKay C, Schuetz E, van Deursen JM, Stravopodis D, Wang D, Brown M, Bodner S, Grosveld G, Ihle JN. Stat5a and Stat5b proteins have essential and nonessential, or redundant, roles in cytokine responses. *Cell* 93: 841–850, 1998.

The Hemodilution in Stroke Study Group. (1989). Hypervolemic hemodilution treatment of acute stroke. Results of a randomized multicenter trial using pentastarch. Stroke *20* , 317 - 323.

Thompson JE, Phillips RJ, Erdjument-Bromage H, Tempst P, Ghosh S (1995) IκB-β regulates the persistent response in a

Thornalley PJ (1998) Cell activation by glycated proteins. AGE receptors, receptor recognition factors and functional classification of AGEs. Cell Mol Biol (Noisy-le-grand) 44:1013–1023

Thornalley PJ (1998) Glutathione-dependent detoxification of alpha-oxoaldehydes by the glyoxalase system: involvement in disease mechanisms and antiproliferative activity of glyoxalase I inhibitors. Chem Biol Interact 111:137–151

Thornalley PJ, Langborg A, Minhas HS (1999) Formation of glyoxal, methylglyoxal and 3-deoxyglucosone in the glycation of proteins by glucose. Biochem J 344(Pt 1):109–116

Tilghman, S.M. and Belayew, A. (1982). Transcriptional control of the murine albumin/alpha-fetoprotein locus during development. Proc. Natl. Acad. Sci. USA *79* , 5254 - 5257.

Tobias PS, Curtiss LK (2007) Toll-like receptors in atherosclerosis. Biochem Soc Trans 35:1453–1455.

Tracey KJ, Andersson J, Palmblad JE (2003) High mobility group 1 B-box mediates activation of human endothelium. J Intern Med 254:375–385

Treutiger CJ, Mullins GE, Johansson AS, Rouhiainen A, Rauvala HM, Erlandsson-Harris H, Andersson U, Yang H,

Truettner J, Busto R, Zhao W, Ginsberg MD, Perez-Pinzon MA (2002) Effect of ischemic preconditioning on the expression of putative neuroprotective genes in the rat brain. Brain Res Mol Brain Res 103:106–115.

Tsukumo DM, Carvalho-Filho MA, Carvalheira JB, Prada PO, Hirabara SM, Schenka AA, Araujo EP, Vassallo J, Curi R, Velloso LA, Saad MJ (2007) Loss-of-function mutation in Toll-like receptor 4 prevents dietinduced obesity and insulin resistance. Diabetes 56:1986–1998.

Uchiba M, Okajima K, Murakami K, Okabe H, Takatsuki K: Attenuation of endotoxin-induced pulmonary vascular injury by antithrombin III. Am J Physiol 1996;270:L921-L930.

Uchiba M, Okajima K, Murakami K: Effects of various doses of antithrombin on endotoxin-induced endothelial cell injury and coagulation abnormalities in rats. Thromb Res 1998;89:233-241.

van Vliet, E.A., da Costa Araujo, S., Redeker, S., van Schaik, R., Aronica, E., and Gorter, J.A. (2007). Blood-brain barrier leakage may lead to progression of temporal lobe epilepsy. Brain *130*, 521 - 534.

Veldhuis W, Derksen J, Floris S, van der Meide P, de Vries H, Schepers J, Vos I, Dijkstra C, Kappelle L, Nicolay K, Bar P (2003a) Interferon-beta blocks infiltration of inflammatory cells and reduces infarct volume after ischemic stroke in the rat. J Cereb Blood Flow Metab 23:1029–1039.

Veldhuis WB, Floris S, van der Meide PH, Vos IM, de Vries HE, Dijkstra CD, Bar PR, Nicolay K (2003b) Interferon-beta prevents cytokine-induced neutrophil infiltration and attenuates blood-brain barrier disruption. J Cereb Blood Flow Metab 23:1060–1069.

Villa P, Bigini P, Mennini T, Agnello D, Laragione T, Cagnotto A, Viviani B, Marinovich M, Cerami A, Coleman TR, Brines M, Ghezzi P. Erythropoietin selectively attenuates cytokine production and inflammation in cerebral ischemia by targeting neuronal apoptosis. *J Exp Med* 198: 971–975, 2003.

Vlassara H, Brownlee M, Cerami A (1985) High affinity receptor mediated uptake and degradation of glucose modified proteins: a potential mechanism for the removal of senescent macromolecules. Proc Natl Acad Sci U S A 82:5588–5592

Vlassara H, Bucala R, Striker L (1994) Pathogenetic effects of advanced glycosylation: biochemical, biologic and clinical implications for diabetes and aging. Lab Invest 70:138–151

Vogel SN, Fitzgerald KA, Fenton MJ (2003) TLRs: differential adapter utilization by toll-like receptors mediates TLR- specific patterns of gene expression. Mol Intervent 3:466–477.

Wang H, Bloom O, Zhang M, Vishnubhakat JM, Ombellino M, Che J, Frazier A, Yang H, Ivanova S, Borovikova L, Manogue KR, Faist E, Abraham E, Andersson J, Andersson U, Molina PE., Abumrad NN, Sama A, Tracey KJ (1999) HMG-1 as a late mediator of endotoxin lethality in mice. Science 285:248–251

Wang L, Zhang Z, Wang Y, Zhang R, Chopp M. Treatment of stroke with erythropoietin enhances neurogenesis and angiogenesis and improves neurological function in rats. *Stroke* 35: 1732–1737, 2004.

Wautier MP, Chappey O, Corda S, Stern DM, Schmidt AM, Wautier JL (2001) Activation of NADPH oxidase by AGE links oxidant stress to altered gene expression via RAGE. Am J Physiol Endocrinol Metab 280:E685–E694

Wendt TM, Tanji N, Kislinger TR, Qu W, Lu Y, Bucciarelli LG, Rong L, Bierhaus A, Nawroth PP, Moser B, Markowitz GS, Stein G, Dágati V, Stern DM, Schmidt AM (2003) RAGE drives the development of glomerulosclerosis and implicates podocyte activation in the pathogenesis of diabetic nephropathy. Am J Pathol 162:1123–1137

Wenger RH. Cellular adaptation to hypoxia: O2-sensing protein hydroxylases, hypoxia-inducible transcription factors, and O2-regulated gene expression. *FASEB J* 16: 1151–1162, 2002.

Wenger RH. Mammalian oxygen sensing, signalling and gene regulation. *J Exp Biol* 203: 1253–1263, 2000.

Witko-Sarsat V, Rieu P, Descamps-Latscha B, Lesavre P, Halbwachs-Mecarelli L. Neutrophils: molecules, functions and pathophysiological aspects. *Lab Invest* 80: 617–653, 2000.

Wood, J.H. and Kee, D.B., Jr. (1985). Hemorheology of the cerebral circulation in stroke. Stroke *16* , 765 - 772.

Wu LY, Ding AS, Zhao T, Ma ZM, Wang FZ, Fan M (2004) Involvement of increased stability of mitochondrial membrane potential and overexpression of Bcl-2 in enhanced anoxic tolerance induced by hypoxic preconditioning in cultured hypothalamic neurons. Brain Res 999:149–154.

Yadav JS, Wholey MH, Kuntz RE, Fayad P, Katzen BT, Mishkel GJ, Bajwa TK, Whitlow P, Strickman NE, Jaff MR, Popma JJ, Snead DB, Cutlip DE, Firth BG, Ouriel K (2004) Protected carotid-artery stenting versus endarterectomy in high-risk patients. N Engl J Med 351:1493–1501.

Yajima N, Yamamoto Y, Yamamoto H, Takeuchi M, Yaghihashi S (2004) Peripheral neuropathy in diabetic mice overexpressing receptor for advanced glycation endproducts (RAGE). Collected abstracts of the 8th International Symposium on the Maillard reaction (Charleston, SC): no. SXI-7; 55

Yamaji R, Okada T, Moriya M, Naito M, Tsuruo T, Miyatake K, Nakano Y. Brain capillary endothelial cells express two forms of erythropoietin receptor mRNA. *Eur J Biochem* 239: 494–500, 1996.

Yamamoto Y, Kazio I, Doi T et al (2001) Development and prevention of advanced diabetic nephropathy in RAGE- overexpressing mice. J Clin Invest 108:261–268

Yamashiro K, Kiryu J, Tsujikawa A, Honjo M, Nonaka A, Miyamoto K, Honda Y, Tanihara H, Ogura Y: Inhibitory effects of antithrombin III against leukocyte rolling and infiltration during endotoxin-induced uveitis in rats. Invest Ophthalmol Vis Sci 2001;42:1553-1560.

Yamauchi T, Umeda F, Inoguchi T, Nawata H: Antithrombin III stimulates prostecyclin production by cultured aortic endothelial cells. Biochem Biophys Res Commun 1989;163:1404-1411.

Yan SD, Chen X, Fu J, Chen M, Zhu H, Roher A, Slattery T, Zhao L, Nagashima M, Morser J, Migheli A, Nawroth P, Stern D, Schmidt AM (1996) RAGE and amyloid-beta peptide neurotoxicity in Alzheimer's disease. Nature 382:685–691

Yan SD, Zhu H, Zhu A, Golabek A, Du H, Roher A, Yu J, Soto C, Schmidt AM, Stern D, Kindy M (2000) Receptor dependent cell stress and amyloid accumulation in systemic amyloidosis. Nat Med 6:643–651

Yao, X., Miao, W., Li, M., Wang, M., Ma, J., Wang, Y., Miao, L., and Feng, H. (2010). Protective effect of albumin on VEGF and brain edema in acute ischemia in rats. Neurosci. Lett. *472* , 179 -183.

Yasuda Y, Masuda S, Chikuma M, Inoue K, Nagao M, Sasaki R. Estrogen-dependent production of erythropoietin in uterus and its implication in uterine angiogenesis. *J Biol Chem* 273: 25381–25387, 1998.

Yeh CH, Sturgis L, Haidacher J, Zhang XN, Sherwood SJ, Bjercke RJ, Juhasz O, Crow MT, Tilton RG, Denner L (2001) Requirement for p38 and p44/p42 mitogen-activated protein kinases in RAGE-mediated nuclear factor-kappaB transcriptional activation and cytokine secretion. Diabetes 50:1495–1504

Yeh HJ, He YY, Xu J, Hsu CY, Deuel TF (1998) Upregulation of pleiotrophin gene expression in developing microvasculature, macrophages, and astrocytes after acute ischemic brain injury. J Neurosci 18:3699–3707.

Yu X, Shacka JJ, Eells JB, Suarez-Quian C, Przygodzki RM, Beleslin-Cokic B, Lin CS, Nikodem VM, Hempstead B, Flanders KC, Costantini F, Noguchi CT. Erythropoietin receptor signalling is required for normal brain development. *Development* 129: 505–516, 2002.

Yusuf S, Reddy S, Ounpuu S, Anand S (2001a) Global burden of cardiovascular diseases: part I: general considerations, the epidemiologic transition, risk factors, and impact of urbanization. Circulation 104:2746–2753.

Yusuf S, Reddy S, Ounpuu S, Anand S (2001b) Global burden of cardiovascular diseases: part II: variations in cardiovascular disease by specific ethnic groups and geographic regions and prevention strategies. Circulation 104:2855–2864.

Zarember KA, Godowski PJ (2002) Tissue expression of human Toll-like receptors and differential regulation of Toll-like receptor mRNAs in leukocytes in response to microbes, their products, and cytokines. J Immunol 168:554–561.

Zhai Y, Shen XD, O'Connell R, Gao F, Lassman C, Busuttil RW, Cheng G, Kupiec-Weglinski JW (2004) Cutting edge: TLR4 activation mediates liver ischemia/reperfusion inflammatory response via IFN regulatory factor 3- dependent MyD88-independent pathway. J Immunol 173:7115–7119.

Zhan RZ, Fujihara H, Baba H, Yamakura T, Shimoji K (2002) Ischemic preconditioning is capable of inducing mitochondrial tolerance in the rat brain. Anesthesiology 97:896–901.

Zhang F, Wang S, Cao G, Gao Y, Chen J. Signal transducers and activators of transcription 5 contributes to erythropoietin-mediated neuroprotection against hippocampal neuronal death after transient global cerebral ischemia. *Neurobiol Dis* 25: 45–53, 2007.

Zhang W, Potrovita I, Tarabin V, Herrmann O, Beer V, Weih F, Schneider A, Schwaninger M (2005) Neuronal activation of NFkappaB contributes to cell death in cerebral ischemia. J Cereb Blood Flow Metab 25:30–40.

Zhang X, Shan P, Jiang G, Cohn L, Lee PJ (2006) Toll-like receptor 4 deficiency causes pulmonary emphysema. J Clin Invest 116: 3050–3059.

Zhou ML, Shi JX, Hang CH, Zhang FF, Gao J, Yin HX (2007) Expression of Toll-like receptor 4 in the brain in a rabbit experimental subarachnoid haemorrhage model. Inflamm Res 56:93–97.

Ziegler G, Harhausen D, Schepers C, Hoffmann O, Rohr C, Prinz V, Konig J, Lehrach H, Nietfeld W, Trendelenburg G (2007) TLR2 has a detrimental role in mouse transient focal cerebral ischemia. Biochem Biophys Res Comm 359:574–579.

20

Time-Window of Progesterone Neuroprotection After Stroke and Its Underlying Molecular Mechanisms

Weiyan Cai[1], Masahiro Sokabe[2] and Ling Chen[1,2]
[1]*Department of Physiology, Nanjing Medical University, Jiangsu,*
[2]*Department of Physiology, Nagoya University Graduate School of Medicine,*
Tsurumai, Nagoya,
[1]*China,*
[2]*Japan*

1. Introduction

Evidence exists for a gender difference in the vulnerability to either stroke or traumatic brain injury (TBI) in humans. For example, pre-menopausal women with the high serum levels of ovarian hormones estrogen (E2) and progesterone (P4) have a lower risk of stroke (Kannel et al., 1994; Sacco et al., 1997) and a better outcome following stroke (Thorvaldsen et al., 1995) or TBI (Groswasser et al., 1998) relative to men of the same age. After menopause, incidence of stroke in women increases abruptly (Wenger et al., 1993) coincident with decreases in the circulating levels of the ovarian steroid hormones, estrogen (E2) and progesterone (P4). Although clinical trial for TBI with P4 treatment has been well tolerated and giving improved outcomes (Wright et al., 2007; Stein et al., 2008), clinical trial with P4 treatment after cerebral stroke has yet to be initiated. There is increasing evidence that P4 exerts a potent neuroprotective effect against ischemia-induced brain injury in experimental models (Chen et al., 1999; Kumon et al., 2000; Morali et al., 2005; Sayeed et al., 2006) when administered either before insult or after the onset of reperfusion (Murphy et al., 2002; Sayeed et al., 2007). Furthermore, the administration of P4 promotes functional recovery after cerebral ischemia (Gibson & Murphy, 2004; Sayeed et al., 2007). Important enough, a single injection of P4 (4 mg/kg) conducted even 2 h after transient focal brain ischemia reduced cortical infarct volumes (Jiang et al., 1996). Our recent study (Cai et al., 2008) has demonstrated that in male rats a single injection of P4 (4 mg/kg) at 1 h or 48 h prior to an experimental stroke shows protective effects against the ischemia-induced neuronal death and the deficits in spatial cognition and LTP induction. However, to date no systematic study has conducted concerning the effects of P4 against brain injury beyond 6 h following the onset of ischemia (Gibson et al., 2008). Therefore, the present study focused on the effective time-window of neuroprotection by P4 treatment, which would give useful information in treating stroke.

Effects of P4 on the brain generally involve three principle mechanisms, including regulation of gene expression, activation of intracellular signal cascades and modulation of neurotransmitter systems. P4 has been well known to affect transcription processes through the action on the classical nuclear progesterone's receptor (P4R) followed by multiple interactions with DNA and sequence-specific transcription factors (Beato et al., 1995; Guerra-Araiza et al., 2003). The activation of P4R regulates the expression of anti-apoptotic proteins such as bcl-2, and pro-apoptotic genes including bax and bad and caspase-3 (Schlesinger and Saito, 2006). On the transcriptional level, P4 reduces both the nuclear concentration of NFκB and expression of NFκB target genes. P4 has been found to influence the activity of many signaling pathways so-called "nongenomic mechanisms" *via* a membrane-associated P4R (mP4R) that lacks functional DNA-binding domain (Guerra-Araiza et al., 2009). Increasing evidence indicates that P4R activates Src-ERK signaling pathway which serves as an indicator of growth factor activity in mammalian breast cancer cells (Boonyaratanakornkit et al., 2008; Faivre and Lange, 2007). Cai et al. (2008) has demonstrated that P4 triggers P4R-mediated long-lasting (> 48 h) phosphorylation of ERK1/2 and enhances the translocation of phosphorelated ERK2 into the nucleus. In addition, rapid effects of P4 is suggested to be mediated by membrane-associated P4-binding protein 25-Dx (Meffre et al., 2005) to increase the level of phosphorylated Akt in neuronal cells (Singh et al., 2001). The membrane-associated P4R component 1 (PGRMC1) has been reported to elevate the level of Akt phosphorylation in breast cancer (Neubauer et al., 2008). P4 increases the phosphorylation of ERK and Akt, and the expression of the regulatory (p85) subunits of phosphoinositide-3 kinase (PI3K) in the brain (Guerra-Araiza et al., 2009). Furthermore, the P4's metabolite allopregnanolone (ALLO) potentiates the GABAergic synapse activity (Ardeshiri et al., 2006). Finally, much attention has recently been attracted to the antagonizing effects of P4 on sigma-1 (σ_1) receptor (Maurice et al., 2006; Monnet & Maurice, 2006).

The objective of the present study was to determine the P4-neuroprotective effect and its effective therapeutic time-window after transient cerebral ischemia. To this end, male animals subjected to 60 min middle cerebral artery occlusion (MCAO) were given a pair of intraperitoneal injections of P4 (4 mg/kg) separated by 8 h starting at 1, 24, 48, 72 or 96 h after the initiation of cerebral ischemia by middle cerebral artery occlusion (MCAO), and the size of brain infarct, loss of pyramidal neurons in the hippocampal CA1 and cognitive performance of the animals were assessed on 7th day after MCAO. Using pharmacologic tools and western blot analysis, molecular mechanisms underlying the P4-neuroprotective effects against ischemia-induced cerebral injury were also investigated.

2. Materials and methods

2.1 Experimental animals

The present studies were approved by Animal Care and Ethical Committee of Nanjing Medical University. All procedures were in accordance with the guidelines of Institute for Laboratory Animal Research of Nanjing Medical University. Male Sprague-Dawley rats (200-250g, Oriental Bio Service Inc., Nanjing, China) before experiments were used throughout the study. We chose to use only adult male rats in the present study to avoide influence of the E2 effects (Nilsen and Brinton, 2003). Animal rooms were maintained on a 12:12 light-dark cycle starting at AM 7:00 and kept at a temperature of 22-23°C. The animals were permitted free access to food and tap water. All efforts were made to minimize animal suffering and to reduce the number of animals used.

2.2 Preparation of focal cerebral ischemia model

Focal cerebral ischemia was induced by middle cerebral artery occlusion (MCAO). Rats were anesthetized with a mixture of 70% N_2O and 30% O_2 containing 2.5% isoflurane, and were maintained by the inhalation of 1.5% isoflurane during the operation. Briefly, a heat-blunted black monofilament surgical suture (4/0 G) was inserted into the internal carotid artery to occlude the origin of MCA. Adequacy of vascular occlusion and reperfusion was monitored in the front parietal cortex of the occluded side with a multi-channel laser Doppler flow-meter (PF5050 Q4, Perimed, Jarfalla, Sweden). Body and head temperatures were controlled at 37±0.5°C using a water pads. Arterial blood pressure and gases were monitored through a femoral catheter. After 60 min of occlusion, the filament was withdrawn to allow for reperfusion. Sham-operated (sham-op) animals were treated identically, except that MCAs were not occluded.

2.3 Drug administration

P4 was dissolved in dimethylsulfoxide (DMSO), then in sesame oil to a final concentration of 1% DMSO. P4 (4 mg/kg) was intraperitonealy (i.p.) injected. Two injections of P4 with 8 h interval were given starting at 1, 24, 48, 72 or 96 h after the initiation of MCAO (post-MCAO). We selected this low dosage because P4 at this dosage is reported to significantly reduce the ischemic damage and regulate anti-apoptotic gene expression following TBI in rats (Stein, 2008). In addition, our study (Cai et al., 2008) determined that the treatment with the same dosage of P4 increases ERK1/2 phosphorylation.

To analyze the molecular mechanisms underlying the P4-actions, the P4R antagonist RU486 (3 mg/kg) and the 5α-reductase inhibitor finasteride (20 mg/kg) (Finn et al., 2006) were given by intraperitoneal injection (i.p.) at 30 min before each administration of P4. The MEK inhibitor U0126 (0.5 nmol) and the PI3K inhibitor LY294002 (0.3 nmol) were injected into the cerebroventricle (i.c.v.) at 30 min before each injections of P4. For i.c.v. implantation, rats were anaesthetized with ketamine (80 mg/kg i.p.). A guide cannula (10 mm length, 22 gauge) aiming above the right lateral ventricle was implanted. The inhibitors or vehicle were injected with a stepper-motorized micro-syringe (Stoelting, Wood Dale, IL, USA) at a rate of 0.5 µl/min. The drugs were prepared freshly on the day of experiment (final volume = 5µl/rat). Control rats were given an equal volume of vehicle.

2.4 Histological examination

2.4.1 Infarct volume measuring

Brains were removed on 7th day post-MCAO, sectioned into 5 equidistant slices (2.0-mm-thick), and incubated in a 2% 2,3,5-triphenyle-tetrazoliumchloride (TTC) solution (15 min) to visualize infarcted tissue. Measurements were performed by manually outlining the margins of the infarcted areas. Unstained areas of brain sections were defined as infarcted using the image analysis software NIH-Image 3.12. Briefly, the infarcted area on the ipsilateral side was indirectly measured by subtracting the noninfarcted area in the ipsilateral hemisphere from the total nonischaemic area of the contralateral (nonischaemic) hemisphere. Hemispheric infarcted areas were calculated separately on each coronal slice and scored from 1 to 5, and each such area was defined as a percentage of the affected hemisphere. The infarction volume did not differ significantly across the samples in MCAO-groups ($P > 0.05$).

2.4.2 Pyramidal cells counting

Rats were deeply anesthetized with pentobarbital (50 mg/kg), transcardially perfused with 4% paraformaldehyde at 7th day post-MCAO. The brains were removed, post-fixed for 24 h, and then processed for paraffin embedding. Coronal sections (4-μm-thick) including the dorsal hippocampus were cut and stained with toluidine blue. Healthy pyramidal cells showing a round cell body with a plainly stained nucleus were counted by eye using a conventional light microscope (PD70) with a 100×objective. The number of surviving CA1 pyramidal cells per 1 mm length along the extent of pyramidal layer were counted as neuronal density (cells/mm) (Cai et al., 2008). We also made supplemental examinations on several slices stained with trypan blue that stains dead cells, and obtained essentially the same result as that determined by eye with hematoxylin and eosin (HE) stained slices.

2.5 Behavioral analysis

2.5.1 Rota rod test

The Rota rod test was used to assess the sensorimotor coordination of rodent on 7th day post-MCAO (see Figure 1A) using an accelerating treadmill (TSE Systems, Germany; 3 cm diameter). For Rota rod training sessions, animals were habituated to the Rota rod and trained to remain on the rotating drum (constant speed 6 rpm) for a minimum of 90 s to provide a preoperative baseline. Animals not achieving baseline criteria were excluded from further study. In the testing sessions, animals were placed on the Rota rod, and the rotational speed was set to accelerate from 6 to 19 rpm over 180 s. The latency time to fall (time on rod), namely the time when the animal first fell off the drum, was recorded.

2.5.2 Morris Water Maze (MWM) test

Morris water maze test was performed from 4th day post-MCAO for consecutive 4 days (see Figure 2A) using a swimming pool (diameter: 180 cm; height: 30 cm) filled with water (20°C) to a depth of 15 cm. A transparent plexiglass platform (7 cm in diameter) was submerged with the top located 1 cm below the water surface. Swimming paths were analyzed by a computer system with a video camera (AXIS-90 Target/2; Neuroscience). After reaching the platform, rat was allowed to remain on it for 30 sec. If the rat did not find the platform within 90 sec, the rat was put on the platform for 30 sec. The escape-latency to reach hidden-platform was measured from three trials to provide a single value for each rat.

2.6 Western blot analysis

Rats were decapitated under deep anesthesia with ethyl ether. The hippocampus in ischemic hemisphere was taken quickly, then homogenized in a lysis buffer containing 50 mM TriseHCl (pH 7.5), 150 mM NaCl, 5 mM EDTA, 10 mM NaF, 1 mM sodium orthovanadate, 1% Triton X-100, 0.5% sodium deoxycholate, 1 mM phenylmethylsulfonyl fluoride and protease inhibitor cocktail (Complete; Roche, Mannheim, Germany). Protein concentration was determined with BCA Protein Assay Kit (Pierce, Rochford, IL, USA). Total proteins (20 μg) were separated by SDS-polyacrylamide gel electrophoresis (SDS-PAGE) and transferred to a polyphorylated difluoride (PVDF) membrane. The membranes were incubated with 5% bovine serum albumin or 5% nonfat dried milk in tris-buffered saline containing 0.1% Tween 20 (TBST) for 60 min at room temperature, and then were incubated with a mouse monoclonal anti-phospho-ERK1/2 antibody (diluted 1:2500, Cell Signaling, Beverly, MA) at 4°C overnight. After being washed with TBST for three times, the membranes were incubated with an HRP-labeled secondary antibody, and developed using the ECL detection Kit (Amersham Biosciences, Piscataway, NJ). Following visualization, the blots were stripped by incubation in stripping buffer (Restore, Pierce Chemical Co, Rockford IL) for 5 min, re-blocked for 60 min with 5% nonfat dried milk at room temperature, then incubated with anti-total ERK1/2 (diluted 1:5000, Cell Signaling, Beverly, MA). In each experiment, levels of both ERK1/2 and phosphorelated ERK1/2 (phospho-ERK1/2) were measured in the hippocampus of ischemic hemisphere in MCAO-rats and sham-op rats (control). For each animal, phospho-ERK1/2 was normalized by respective ERK1/2 protein. Each experimental group contained 12 rats. The Western blot bands were scanned and analyzed with the image analysis software package, NIH Image.

2.7 Data analysis/statistics

Data were retrieved and processed with the software Microcal Origin 6.1. The group data are expressed as the means ± standard error (SE). For comparison between two groups the 2-sided student t-test was used. For comparison between more than 2 groups one-way analysis of variance (ANOVA) followed by the Bonferroni's post hoc test was performed. Statistical analysis was performed using the software State7 (STATA Corporation, USA). For the analysis of Morris water maze test, statistical differences were determined by an ANOVA with repeated measures, followed by the Bonferroni post hoc test. Statistical analysis was performed using the State7 software (Stata Corporation, USA). Differences at $P<0.05$ were considered statistically significant.

3. Results

3.1 Effective time-window of P4 against ischemic brain infarct and motor dysfunction

To examine the effects of P4 on ischemia-induced brain infarction, a pair of injections (i.p.) of P4 (4 mg/kg) with an 8 h interval were given starting at 1, 24, 48, 72 or 96 h post-MCAO (Figure 1A). On 7th day post-MCAO the results of TTC staining showed that the 60 min MCAO caused approximately 34% brain infarction mainly in the striatum and the frontoparietal cortex (Figure 1B). In comparison with vehicle-treated MCAO-rats, infarct volumes were significantly decreased by the administration of P4 at 1 and 24 h ($P<0.01$, n=12) or 48 and 72 h post-MCAO ($P<0.05$, n=12), but not at 96 h ($P>0.05$, n=12). Similarly, the performance of rota rod test on 7th day post-MCAO perfectly restored in MCAO-rats treated with P4 at 1, 24, 48 ($P<0.01$, n=12) and 72 h post-MCAO ($P<0.05$, n=12; Figure 1C) compared to vehicle-treated MCAO-rats. By contrast, P4 when administered at 96 h post-MCAO had no effect on the ischemia-induced motor impairment ($P>0.05$, n=12). The results indicate that the administration of P4 after stroke exerts a powerful neuroprotection against ischemia-induced brain damages with a wide effective time-window up to 72 h.

3.2 Effective time-window of P4 against ischemic death of neuronal cells and cognitive impairment

Consistent with the previous report (Cai et al., 2008), the number of hippocampal CA1 pyramidal neurons in ischemic hemisphere decreased to approximately 50% of sham-op hemisphere on 7th day post-MCAO ($P<0.01$, n=8; Figure 2B). To examine the effects of P4 on ischemia-induced death of pyramidal neurons and impairment of spatial memory, a pair of injections (i.p.) of P4 (4 mg/kg) with an 8 h interval was given at 1, 24, 48, 72 or 96 h

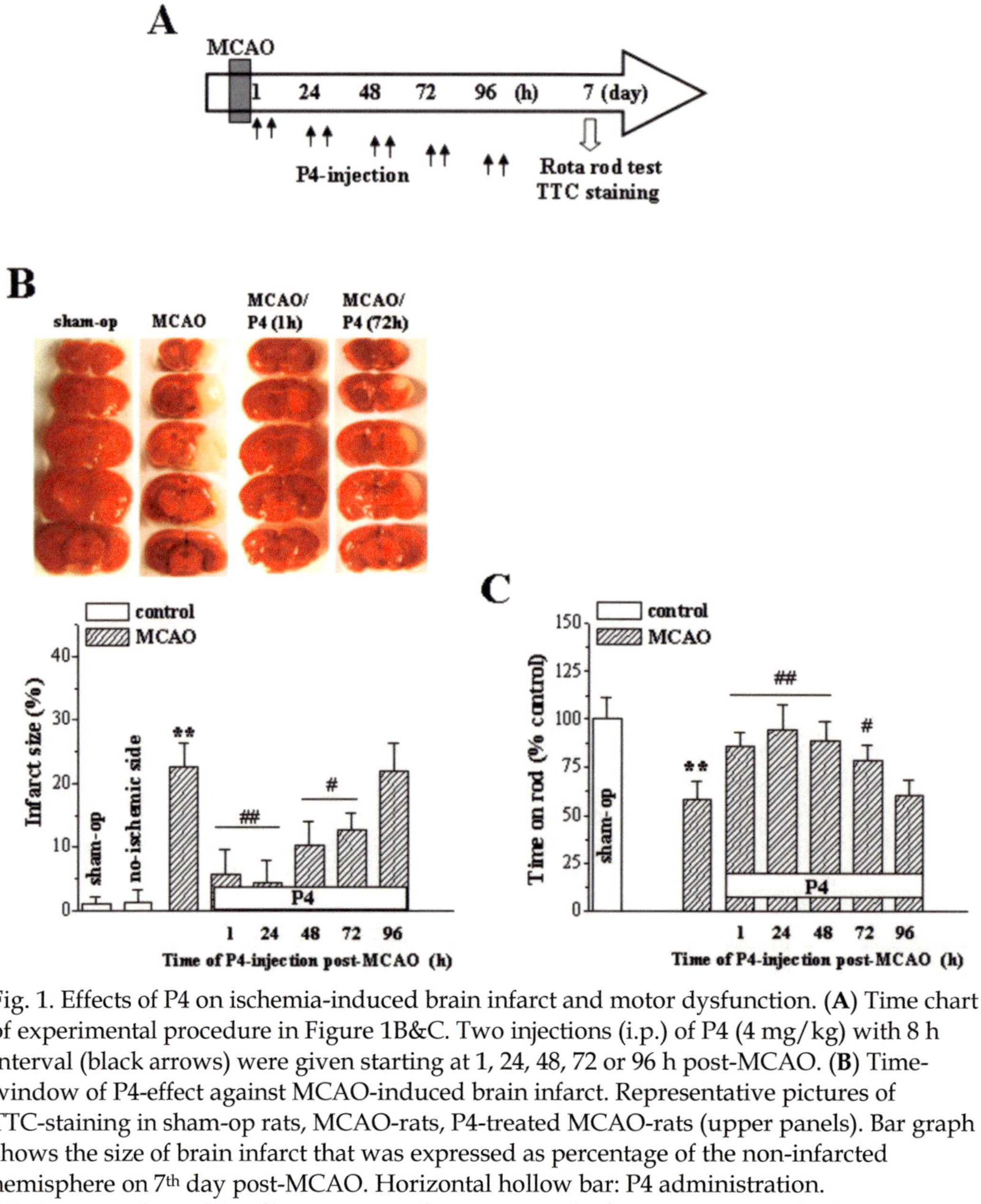

Fig. 1. Effects of P4 on ischemia-induced brain infarct and motor dysfunction. (**A**) Time chart of experimental procedure in Figure 1B&C. Two injections (i.p.) of P4 (4 mg/kg) with 8 h interval (black arrows) were given starting at 1, 24, 48, 72 or 96 h post-MCAO. (**B**) Time-window of P4-effect against MCAO-induced brain infarct. Representative pictures of TTC-staining in sham-op rats, MCAO-rats, P4-treated MCAO-rats (upper panels). Bar graph shows the size of brain infarct that was expressed as percentage of the non-infarcted hemisphere on 7th day post-MCAO. Horizontal hollow bar: P4 administration.
(**C**) Time-window of P4-effect against ischemic motor dysfunction. Bar graph shows time on rod in sham-op (open bar) and MCAO-rats (hatched bars) on 7th day post-MCAO. **P<0.01 vs. sham-op rats; #P<0.05 and ##P<0.01 vs. MCAO-rats.

post-MCAO. The number of dead pyramidal cells was significantly reduced by the treatment with P4 at 1, 24 and 48 h (P<0.01, n=8) or 72 h post-MCAO (P<0.05, n=8) compared to vehicle-treated MCAO-rats. However, the administration of P4 at 96 h post-MCAO exerted no significant effect in reducing the number of ischemia-induced loss of

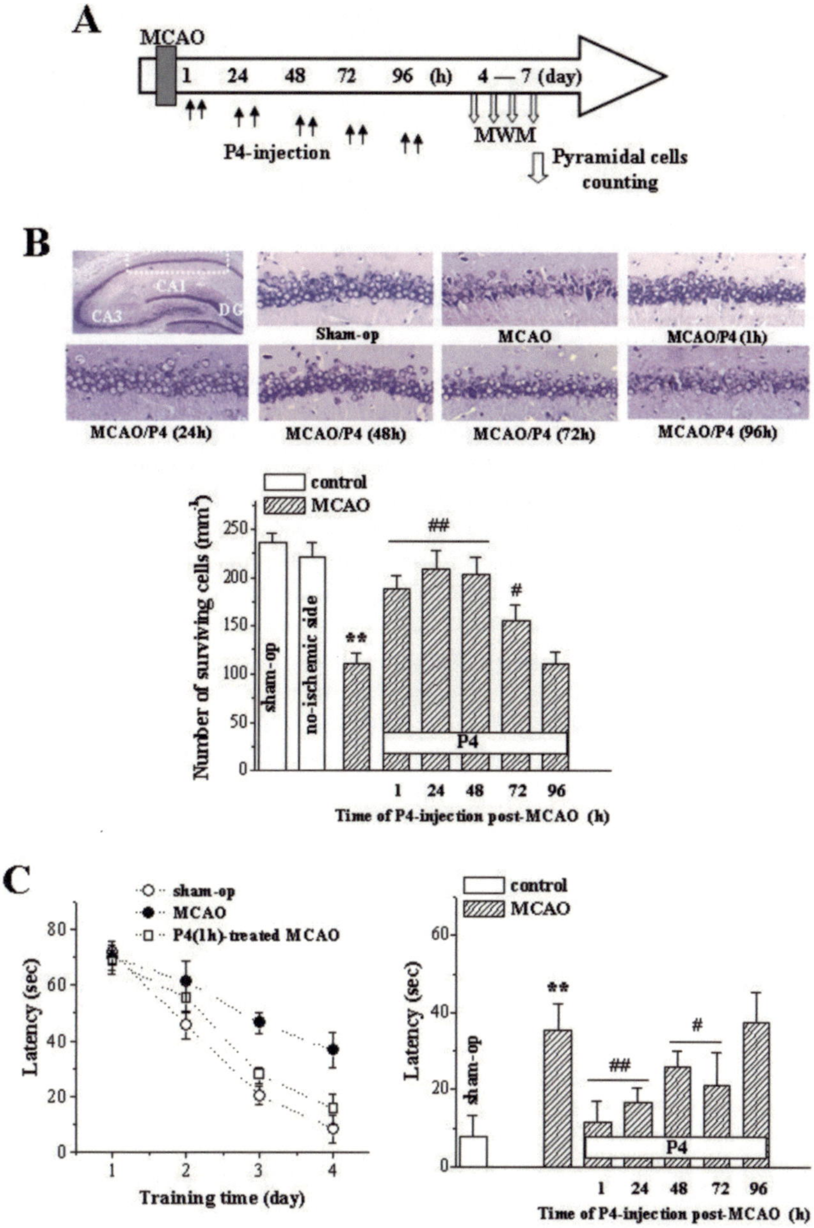

Fig. 2. Effects of P4 on ischemia-induced neuronal cell death and cognitive impairment. (**A**) Time chart of experimental procedure in Figure 2B&C. Two injections (i.p.) of P4 (4 mg/kg) with 8 h interval (black arrows) were given starting at 1, 24, 48, 72 or 96 h post-MCAO. (**B**) Time-window of P4-effect against MCAO-induced neuronal cell death. Representative pictures of hippocampal CA1 region in sham-op rats, MCAO-rats, P4-treated MCAO-rats (upper panels). Scale bar=100μm. Bar graph shows density of surviving neurons in the hippocampal CA1 on 7th day post-MCAO. Horizontal hollow bar: P4 administration. (**C**) Time-window of P4-effect against MCAO-induced deficits in spatial memory. Typical

trials of "Morris" water maze test (left panel) show latency (sec) to reach the hidden-platform against training time (day, day 4-7 post-MCAO) in sham-op rats, MCAO-rats, P4 (1h post-MCAO)-treated MCAO-rats. Bar graph shows the mean latency (±SEM) to reach the hidden-platform on 4th day post-training. **P<0.01 vs. sham-op rats; #P<0.05 and ##P<0.01 vs. MCAO-rats.

pyramidal cells (P>0.05, n=8). The P4 administration per se caused no observable change in CA1 pyramidal neurons on 7th day after sham-op. Spatial learning and memory function was examined by the Morris water maze test from 4th day post-MCAO for consecutive 4 days (Figure 2A). In comparison with sham-op rats, the escape-latency to reach the hidden-platform on 7th day post-MCAO increased approximately 2-fold (P<0.01, n=8; Figure 2C). The behavior of acquisition performance coincided with the histological changes; the prolongation of escape-latency was perfectly improved by the treatment with P4 at 1, 24 and 48 h post-MCAO (P<0.01, n=8), while was partially reduced by the injection of P4 at 72 h post-MCAO (P<0.05, n=8). By contrast, the administration of P4 at 96 h post-MCAO failed to affect the prolonged escape-latency (P>0.05, n=8). Both the histological and behavioral examinations here strongly suggest that the effective time-window of the neuroprotection by the P4 treatment is spanning from 1 h to 72 h post-MCAO. In the following sections, we describe the results on the analyses of the molecular mechanisms underlying the P4 affording neuroprotective effects on ischemia-induced death of pyramidal cells.

3.3 P4-neuroprotection at 1 h post-MCAO is mediated by its metabolite ALLO

A recent study (Ciriza et al., 2006) has revealed that the neuroprotection by P4 after ischemic brain injury is abolished by finasteride, a 5α-reductase inhibitor that inhibits the conversion of P4 to allopregnanolone (ALLO). To determine whether P4 exerts neuroprotection through its metabolite ALLO, finasteride (20 mg/kg i.p.) was given at 30 min prior to every P4-injection. The results showed that the pre-treatment with finasteride partially attenuated the neuroprotection of P4 at 1 h post-MCAO against MCAO-induced neuronal death (P<0.05, n=8; Figure 3A) and prolongation of escape-latency (P<0.05, n=8; Figure 3B), but it did not

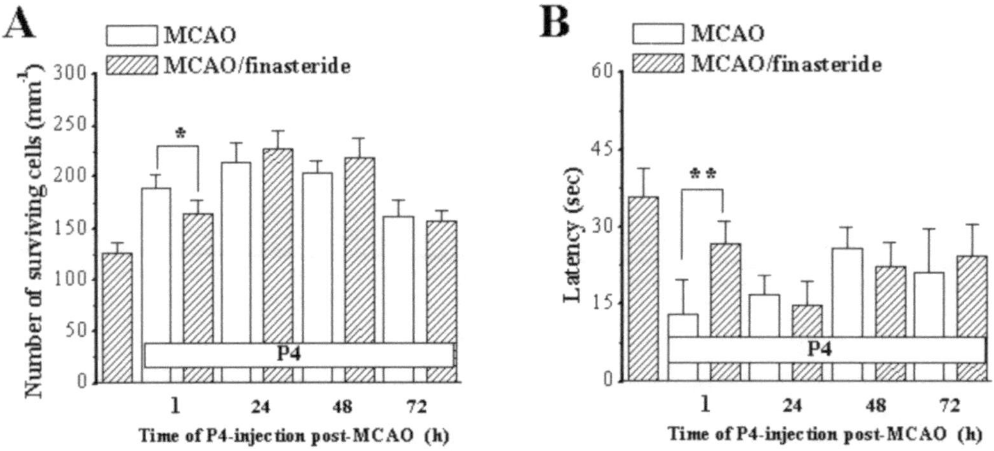

Fig. 3. Effects of finasteride, a 5α-reductase inhibitor, on the neuroprotection of P4 against MCAO-induced neuronal cell death (**A**) and cognitive impairment (**B**). Horizontal hollow bar: P4 administration. Animals were treated with finasteride at 30 min before every P4-injection. Note that the P4-neuroprotection at 1 h post-MCAO is partially blocked by

finasteride. *P<0.05 and *P<0.01 vs. P4-treated MCAO-rats at 1 h post-MCAO.
affect the neuroprotection by P4 at 24, 48 or 72 h post-MCAO (P>0.05, n=8). The results indicate that the neuroprotection by P4 at 1 h post-MCAO is, if not all, caused by a protective action of its metabolite ALLO against ischemia-induced brain damage.

3.4 P4-neuroprotection at 24 and 48 h post-MCAO is mediated by P4R activation

The neuroprotection by P4 administered at 48 h pre-MCAO has been known to depend on P4R function (Faivre and Lange, 2007). To test this possibility in our case, the nuclear P4R blocker RU486 (3 mg/kg, i.p.) was given at 30 min prior to each P4 injection. The results showed that the pre-treatment with RU486 abolished the neuroprotective effects of P4 at 24 and 48 h post-MCAO against ischemia-induced neuronal death (P<0.01, n=8; Figure 4A) and spatial memory impairment (P<0.01, n=8; Figure 4B), whereas it failed to affect the neuroprotection by P4 at 1 or 72 h post-MCAO (P>0.05, n=8). Meanwhile, in the absence of P4 the administration of RU486 at 24 or 48 h post-MCAO had no effect on either neuronal death (P>0.05, n=8) or spatial cognitive function (P>0.05, n=8). These results suggest that the neuroprotective effect of P4 administered at 24 and 48 h post-MCAO involves the P4R-mediated mechanism.

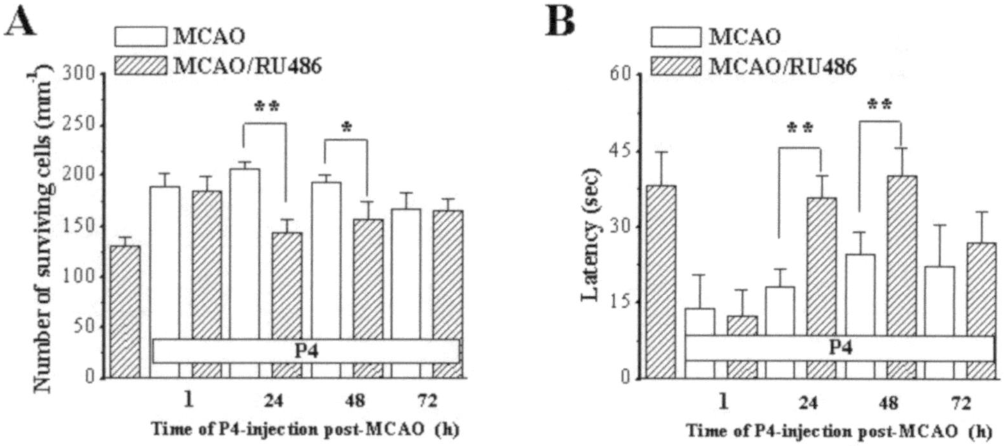

Fig. 4. Effects of RU486, a R4R antagonist, on the neuroprotection of P4 against MCAO-induced neuronal cell death (**A**) and cognitive impairment (**B**). Horizontal hollow bar: P4 administration. Animals were treated with RU486 at 30 min before every time P4-injection. Note that the P4-neuroprotection at 24 and 48 h post-MCAO is blocked by RU486. *P<0.05 and *P<0.01 vs. P4-treated MCAO-rats at 24 and 48 h post-MCAO.

3.5 P4-neuroprotection at 24 and 48 h post-MCAO depends on P4R-ERK signaling

As P4R-mediated ERK1/2 activation protects the ischemic brain damage (Cai et al., 2008), the experiment was designed to explore the involvement of ERK1/2 in the P4R-dependent neuroprotection after MCAO. Expectedly, the ERK kinase (MEK) inhibitor U0126 (0.3 nmol, i.c.v.) blocked the neuroprotection by P4 at 24 and 48 h against MCAO-induced neuronal death (P<0.01, n=8; Figure 5A) and spatial memory impairment (P4 at 24 h post-MCAO, P<0.01, n=8; P4 at 48 h post-MCAO, P<0.05, n=8; Figure 5B), whereas it failed to affect the

P4R-independent neuroprotection exerted by P4 administered at 1 or 72 h post-MCAO (P>0.05, n=8). These results indicate that the P4R-mediated neuroprotection is highly coupled with ERK1/2 signaling pathway.

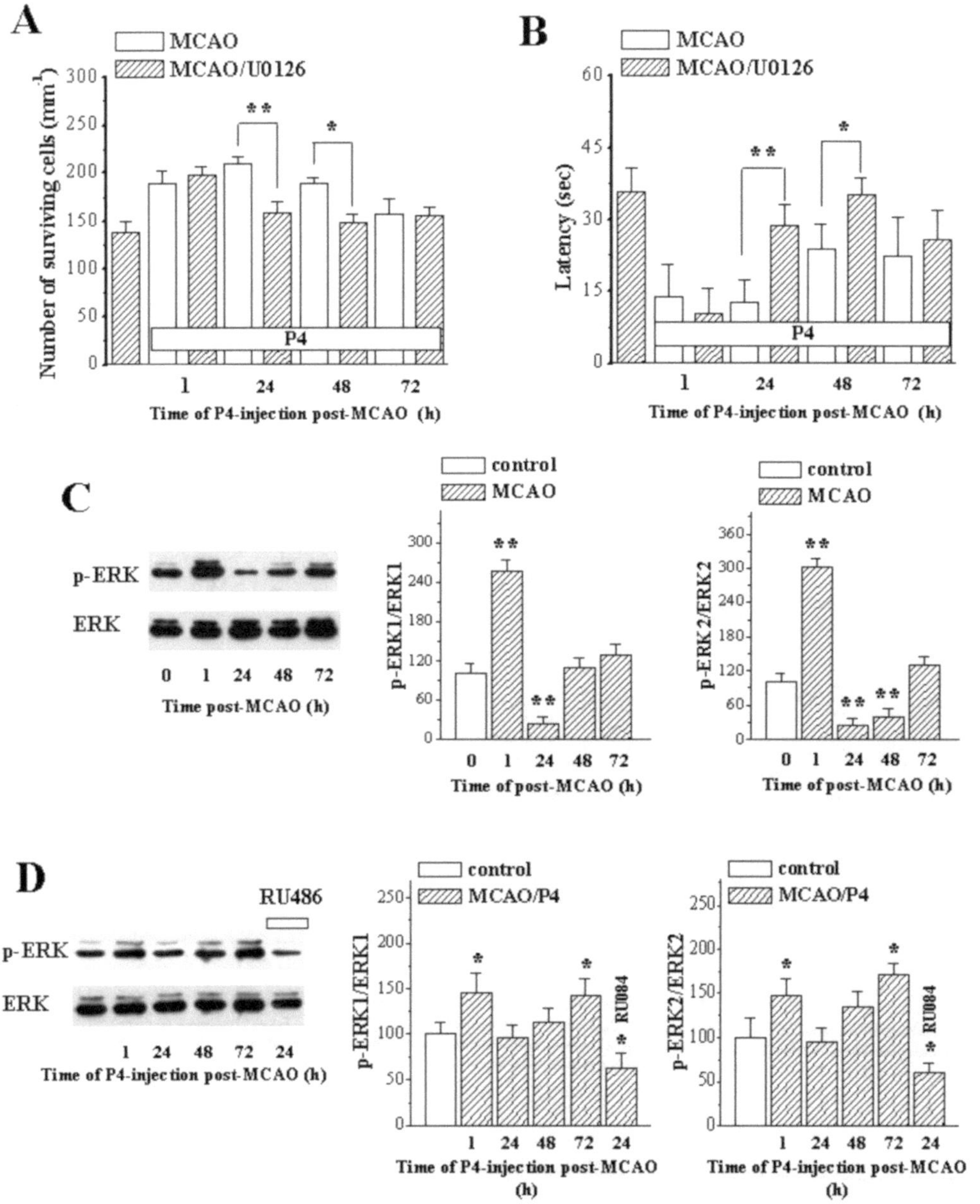

Fig. 5. Effects of U0126, a MEK inhibitor, on the neuroprotection of P4 against MCAO-induced neuronal cell death (**A**) and cognitive impairment (**B**). Horizontal hollow bar: P4 administration. Animals were treated with U0126 at 30 min before every time P4-injection. Note that the phospho-ERK1/2 at 24 and 48 h post-MCAO is blocked by U0126. *P<0.05 and *P<0.01 vs. P4-treated MCAO-rats at 24 and 48 h post-MCAO. (**C**) Kinetics of hippocampal

phospho-ERK1/2 at 1, 24, 48 and 72 h post-MCAO. Representative western blots represent ERK1/2 phosphorylation immunoreactivity obtained from whole-cell lysates. Level of phospho-ERK1/2 is expressed as a percentage of phospho-ERK1/2 in sham-op rats. (**D**) Effect of P4 on phospho-ERK1/2 at 1, 24, 48 and 72 h post-MCAO. P4 was given at 30 min before harvested hippocampus. Values of phospho-ERK1/2 were normalized by phospho-ERK1/2 in sham-op rats. *P<0.05 and **P<0.01 vs. sham-op group; #<0.05 vs. MCAO-rats treated with P4 at 24 h post-MCAO. Horizontal axis: Time of post-MCAO p4 injection.

Emerging evidence indicates that transient cerebral ischemia promotes the dephosphorylation of ERK1/2 (Jover-Mengual et al., 2007). To confirm this, kinetics of hippocampal ERK1/2 phosphorylation (phospho-ERK1/2) after MCAO was measured using Western blot analysis. In comparison with that before MCAO, the level of phospho-ERK1/2 was largely increased at 1 h post-MCAO (P<0.05, n=12; Figure 5C), followed by a persistent decrease at 24 h and 48 h post-MCAO (P<0.05, n=12), then returned to the basal level at 72 h post-MCAO (P>0.05, n=12). To investigate the effects of P4 on the changes in ERK1/2 phosphorylation after MCAO, the MCAO-rats were given a single injection of P4 at 1, 24, 48 or 72 h post-MCAO. Thirty minutes after the P4-injection hippocampal preparations were harvested to measure phospho-ERK1/2. As shown in Figure 5D, the treatment with P4 slightly attenuated the increased phospho-ERK1/2 at 1 h post-MCAO (P<0.05, n=12), perfectly rescued the reduction of phospho-ERK1/2 at 24 and 48 h post-MCAO (P<0.01, n=12), and elevated the level of phospho-ERK1/2 at 72 h post-MCAO (P<0.05, n=12). The P4R antagonist RU486 could block the protective effect of P4 on the reduction of phospho-ERK1/2 at 24 h post-MCAO (P<0.05 vs. P4-treated MCAO-rats, n=12). These observations clearly indicate that the P4R-dependent neuroprotection against ischemia-induced brain damage is mediated, at least in part, through the regulation of ERK1/2 activity.

3.6 P4-neuroprotection at 24–72 h post-MCAO requires PI3K signaling

As P4 increases the level of Akt-phosphorylation, a partial process of PI3K signaling (Guerra-Araiza et al., 2009), the specific PI3K inhibitor LY294002 (0.3 nmol) was injected into the cereboventricle (i.c.v.) at 30 min prior to P4 injection to examine the involvement of PI3K-Akt signaling pathway in the P4-neuroprotection. The results showed that the pre-treatment with LY294002 partially attenuated the neuroprotection of P4 at 24 and 48 h post-MCAO (P<0.05, n=8; Figure 6A) and completely abolished the neuroprotection of P4 at 72 h post-MCAO (P<0.01, n=8), whereas it had no effect on the neuroprotection of P4 at 1 h post-MCAO (P>0.05, n=8). Furthermore, the pre-treatment with LY294002 blocked the P4-improved impairment of spatial memory when administered at 24, 48 and 72 h post-MCAO (P<0.05, n=8; Figure 6B). The results indicate that the PI3K-Akt signaling is involved in the P4R-dependent and P4R-independent neuroprotections by P4, depending on the timing of P4 injection.

4. Discussion

The present study provides evidence that the treatment with P4 after transient brain ischemia exerts a powerful neuroprotection with a wide effective time-window up to 72 h post-MCAO. The neuroprotective effects of P4 were mediated by different molecular mechanisms depending on the timing of P4 administration after ischemia. The neuroprotection by P4 at 1 h post-MCAO appeared to be caused through P4's metabolite allopregnanolone (ALLO) because the protection was significantly attenuated by the 5α-reductase inhibitor finasteride. The neuroprotection of P4 at 24 and 48 h post-MCAO appeared to be P4R-dependent through rescuing the down-regulation of ERK1/2 phosphorylation after stroke. The neuroprotective effects of P4 at 72 h post-MCAO required PI3K activation in a P4R-independent way.

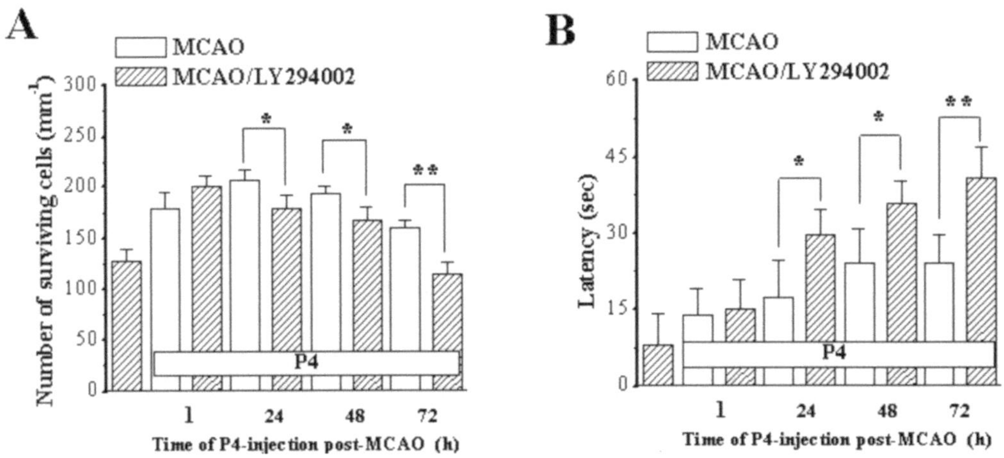

Fig. 6. Involvement of PI3K in P4-neuroprotection. Animals were treated with the specific PI3K inhibitor LY294002 (LY) at 30 min before administration of P4. Horizontal hollow bar: P4 administration. Note that the P4-neuroprotection at 24–72 hr post-MCAO requires PI3K signaling. *P<0.05 and **P<0.01 vs. MCAO-rats treated with P4 at 24, 48 and 72 hr post-MCAO.

4.1 Anti-excitotoxic effect of P4's metabolite ALLO at 1 h after MCAO

One recent report indicates that either P4 or ALLO when administered at 2 h post-MCAO is effective in reducing the infarct volume after focal brain ischemia, where ALLO shows more effective neuroprotection than its parent compound (Sayeed et al., 2007). Similarly, our results in the present study showed that the neuroprotection of P4 at 1 h post-MCAO was sensitive to the 5α-reductase inhibitor fenasteride. Thus, it is proposed that the acute neuroprotection of P4 within 1−2 h ischemia/reperfusion is caused by ALLO, a positive regulator of GABAA receptor (Belelli & Lambert, 2005). This notion is supported by an earlier study (Ardeshiri et al., 2006) showing that the GABAA receptor antagonist picrotoxin could prevent the neuroprotection afforded by P4. The P4 neuroprotection mainly focuses on some populations of neurons that are sensitive to excitotoxicty, including the pyramidal neurons in the hippocampus and cerebral cortex, Purkinje cells in the cerebellum, as well as the neurons in the dorsal striatum and the caudate nucleus (Monnet and Maurice, 2006; Schumacher et al., 2007). Immediately after ischemia, excessive presynaptic glutamate releases result in the accumulation of extracellular glutamate to reach concentrations that induce over-activation of glutamate receptors called excitotoxicity (Jabaudon et al., 2000; Phillis and O'Regan, 2003). The process of excitotoxicity has been demonstrated in several experimental models of cerebral ischemia (Butcher et al., 1990). Therefore, it is highly likely that P4 and ALLO at 1 h post-MCAO prevent the brain injury by suppressing over-excitation of pyramidal neurons through the activation of $GABA_A$ receptors.

However, we noted that the treatment with finasteride could not completely block the P4-neuroprotection at 1 h post-MCAO (see Figure 3A). Excessive presynaptic glutamate releases after cerebral ischemia lead to neuronal death mainly by excessive calcium entry through N-methyl-D-aspartate receptor (NMDAr). Our recent study (Cai et al., 2008) has revealed that P4, as a potential σ_1 receptor antagonist (Monnet and Maurice, 2006), reduces Ca^{2+} influx across NMDAr-channels to protect hippocampal neurons from ischemia-induced cell death. In addition, at 1 h after brain ischemia the activation of $\sigma 1$ receptor by PRE-084, a σ_1 receptor agonist, exacerbates ischemia-induced neuronal cell death in an NMDAr-dependent manner (Li et al., 2009). However, conflicting results have reported that the activation of σ_1 receptor enhances presynaptic glutamate release in the hippocampal CA1 (Meyer et al., 2002), and promotes the Ca^{2+} influx across NMDAr-channels (Monnet et al., 2003) and the Ca^{2+} efflux from calcium pools via inositol 1,4,5-trisphosphate receptors (Su and Hayashi, 2003). This discrepancy may be due to the difference in experimental condition or timing of P4 action. Further studies are required to directly observe the P4 effects on NMDAr-Ca^{2+} influx in an acute phase after stroke.

4.2 P4R-dependent ERK activation at 24—48 h after stroke

Our results revealed that the P4R-mediated ERK1/2 signaling was involved in the neuroprotection by P4 at 24—48 h post-MCAO. P4R ligand has been demonstrated to induce a transient (5—10 min after P4-application) activation of Src-Ras-ERK1/2 and a persistent (6—72 h) ERK1/2 activation (Faivre and Lange, 2007). Recently, Cai et al. (2008) provided in vivo evidence that P4 acts on P4R to trigger a long-lasting (> 48 hr) phosphorylation of ERK1/2, resulting in a promoted translocation of phosphorelated ERK2 into the nucleus. The translocation of ERK1/2 is a pivotal and necessary process for the activation of cAMP response element binding protein (CREB) (Nilsen and Brinton, 2003). The ERK1/2-CREB signaling has been implicated to play a critical role in the brain ischemic tolerance (Gonzalez-Zulueta et al., 2000) and neuronal cell survival (Singh, 2005; 2006). The CREB cascade can increase the expression of anti-apoptotic molecules such as Bcl-2 and Bcl-XL (Yao et al., 2005) and decrease the expression of pro-apoptotic molecules such as Bax, Bad and caspase-3 (Djebaili et al., 2004). Consistent with the results reported by Jover-Mengual et al. (2007), we in the present study showed a decreased activity of ERK1/2 at 24 and 48 h post-MCAO. More importantly, the activation of P4R at 24—48 h after ischemia could rescue the down-regulation of ERK1/2. Therefore, it is highly likely that the P4R-dependent neuroprotection is closely coupled with ERK1/2 signaling.

On the other hand, western blot analysis showed a transient elevation of ERK1/2 phosphorylation at 1 h post-MCAO. The elevation of ERK1/2 activity immediately after stroke has also been observed in humans (Slevin et al., 2000) and a rat model of cerebral ischemia (Wang et al., 2003), in which increased intracellular Ca^{2+} levels ($[Ca^{2+}]_i$) after ischemia seem to lead hyper-activation of ERK1/2. Alessandrini et al. (1999) and Namura et al. (2001) provided evidence for a neuroprotective role of MEK inhibitor following transient ischemia as manifested by the reduction of infarct size and improvement of functional outcome. The neuroprotection by MEK-inhibition in ischemic brain is associated with an activation of potential anti-apoptotic pathway that suppresses caspase-3 activation and apoptosis (Wang et al., 2003). To our surprise, we observed that the treatment with P4 could attenuate the elevation of ERK1/2 phosphorylation at 1 h post-MCAO. Because the neuroprotection by P4 at 1 h post-MCAO was P4R-independent, it is proposed that P4 prevents ischemia-increased $[Ca^{2+}]_i$ by antagonizing σ_1 receptor, which may stabilize the ERK1/2 activation.

4.3 PI3K signaling is required for P4R-independent and P4R-dependnet neuroprotections

P4 has been reported to enhance the phosphorylation of Akt/PKB (Singh et al., 2001; Kuolen et al., 2008) in the hippocampus and cerebellum (Guerra-Araiza et al., 2009). On the other hand, PI3K signaling is believed to suppress apoptotic cell death via its downstream effectors, such as Akt/PKB, to inhibit the Bcl2 family protein Bad (Noshita et al., 2001). Using the specific PI3K inhibitor LY294002, the present study provided in vivo evidence that the PI3K signaling is required for the P4-neuroprotection at 24−72 h post-MCAO against ischemia-induced brain damage. In human breast cancer cells, P4 induces rapid and transient activation of PI3K-Akt pathway in a P4R-dependent manner (Migliaccio et al., 1998; Castoria et al., 2001). It was reported that progestins rapidly activated PI3K-Akt pathway via P4R (Vallejo et al., 2005; Ballare et al., 2006). However, our results here showed that the PI3K-mediated neuroprotection by P4 administered at 72 h post-MCAO is P4R-independent. P4 is reportedly to regulate PI3K signaling pathway through its metabolites (Guerra-Araiza et al., 2009), but our data determined that the neuroprotection of P4 at 24−72 h post-MCAO was insensitive to the inhibition of 5α-reductase by fenasteride. P4-binding membrane protein 25-Dx (also known as PGRMC1) in the brain (Krebs et al., 2000; Sakamoto et al., 2004) is involved in the anti-apoptotic actions of P4 (Peluso et al., 2006, 2008). Further studies are needed to elucidate whether P4 cascades PI3K signaling after stroke through P4-binding 25-Dx mechanisms.

4.4 Clinical significance

P4 treatment after ischemia at relatively a low dose (4 mg/kg) exerts powerful neuroprotective effects with a wide, at least up to 72 h post ischemia, effective time-window, which would provide a great benefit in treating stroke. The present study provides evidence that the P4 neuroprotection has a wide effective time-window that is realized by a time dependent multiple neuroprotective mechanisms after ischemia. The results shown here not only help to understand the correlation between the declined level of P4 and the abruptly increasing incidence of stroke following the menopause, but also provide a novel the therapeutic opportunity of P4 against the ischemic brain injury.

5. Acknowledgments

This work was supported by grants for NSFC (30872725; 81071027; 31171440) to Chen L.
We declare that there is no competing financial that could be construed as influencing the results or interpretation of the reported study.

6. References

Alessandrini A, Namura S, Moskowitz MA & Bonventre JV. (1999). MEK1 protein kinase inhibition protects against damage resulting from focal cerebral ischemia. *Proc Natl Acad Sci USA*, vol. 96, pp. 12866–12869

Ardeshiri A, Kelley MH, Korner IP, Hurn PD & Herson PS. (2006). Mechanism of progesterone neuroprotection of rat cerebellar Purkinje cells following oxygen-glucose deprivation. *Eur J Neurosci*, vol. 24, pp. 2567–2574

Ballare C, Vallejo G ,Vicent GP, Saragüeta P & Beato M. (2006). Progesterone signaling in breast and endometrium. *J Steroid Biochem Mol Biol* vol. 102, pp. 2–10

Beato M, Herrlich P & Schutz G. (1995). Steroid hormone receptors: many actors in search of a plot. *Cell*, vol. 83, pp. 851–857

Belelli D & Lambert JJ. (2005). Neurosteroids: endogenous regulators of the GABA (A) receptor. *Nat Rev Neurosci vol.* 6, pp. 565–575

Boonyaratanakornkit V, Bi Y, Rudd M & Edwards DP. (2008). The role and mechanism of progesterone receptor activation of extra-nuclear signaling pathways in regulating gene transcription and cell cycle progression. *Steroids*, vol. 73, pp. 922–928

Butcher SP, Bullock R, Graham DI & McCulloch J. (1990). Correlation between amino acid release and neuropathologic outcome in rat brain following middle cerebral artery occlusion. *Stroke*, vol. 21, pp. 1727-1733

Cai W, Zhu Y, Furuya K, Li Z, Sokabe M & Chen L. (2008). Two different molecular mechanisms underlying progesterone neuroprotection against ischemic brain damage. *Neuropharmacology*, vol. 55, pp. 127–138

Castoria G, Migliaccio A, Bilancio A, Di Domenico M, de Falco A, Lombardi M, Fiorentino R, Varricchio L, Barone MV & Auricchio F. (2001). PI3-kinase in concert with Src promotes the S-phase entry of oestradiol-stimulated MCF-7 cells. *EMBO J*, vol. 20, pp. 6050–6059

Chen J, Chopp M & Li Y. (1999). Neuroprotective effects of progesterone after transient middle cerebral artery occlusion in rat. *J Neurol Sci*, vol. 171, pp. 24–30

Ciriza I, Carrero P, Frye CA & Garcia-Segura LM. (2006). Reduced metabolites mediate neuroprotective effects of progesterone in the adult rat hippocampus. The synthetic progestin medroxyprogesterone acetate (Provera) is not neuroprotective. *J Neurobiol*, vol. 66, pp. 916–928

Djebaili M, Hoffman SW & Stein DG. (2004). Allopregnanolone and progesterone decrease cell death and cognitive deficits after a contusion of the rat pre-frontal cortex. *Neuroscience*, vol. 123, pp. 349–359

Faivre EJ & Lange CA. (2007). Progesterone receptors upregulate Wnt-1 to induce epidermal growth factor receptor transactivation and c-Src-dependent sustained activation of Erk1/2 mitogen-activated protein kinase in breast cancer cells. *Mol Cell Biol*, vol. 27, pp. 466–480

Finn DA, Beadles-Bohling AS, Beckley HE, Ford MM, Gililland KR, Gorin-Meyer RE & Wiren KM. (2006). A new look at the 5alpha-reductase inhibitor finasteride. *J compilation* ,vol. 12, pp. 53–76

Gibson CL & Murphy SP. (2004). Progesterone enhances functional recovery after middle cerebral artery occlusion in male mice. *J Cereb Blood Flow Metab*, vol. 24, pp. 805–813

Gibson CL, Gray LJ, Bath PM & Murphy SP. (2008). Progesterone for the treatment of experimental brain injury; a systematic review. *Brain*, vol. 13, pp. 318-328

Gonzalez-Zulueta M, Feldman AB, Klesse LJ, Kalb RG, Dillman JF, Parada LF, Dawson TM & Dawson VL. (2000). Requirement for nitric oxide activation of p21(ras)/extracellular regulated kinase in neuronal ischemic preconditioning. *Proc Natl Acad Sci USA*, vol. 97, pp. 436–441

Groswasser Z, Cohen M & Keren O. (1998). Female TBI patients recover better than males. *Brain Inj*, vol. 12, pp. 805–808

Guerra-Araiza C, Amorim MA, Pinto-Almazán R, González-Arenas A, Campos MG & Garcia-Segura LM. (2009). Regulation of the phosphoinositide-3 kinase and mitogen-activated protein kinase signaling pathways by progesterone and its reduced metabolites in the rat brain. *J Neurosci Res*, vol. 87, pp. 470-481

Guerra-Araiza C, Villamar-Cruz O, González-Arenas A, Chavira R & Camacho-Arroyo I. (2003). Changes in progesterone receptor isoforms content in the rat brain during the oestrous cycle and after oestradiol and progesterone treatments. *J Neuroendocrinol*, vol. 15, pp. 984–990

Jabaudon D, Scanziani M, Gähwiler BH & Gerber U. (2000). Acute decrease in net glutamate uptake during energy deprivation. *Proc Natl Acad Sci U S A*, vol. 97, pp. 5610-5615

Jiang N, Chopp M, Stein D & Feit H. (1996). Progesterone is neuroprotective after transient middle cerebral artery occlusion in male rats. *Brain Res*, vol. 30, pp. 101–107

Jover-Mengual T, Zukin RS & Etgen AM. (2007). MAPK signaling is critical to estradiol protection of CA1 neurons in global ischemia. *Endocrinology*, vol. 148, pp. 1131–1143

Kannel WB, Ho K & Thom T. (1994). Changing epidemiological features of cardiac failure. *Br Heart J* , vol. 72, pp. 3–9

Koulen P, Madry C,Duncan RS, Hwang JY, Nixon E, McClung N, Gregg EV & Singh M. (2008). Progesterone potentiates IP(3)-mediated calcium signaling through Akt/PKB. *Cell Physiol Biochem*, vol. 21, pp. 161–172

Krebs CJ, Jarvis ED, Chan J, Lydon JP, Ogawa S & Pfaff DW. (2000). A membrane-associated progesterone-binding protein, 25-Dx, is regulated by progesterone in brain regions involved in female reproductive behaviors. *Proc Natl Acad Sci USA* , vol. 97, pp. 12816–12821

Kumon Y, Kim SC, Tompkins P, Stevens A, Sakaki S & Loftus CM. (2000). Neuroprotective effect of postischemic administration of progesterone in spontaneously hypertensive rats with focal cerebral ischemia. *J Neurosurg* , vol. 92, pp. 848–852

Li Z, Cui S, Zhang Z, Zhou R, Ge Y, Sokabe M & Chen L. (2009). DHEA-neuroprotection and -neurotoxicity after transient cerebral ischemia in rats. *J Cereb Blood Flow Metab*, vol. 29, pp. 287-296

Maurice T, Gregoire C & Espallergues J. (2006). Neuro(active)steroids actions at the neuromodulatory sigma(1) receptor: Biochemical and physiological evidences, consequences in neuroprotection. *Pharmacol Biochem Behav*, vol. 84, pp. 581–597

Meffre D, Delespierre B, Gouézou M, Leclerc P, Vinson GP, Schumacher M, Stein DG & Guennoun R. (2005). The membrane-associated progesterone-binding protein 25-Dx is expressed in brain regions involved in water homeostasis and is up-regulated after traumatic brain injury. *J Neurochem*, vol. 93, pp. 1314–1326

Meyer DA, Carta M, Partridge LD, Covey DF & Valenzuela CF. (2002). Neurosteroids enhance spontaneous glutamate release in hippocampal neurons. Possible role of metabotropic sigma1-like receptors. *J Biol Chem*, vol. 277, pp. 28725–28732

Migliaccio A, Piccolo D, Castoria G, Di Domenico M, Bilancio A, Lombardi M, Gong W, Beato M & Auricchio F. (1998). Activation of the Src/p21ras/Erk pathway by progesterone receptor via cross-talk with estrogen receptor. *EMBO J*, vol. 17, pp. 2008–2018

Monnet FP & Maurice T. (2006). The sigma1 protein as a target for the non-genomic effects of neruo(active)steroids: molecular, physiological, and behavioral aspects. *J Pharmacol Sci*, vol. 100, pp. 93–118

Monnet FP, Morin-Surun MP, Leger J & Combettes L. (2003). Protein kinase C-dependent potentiation of intracellular calcium influx by σ1 receptor agonists in rat hippocampal neurons. *J Pharmacol Exp Ther*, vol. 307, pp. 705–712

Morali G, Letechipia-Vallejo G, Lopez-Loeza E, Montes P, Hernández-Morales L & Cervantes M. (2005). Post-ischemic administration of progesterone in rats exerts neuroprotective effects on the hippocampus. *Neurosci Lett*, vol. 382, pp. 286–290

Murphy SJ, Littleton-Kearney MT & Hurn PD. (2002). Progesterone administration during reperfusion, but not preischemia alone, reduces injury in ovariectomized rats. *J Cereb Blood Flow Metab*, vol. 22, pp. 1181–1188

Namura S, Iihara K, Takami S, Nagata I, Kikuchi H, Matsushita K, Moskowitz MA, Bonventre JV & Alessandrini A. (2001). Intravenous administration of MEK inhibitor U0126 affords brain protection against forebrain ischemia and focal cerebral ischemia. *Proc Natl Acad Sci USA*, vol. 98, pp. 11569–11574

Neubauer H, Clare SE, Wozny W, Schwall GP, Poznanovic S, Stegmann W, Vogel U, Sotlar K, Wallwiener D, Kurek R, Fehm T & Cahill MA. (2008). Breast cancer proteomics reveals correlation between estrogen receptor status and differential phosphorylation of PGRMC1. *Breast Cancer Res*, vol. 15, pp. R85.

Nilsen J & Brinton RD. (2003). Divergent impact of progesterone and medroxyprogesterone acetate (Provera) on nuclear mitogen-activated protein kinase signaling. *Proc Natl Acad Sci USA*, vol. 100, pp. 10506–10511

Noshita N, Lewén A, Sugawara T & Chan PH. (2001). Evidence of phosphorylation of Akt and neuronal survival after transient focal cerebral ischemia in mice. *J Cereb Blood Flow Metab*, vol. 21, pp. 1442–1450

Peluso JJ, Pappalardo A, Losel R & Wehling M. (2006). Progesterone membrane receptor component 1 expression in the immature rat ovary and its role in mediating progesterone's antiapoptotic action. *Endocrinology*, vol.147, pp. 3133–3140

Peluso JJ, Romak J & Liu X. (2008). Progesterone receptor membrane component-1 (PGRMC1) is the mediator of progesterone's antiapoptotic action in spontaneously immortalized granulosa cells as revealed by PGRMC1 small interfering ribonucleic acid treatment and functional analysis of PGRMC1 mutations. *Endocrinology* , vol. 149, pp. 534–543

Phillis JW & O'Regan MH. (2003). Characterization of modes of release of amino acids in the ischemic/reperfused rat cerebral cortex. *Neurochem Int*, vol. 43, pp. 461-467.

Sacco RL. (1998). Identifying patient populations at high risk for stroke. *Neurology*, vol. 51, pp. 27–30

Sakamoto H, Ukena K, Takemori H, Okamoto M, Kawata M & Tsutsui K. (2004). Expression and localization of 25-Dx, a membraneassociated putative progesterone-binding protein, in the developing Purkinje cell. *Neuroscience*, vol. 126, pp. 325–334

Sayeed I, Guo Q, Hoffman SW & Stein DG. (2006). Allopregnanolone, a progesterone metabolite, is more effective than progesterone in reducing cortical infarct volume after transient middle cerebral artery occlusion. *Ann Emerg Med*, vol. 47, pp. 381–389

Sayeed I, Wali B & Stein DG. (2007). Progesterone inhibits ischemic brain injury in a rat model of permanent middle cerebral artery occlusion. *Restor Neurol Neurosci*, vol. 25, pp. 151–159

Schlesinger PH & Saito M. (2006). The Bax pore in liposomes, Biophysics. *Cell Death Differ*, vol. 13, pp. 1403-1408

Schumacher M, Guennoun R, Stein DG & De Nicola AF. (2007). Progesterone: therapeutic opportunities for neuroprotection and myelin repair. *Pharmacol Ther*, vol. 116, pp. 77-106

Singh M. (2001). Ovarian hormones elicit phosphorylation of Akt and extracellular-signal regulated kinase in explants of the cerebral cortex. *Endocrine*, vol. 14, pp. 407–415

Singh M. (2005). Mechanisms of progesterone-induced neuroprotection. *Ann NY Acad Sci USA*, vol. 1052, pp. 145–151

Singh M. (2006). Progesterone-induced neuroprotection. *Endocrinology*, vol. 29, pp. 271–274

Slevin M, Krupinski J, Slowik A, Rubio F, Szczudlik A & Gaffney J. (2000). Activation of MAP kinase (ERK-1/ERK-2), tyrosine kinase and VEGF in the human brain following acute ischaemic stroke. *Neuroreport*, vol. 11, pp. 2759–2764

Stein DG. (2008). Progesterone exerts neuroprotective effects after brain injury. *Brain Res Rev*, vol. 57, pp. 386-397.

Su TP & Hayashi T. (2003). Understanding the molecular mechanism of sigma-1 receptors: towards a hypothesis that sigma-1 receptors are intracellular amplifiers for signal transduction. *Curr Med Chem*, vol. 10, pp. 2073–2080

Thorvaldsen P, Asplund K, Kuulasmaa K, Rajakangas AM & Schroll M. (1995). Stroke incidence, case fatality, and mortality in the WHO MONICA project. *Stroke*, vol. 26, pp. 361–367

Vallejo G, Ballare C, Baranao JL, Beato M & Saragüeta P. (2005). Progestin activation of nongenomic pathways via cross talk of progesterone receptor with estrogen receptor-induces proliferation of endometrial stromal cells. *Mol Endocrinol*, vol. 19, pp. 3023–3037

Wang Z, Chen X, Zhou L, Wu D, Che X & Yang G. (2003). Effects of extracellular signal-regulated kinase (ERK) on focal cerebral ischemia. *Chin Med J (Engl)*, vol. 116, pp. 1497–503

Wenger NK, Speroff L & Packard B. (1993). Cardiovascular health and disease in women. *N Engl J Med*, vol. 329, pp. 247–256.

Wright DW, Kellermann AL, Hertzberg VS, Clark PL, Frankel M, Goldstein FC, Salomone JP, Dent LL, Harris OA, Ander DS, Lowery DW, Patel MM, Denson DD, Gordon AB, Wald MM, Gupta S, Hoffman SW & Stein DG. (2007). ProTECT: a randomized clinical trial of progesterone for acute traumatic brain injury. *Ann Emerg Med*, vol. 49, pp. 391–402

Yao XL, Liu J, Lee E, Ling GS & McCabe JT. (2005). Progesterone differentially regulates pro- and anti-apoptotic gene expression in cerebral cortex following traumatic brain injury in rats. *J Neurotrauma*, vol. 22, pp. 656–668

21

The Na^+/H^+ Exchanger-1 as a New Molecular Target in Stroke Interventions

Vishal Chanana[1], Dandan Sun[2] and Peter Ferrazzano[1,3]
[1]*Waisman Center, University of Wisconsin, Madison, WI*
[2]*Dept. of Neurology, University of Pittsburgh, Pittsburgh, PA*
[3]*Dept. of Pediatrics, University of Wisconsin, Madison, WI*
USA

1. Introduction

Loss of ion homeostasis plays an important role in the pathogenesis of ischemic cell damage. Ischemia induces accumulation of intracellular Na^+ ($[Na^+]_i$) and Ca^{2+} ($[Ca^{2+}]_i$), and subsequent activation of proteases, phospholipases, and formation of oxygen and nitrogen free radicals. The Na^+/H^+ exchanger (NHEs) family is a group of secondary active membrane transport proteins that catalyze the electroneutral exchange of Na^+ for H^+ and is important in restoring intracellular pH (pH_i) after ischemia-induced intracellular acidosis. Nine isoforms of NHE (NHE1-9) have been identified in mammalian tissues (Orlowski & Grinstein, 2004). These isoforms differ in their tissue expression, subcellular distribution, kinetic properties, inhibitor sensitivity, and physiological functions. NHE-1 is ubiquitously expressed on the plasma membrane of virtually all mammalian cell types (Sardet et al., 1989). NHE-2-4 are expressed on the plasma membrane, predominantly in the epithelia of the kidney and gastrointestinal tract (Orlowski & Grinstein, 2004). NHE-3 is the only isoform known to recycle between the plasma membrane and the endosomal compartment (D'Souza et al., 1998). NHE-5 expression is concentrated in neurons (Attaphitaya et al., 1999) and may modulate the pH of synaptic vesicles (Szaszi et al., 2002). NHE-6 and NHE-9 are expressed predominantly in endosomal vesicles (Nakamura et al., 2005) and NHE-7 localizes to the trans-Golgi network and associated endosomes (Numata & Orlowski, 2001). NHE-8 has been localized to the plasma membrane of renal proximal tubule epithelial cells, and to endosomal vesicles and the trans-Golgi network (Goyal et al., 2003; Nakamura et al., 2005).

NHE-1 is the most extensively studied isoform, and the most abundant isoform in the CNS (Ma & Haddad, 1997; Orlowski et al., 1992). Research over the past two decades has expanded our understanding of the role of NHE-1 beyond that of simply maintenance of ion homeostasis and cell volume, to an emerging picture of a regulator of many cell functions. NHE-1 plays a role in regulation of cell proliferation, migration (Bussolino et al., 1989), and the microglial respiratory burst (Liu et al., 2010). NHE-1 protein consists of 815 amino acids with a calculated molecular weight of 85 kDa. However, NHE-1 has an apparent size of ~110 kDa due to its N- and O- linked glycosylation in the extracellular loop 1. NHE-1 has two large functional domains, the highly conserved amphipathic N-terminal domain (~500 amino acids), which is responsible for cation translocation, and a less conserved hydrophilic cytoplasmic C-terminal domain (~315 amino acids), which is crucial for modulating NHE-1 activity (Putney et al., 2002). Activation of NHE-1 has been shown to be a pivotal event in cell damage induced by ischemia and reperfusion in the brain (Horikawa et al., 2001; Hwang et al., 2008; Luo et al., 2005), heart (Liu et al., 1997; Murphy et al., 1991; Wang et al., 2003), liver (Gores et al., 1989), and lungs (Rios et al., 2005). Here we will review recent findings implicating NHE-1 activation as a critical event in the pathogenesis of cellular dysfunction after cerebral ischemia, and the growing evidence supporting the use of NHE inhibitors as neuroprotective agents following cerebral ischemia.

2. Na^+/H^+ Exchanger isoform-1 (NHE-1) in cerebral ischemia

Ischemia and reperfusion injury is a complex and incompletely understood phenomenon. Ischemia deprives the cell of the energy required for normal cell function and leads to loss of ionic homeostasis within the cell due to opening of ionotropic glutamate receptors (Nishizawa, 2001) and acid sensing non-glutamate-dependent channels (Xiong et al., 2004), as well as activation of ion transport proteins such as NHE-1, $Na^+/K^+/Cl^-$ cotransporter (NKCCl) (Chen et al., 2005), and the Na^+/Ca^{2+} exchanger (NCXs) (Hoyt et al., 1998). Reperfusion triggers a cascade of intracellular events including release of reactive oxygen species (ROS) and inflammatory mediators, which exacerbate injury and promote cell death. Ischemia and reperfusion induces intracellular acidosis due to a shift from aerobic to anaerobic glycolysis, and leads to an increase in $[Na^+]_i$ and $[Ca^{2+}]_i$ by mechanisms that include the activation of acid responsive ion transporters (Yao & Haddad, 2004). Recent findings from our group and others highlight the important role of NHE-1 in pH_i regulation after cerebral ischemia and reperfusion.

2.1 NHE-1 mediated intracellular pH regulation

To regulate and maintain constant pH_i, eukaryotic cells express plasma membrane ion transporters such as NHE-1 that protect cells from internal acidification by exchanging extracellular Na^+ for intracellular H^+ (Luo et al., 2005). At physiological pH_i, NHE-1 is essentially inactive, despite the large inward Na^+ gradient established by Na^+/K^+- ATPase. However, upon exposure to intracellular acidification, NHE-1 is rapidly activated and uses the electrochemical gradient of Na^+ to pump H^+ out of the cell and restore pH_i. Upon restoration of pH_i, NHE-1 activity returns to steady state levels (Pedersen, 2006). Extracellular acidification (low pH_o) or removal of extracellular sodium suppresses this gradient-driven Na^+/H^+ exchange (Bobulescu et al., 2005). While NHE-1 serves to maintain homeostasis in the face of normal pH_i fluctuations (which result from changes in metabolic activity), profound acidosis after anoxia can induce a NHE-1 mediated parodoxic alkalinization, a so-called "overshoot" of pH_i restoration. We reported that post-anoxia alkalinization is ablated by pharmacological inhibition of NHE-1 and removal of extracellular sodium (Kintner et al., 2005). Protein kinase inhibitors attenuate this alkalinization, suggesting that activation of NHE-1 involves protein phosphorylation and multiple up-stream regulatory pathways such as extracellular signal-regulated kinases (ERK 1/2), protein kinase A (PKA), and protein kinase C (PKC) (Kintner et al., 2005; Luo et al., 2007; Yao et al., 2001).

2.2 Ionic homeostasis and brain cell function

Secondary active ion transport proteins are important in maintaining steady-state intracellular ion concentrations. NHE-1 plays an important role in regulation of many cellular processes in addition to pH_i and cell volume regulation, such as cell growth, proliferation and differentiation, cell migration and adhesion, cellular immunity, and as cytoskeletal scaffolding for the assembly of intracellular signaling complexes (De Vito, 2006; Luo & Sun, 2007; Luo et al., 2005; Meima et al., 2007; Orlowski & Grinstein, 2004; Pedersen et al., 2006; Xue & Haddad, 2010). Due to their high metabolic rate and rapid changes in metabolic demand, neurons are exposed to frequent fluctuations in pH_i, making efficient acid extrusion mechanisms essential for normal neuronal function. Neurons and astrocytes from mice deficient in the NHE-1 protein (NHE-$1^{-/-}$) demonstrate decreased basal pH_i and are unable to recover from an acid load (Luo et al., 2005). NHE-1 is the predominant NHE isoform in the CNS (Ma & Haddad, 1997; Orlowski et al., 1992), and as evidence of its importance in normal neurologic function, NHE-$1^{-/-}$ mice exhibit severe neurologic defects and seizures (Bell et al., 1999; Gu et al., 2001).

2.3 Role of NHE-1 in cellular dysfunction and cerebral injury during *in vivo* ischemia

Results from *in vivo* experimental studies support the importance of ion transport proteins in ischemia-mediated loss of ion homeostasis. NHE-1 activity in astrocytes (Cengiz et al., 2010), neurons (Manhas et al., 2010), and microglia (Shi et al., 2011) is stimulated following cerebral ischemia. Excessive stimulation of NHE-1 leads to intracellular Na^+ overload, and in turn causes a rise in intracellular Ca^{2+} due to increased Ca^{2+} influx via reversal of the Na/Ca exchanger. Thus, NHE-1 activity contributes to cerebral ischemic damage in part by disruption of intracellular Na^+ and Ca^{2+} homeostasis, an event which is characterized by rapid influx of Ca^{2+} and subsequent cell death.

2.3.1 Global ischemia

Global cerebral ischemia entails diminution in cerebral blood flow (CBF) over the entire brain, and is encountered clinically in cardiac arrest. On restoration of CBF, a secondary reperfusion brain injury may occur due to altered ionic homeostasis, increases in ROS, cerebral edema, and inflammatory cascades (Schaller & Graf, 2004). The contribution of NHE-1 activity to global cerebral ischemia has been reported in a number of animal models. In a gerbil model of transient forebrain ischemia, NHE-1 immunoreactivity was markedly increased in CA1 pyramidal neurons as well as in glial cells 4 days following injury, and inhibition of NHE protected CA1 pyramidal neurons and attenuated the activation of astrocytes and microglia (Hwang et al., 2008). Yorkshire-Duroc pigs treated with cariporide (HOE 642), a potent and selective inhibitor of NHE-1, at the onset of a 90 min deep hypothermic circulatory arrest demonstrated improved neurologic recovery (Castellá et al., 2005). Similarly, inhibition of NHE-1 with N-[aminoiminomethyl]-1-methyl-1H-indole-2-carboxamide methanesulfonate (SM-20220) improved neurologic function in a gerbil model of transient global cerebral ischemia (Kuribayashi et al., 2000). Administration of the NHE-1 inhibitor ethylisopropylamiloride (EIPA) prior to bilateral carotid artery occlusion in gerbils resulted in decreased hippocampal neuronal cell death and improved neurologic function (Phillis et al., 1999).

2.3.2 Focal ischemia

Unlike global cerebral ischemia, focal cerebral ischemia entails reduction in regional CBF in a specific vascular territory and is usually encountered clinically as an "ischemic stroke" due to thromboembolic or vaso-occlusive disease. An abundance of *in vivo* studies support the importance of NHE-1 in focal ischemia. The NHE-1 inhibitor SM-20220 reduces infarct size in both transient and permanent focal ischemia models (Kuribayashi et al., 1999). Another NHE inhibitor, Sabiporide, reduces infarct size and edema volume when administered before or after ischemia (Park et al., 2005).

Our investigations into the role of NHE-1 in cerebral ischemia have used both genetic and pharmacologic inhibition of NHE-1 in a mouse transient middle cerebral artery occlusion model (MCAO). Mice treated with HOE 642, a potent and selective inhibitor of NHE-1, prior to MCAO demonstrated a 35% reduction in infarct volume compared to vehicle treated controls. NHE-1 heterozygous mice (NHE-1$^{+/-}$), which demonstrate a ~ 70% reduction in NHE-1 protein expression, exhibited a similar reduction in infarct volumes, establishing the importance of NHE-1 over other NHE isoforms in the CNS (Luo et al., 2005; Wang et al., 2008). With T2-weighted and Diffusion Weighted MRI, we further confirmed that NHE-1$^{+/+}$ mice treated with HOE 642 immediately prior to reperfusion or 60 minutes post-reperfusiion, exhibited a significant reduction in infarct volume compared to NHE-1$^{+/+}$ vehicle control mice. NHE-1$^{+/-}$ mice demonstrated a significant reduction in infarct volume on T2 MRI at 72 hours after injury (Ferrazzano et al., 2011). These findings suggest that elevated NHE-1 activity contributes to neuronal injury following ischemia and reperfusion. We subsequently revealed that focal cerebral ischemia triggers a transient stimulation of the extracellular signal-regulated kinase/p90 ribosomal S6 kinase (ERK/p90^{RSK}) pathway that contributes to ischemic damage in part via phosphorylation of NHE-1 protein (Manhas et al., 2010). The NHE-1-mediated $[Na^+]_i$ overload causes reverse function of the Na^+/Ca^{2+} exchanger, elevating $[Ca^{2+}]_i$ and enhancing the p38 mitogen-activated protein kinase (MAPK) and/or nuclear factor kappa-light-chain-enhancer of activated B cells (NF-kB) (Liu et al., 2010). NHE-1 activity also plays a detrimental role in mitochondrial Ca^{2+} overload and mitochondrial dysfunction after ischemia as evidenced by attenuation of ischemia-induced cytochrome C release from mitochondria after NHE-1 inhibition (Wang et al., 2008). Interestingly, when NHE-1 activity is blocked either pharmacologically or by genetic knockdown, microglia activation and proinflammatory cytokine formation is significantly reduced in ischemic brains after MCAO (Shi et al., 2011). Taken together, these results strongly support that NHE-1 is activated after cerebral ischemia and worsens ischemic brain injury.

2.3.3 Hypoxia/Ischemia

Hypoxia-ischemia (HI) is a common cause of brain injury in neonates (Ferriero, 2004). We recently investigated the role of NHE-1 using a mouse model of neonatal hypoxia-ischemia as described by Vannucci (Vannucci & Vannucci, 2005). In these studies, post-natal day 9 mice (P9) underwent unilateral carotid artery ligation and subsequent exposure to 55 minutes of 8% O_2. Following carotid ligation, mice were treated with HOE 642 either immediately before or 10 minutes following exposure to hypoxia (Cengiz et al., 2010). Following HI, vehicle-treated control brains exhibited astrogliosis in the ipsilateral hippocampus, and reactive astrocytes expressed an abundant level of NHE-1. Inhibition of NHE-1 before or after HI resulted in decreased neurodegeneration in striatum, thalamus and hippocampus and improved performance on tests of motor learning and memory (Cengiz et al., 2010). These findings suggest that NHE-1 mediated disruption of ionic homeostasis can contribute to CA1 pyramidal neuronal injury after neonatal HI. Moreover, T2 weighted and Diffusion Tensor (DTI) MRI revealed that NHE-1 inhibition with HOE 642 after HI resulted in improved white matter injury in the corpus callosum, which correlated with improvements in memory and learning (Cengiz et al., 2011).

2.4 Role of NHE-1 in cellular dysfunction during *in vitro* ischemia

Extensive *in vitro* studies have established that ischemia stimulates NHE-1 by reduction in pH_i or via signaling pathways such as ERK-$p90^{rsk}$, PKA or PKC (Dunbar & Caplan, 2001; Herrera et al., 1994; Kintner et al., 2007a; Li et al., 2004). The role of NHE-1 in cerebral ischemia has been mainly examined in two types of *in vitro* ischemic models, oxygen glucose deprivation/reoxygenation (OGD/REOX) or the hypoxic, acidic, ion-shifted Ringers's solution (HAIR). Superfused brain slices also represent a useful preparation to study acid-base disturbance that occurs in the mammalian brain during *in vitro* ischemic conditions.

2.4.1 Cell cultures

NHE-1 activity is stimulated during *in vitro* ischemia and subsequent reoxygenation and contributes substantially to neuronal and glial cell injury. Acutely isolated CA1 neurons exhibit a tri-phasic response to 5 minutes of anoxia. During anoxia, an initial acidification progresses to alkalinization that is followed by further alkalinization on exposure to reoxygenation. This alkalinization is attenuated by reduction of external pH, removal of extracellular sodium, or inhibition of NHE-1 (Sheldon & Church, 2002; Yao et al., 2001). Additionally, inhibition of PKA can block post-anoxia alkalinization, suggesting cAMP-dependent signaling pathways for NHE-1 activation (Sheldon & Church, 2002).

We have demonstrated that NHE-1 is essential in pH_i regulation using an internal acid load in cultured cortical neurons (Luo et al., 2005). Additionally, we found that activation of NHE-1 after OGD/REOX results in a significant increase in neuronal $[Na^+]_i$. This rise in $[Na^+]_i$ following OGD is significantly attenuated in HOE 642-treated or NHE-$1^{-/-}$ neurons, and cell death is reduced (Luo et al., 2005). In a separate study, we demonstrated that NHE-1-mediated Na^+ entry leads to reverse activation of the Na^+/Ca^{2+} exchanger (NCX_{rev}) and rise in $[Ca^{2+}]_i$, which contribute to the selective dendritic vulnerability to *in vitro* ischemia (Kintner et al., 2010). Taken together, our studies suggest that NHE-1 activity in neurons is significantly stimulated in response to the metabolic acidification associated with an ischemic insult. This ischemia-induced increase in NHE-1 activity causes intracellular Na^+ and Ca^{2+} overload, and eventually leads to cell death.

In another series of studies, we examined the role of NHE-1 in ischemic astrocyte damage using OGD/REOX in cultured cortical astrocytes and found that NHE-1 is the primary pH regulatory mechanism after ischemia. Astrocyte NHE-1 activity is increased by ~ 1.8 fold during REOX (Kintner et al., 2004), and depends on ERK1/2 signaling pathways (Kintner et al., 2005). OGD/REOX results in a drop in pH_i by 0.29 pH units (Kintner et al., 2004), and inhibition of NHE-1 results in a further decrease of pH_i. Additionally, we observed that OGD/REOX triggers a ~5-fold increase in $[Na^+]_i$ and 26% increase in astrocyte cell volume. This increase in $[Na^+]_i$ and cell swelling are significantly reduced either with HOE 642 treatment or in NHE-$1^{-/-}$ astrocytes (Kintner et al., 2004). Using the HAIR model in astrocytes, we found a similar increase in $[Na^+]_i$ which could be abolished by the NHE-1 inhibitor HOE 642 (Kintner et al., 2007b). It has been reported that the expected rise in $[Ca^{2+}]_i$ after HAIR exposure is inhibited by NHE-1 inhibition with HOE 694 (Bondarenko et al., 2005). Taken together, these results indicate that NHE-1 activity raises $[Na^+]_i$ which fosters reversal of the Na^+/Ca^+ exchanger leading to increased intracellular Ca^{2+} and astrocyte cell death.

More recently, new evidence supports a role of NHE-1 in microglial pH_i regulation. Microglia activation by lipopolysaccharide (LPS), phorbol myristate acetate (PMA), or OGD/REOX triggers a concurrent stimulation of NHE-1 and NADPH oxidase (Liu et al., 2010). The elevation in NHE-1-mediated H^+ extrusion prevents intracellular acidosis, allowing for sustained NADPH oxidase function (Liu et al., 2010). Moreover, the coupling of NHE-1 activation with NCX_{rev} activates $[Na^+]_i$ and $[Ca^{2+}]_i$ dependent signaling, which promotes the microglial respiratory burst and production of proinflammatory cytokines (Liu et al., 2010).

2.4.2 Brain slice

Few studies have used brain slice preparations to examine acid-base homeostatic disturbances during ischemia. In hippocampal slices, hypoxia induces a significant drop in both pH_i and pH_o, and a brief alkaline peak is also occasionally observed (Fujiwara et al., 1992; Melzian et al., 1996; Roberts & Chih, 1997). In slice preparations from various brain regions, hypoxia causes acidosis with an approximately 0.8-1.2 pH_i unit drop (Ballanyi et al, 1996; Knopfel et al., 1998; Pirttila & Kauppinen, 1994). Cytosolic calcium changes are observed during ischemia in cortical brain slices that can be only partially inhibited by combined blockade of ion channels (Bickler and Hansen, 1994). Only one report shows a direct involvement of NHE mediated pH_i regulation in slice preparations. In brainstem slices from neonatal rats exposed to 10 minutes of anoxia, intracellular pH drops by 0.1-0.3 pH units in neurons. Inhibition of NHE with amiloride increases this anoxia-induced intracellular acidification (Chambers-Kersh et al., 2000).

2.5 NHE-1 inhibitors and potential therapies

Despite decades of research, the effective treatment and prevention of cerebral ischemic injury remains challenging. Inhibition of NHE-1 with either pharmacological agents or genetic ablation has been demonstrated to significantly reduce brain damage after ischemic insult, in both *in vitro* and *in vivo* models. These encouraging findings suggest the potential use of NHE inhibitors as neuroprotective therapies after cerebral ischemia.

2.5.1 Pharmacological approach

Two major classes of pharmacological agents are currently used to inhibit NHE-1 activity (Putney et al., 2002). The first class of drugs includes amiloride and its 5' alkyl-substituted derivatives (Counillon et al., 1993; Yu et al., 1993), such as ethylisopropylamiloride (EIPA), dimethylamiloride (DMA), 5-*N* (methylpropyl)amiloride (MPA), 5-(N-methyl-N-isobutyl)-amiloride (MIBA), and 5-(N, N-hexamethylene) amiloride (HMA). These agents are more effective inhibitors of NHE-1 than amiloride but have relatively weak selectivity toward NHE-1. The simultaneous replacement of the pyrazine ring by a phenyl and of the 6-chloro by sulfomethyl leads to another class of inhibitors that includes the benzoylguanidines and derivatives such as HOE 694 (Counillon et al., 1993) and HOE 642 (cariporide) (Scholz et al.,

1995). Both classes are more specific for NHE-1 than NHE-3, with the amiloride compounds demonstrating ~10^2-fold increased specificity and the HOE compounds ~10^3- to 10^5-fold more NHE-1 specificity. The HOE compounds are viewed as the most promising agents for treatment of ischemia-reperfusion injury due to their selectivity for NHE-1, and excellent solubility, resorption, and bioavailability profiles (Scholz et al., 1999; Baumgarth et al., 1997; Xue & Haddad, 2010). HOE compounds are competitive inhibitors of Na^+ binding at the extracellular cation-binding site (Baumgarth et al., 1997; Counillon et al., 1993; Kinsella & Aronson, 1981; Mahnensmith & Aronson, 1985), while the amiloride derivatives also act non-competitively (Warnock et al., 1988). More recently, several new molecules have been designed as potential NHE blockers based on the bicyclic template, including SM-20220, SM-20550, BMS-284640, T-162559, and TY-12533, which have also shown promising results in *in vivo* studies of cerebral ischemia (Kitayama et al., 2001). The IC_{50} for the human NHE-1 are as follows: Amiloride = 10.7 μM, Cariporide = 0.08 μM, T-165229 = 13 nM. Importantly, the NHE inhibitors HOE 642 and SM-20220 not only reduce cell death and edema, but also improve neurological function in *in vivo* ischemia models, and have demonstrated benefits when administered after ischemia (Kintner et al., 2007b; Kuribayashi et al., 2000).

2.5.2 Transgenic approach

While pharmacological studies indicate that NHE-1 plays a central role in cerebral ischemia-reperfusion injury, the use of pharmacologic inhibitors to study ion transport function raises questions regarding dosing, absorption, species specific T1/2, and non-specific effects. For this reason, confirmation by an alternative method using NHE-1 knockdown mice is warranted. NHE-1$^{-/-}$ mice exhibit neurologic abnormalities, seizures, ataxia, and growth retardation, and do not survive into adulthood (Bell et al., 1999; Gu et al., 2001). Therefore, NHE-1$^{-/-}$ mice are useful for cultures of NHE-1 null neurons, astrocytes and microglia, but cannot be used for *in vivo* studies. NHE-1$^{+/-}$ mice express <50% of NHE-1 protein levels, and are useful for *in vivo* studies of the role of NHE function after cerebral ischemia. A marked decrease of infarct volume, microglial activation and proinflammatory cytokine formation is found in NHE-1$^{+/-}$ mice after MCAO (Luo et al., 2005). NHE-1 $^{+/-}$ and NHE-1 $^{-/-}$ cortical neurons and astrocytes demonstrate decreased cell death after OGD/REOX (Luo et al., 2005).

The fact that NHE-1 inhibitors applied during or after cerebral ischemia protect the brain against ischemic damage is now well established in animal studies. Despite the uniformity of results from animal models, a number of challenges remain before NHE-1 inhibitors can be translated into clinical use. Questions regarding safety, optimal dose, and timing of administration remain to be addressed, and large animal studies demonstrating improved functional outcomes are still lacking.

3. Conclusion

NHE-1 plays a pivotal role in maintaining tissue ionic homeostasis under normal physiological conditions. However, excessive stimulation of NHE-1 appears to be a major contributor to cellular damage in ischemic conditions. The proposed mechanism for injury induced by NHE-1 activation includes accumulation of $[Na^+]_i$, subsequent $[Ca^{2+}]_i$ overload via reverse activation of the Na^+/Ca^{2+} exchanger, and eventual cell death. Additionally, activation of MAPKs, and release of excitatory amino acids and ROS also contribute to cell damage and death after ischemia. NHE-1 inhibitors have been demonstrated to be neuroprotective in both *in vitro* and *in vivo* ischemia models, making NHE-1 an attractive therapeutic target for cerebral ischemia. Thus, mechanisms of NHE-1 activation in ischemia continue to present an interesting focus for future research in this field.

4. Acknowledgment

This work was supported by NIH grants R01NS48216 and R01NS38118 (D. Sun), 1UL1RR025011 from the Clinical and Translational Science Award (CTSA) program of the National Center for Research Resources (NCRR) (P. Ferrazzano), and P30HD03352 (Waisman Center).

5. References

Attaphitaya, S., Park, K. & Melvin, J.E. (1999). Molecular cloning and functional expression of a rat Na^+/H^+ exchanger (NHE5) highly expressed in brain. *Journal of Biological Chemistry,* 274, 4383-4388.

Ballanyi, K., Doutheil, J. & Brockhaus, J. (1996). Membrane potentials and microenvironment of rat dorsal vagal cells in vitro during energy depletion. *Journal of Physiology,* 495, 769–784.

Baumgarth, M., Beier, N. & Gericke, R. (1997). (2-Methyl-5-(methylsulfonyl)benzoyl) guanidine Na^+/H^+ antiporter inhibitors. *Journal of Medicinal Chemistry,* 40, 2017–2034.

Bell, S.M., Schreiner, C.M., Schultheis, P.J., Miller, M.L., Evans, R.L., Vorhees, C.V., Shull, G.E. & Scott, W.J. (1999). Targeted disruption of the murine *Nhe1* locus induces ataxia, growth retardation, and seizures. *American Journal of Physiology,* 276, C788 – C795.

Bickler, P.E. & Hansen, B.M. (1994). Causes of calcium accumulation in rat cortical brain slices during hypoxia and ischemia: role of ion channels and membrane damage. *Brain Research,* 665, 269-276.

Bobulescu, I.A., Di Sole, F. & Moe, O.W. (2005). Na^+/H^+ exchangers: physiology and link to hypertension and organ ischemia. *Current Opinion in Nephrology and Hypertension,* 14: 485-494.

Bondarenko, A., Svichar, N. & Chesler, M. (2005). Role of Na^+-H^+ and Na^+-Ca^{2+} exchange in hypoxia-related acute astrocyte death. *Glia,* 49, 143-152.

Bussolino, F., Wang, J.M., Turrini, F., Alessi, D., Ghigo, D., Costamagna, C., Pescarmona, G., Mantovani, A. & Bosia, A. (1989). Stimulation of the Na^+/H^+ exchanger in human endothelial cells activated by granulocyte- and granulocyte- macrophage-colony-stimulating factor. Evidence for a role in proliferation and migration. *Journal of Biological Chemistry,* 264, 18284–18287.

Castellá, M., Buckberg, G.D. & Tan, G. (2005). Neurologic preservation by Na^+-H^+ exchange inhibition prior to 90 minutes of hypothermic circulatory arrest. The *Annals of Thoracic Surgery,* 79, 646-654.

Cengiz, P., Kleman, N., Uluc, K., Kendigelen, P., Hagemann, T., Akture, E., Messing, A., Ferrazzano, P. & Sun, D. (2010). Inhibition of Na^+/H^+ exchanger isoform 1 is neuroprotective in neonatal hypoxic ischemic brain injury. *Anitoxidants and Redox Signaling,* 14, 1803-1813.

Cengiz, P., Uluc, K., Kendigelen, P., Akture, E., Hutchinson, E., Song, C., Zhang, L., Lee, J., Budoff, G., Meyerand, E., Sun, D. & Ferrazzano, P. (2011). Chronic neurological deficits in mice after perinatal hypoxia and ischemia correlate with hemispheric tissue loss and white matter inury detected by MRI. *Developmental Neuroscience,* (in press).

Chambers-Kersh, L., Ritucci, N.A., Dean, J.B. & Putnam, R.W. (2000). Response of intracellular pH to acute anoxia in individual neurons from chemosensitive and nonchemosensitive regions of the medulla. *Advances in Experimental Medicine and Biology,* 475, 453–464.

Chen, H., Luo, J., Kintner, D.B., Shull, G.E. & Sun, D. (2005). Na+-dependent chloride transporter (NKCC1)-null mice exhibit less gray and white matter damage after focal cerebral ischemia. *Journal of Cerebral Blood Flow and Metabolism,* 25, 54-66.

Counillon, L., Scholz, W., Lang, H.J. & Pouyssegur, J. (1993). Pharmacological characterization of stably transfected Na^+/H^+ antiporter isoforms using amiloride analogs and a new inhibitor exhibiting antiischemic properties. *Molecular Pharmacology,* 44, 1041–1045.

De Vito, P. (2006). The sodium/hydrogen exchanger: a possible mediator of immunity. *Cell Immunology,* 240, 69–85.

D'Souza, S., Garcia-Cabado, A., Yu, F., Teter, K., Lukacs, G., Skorecki, K., Moore, H.P., Orlowski, J. & Grinstein, S. (1998). The epithelial sodiumhydrogen antiporter Na^+/H^+ exchanger 3 accumulates and is functional in recycling endosomes. *Journal of Biological Chemistry,* 273, 2035-2043.

Dunbar, L.A. & Caplan, M.J. (2001). Ion pumps in polarized cells: sorting and regulation of the Na^+, K^+- and H^+, K^+-ATPases. *Journal of Biological Chemistry,* 276, 29617–29620.

Ferrazzano, P., Shi, Y., Manhas, N., Wang, Y., Hutchinson, B., Chen, X., Chanana, V., Gerdts, J., Meyerand, M.E. & Sun, D. (2011). Inhibiting the Na^+/H^+ exchanger reduces reperfusion injury: a small animal MRI study. *Frontiers in BioScience,* 3, 81-88.

Ferriero, D.M. (2004). Neonatal brain injury. *The New England Journal of Medicine,* 351, 1985-1995.

Fujiwara, N., Abe, T., Endoh, H., Warashina, A. & Shimoji, K. (1992). Changes in intracellular pH of mouse hippocampal slices responding to hypoxia and/or glucose depletion. *Brain Research,* 572, 335–339.

Gores, G.J., Nieminen, A.L., Wray, B.E., Herman, B. & Lemasters, J.J. (1989). Intracellular pH during "chemical hypoxia" in cultured rat hepatocytes. Protection by intracellular acidosis against the onset of cell death. *Journal of Clinical Investigation,* 83, 386–396.

Goyal, S., Heuvel, V.G. & Aronson, P.S. (2003). Renal expression of novel Na^+/H^+ exchanger isoform NHE8. *American Journal of Physiology Renal Physiology,* 284, F467-F473.

Gu, X.Q., Yao, H. & Haddad, G.G. (2001). Increased neuronal excitability and seizures in the Na^+/H^+ exchanger null mutant mouse. *American Journal of Physiology Cell Physiology,* 281, C496–C503.

Herrera, V.L., Cova, T., Sassoon, D. & Ruiz-Opazo, N. (1994). Developmental cell-specific regulation of $Na^{(+)}$-$K^{(+)}$-ATPase alpha 1-, alpha 2-, and alpha 3-isoform gene expression. *American Journal of Physiology*, 266, C1301–C1312.

Horikawa, N., Nishioka, M., Itoh, N., Kuribayashi, Y., Matsui, K. & Ohashi, N. (2001) The Na^+/H^+ exchanger SM-20220 attenuates ischemic injury in *in vitro* and *in vivo* models. *Pharmacology*, 63, 76–81.

Hoyt, K.R., Arden, S.R., Aizenman, E. & Reynolds, I.J. (1998). Reverse Na^+/Ca^{2+} exchange contributes to glutamate-induced intracellular Ca^{2+} concentration increases in cultured rat forebrain neurons. *Molecular Pharmacology*, 53, 742-749.

Hwang, I.K., Yoo, K.Y., An, S.J., Li, H., Lee, C.H., Choi, J.H., Lee, J.Y., Lee, B.H., Kim, Y.M., Kwon, Y.G. & Won, M.H. (2008). Late expression of Na^+/H^+ exchanger 1 (NHE1) and neuroprotective effects of NHE inhibitor in the gerbil hippocampal CA1 region induced by transient ischemia. *Experimental Neurology*, 212, 314-323.

Kinsella, J.L. & Aronson, P.S. (1981). Amiloride inhibition of the Na^+-H^+ exchanger in renal microvillus membrane vesicles. *American Journal of Physiology*, 241, F374–F379.

Kintner, D.B., G. Su, G., Lenart, B., Ballard, A.J., Meyer, J.W., Ng, L.L., Shull, G.E. & Sun, D. (2004). Increased tolerance to oxygen and glucose deprivation in astrocytes from Na^+/H^+ exchanger isoform 1 null mice. *American Journal of Physiology Cell Physiology*, 287, C12-C21.

Kintner, D.B., Look, A., Shull, G.E. & Sun, D. (2005). Stimulation of astrocyte Na^+/H^+ exchange activity in response to *in vitro* ischemia in part depends on activation of extracellular signal-regulatory kinase. *American Journal of Physiology Cell Physiology*, 289, C934-C945.

Kintner, D.B., Luo, J., Gerdts, J., Ballard, A.J., Shull, G.E. & Sun, D. (2007a). Role of Na^+-K^+-Cl^- cotransport and Na^+/Ca^{2+} exchange in mitochondrial dysfunction in astrocytes following *in vitro* ischemia. *American Journal of Physiology Cell Physiology*, 292, C1113–C1122.

Kintner, D.B., Wang, Y. & Sun, D. (2007b). The role of membrane ion transport proteins in cerebral ischemic damage. *Frontiers in Bioscience*, 12, 762-770.

Kintner, D.B., Chen, X., Currie, J., Chanana, V., Ferrazzano, P., Baba, A., Matsuda, T., Cohen, M., Orlowski, J., Chiu, S.Y., Taunton, J. & Sun, D. (2010). Excessive Na^+/H^+ exchange in disruption of dendritic Na^+ and Ca^{2+} homeostasis and mitochondrial dysfunction following *in vitro* ischemia. *Journal of Biological Chemistry*, 285, 35155-35168.

Kitayama, J., Kitazono, T., Yao, H., Ooboshi, H., Takaba, H., Ago, T., Fujishima, M. & Ibayashi, S. (2001). Inhibition of Na^+/H^+ exchanger reduces infarct volume of focal cerebral ischemia in rats. *Brain Research*, 922, 223-228.

Knopfel, T. Tozzi, A., Pisani, A., Calabresi, P. & Bernardi, G. (1998). Hypoxic and hypoglycaemic changes of intracellular pH in cerebral cortical pyramidal neurons. *Neuroreport*, 9, 1447–1450.

Kuribayashi, Y., Horikawa, N., Itoh, N., Kitano, M. & Ohashi, N. (1999). Delayed treatment of Na^+/H^+ exchange inhibitor SM-20220 reduces infarct size in both transient and permanent middle cerebral artery occlusion in rats. *International Journal of Tissue Reactions*, 21, 29-33.

Kuribayashi, Y., Itoh, N., Horikawa, N. & Ohashi, N. (2000). SM-20220, a potent Na^+/H^+ exchange inhibitor, improves consciousness recovery and neurological outcome following transient cerebral ischaemia in gerbils. *Journal of Pharmacy and Pharmacology*, 52, 441-444.

Li, C., Grosdidier, A., Crambert, G., Horisberger, J.D., Michielin, O. & Geering, K. (2004). Structural and functional interaction sites between Na,K-ATPase and FXYD proteins. *Journal of Biological Chemistry*, 279, 38895–38902.

Liu, H., Cala, P.M. & Anderson, S.E. (1997). Ethylisopropylamiloride diminishes changes in intracellular Na, Ca and pH in ischemic newborn myocardium. *Journal of Molecular and Cellular Cardiology*, 29, 2077–2086.

Liu, Y., Kintner, D.B., Chanana, V., Algharabli, J., Chen, X., Gao, Y., Chen, J., Ferrazzano, P., Olson, J.K. & Sun, D. (2010). Activation of microglia depends on Na^+/H^+ exchange-mediated H^+ homeostasis. *Journal of Neuroscience*, 30, 15210–15220.

Luo, J. & Sun, D. (2007). Physiology and Pathophysiology of Na^+/H^+ Exchange Isoform 1 in the Central Nervous System. *Current Neurovascular Research*, 4, 205-215.

Luo, J., Chen, H., Kintner, D.B., Shull, G.E. & Sun, D. (2005). Decreased neuronal death in Na^+/H^+ exchanger isoform 1-null mice after *in vitro* and *in vivo* ischemia. *Journal of Neuroscience*, 25, 11256-11268.

Luo, J., Kintner, D.B., Shull, G.E. & Sun, D. (2007). ERK1/2-p90^{RSK}-mediated Phosphorylation of Na+/H+ Exchanger Isoform 1, a role in ishcemic neuronal death. Journal of Biological Chemistry, 282, 28274-28284.

Ma, E. & Haddad, G.G. (1997). Expression and localization of Na^+/H^+exchangers in rat central nervous system. *Neuroscience*, 79, 591–603.

Mahnensmith, R.L. & Aronson, P.S. (1985). Interrelationships among quinidine, amiloride, and lithium as inhibitors of the renal Na^+-H^+ exchanger. *Journal of Biological Chemistry*, 260, 586–592.

Manhas, N., Shi, Y., Taunton, J. & Sun, D. (2010). p90$^{(RSK)}$ activation contributes to cerebral ischemic damage via phosphorylation of $Na^{(+)}/H^{(+)}$ exchanger isoform 1. *Journal of Neurochemistry*, 114, 1476-1486.

Meima, M.E., Mackley, J.R. & Barber, D.L. (2007). Beyond ion translocation: structural functionsof the sodium-hydrogen exchanger isoform-1. *Current Opinion in Nephrology and Hypertension*, 16, 365–372.

Melzian, D., Scheufler, E., Grieshaber, M. & Tegtmeier, F. (1996). Tissue swelling and intracellular pH in the CA1 region of anoxic rat hippocampus. *Journal of Neuroscience Methods*, 65, 183–187.

Murphy, E., Perlman, M., London, R.E. & Steenbergen, C. (1991). Amiloride delays the ischemia-induced rise in cytosolic free calcium. *Circulation Research*, 68, 1250–1258.

Nakamura, N., Tanaka, S., Teko, Y., Mitsui, K. & Kanazawa, H. (2005). Four Na^+/H^+ exchanger isoforms are distributed to golgi and post-golgi compartments and are involved in organelle pH regulation. *Journal of Biological Chemistry*, 280, 1561-1572.

Nishizawa, Y. (2001). Glutamate release and neuronal damage in ischemia. *Life Sciences*, 69, 369-381.

Numata, M. & Orlowski, J. (2001). Molecular cloning and characterization of a novel (Na^+,K^+)/H^+ exchanger localized to the trans-Golgi network. *Journal of Biological Chemistry*, 276, 17387-17394.

Orlowski, J. & Grinstein, S. (2004). Diversity of the mammalian sodium/proton exchanger SLC9 gene family. *Pflugers Arch- European Journal of Physiology*, 447, 549-565.

Orlowski, J., Kandasamy, R.A. and Shull, G.E. (1992). Molecular cloning of putative members of the Na/H exchanger gene family. cDNA cloning, deduced amino acid sequence, and mRNA tissue expression of the rat Na/H exchanger NHE-1 and two structurally related proteins. *Journal of Biological Chemistry*, 267, 9331–9339.

Park, H.S., Lee, B.K., Park, S., Kim, S.U., Lee, S.H., Baik, E.J., Lee, S., Yi, K.Y., Yoo, S.E., Moon, C.H. & Jung, Y.S. (2005). Effects of sabiporide, a specific Na^+/H^+ exchanger inhibitor, on neuronal cell death and brain ischemia. *Brain Research*, 1061, 67-71.

Pedersen, S.F. (2006). The Na^+/H^+ exchanger NHE1 in stress-induced signal transduction: implications for cell proliferation and cell death. *Pflugers Archiv - European Journal of Physiology*, 452, 249–259.

Pedersen, S.F., O'Donnell, M.E., Anderson, S.E. & Cala, P.M. (2006). Physiology and pathophysiology of Na^+/H^+ exchange and Na^+-K^+-$2Cl^-$ cotransport in the heart, brain, and blood. *American Journal of Physiology-Regulatory, Integrative and Comparative Physiology*, 291, R1–R25.

Phillis, J.W., Estevez, A.Y., Guyot, L.L. & O'Regan, M.H. (1999). 5-(N-Ethyl-N-isopropyl)-amiloride, an Na^+-H^+ exchange inhibitor, protects gerbil hippocampal neurons from ischemic injury. *Brain Research*, 839, 199-202.

Pirttila, T.R. & Kauppinen, R.A. (1994). Regulation of intracellular pH in guinea pig cerebral cortex ex vivo studied by ^{31}P and ^{1}H nuclear magnetic resonance spectroscopy: role of extracellular bicarbonate and chloride. *Journal of Neurochemistry*, 62, 656–664.

Putney, L.K., Denker, S.P. & Barber, DL. (2002). The changing face of the Na^+/H^+ exchanger, NHE1: structure, regulation, and cellular actions. *Annual Reviw of Pharmacology and Toxicology*, 42, 527-552.

Rios, E.J., Fallon, M., Wang, J. & Shimoda, L.A. (2005). Chronic hypoxia elevates intracellular pH and activates Na^+/H^+ exchange in pulmonary arterial smooth muscle cells. *American Journal of Physiology Lung Cellular and Molecular Physiology*, 289, L867–L874.

Roberts Jr., E.L. & Chih, C.P. (1997). The influence of age of pH regulation in hippocampal slices before, during, and after anoxia. *Journal of Cerebral Blood Flow and Metabolism*, 17, 560–566.

Sardet, C., Franchi, A. & Pouyssegur, J. (1989). Molecular cloning, primary structure, and expression of the human growth factor-activatable Na^+/H^+ antiporter. *Cell*, 56, 271-280.

Schaller, B. & Graf, R. (2004). Cerebral ischemia and reperfusion: The pathophysiologic concept as a basis for clinical therapy. *Journal of Cerebral Blood Flow & Metabolism,* 24, 351-371.

Scholz, W., Albus, U., Counillon, L., Gogelein, H., Lang, H.J. , Linz, W., Weichert, A. & Scholkens, B.A. (1995). Protective effects of HOE642, a selective sodium-hydrogen exchange subtype 1 inhibitor, on cardiac ischaemia and reperfusion. *Cardiovascular Research,* 29, 260–268.

Scholz, W., Jessel, A. & Albus, U. (1999). Development of the Na^+/H^+ exchange inhibitor cariporide as a cardioprotective drug: from the laboratory to the GUARDIAN trial. *Journal of Thrombosis and Thrombolysis,* 8, 61–70.

Sheldon, C. & Church, J. (2002). Intracellular pH response to anoxia in acutely dissociated adult rat hippocampal CA1 neurons. *Journal of Neurophysiology,* 87, 2209-2224.

Shi, Y., Chanana, V., Watters, J.J., Ferrazzano, P. & Sun, D. (2011). Role of sodium/hydrogen exchanger isoform 1 in microglial activation and proinflammatory responses in ischemic brains. *Journal of Neurochemistry,* (in press).

Szaszi, K., Paulsen, A., Szabo, E.Z., Numata, M., Grinstein, S. & Orlowski, J. (2002). Clathrin-mediated endocytosis and recycling of the neuronspecific Na^+/H^+ exchanger NHE5 isoform. Regulation by phosphatidylinositol 3'-kinase and the actin cytoskeleton. *Journal of Biological Chemistry,* 277, 42623-42632.

Vannucci, R.C. & Vannucci, S.J. (2005). Perinatal hypoxic-ischemic brain damage: evolution of an animal model. *Developmental Neuroscience,* 27, 81-86.

Wang, Y., Meyer, J.W., Ashraf, M. & Shull, G.E. (2003). Mice with a null mutation in the NHE1 Na^+/H^+ exchanger are resistant to cardiac ischemia-reperfusion injury. *Circulation Research,* 93, 776–782.

Wang, Y., Luo, J., Chen, X., Chen, H., Cramer, S.W. and Sun, D. (2008). Gene inactivation of Na^+/H^+ exchanger isoform 1 attenuates apoptosis and mitochondrial damage following transient focal cerebral ischemia. *European Journal of Neuroscience,* 28, 51–61.

Warnock, D.G., Yang, W.C., Huang, Z.Q. & Cragoe, E.J. Jr. (1988). Interactions of chloride and amiloride with the renal Na^+/H^+ antiporter. *Journal of Biological Chemistry,*263, 7216–7221.

Xiong, Z.G., Zhu, X.M., Chu, X.P., Minami, M., Hey, J., Wei, W.L., MacDonald, J.F., Wemmie, J.A., Price, M.P., Welsh, M.J. & Simon, R.P. (2004). Neuroprotection in ischemia: blocking calcium-permeable acid-sensing ion channels. *Cell,* 118, 687-698.

Xue, J. & Haddad, G.G. (2010). The Na^+/H^+ exchanger: A target for therapeutic intervention in cerebral ischemia, In: *New strategies in stroke intervention: Ionic transporters, pumps, and new channels,* Annunziato, L. pp. (113-128), Human press, a part of Springer Science, ISBN 978-1-60761-279-7, New York, USA

Yao, H. & Haddad, G.G. (2004). Calcium and pH homeostasis in neurons during hypoxia and ischemia. *Cell Calcium,* 36, 247-255.

Yao, H., Gu, X.Q., Douglas, R.M. & Haddad, G.G. (2001). Role of Na^+/H^+ exchanger during O_2 deprivation in mouse CA1 neurons. *American Journal of Physiology Cell Physiology,* 281, C1205-C1210.

Yu, F.H., Shull, G.E. & Orlowski, J. (1993). Functional properties of the rat Na/H exchanger NHE-2 isoform expressed in Na/H exchanger-deficient Chinese hamster ovary cells. *Journal of Biological Chemistry*, 268, 25536–25541.

22

PPAR Agonism as New Pharmacological Approach to the Management of Acute Ischemic Stroke

Elisa Benetti[1], Nimesh Patel[2] and Massimo Collino[1]
[1]*Dipartimento di Scienza e Tecnologia del Farmaco, University of Turin, Turin,*
[2]*Centre for Translational Medicine and Therapeutics, Queen Mary University of London, The William Harvey Research Institute, London,*
[1]*Italy*
[2]*UK*

1. Introduction

Despite increasing knowledge of the biochemical mechanisms that occur in the brain following an ischemic insult and the availability of several diverse animal models of stroke, there are still no drugs that can be given to stroke patients soon after the onset of symptoms to minimize the subsequent neurological damage. To date, the thrombolytic compound recombinant tissue Plasminogen Activator (rt-PA) remains the only approved drug for the treatment of stroke. At present, intravenous administration of rt-PA is the only proven effective treatment to re-establish cerebral blood flow in the case of acute vessel occlusion, but unfortunately, only few patients with acute ischemic stroke are qualified to receive this drug. The failure of rt-PA to achieve rapid reperfusion in many patients and its bleeding risk have prompted the development of fibrinolytic agents with greater fibrin specificity and better risk-benefit profiles, such as tenecteplase or desmoteplase, which are now under active investigation. Early restoration of blood flow remains the treatment of choice for limiting brain injury following stroke, but a second fundamental goal of intervention is to protect neurons by interrupting or slowing the ischemic cascade. Current research is being done to develop neuroprotective agents that are able to block amino acid pathways and decrease neurotransmitter activity of injured tissue. Drugs blocking voltage-dependent calcium channels were effective in stroke rodent models but the results of clinical trials have been often discouraging. Overactivation of the N-methyl-D-aspartate receptor (NMDAR) is crucial for neuronal death after stroke. Several compounds that interfere with glutamate receptor activation have been developed and tested, in particular noncompetitive NMDA antagonists. However, their clinical use is limited by intolerable side effects, including some psycomimetic symptoms, as these blockers may also impair some key brain functions mediated by the same receptor. Accumulating evidence strongly suggests that apoptosis contributes to neuronal cell death in stroke injury and currently several caspase inhibitors are under investigation, but to date the efficacy of antiapoptotic agents in human stroke patients has not yet been tested. Anti-inflammatory approaches to stroke treatment intended to block cell-mediated inflammation with different strategies such as humanized antibodies against ICAM-1, inhibitors of interleukin-1 beta or a interleukin-1 receptor antagonist. However, there have been no successful clinical trials of these anti-inflammatory agents so far.

The complexity of events in cerebral ischemia and the disappointing results from human clinical stroke trials using a single agent suggest that perhaps to treat the stroke a new pleiotropic approach is required. In the pharmacological perspective, the evaluation of drugs with multiple effects on the ischemic cascade may be more effective in reducing infarct size and improving outcome in respect to single target strategy, because the ischemic cascade is diverse and it is likely that many different mechanisms of ischemia induced cell death occur simultaneously. Therefore, the development of neuroprotective drugs with multiple effects on the ischemic cascade is potentially more appealing than drugs acting on only one component of the cascade, if the safety profile is reasonable and the preclinical assessment package fulfils recent recommendations. Most recent discoveries portray Peroxisome Proliferator-Activated Receptors (PPARs) as promising pharmacological targets for the treatment of acute ischemic stroke, thanks to their ability to simultaneously interfere with several mechanisms that underlie the pathophysiology of brain ischemia, thus leading to an interesting protective strategy to counteract the multiple deleterious effects of ischemic injury.

2. PPAR

Peroxisome Proliferator-Activated Receptors (PPARs) are members of the nuclear hormone receptor (NHR) superfamily of ligand-activated transcription factors. There are three PPAR subtypes: α, β/δ and γ, named also NR1C1, NR1C2 and NR1C3, respectively, according to the unified nomenclature of nuclear receptors (Nuclear Receptors Nomenclature Committee, 1999). The three isoforms are the products of distinct genes: the human PPARα gene was mapped on chromosome 22 in the general region 22q12–q13.1, the PPARγ gene is located on chromosome 3 at position 3p25, whereas PPARβ/δ has been assigned to chromosome 6, at position 6p21.1–p21.2 (Sher, Yi et al. 1993; Greene, Blumberg et al. 1995; Yoshikawa, Brkanac et al. 1996). PPARs were originally identified by Isseman and Green (Issemann and Green 1990) after screening the rat liver cDNA library with a cDNA sequence located in the highly conserved C domain of NHRs. The name PPAR is derived from the fact that activation of PPARα, the first member of the PPAR family to be cloned, results in peroxisome proliferation in rodent hepatocytes (Desvergne and Wahli 1999). Activation of neither PPARβ/δ nor PPARγ, however, elicits this response and, interestingly, the phenomenon of peroxisome proliferation does not occur in humans. The molecular basis for this difference between species is not yet clear. With respect to the PPARγ isotype, alternative splicing and promoter use results in the formation of two further isoforms: PPARγ1 and PPARγ2. In particular, differential promoter usage and alternate splicing of the gene generates three mRNA isoforms. PPARγ1 and PPARγ3 mRNA both encode the PPARγ1 protein product which is expressed in most tissues, whereas PPARγ2 mRNA encodes the PPARγ2 protein, which contains an additional 28 amino acids at the amino terminus and is specific to adipocytes (Gurnell 2003). PPARβ/δ was initially reported as PPARβ in Xenopus laevis and NUC1 in humans (Schmidt, Endo et al. 1992). Subsequently, a similar transcript was cloned from mice and termed PPARδ (Amri, Bonino et al. 1995). Though now recognised as homologues for each other, it was not originally certain whether PPARβ from Xenopus was identical to murine PPARδ, hence the terminology PPARβ/δ.

All members of this superfamily share the typical domain organization of nuclear receptors (Figure 1). The N-terminal A/B domain contains a ligand-independent transactivation function. In the α and γ isotypes, the activity of this domain can be regulated by Mitogen-Activated Protein Kinase (MAPK) phosphorylation (Hu, Kim et al. 1996). The C domain is the DNA binding domain with its typical two zinc-finger-like motifs, as previously described for the steroid receptors, and the D domain is the co-factor docking domain (Schwabe, Neuhaus et al. 1990). The E/F domain is the ligand binding domain, it contains a ligand-dependent trans-activation function (AF)-2 (Fajas, Auboeuf et al. 1997), and is able to interact with transcriptional coactivators such as steroid receptor coactivator (SRC)-1 (Onate, Tsai et al. 1995) and CREB-binding protein (CBP) (Amri, Bonino et al. 1995).

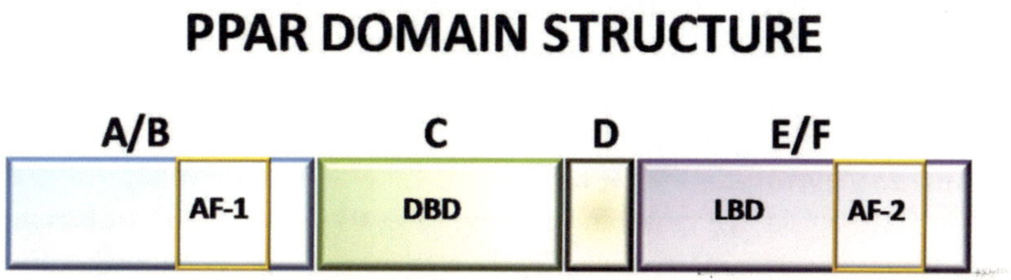

ISOFORMS	ENCODING GENE	AMINO ACID IDENTITY (% vs α) DBD	LBD	AMINO ACID NUMBER
α (NR1C1)	22q12-q13.1	-	-	468
β/δ (NR1C2)	6p21.1-p21.2	86%	70%	441
γ (NR1C3)	3p25	83%	68%	477

Fig. 1. Schematic representation of the domain organization of human PPAR isoforms. The A/B domain contains the Activation Function 1 (AF-1) which has a ligand-independent transcriptional activity. The C domain corresponds to the DNA Binding Domain (DBD). The D domain is the co-factor docking domain. The E/F domain contains the Ligand Binding Domain (LBD) and carries the Activation Function 2 (AF-2), which has a ligand-dependent transcriptional activity. The human chromosome regions in which disting genes encoding for PPAR isoforms are mapped, the percentage of amino acid sequence identity (in comparison with PPARα) and the amino acid number of different isoforms are reported in the Table.

The highest PPARα expression has been found in the liver and in tissues with high fatty acid catabolism, such as the kidney, heart, skeletal muscle, and brown fat (Lefebvre, Chinetti et al. 2006). PPARα mainly regulates energy homeostasis, activating fatty acid catabolism and stimulating gluconeogenesis (Kersten, Seydoux et al. 1999). This increased fatty acid oxidation in response to PPARα activation with a selective agonist, WY14643, results in lower circulating triglyceride levels and reduction of lipid storage in liver, muscle, and adipose tissue (Chou, Haluzik et al. 2002), which is associated with improved insulin sensitivity (Kim, Haluzik et al. 2003). Consequently, fibrates (fenofibrate, bezafibrate, gemfibrozil), which are synthetic agonists for PPARα, are in wide clinical use for the treatment of dyslipidaemias.

PPARγ is expressed in white and brown adipose tissue, gut, and immune cells (Feige, Gelman et al. 2006). It is involved in adipocyte differentiation and lipid storage in white adipose tissue (Rosen, Sarraf et al. 1999). Furthermore, PPARγ is involved in glucose metabolism via an improvement of insulin sensitivity (Hevener, He et al. 2003). Therefore, synthetic PPARγ agonists (thiazolidinediones) are in clinical use as insulin sensitizers to treat patients with type-2 diabetes.

PPARβ/δ remained an enigma for almost a decade after its cloning in 1992. It has been reported to be ubiquitously expressed in almost every tissue and, in the past, this widespread tissue expression has suggested a possible "general housekeeping" role for PPARβ/δ (Kliewer, Forman et al. 1994). More recently, the use of transgenic mouse models and the availability of high-affinity synthetic ligands has led researchers to a better understanding of its physiological role. Specifically, increasing evidence has shown a particular role for PPARβ/δ in insulin sensitivity regulation, lipid metabolism and the inflammation response. However, in contrast to PPARα and γ, PPARβ/δ agonists are not yet in clinical use.

2.1 Endogenous and synthetic PPAR ligands

Although many fatty acids are capable of activating all three PPAR isoforms, some fatty acids are also specific for a particular PPAR isoform. X-ray crystallography studies of PPARβ/δ revealed an exceptionally large ligand-binding pocket of approximately 1,300 Å3, similar to that of PPARγ but much larger than the pockets of other nuclear receptors (Xu, Lambert et al. 1999). The increased dimension is believed to accommodate the binding of various fatty acids or other amphipathic acids to PPARβ/δ via hydrogen bonds and hydrophobic interactions. The long-chain polyunsaturated fatty acids and their oxidized derivatives, especially eicosanoids such as 8-S-hydroxyeicosatetraenoic acid (8-S-HETE), leukotriene B4 (LTB4) and arachidonate monooxygenase metabolite epoxyeicosatrienoic acids have been shown to potently activate PPARα with high affinity (Theocharisa, Margeli et al. 2003; Feige, Gelman et al. 2006). PPARγ can be activated by several prostanoids, such as 15-deoxy-Δ12,14-prostaglandin J2 (15d-PGJ2) and 12- and 15-hydroxy-eicosatetraenoic acid (12- and 15-HETE), which are derivatives of arachidonic acid synthesized through the lipoxygenase pathway, as well as modified oxidised lipids, 9- and 13-hydroxyoctadecadienoic acids (9- and 13-HODE) (Willson, Brown et al. 2000; Theocharisa, Margeli et al. 2003). PPARβ/δ agonists include linoleic acid, oleic acid, arachidonic acid and eicosapentaenoic acid (EPA), which have been shown to co-crystallize within the ligand binding domain of this nuclear receptor (Xu, Lambert et al. 1999). A number of eicosanoids, including prostaglandin (PG)A1 and PGD2, and carbaprostacyclin, a semi-synthetic prostaglandin, have micromolar affinities for PPARβ/δ (Forman, Chen et al. 1997). Recently, cows milk, ice cream, butter, and yoghurt were described as activators of PPARβ/δ in reporter assays, but a specific common compound was not identified (Suhara, Koide et al. 2009).

With respect to the synthetic ligands, fibrates (e.g. fenofibrate, clofibrate), which are hypolipidaemic drugs, are well-known ligands for PPARα (Willson, Brown et al. 2000). Fibrates are capable of activating PPARα at pharmacological doses leading to increased expression of lipid metabolizing enzymes that effectively lower serum lipid levels in humans. In contrast to the well-documented therapeutic effect, there is also evidence of liver toxicity induced by activation of PPARα, mainly hepatocarcinogenesis. The most serious safety risk associated with fibrates, although rare, is myopathy and rhabdomyolysis. Studies suggest that the mechanism of myotoxicity through fibrates is not entirely clear, because complex and multifactorial mechanisms are involved, including genetic predisposition, pharmacokinetics, drug interactions, and dose. It is of interest to note that increased expression of lipoprotein lipase, which is a known PPARα target gene, in skeletal muscle leads to severe myopathy in mice.

The most widely used PPARγ agonists belong to the thiazolidinedione (TZD) or glitazone class of anti-diabetic drugs used in the treatment of type-2 diabetes. Troglitazone, the first TZD approved for this use, was withdrawn from the market in March 2000 following the emergence of a serious hepatotoxicity in some patients. Since troglitazone induces CYP3A4, it has been hypothesized that potentially toxic quinones derived from CYP3A4-dependent metabolism could cause liver damage (Yamamoto, Yamazaki et al. 2002). Rosiglitazone and pioglitazone are the only available thiazolidinediones in North America, but meta-analyses of randomised controlled trials have suggested an increased risk of ischaemic cardiovascular events with rosiglitazone (Nissen and Wolski ; Singh, Loke et al. 2007). In contrast, meta-analysis of trials of pioglitazone indicates the possibility of an ischaemic cardiovascular benefit (Lincoff, Wolski et al. 2007). Robust evidence also shows that both drugs increase the risk of congestive heart failure and fractures, but whether any meaningful difference exists in the magnitude of risk between the two thiazolidinediones is not known (Singh, Loke et al. 2007; Loke, Singh et al. 2009). The European Medicines Agency has recommended the suspension of marketing authorisation for rosiglitazone, whereas the US Food and Drug Administration has allowed the continued marketing of rosiglitazone with additional restrictions.

On the contrary, there are no PPARβ/δ drugs in clinical use yet. However several selective PPARβ/δ ligands have been recently designed, including GW0742, GW2433, GW9578, L-783483, L-165041, or GW501516 (Berger, Leibowitz et al. 1999; Lim and Dey 2000; Martens, Visseren et al. 2002). As yet only one selective PPARβ/δ antagonist has been described GSK0660. In skeletal muscle myoblast cells in culture, GSK0660 inhibited GW0742 induction of established PPARβ/δ target genes (carnitine palmitoyltransferase 1A, angiopoietin-like 4 protein and pyruvate dehydrogenase kinase-4)(Shearer, Steger et al. 2008).

2.2 Molecular mechanisms of PPAR activation

There are at least three primary mechanisms by which PPARs can regulate biological functions: transcriptional transactivation, transcriptional transrepression and ligand-independent transrepression (Figure 2).

2.2.1 Mechanism of transcriptional transactivation

PPARs function as heterodimers with their obligatory partner the Retinoid X Receptor (RXR). Like other NHRs, the PPAR/RXR heterodimer most likely recruits co-factor complexes - either co-activators or co-repressors - that modulate its transcriptional activity (Shi, Hon et al. 2002). The PPAR/RXR heterodimer then binds to sequence specific PPAR Response Elements (PPREs), located in the 5′-flanking region of target genes, thereby acting as a transcriptional regulator (Palmer, Hsu et al. 1995). The PPRE consists of two direct repeats of the consensus sequence AGGTCA separated by a single nucleotide, which constitutes a DR-1 motif. PPAR binds 5′ of RXR on the DR-1 motif and the 5′-flanking

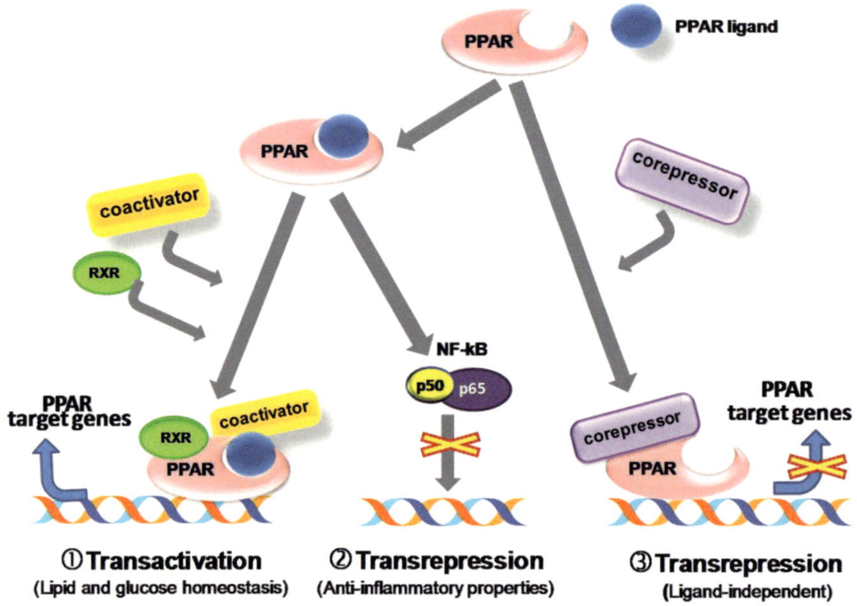

Fig. 2. Molecular mechanisms of PPAR activation. After ligand binding, PPAR undergoes conformational changes, which lead to recruitment of Retinoid X Receptor (RXR) and coactivators. The resultant heterodimer binds to specific DNA response elements called PPAR response elements, causing target gene transcription (Transactivation). A second mechanism (Transrepression) involves interfering with other transcription-factor pathways by negatively regulating the expression of pro-inflammatory genes. Lastly, PPAR may repress the transcription of direct target genes in the absence of ligands (ligand-independent Transrepression) recruiting corepressor complexes that mediate active repression.

sequence conveys the selectivity of binding between different PPAR isotypes (Juge-Aubry, Pernin et al. 1997). In the absence of a ligand, to prevent PPAR/RXR binding to DNA, high-affinity complexes are formed between the inactive PPAR/RXR heterodimers and co-repressor molecules, such as nuclear receptor co-repressor or silencing mediator for retinoic receptors. In response to ligand binding, PPAR undergoes a conformational change, leading to release of auxiliary proteins and co-repressors and recruitment of co-activators that contain histone acetylase activity. Acetylation of histones by co-activators bound to the ligand-PPAR complex leads to nucleosome remodelling, allowing for recruitment of RNA polymerase II causing target gene transcription. The search for PPAR target genes with identified PPREs has led to the identification of several genes involved in lipid metabolism, oxidative stress and inflammatory response, as widely documented in the literature.

2.2.2 Mechanism of transcriptional transrepression

PPARs can also negatively regulate gene expression in a ligand-dependent manner by inhibiting the activities of other transcription factors, such as Activated Protein-1 (AP-1), Nuclear Factor-κB (NF-κB) and Nuclear Factor of Activated T cells (NFAT) (ligand-dependent transrepression). In contrast to transcriptional activation, which usually involves the binding of PPARs to specific response elements in the promoter or enhancer regions of target genes, transrepression does not involve binding to typical receptor specific response elements (Pascual and Glass 2006). Several lines of evidence suggest that PPARs may exert anti-inflammatory effects by negatively regulating the expression of pro-inflammatory genes. To date, several mechanisms have been suggested to account for this activity, but despite intensive investigation, unifying principles remain to be elucidated.

Firstly, competition for limited amounts of essential, shared transcriptional co-activators may play a role in transrepression. The activated PPAR/RXR heterodimer reduces the availability of co-activators required for gene induction by other transcriptional factors. Thus, without distinct co-factors, transcription factors cannot cause gene expression.

Secondly, PPAR/RXR complexes may cause a functional inhibition by directly binding to transcription factors, preventing them from inducing gene transcription or inducing the expression of inhibitory proteins, such as the protein inhibitor of kappa B (IκB)α, which sequesters the NF-κB subunits in the cytoplasm and consequently reduces their DNA binding activity (Delerive, Martin-Nizard et al. 1999).

Thirdly, PPAR/RXR heterodimers may also inhibit phosphorylation and activation of several members of the MAPK family. In general very little is known about the molecular mechanisms by which PPARs and their ligands modulate kinase activities.

Recent studies have suggested another mechanism based on co-repressor-dependent transrepression by PPARs. Evidence has been presented in which PPARβ/δ controls the inflammatory status of macrophages based on its association with the transcriptional repressor BCL-6 (Lee, Chawla et al. 2003). Free BCL-6 suppresses the expression of multiple proinflammatory cytokines and chemokines. PPARβ/δ, but not PPARα and PPARγ, exhibits BCL-6 binding ability (Barish, Atkins et al. 2008; Takata, Liu et al. 2008). In the absence of a ligand, PPARβ/δ sequesters BCL-6 from inflammatory response genes. In contrast, in the presence of a ligand, PPARβ/δ releases the repressor, which now distributes to NF-κB-dependent promoters and exerts anti-inflammatory effects by repressing transcription from these genes.

2.2.3 Mechanism of ligand-independent transrepression

PPARs may repress the transcription of direct target genes in the absence of ligands (ligand-independent repression). PPARs bind to response elements in the absence of any ligand and recruit co-repressor complexes that mediate active repression. The co-repressors are capable of fully repressing PPAR-mediated transactivation induced either by ligands or by cAMP-regulated signalling pathways. This suggests co-repressors as general antagonists of the various stimuli inducing PPAR-mediated transactivation. Co-repressors can display different ligand selectivity: the nuclear receptor co-repressor NCoR interacted strongly with the ligand-binding domain of PPARβ/δ, whereas interactions with the ligand-binding domains of PPARγ and PPARα were significantly weaker (Krogsdam, Nielsen et al. 2002).

Very recently, a team of Harvard Medical School researchers has shown that PPARγ is phosphorylated at Ser273 by cyclin dependent kinase 5 (CDK5) during obesity which results in deregulation of a subset of genes; including a number of key metabolic regulators, such as adipsin, the first fat cell-selective gene whose expression is altered in obesity and adiponectin, a central regulator of insulin sensitivity *in vivo* (Choi, Banks et al.). Ser273 phosphorylation did not alter the chromatin occupancy of PPARγ, suggesting that other mechanisms, such as differential recruitment of co-regulators, may cause these differences in target gene expression. PPARγ ligands inhibited Ser273 phosphorylation and reversed associated changes in gene expression. Critically, the extent to which PPARγ ligands inhibit CDK5-mediated phosphorylation of PPARγ is not correlated with the extent to which they exert PPAR agonism, suggesting that these compounds have two distinct and separable activities. Whether or not similar mechanisms of receptor phosphorylation lead to changes in gene expression also in the other two PPAR isoforms -α and β/δ is a very important question, so far not yet addressed.

3. PPAR in the brain

All three PPAR isotypes are co-expressed in the nervous system during late rat embryogenesis. Their expression peaks in the central nervous system at mid-gestation. Whereas PPARβ/δ remains highly expressed in this tissue, the expression of PPARα and PPARγ decreases postnatally in the brain (Braissant, Foufelle et al. 1996). While PPARβ/δ has been found in neurons of numerous brain areas of adult rodents, PPARα and PPARγ have been localized to more restricted areas of the brain (Moreno, Farioli-Vecchioli et al. 2004). The localization of PPARs has also been investigated in purified cultures of neural cells. PPARβ/δ is expressed in immature oligodendrocytes where its activation promotes differentiation, myelin maturation and turnover. The PPARγ isotype is the dominant isoform in microglia. Astrocytes possess all three PPAR isotypes, although to different degrees depending on the brain area and animal age (Cristiano, Bernardo et al. 2001). The role of PPARs in the CNS is mainly related to lipid metabolism; however, these receptors have been implicated in neural cell differentiation and death as well as in inflammation and neurodegeneration. The expression of PPARγ in the brain has been extensively studied in relation to inflammation and neurodegeneration. PPARα has been suggested to be involved in acetylcholine metabolism, excitatory amino acid neurotransmission and oxidative stress defence. PPARβ/δ seems to play a critical role in regulating myelinogenesis and differentiation of cells within the CNS (Peters, Lee et al. 2000).

4. PPARs and cerebral ischemia

4.1 Experimental data on the effects of PPAR ligands in ischemic stroke

Although the relevance of animal models to the development of therapies for acute stroke has been often questioned, evidence demonstrates that animal models of stroke do have clinical relevance and are useful in the development of drugs that attenuate the ischemic damage. The characteristics of brain injury depends on the severity and the duration of cerebral blood flow reduction but it can be significantly exacerbated by the following phase of reperfusion; for this reason several animal models of the so-called "cerebral ischemia/reperfusion injury (IRI)" have been developed, demonstrating that often reperfusion after a long ischemic period may cause a larger infarct than that associated with permanent vessel occlusion. In general, the role of neuroprotective agents is to interfere with one or more of the mechanisms involved in the "IRI cascade" and thereby limit the resultant tissue damage. It seem reasonable to assume that drugs that work on a specific biochemical mechanism must be given at the time that the mechanism is active, mainly during ischemia and/or reperfusion. Accordingly, in general, two different experimental paradigms can be identified: prophylactic administration, aimed to evaluate drug effects on stroke prevention, and therapeutic administration, when the drug is administered during reperfusion to test its potential beneficial effects on IRI after stroke had occurred. A role for PPARs in reducing IRI has been first established in animal models of acute myocardial infarction (Yue Tl, Chen et al. 2001). More recently, good evidence supporting the beneficial role of PPAR in stroke has been provided by several *in vivo* experimental models of cerebral IRI, evaluating the effects of both prophylactic and therapeutic administration of PPAR agonists. It has been demonstrated that a 14-day preventive treatment with fenofibrate reduced susceptibility to stroke in apolipoprotein E-deficient mice as well as decreased cerebral infarct volume in wild-type littermates (Deplanque, Gele et al. 2003). The authors demonstrated that fenofibrate administration was associated with a decrease in cerebral oxidative stress depending on the increase in activity of several anti-oxidant enzymes and with a reduced expression of adhesion molecules. In another study, it was confirmed that two different PPARα agonists, fenofibrate and WY14643, provided similar brain protection when administered 3 or 7 days, respectively, before the induction of cerebral ischemia (Inoue, Jiang et al. 2003). More recently, we have found that PPARα agonists may also reduce cerebral I/R injury when administered just before ischemia or during reperfusion (Collino, Aragno et al. 2006). We showed that the potential neuroprotective effects of PPARα agonists is manifested by modulation of protein S100B levels in the rat CNS. S100B is a calcium-binding protein, mainly expressed in the brain and recent preclinical and clinical studies indicate that increased S100B levels is a reliable indicator of infarct size in acute ischemic stroke (Buyukuysal 2005; Foerch, Singer et al. 2005). Pre-treatment of rats with the selective PPARα agonist, WY14643, prior to cerebral ischemia causes a marked reduction of S100B levels in the rat hippocampus. This protective effect is reversed by administration of the PPARα antagonist, MK886, thus confirming the involvement of PPARα activation in neuroprotection. Similarly, fenofibrate pretreatment for 14 days significantly reduced the cerebral infarct volume in an experimental model of Middle Cerebral Artery Occlusion (MCAO), although its withdrawal 3 days before induction of cerebral ischemia decreased the neuroprotective effect (Ouk, Laprais et al. 2009). Also prophylactic administration of gemfibrozil resulted in reduction of infarct size 24 h after MCAO and increased cortical blood flow in the ischemic hemisphere (Guo, Wang et al. 2009). However, the principal focus of studies of PPAR agonists has been on agonists of the PPARγ isoform. Emerging studies have reported the protective effects of PPARγ agonist administration in animal models of cerebral IRI (Sundararajan, Gamboa et al. 2005; Collino, Aragno et al. 2006; Allahtavakoli, Shabanzadeh et al. 2007) and in models of permanent ischemia (Sayan-Ozacmak, Ozacmak et al.; Zhang, Xu et al.). The effect of delayed post ischemia administration of a PPARγ agonist, rosiglitazone, has been recently evaluated, demonstrating that post-treatment with rosiglitazone, 24 h after stroke induction, may reduce ischemic injury, improve neurological outcome, and prevent neutrophilia, thus supporting an extended therapeutic window for the treatment of ischemic stroke (Allahtavakoli, Moloudi et al. 2009). Recent experimental data confirmed that PPARγ agonists are protective at clinically relevant doses, independent of any effects on systemic blood pressure or cerebral blood flow and, most notably, the timing of reperfusion relative to drug administration, may significantly influence the ability of PPARγ agonists to reduce infarction volume and improve neurologic function following ischemic injury (Gamboa, Blankenship et al.). The relevance of PPARγ as an endogenous protective factor was also shown by the fact that treatment with a PPARγ antagonist increased infarct size (Victor, Wanderi et al. 2006). Moreover, it was demonstrated that in primary cortical neurons of PPARγ KO mice exposed to ischemia there was a reduced expression of numerous key gene products (including superoxide dismutase-1, catalase, and glutathione S-transferase) along with an increased damage. PPARγ mRNA is up-regulated in ischemic brain, especially in the peri-infarct area. Increased PPARγ mRNA was detected in the infarcted brain as early as 6 h following focal ischemia (Ou, Zhao et al. 2006), and PPARγ immunopositive neurons were detected between 4 h and 14 days, whereas in neurons and microglia only transiently at 12 h in the post-ischemic brain (Zhao, Patzer et al. 2005; Victor, Wanderi et al. 2006). The beneficial role of PPARβ/δ in stroke has been demonstrated by two different studies in which PPARβ/δ knockout mice subjected to cerebral IRI showed significantly larger infarct size than wild-type littermates (Pialat, Cho et al. 2007). This finding is confirmed by another study demonstrating that intracerebroventricular administration of high affinity PPARβ/δ agonists such as L-165041 and GW501516 significantly decreased the infarct volume at 24 h of reperfusion after cerebral ischemia in rats (Iwashita, Muramatsu et al. 2007).

4.2 Clinical evidence of beneficial effects of PPAR ligands in ischemic stroke

Although various PPAR agonists applied before the onset of ischemia can effectively protect the brain in animal models of acute IRI, these treatments are seldom possible in the clinical setting of stroke because patients with stroke present after onset of the ischemic attack. Neuroprotective interventions applied after the onset of ischemia would thus seem to have greater clinical potential. Although some preclinical data provide evidence that administration of PPAR agonists during reperfusion decreases cerebral IRI, to date, there are no clinical data on the therapeutic efficacy of PPAR agonists administration after the onset of the ischemic event. Nevertheless, it must be noted that there may be subgroups of patients at high risk for stroke that could benefit from taking neuroprotective agents as prophylactic treatment. As already mentioned, pioglitazone and rosiglitazone (the TZD class of PPARγ agonists) have proven to be beneficial in type-2 diabetes mellitus patients. Diabetics are at an increased risk of stroke incidence and stroke causes more damage in diabetics compared to normoglycemic individuals. For this reason, such patients might benefit from taking an antidiabetic medication with neuroprotective properties, which might lessen the incidence and/or the severity of acute ischemic stroke. However, it's important to assess whether the potential benefits of taking an oral neuroprotective drug chronically outweighs the risks, including potential side effects. The use of a PPARγ agonist, specifically pioglitazone, as a preventive approach to ischemic brain injury has been recently addressed by two large clinical trials: the Prospective Pioglitazone Clinical Trial in Macrovascular Events (PROactive) and the Insulin Resistance Intervention after Stroke Trial (IRIS trial). The PROactive study has demonstrated that pioglitazone significantly reduces the combined risk of heart attacks, strokes and death by 16% in high risk patients with type-2 diabetes (Dormandy, Charbonnel et al. 2005). Enhanced functional recovery was also reported in a small group of stroke patients with type-2 diabetes treated with pioglitazone (Lee, Olson et al. 2006). However, it remain unclear whether the suggested beneficial effects of pioglitazone are mediated by insulin sensitization or by additional observed reductions in risk factors, such as hyperthension and dyslipidemia. This question and that related to the potential beneficial effects of pioglitazone in non-diabetic patients with stroke will be addressed by the IRIS trial, a randomized, double-blind, placebo-controlled trial on more than 3000 non-diabetic subjects who are insulin resistant and have had a recent transient ischemic attack or ischemic stroke. The IRIS study (ClinicalTrials.gov Identifier: NCT00091949) began on February 2005 and it is still recruiting patients. Interestingly, high plasma levels of 15d-PGJ2 (the natural ligand for PPARγ) have been associated with good neurological outcome and smaller infarct volume in patients with an acute atherothrombotic stroke (Blanco, Moro et al. 2005). Moreover, a recent report suggests that the Pro12Ala polymorphism of PPARγ2 is associated with a reduced risk for ischemic stroke (Lee, Olson et al. 2006), further supporting the importance of PPARs in cerebral ischemia. Nevertheless, as TZDs are hampered by adverse effects related to increased weight gain, fluid overload, and congestive heart failure, the risks associated with chronic TZD administration needs to be better elucidated.

Abnormal levels of serum lipids, including triglycerides, low density lipoprotein (LDL) and high density lipoprotein (HDL), are regarded as other important risk factors for cerebrovascular disease, including stroke. The association between hypercholesterolemia and stroke has become more apparent because of data from prospective cohort studies that show higher risks of ischemic stroke with increasing levels of total cholesterol in both men and women. Increased HDL cholesterol levels have a protective effect against the occurrence of ischemic stroke and elevated triglyceride levels have also been reported as a risk factor for stroke. Overall, elevated total cholesterol confers an approximately two-fold relative increase in stroke risk for men and women. As fibrates are used as lipid-lowering agents, it has been supposed that these PPARα agonists could also protect the brain against noxious biological reactions induced by cerebral IRI. A recent systematic meta-analysis of randomized clinical trials shows that fibrates do not significantly reduce the odds of stroke (Saha, Kizhakepunnur et al. 2007). However, data from large trials specifically investigating the role of fibrates in stroke event reduction are needed to conclusively elucidate their potential neuroprotective role. For instance, a large clinical trial, named Action to Control Cardiovascular Risk in Diabetes (ACCORD) is currently testing the ability of fenofibrate to decrease stroke incidence in high-risk patients with type-2 diabetes (ACCORD study group 2007).

5. Molecular mechanisms of beneficial effects of PPARs against cerebral ischemia

Cerebral IRI is known to induce generation of ROS, as well as the expression of cytokines, adhesion molecules and enzymes involved in the inflammatory response, and is known to be regulated by oxygen- or redox-sensitive mechanisms. Recent studies have confirmed the pivotal role of both oxidative stress and inflammatory response in the pathogenesis of acute ischemic stroke. Through various mechanisms PPARs can regulate both inflammatory and oxidative pathways and PPAR agonist-induced neuroprotection seems to be specific for injuries in which inflammation or free radical generation are the main causes of cell damage. For instance, PPARα activation can induce expression and activation of antioxidant enzymes, such as superoxide dismutase (SOD) and glutathione peroxidase (GSH). We have demonstrated that administration of a highly selective PPARα agonist, WY14643, 30 min prior to IRI, decreased ROS production and lipid peroxidation in rats subjected to IRI and, at the same time, offered protection against GSH depletion (Collino, Aragno et al. 2006). Similar results on oxidative stress modulation have been reported when another PPARα agonist, fenofibrate, was tested in a mouse model of middle cerebral artery occlusion (Deplanque, Gele et al. 2003). Interestingly, PPARγ KO mice have been found to exhibit significant increases in oxidative stress and lipid peroxidation much earlier in their life than wild-type littermates (Poynter and Daynes 1998). The PPAR-induced protective effect on oxidative stress could be related to a direct effect on antioxidant enzyme expression, as the catalase and SOD gene promoters contain the PPRE. In fact, rats that have been treated with a diet containing PPARα ligands, WY14643 or fenofibrate, have demonstrated an enhanced expression of antioxidant enzymes such as SOD and catalase (Toyama, Nakamura et al. 2004). Based on gene expression microarray experiments, Coleman and colleagues (Coleman, Prabhu et al. 2007) have demonstrated that PPARβ/δ activation increased mRNA for aldheyde dehydrogenase and glutathione-S-transferase, thus protecting the cell from oxidative damage. In normotensive and hypertensive animals treated with rosiglitazone, ischemic hemispheres showed increased catalase and Cu/Zn-SOD activity in the peri-infarct region (Tureyen, Kapadia et al. 2007) and the level of Cu/Zn-SOD was demonstrated to increase in the ischemic cortex of animals treated with pioglitazone for 4 days prior to focal cerebral ischemia (Shimazu, Inoue et al. 2005). As we have recently shown, treatment of rats with either pioglitazone or rosiglitazone before occlusion of the common carotid artery decreased the production of ROS and nitrite, decreased lipid peroxidation and reversed the depleted stores of glutathione in the hippocampus (Collino, Aragno et al. 2006). These findings are supported by data from an *in vitro* model demonstrating that pre-treatment with PPARγ agonists protected an immortalized mouse hippocampal cell line against oxidative stress induced by glutamate or hydrogen peroxide (Aoun, Watson et al. 2003). Moreover, PPARγ agonists attenuate the expression of iNOS in inflammatory cells, which is an important source of nitric oxide (NO). NO may react with ROS to produce peroxynitrites, with deleterious effects on neuronal survival. Thus, iNOS inhibition may represent a further mechanism for neuroprotection by PPAR agonists. Mitochondria are the major source of ROS, which are mainly generated at complexes I and III of the respiratory chain. There is now evidence indicating that rosiglitazone and pioglitazone exert direct and rapid effects on mitochondrial respiration, inhibiting complex I and complex III activity (Brunmair, Lest et al. 2004). As PPARγ agonists partially disrupt the mitochondrial respiratory chain, both electron transport and superoxide anion generation are affected. Moreover, a novel mitochondrial target protein for PPARγ agonists ("mitoNEET") has recently been identified (Colca, McDonald et al. 2004). MitoNEET was found associated with components of complex III, suggesting how binding of PPARγ agonists to mitoNEET could selectively block different mitochondrial targets. The ability of PPARγ agonists to influence mitochondrial function might contribute to their inhibitory effects on ROS generation that is evoked by IRI.

Another mechanism through which PPAR agonists may provide neuroprotection is by down-regulating the inflammatory response associated with IRI. Depending on the affected tissue and which PPAR isoforms are involved, PPAR agonists can differently modulate the intensity, duration and consequences of inflammatory events. For instance, ischemia-induced COX-2 overexpression is prevented by PPARγ agonists but not by PPARα agonists (Sundararajan, Gamboa et al. 2005; Collino, Aragno et al. 2006; Collino, Aragno et al. 2006). Activation of PPARγ attenuates the expression of matrix metalloproteinase (MMP)-9 and various inflammatory cytokines in ischemic brain tissue (Pereira, Hurtado et al. 2005). PPARγ is constitutively expressed in macrophages and microglial cells and the systemic treatment of rodents with rosiglitazone reduces the infiltration of these cells into peri-infarct brain regions. Both chronic and acute administration of PPARγ agonists has been demonstrated to prevent cerebral IRI-induced expression of vascular cell adhesion molecule-1 (VCAM-1) and ICAM-1 in two independent studies (Deplanque, Gele et al. 2003; Collino, Aragno et al. 2006). In the brain, the decreased expression of these adhesion molecules might contribute to inhibit the infiltration of the brain ischemic area by neutrophils. Studies addressing the molecular mechanisms of these anti-inflammatory actions demonstrated that the involvement of PPARs in the control of IRI-induced inflammation is mediated mainly through their transrepression capabilities. PPARs can suppress the activities of many distinct families of transcription factors. The range of transcription factors affected and the mechanisms involved may be different for each PPAR isotype, although a common mechanism of PPARα and PPARγ neuroprotection appears to involve inhibition of p38 MAPK activation and NF-κB nuclear translocation. A recent study confirms that PPARγ activation prevents the post-ischemic cerebral expression of pro-inflammatory transcription factors, such as Egr1, C/EBP and NF-κB, possibly by decreasing DNA binding (Tureyen, Kapadia et al. 2007). The inhibitory protein IκBα, which is an indicator of NF-κB transcriptional activity, is remarkably increased in the brain of rats that underwent cerebral ischemia and completely blocked by rosiglitazone and 15d-PGJ2 administration, thus further confirming that both endogenous and synthetic PPARγ ligands inhibit NF-κB signalling (Pereira, Hurtado et al. 2006). Similarly, p38 MAPK and NF-κB activation by cerebral IRI has been demonstrated to be inhibited by pre-treatment with the PPARα agonist WY14643 or the PPARγ agonist pioglitazone. However, as MAPK and NF-κB are functionally interconnected and do not act independently, we cannot rule out the possibility that PPARs affect NF-κB activation by interfering with the MAPK signalling cascade or vice versa.

The generation of ROS is known to be associated with the induction of apoptosis and, in neurons, inhibition of cell death is an important factor to prevent during IRI. PPAR activation may decrease the IRI-induced activation of apoptotic pathways depending on the increase in activity and expression of numerous anti-oxidant enzymes. Moreover, by their anti-inflammatory action on microglia and astrocytes, PPAR agonists prevent the release of neurotoxic agents, which induce neuronal apoptosis. PPARγ agonists may attenuate ischemia-induced reactive oxygen species and subsequently alleviate the post-ischemic degradation of Bcl-2, Bcl-xl, and Akt, by increasing SOD/catalase and decreasing nicotinamide adenine dinucleotide phosphate oxidase levels (Fong, Tsai et al.). Chu and colleagues (Chu, Lee et al. 2006) have demonstrated that rosiglitazone-fed rats had better neurological scores and reduced number of TUNEL-positive cells following transient focal ischemia. Interestingly, these authors also reported an increased vasculature in the rosiglitazone-treated group with increased number of endothelial cells positive for BrdU, suggesting there may be enhanced angiogenesis following PPARγ activation. Administration of a selective PPARγ agonist (L-796449) 10 min prior to permanent cerebral artery occlusion, resulted in decreased apoptosis, measured as reduction of caspase-3 activity (Pereira, Hurtado et al. 2005). Another study confirmed inhibition on caspase-3 activity by both exogenous and endogenous PPARγ agonists, rosiglitazone and 15d-PGJ2, in the ischemic cortex (Lin, Cheung et al. 2006). The same authors observed that rosiglitazone and 15d-PGJ2 exhibit a concentration-dependent paradoxical effect on cytotoxicity, when tested in an *in vitro* model of hydrogen peroxide induced neuronal apoptosis. The drugs induced pro-apoptotic effects when used at concentrations higher that 5 μmol/L but protect neurons from necrosis and apoptosis at concentrations lower than 1 μmol/L. The reason for

this paradoxical action is unclear and further studies are needed to better clarify the effects of PPARs in IRI induced-apoptosis and necrosis.
Recently published data suggest that an increased uptake of cerebral extracellular glutamate levels after ischemia may represent an additional mechanism for the neuroprotection exerted by PPARγ activation (Romera, Hurtado et al. 2007). Both *in vivo* and *in vitro* experiments showed that rosiglitazone administration increased the expression of the GLT1/EAAT2 glutamate transporter in the brain, thus preventing the extracellular glutamate levels from rising to neurotoxic values.

6. Conclusion

Although clinical data are limited, a wide array of evidence obtained in animal models now shows that PPAR activation may be a rational and effective strategy against ischemic brain damage. The beneficial effects of PPAR agonists in experimental models of stroke are mediated by different mechanisms, as expected based on their pleiotropic pharmacological profile. The neuroprotective actions appear to be mainly related to the reduction in oxidative damage as well as anti-inflammatory and anti-apoptotic effects. These results have been essentially obtained with PPARα and PPARγ agonists, while the PPARβ/δ pathway remains largely unexplored, despite a significant interest in this target. Selective activation of different isoforms of PPARs may account for the difference in molecular pathways underlying neuroprotection and these different features still remain far from being completely understood. In conclusion, currently available management protocols for patients with stroke may benefit from the use of PPAR agonists that target detrimental processes associated with IRI. However, several critical issues still need to be resolved. For instance, well-structured clinical trials aimed at evaluating the effects of PPAR ligands on stroke recovery are needed before firm conclusions are drawn about their therapeutic efficacy. A more stringent approach regarding the concentration range of PPAR agonists, especially within the CNS, and the duration of exposure should be applied. Also acceptable water solubility with satisfactory blood-brain barrier penetrability is an important aspect of PPAR agonists that needs to be optimized.

7. References

Allahtavakoli, M., R. Moloudi, et al. (2009). "Delayed post ischemic treatment with Rosiglitazone attenuates infarct volume, neurological deficits and neutrophilia after embolic stroke in rat." *Brain Res* 1271: 121-7.

Allahtavakoli, M., A. Shabanzadeh, et al. (2007). "Combination therapy of rosiglitazone, a peroxisome proliferator-activated receptor-gamma ligand, and NMDA receptor antagonist (MK-801) on experimental embolic stroke in rats." *Basic Clin Pharmacol Toxicol* 101(5): 309-14.

Amri, E. Z., F. Bonino, et al. (1995). "Cloning of a protein that mediates transcriptional effects of fatty acids in preadipocytes. Homology to peroxisome proliferator-activated receptors." *J Biol Chem* 270(5): 2367-71.

Aoun, P., D. G. Watson, et al. (2003). "Neuroprotective effects of PPARgamma agonists against oxidative insults in HT-22 cells." *Eur J Pharmacol* 472(1-2): 65-71.

Barish, G. D., A. R. Atkins, et al. (2008). "PPARdelta regulates multiple proinflammatory pathways to suppress atherosclerosis." *Proc Natl Acad Sci U S A* 105(11): 4271-6.

Berger, J., M. D. Leibowitz, et al. (1999). "Novel peroxisome proliferator-activated receptor (PPAR) gamma and PPARdelta ligands produce distinct biological effects." *J Biol Chem* 274(10): 6718-25.

Blanco, M., M. A. Moro, et al. (2005). "Increased plasma levels of 15-deoxyDelta prostaglandin J2 are associated with good outcome in acute atherothrombotic ischemic stroke." *Stroke* 36(6): 1189-94.

Braissant, O., F. Foufelle, et al. (1996). "Differential expression of peroxisome proliferator-activated receptors (PPARs): tissue distribution of PPAR-alpha, -beta, and -gamma in the adult rat." *Endocrinology* 137(1): 354-66.

Brunmair, B., A. Lest, et al. (2004). "Fenofibrate impairs rat mitochondrial function by inhibition of respiratory complex I." *J Pharmacol Exp Ther* 311(1): 109-14.

Buyukuysal, R. L. (2005). "Protein S100B release from rat brain slices during and after ischemia: comparison with lactate dehydrogenase leakage." *Neurochem Int* 47(8): 580-8.

Choi, J. H., A. S. Banks, et al. (2010). "Anti-diabetic drugs inhibit obesity-linked phosphorylation of PPARgamma by Cdk5." *Nature* 466(7305): 451-6.

Chou, C. J., M. Haluzik, et al. (2002). "WY14,643, a peroxisome proliferator-activated receptor alpha (PPARalpha) agonist, improves hepatic and muscle steatosis and reverses insulin resistance in lipoatrophic A-ZIP/F-1 mice." *J Biol Chem* 277(27): 24484-9.

Chu, K., S. T. Lee, et al. (2006). "Peroxisome proliferator-activated receptor-gamma-agonist, rosiglitazone, promotes angiogenesis after focal cerebral ischemia." *Brain Res* 1093(1): 208-18.

Colca, J. R., W. G. McDonald, et al. (2004). "Identification of a novel mitochondrial protein ("mitoNEET") cross-linked specifically by a thiazolidinedione photoprobe." *Am J Physiol Endocrinol Metab* 286(2): E252-60.

Coleman, J. D., K. S. Prabhu, et al. (2007). "The oxidative stress mediator 4-hydroxynonenal is an intracellular agonist of the nuclear receptor peroxisome proliferator-activated receptor-beta/delta (PPARbeta/delta)." *Free Radic Biol Med* 42(8): 1155-64.

Collino, M., M. Aragno, et al. (2006). "Oxidative stress and inflammatory response evoked by transient cerebral ischemia/reperfusion: effects of the PPAR-alpha agonist WY14643." *Free Radic Biol Med* 41(4): 579-89.

Collino, M., M. Aragno, et al. (2006). "Modulation of the oxidative stress and inflammatory response by PPAR-gamma agonists in the hippocampus of rats exposed to cerebral ischemia/reperfusion." *Eur J Pharmacol* 530(1-2): 70-80.

Cristiano, L., A. Bernardo, et al. (2001). "Peroxisome proliferator-activated receptors (PPARs) and peroxisomes in rat cortical and cerebellar astrocytes." *J Neurocytol* 30(8): 671-83.

Delerive, P., F. Martin-Nizard, et al. (1999). "Peroxisome proliferator-activated receptor activators inhibit thrombin-induced endothelin-1 production in human vascular endothelial cells by inhibiting the activator protein-1 signaling pathway." *Circ Res* 85(5): 394-402.

Deplanque, D., P. Gele, et al. (2003). "Peroxisome proliferator-activated receptor-alpha activation as a mechanism of preventive neuroprotection induced by chronic fenofibrate treatment." *J Neurosci* 23(15): 6264-71.

Desvergne, B. and W. Wahli (1999). "Peroxisome proliferator-activated receptors: nuclear control of metabolism." *Endocr Rev* 20(5): 649-88.

Dormandy, J. A., B. Charbonnel, et al. (2005). "Secondary prevention of macrovascular events in patients with type 2 diabetes in the PROactive Study (PROspective pioglitAzone Clinical Trial In macroVascular Events): a randomised controlled trial." *Lancet* 366(9493): 1279-89.

Fajas, L., D. Auboeuf, et al. (1997). "The organization, promoter analysis, and expression of the human PPARgamma gene." *J Biol Chem* 272(30): 18779-89.

Feige, J. N., L. Gelman, et al. (2006). "From molecular action to physiological outputs: peroxisome proliferator-activated receptors are nuclear receptors at the crossroads of key cellular functions." *Prog Lipid Res* 45(2): 120-59.

Foerch, C., O. C. Singer, et al. (2005). "Evaluation of serum S100B as a surrogate marker for long-term outcome and infarct volume in acute middle cerebral artery infarction." *Arch Neurol* 62(7): 1130-4.

Fong, W. H., H. D. Tsai, et al. (2010). "Anti-apoptotic actions of PPAR-gamma against ischemic stroke." *Mol Neurobiol* 41(2-3): 180-6.

Forman, B. M., J. Chen, et al. (1997). "Hypolipidemic drugs, polyunsaturated fatty acids, and eicosanoids are ligands for peroxisome proliferator-activated receptors alpha and delta." *Proc Natl Acad Sci U S A* 94(9): 4312-7.

Gamboa, J., D. A. Blankenship, et al. (2010). "Extension of the neuroprotective time window for thiazolidinediones in ischemic stroke is dependent on time of reperfusion." *Neuroscience* 170(3): 846-57.

Greene, M. E., B. Blumberg, et al. (1995). "Isolation of the human peroxisome proliferator activated receptor gamma cDNA: expression in hematopoietic cells and chromosomal mapping." *Gene Expr* 4(4-5): 281-99.

Guo, Q., G. Wang, et al. (2009). "Effects of gemfibrozil on outcome after permanent middle cerebral artery occlusion in mice." *Brain Res* 1279: 121-30.

Gurnell, M. (2003). "PPARgamma and metabolism: insights from the study of human genetic variants." *Clin Endocrinol (Oxf)* 59(3): 267-77.

Hevener, A. L., W. He, et al. (2003). "Muscle-specific Pparg deletion causes insulin resistance." *Nat Med* 9(12): 1491-7.

Hu, E., J. B. Kim, et al. (1996). "Inhibition of adipogenesis through MAP kinase-mediated phosphorylation of PPARgamma." *Science* 274(5295): 2100-3.

Inoue, H., X. F. Jiang, et al. (2003). "Brain protection by resveratrol and fenofibrate against stroke requires peroxisome proliferator-activated receptor alpha in mice." *Neurosci Lett* 352(3): 203-6.

Issemann, I. and S. Green (1990). "Activation of a member of the steroid hormone receptor superfamily by peroxisome proliferators." *Nature* 347(6294): 645-50.

Iwashita, A., Y. Muramatsu, et al. (2007). "Neuroprotective efficacy of the peroxisome proliferator-activated receptor delta-selective agonists in vitro and in vivo." *J Pharmacol Exp Ther* 320(3): 1087-96.

Juge-Aubry, C., A. Pernin, et al. (1997). "DNA binding properties of peroxisome proliferator-activated receptor subtypes on various natural peroxisome proliferator response elements. Importance of the 5'-flanking region." *J Biol Chem* 272(40): 25252-9.

Kersten, S., J. Seydoux, et al. (1999). "Peroxisome proliferator-activated receptor alpha mediates the adaptive response to fasting." *J Clin Invest* 103(11): 1489-98.

Kim, H., M. Haluzik, et al. (2003). "Peroxisome proliferator-activated receptor-alpha agonist treatment in a transgenic model of type 2 diabetes reverses the lipotoxic state and improves glucose homeostasis." *Diabetes* 52(7): 1770-8.

Kliewer, S. A., B. M. Forman, et al. (1994). "Differential expression and activation of a family of murine peroxisome proliferator-activated receptors." *Proc Natl Acad Sci U S A* 91(15): 7355-9.

Krogsdam, A. M., C. A. Nielsen, et al. (2002). "Nuclear receptor corepressor-dependent repression of peroxisome-proliferator-activated receptor delta-mediated transactivation." *Biochem J* 363(Pt 1): 157-65.

Lee, C. H., A. Chawla, et al. (2003). "Transcriptional repression of atherogenic inflammation: modulation by PPARdelta." *Science* 302(5644): 453-7.

Lee, C. H., P. Olson, et al. (2006). "PPARdelta regulates glucose metabolism and insulin sensitivity." *Proc Natl Acad Sci U S A* 103(9): 3444-9.

Lefebvre, P., G. Chinetti, et al. (2006). "Sorting out the roles of PPAR alpha in energy metabolism and vascular homeostasis." *J Clin Invest* 116(3): 571-80.

Lim, H. and S. K. Dey (2000). "PPAR delta functions as a prostacyclin receptor in blastocyst implantation." *Trends Endocrinol Metab* 11(4): 137-42.

Lin, T. N., W. M. Cheung, et al. (2006). "15d-prostaglandin J2 protects brain from ischemia-reperfusion injury." *Arterioscler Thromb Vasc Biol* 26(3): 481-7.

Lincoff, A. M., K. Wolski, et al. (2007). "Pioglitazone and risk of cardiovascular events in patients with type 2 diabetes mellitus: a meta-analysis of randomized trials." *JAMA* 298(10): 1180-8.

Loke, Y. K., S. Singh, et al. (2009). "Long-term use of thiazolidinediones and fractures in type 2 diabetes: a meta-analysis." *CMAJ* 180(1): 32-9.

Martens, F. M., F. L. Visseren, et al. (2002). "Metabolic and additional vascular effects of thiazolidinediones." *Drugs* 62(10): 1463-80.

Moreno, S., S. Farioli-Vecchioli, et al. (2004). "Immunolocalization of peroxisome proliferator-activated receptors and retinoid X receptors in the adult rat CNS." *Neuroscience* 123(1): 131-45.

Nissen, S. E. and K. Wolski (2010). "Rosiglitazone revisited: an updated meta-analysis of risk for myocardial infarction and cardiovascular mortality." *Arch Intern Med* 170(14): 1191-1201.

Onate, S. A., S. Y. Tsai, et al. (1995). "Sequence and characterization of a coactivator for the steroid hormone receptor superfamily." *Science* 270(5240): 1354-7.

Ou, Z., X. Zhao, et al. (2006). "Neuronal expression of peroxisome proliferator-activated receptor-gamma (PPARgamma) and 15d-prostaglandin J2--mediated protection of brain after experimental cerebral ischemia in rat." *Brain Res* 1096(1): 196-203.

Ouk, T., M. Laprais, et al. (2009). "Withdrawal of fenofibrate treatment partially abrogates preventive neuroprotection in stroke via loss of vascular protection." *Vascul Pharmacol* 51(5-6): 323-30.

Palmer, C. N., M. H. Hsu, et al. (1995). "Novel sequence determinants in peroxisome proliferator signaling." *J Biol Chem* 270(27): 16114-21.

Pascual, G. and C. K. Glass (2006). "Nuclear receptors versus inflammation: mechanisms of transrepression." *Trends Endocrinol Metab* 17(8): 321-7.

Pereira, M. P., O. Hurtado, et al. (2005). "The nonthiazolidinedione PPARgamma agonist L-796,449 is neuroprotective in experimental stroke." *J Neuropathol Exp Neurol* 64(9): 797-805.

Pereira, M. P., O. Hurtado, et al. (2006). "Rosiglitazone and 15-deoxy-Delta12,14-prostaglandin J2 cause potent neuroprotection after experimental stroke through noncompletely overlapping mechanisms." *J Cereb Blood Flow Metab* 26(2): 218-29.

Peters, J. M., S. S. Lee, et al. (2000). "Growth, adipose, brain, and skin alterations resulting from targeted disruption of the mouse peroxisome proliferator-activated receptor beta(delta)." *Mol Cell Biol* 20(14): 5119-28.

Pialat, J. B., T. H. Cho, et al. (2007). "MRI monitoring of focal cerebral ischemia in peroxisome proliferator-activated receptor (PPAR)-deficient mice." *NMR Biomed* 20(3): 335-42.

Poynter, M. E. and R. A. Daynes (1998). "Peroxisome proliferator-activated receptor alpha activation modulates cellular redox status, represses nuclear factor-kappaB signaling, and reduces inflammatory cytokine production in aging." *J Biol Chem* 273(49): 32833-41.

Romera, C., O. Hurtado, et al. (2007). "Ischemic preconditioning reveals that GLT1/EAAT2 glutamate transporter is a novel PPARgamma target gene involved in neuroprotection." *J Cereb Blood Flow Metab* 27(7): 1327-38.

Rosen, E. D., P. Sarraf, et al. (1999). "PPAR gamma is required for the differentiation of adipose tissue in vivo and in vitro." *Mol Cell* 4(4): 611-7.

Saha, S. A., L. G. Kizhakepunnur, et al. (2007). "The role of fibrates in the prevention of cardiovascular disease--a pooled meta-analysis of long-term randomized placebo-controlled clinical trials." *Am Heart J* 154(5): 943-53.

Sayan-Ozacmak, H., V. H. Ozacmak, et al. (2011). "Neuroprotective Efficacy Of The Peroxisome Proliferator-Activated Receptor-g Ligand In Chronic Cerebral Hypoperfusion." *Curr Neurovasc Res.* 8 (3): 190-9.

Schmidt, A., N. Endo, et al. (1992). "Identification of a new member of the steroid hormone receptor superfamily that is activated by a peroxisome proliferator and fatty acids." *Mol Endocrinol* 6(10): 1634-41.

Schwabe, J. W., D. Neuhaus, et al. (1990). "Solution structure of the DNA-binding domain of the oestrogen receptor." *Nature* 348(6300): 458-61.

Shearer, B. G., D. J. Steger, et al. (2008). "Identification and characterization of a selective peroxisome proliferator-activated receptor beta/delta (NR1C2) antagonist." *Mol Endocrinol* 22(2): 523-9.

Sher, T., H. F. Yi, et al. (1993). "cDNA cloning, chromosomal mapping, and functional characterization of the human peroxisome proliferator activated receptor." *Biochemistry* 32(21): 5598-604.

Shi, Y., M. Hon, et al. (2002). "The peroxisome proliferator-activated receptor delta, an integrator of transcriptional repression and nuclear receptor signaling." *Proc Natl Acad Sci U S A* 99(5): 2613-8.

Shimazu, T., I. Inoue, et al. (2005). "A peroxisome proliferator-activated receptor-gamma agonist reduces infarct size in transient but not in permanent ischemia." *Stroke* 36(2): 353-9.

Singh, S., Y. K. Loke, et al. (2007). "Long-term risk of cardiovascular events with rosiglitazone: a meta-analysis." *JAMA* 298(10): 1189-95.

Suhara, W., H. Koide, et al. (2009). "Cow's milk increases the activities of human nuclear receptors peroxisome proliferator-activated receptors alpha and delta and retinoid X receptor alpha involved in the regulation of energy homeostasis, obesity, and inflammation." *J Dairy Sci* 92(9): 4180-7.

Sundararajan, S., J. L. Gamboa, et al. (2005). "Peroxisome proliferator-activated receptor-gamma ligands reduce inflammation and infarction size in transient focal ischemia." *Neuroscience* 130(3): 685-96.

Takata, Y., J. Liu, et al. (2008). "PPARdelta-mediated antiinflammatory mechanisms inhibit angiotensin II-accelerated atherosclerosis." *Proc Natl Acad Sci U S A* 105(11): 4277-82.

Theocharisa, S., A. Margeli, et al. (2003). "Peroxisome proliferator activated receptor-gamma ligands as potent antineoplastic agents." *Curr Med Chem Anticancer Agents* 3(3): 239-51.

Toyama, T., H. Nakamura, et al. (2004). "PPARalpha ligands activate antioxidant enzymes and suppress hepatic fibrosis in rats." *Biochem Biophys Res Commun* 324(2): 697-704.

Tureyen, K., R. Kapadia, et al. (2007). "Peroxisome proliferator-activated receptor-gamma agonists induce neuroprotection following transient focal ischemia in normotensive, normoglycemic as well as hypertensive and type-2 diabetic rodents." *J Neurochem* 101(1): 41-56.

Victor, N. A., E. W. Wanderi, et al. (2006). "Altered PPARgamma expression and activation after transient focal ischemia in rats." *Eur J Neurosci* 24(6): 1653-63.

Willson, T. M., P. J. Brown, et al. (2000). "The PPARs: from orphan receptors to drug discovery." *J Med Chem* 43(4): 527-50.

Xu, H. E., M. H. Lambert, et al. (1999). "Molecular recognition of fatty acids by peroxisome proliferator-activated receptors." *Mol Cell* 3(3): 397-403.

Yamamoto, Y., H. Yamazaki, et al. (2002). "Formation of a novel quinone epoxide metabolite of troglitazone with cytotoxicity to HepG2 cells." *Drug Metab Dispos* 30(2): 155-60.

Yoshikawa, T., Z. Brkanac, et al. (1996). "Assignment of the human nuclear hormone receptor, NUC1 (PPARD), to chromosome 6p21.1-p21.2." *Genomics* 35(3): 637-8.

Yue Tl, T. L., J. Chen, et al. (2001). "In vivo myocardial protection from ischemia/reperfusion injury by the peroxisome proliferator-activated receptor-gamma agonist rosiglitazone." *Circulation* 104(21): 2588-94.

Zhang, H. L., M. Xu, et al. (2011). "Neuroprotective effects of pioglitazone in a rat model of permanent focal cerebral ischemia are associated with peroxisome proliferator-activated receptor gamma-mediated suppression of nuclear factor-kappaB signaling pathway." *Neuroscience* 176: 381-95.

Zhao, Y., A. Patzer, et al. (2005). "The intracerebral application of the PPARgamma-ligand pioglitazone confers neuroprotection against focal ischaemia in the rat brain." *Eur J Neurosci* 22(1): 278-82.